Liver Disorders in Childhood
Third Edition

To
Ann, Neil and Adrian

Liver Disorders In Childhood

Third Edition

ALEX P. MOWAT
Consultant Paediatric Hepatologist, Department of Child Health, Variety Club
Children's Hospital, King's College Hospital

Professor of Paediatric Hepatology, King's College School of Medicine and Dentistry,
University of London
London

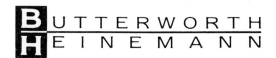

Butterworth-Heinemann
Linacre House, Jordan Hill, Oxford OX2 8DP
225 Wildwood Avenue, Woburn, MA 01801-2041
A division of Reed Educational and Professional Publishing Ltd

A member of the Reed Elsevier plc group

OXFORD   BOSTON   JOHANNESBURG
MELBOURNE   NEW DELHI   SINGAPORE

First published 1979
Second edition 1987
Third edition 1994
Paperback edition 1998

British Library Cataloguing in Publication Data
Mowat, Alex P.
  Liver Disorders in Childhood. - 3Rev.ed
  I. Title
  618.92362

Library of Congress Cataloguing in Publication Data
Mowat, Alex P.
  Liver disorders in childhood/Alex P. Mowat. - 3rd ed.
  p. cm.
  Includes bibliographical references and index.
  1. Liver - Diseases. 2. Pediatric gastroenterology. I. Title
  [DNLM: 1. Liver Diseases - in infancy & childhood, WS 310 M936L
  1993]
  RJ456.L5M68   93-31532
  618.9'362 - dc20   CIP

ISBN 0 7506 4200 9

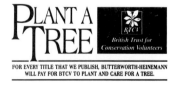

FOR EVERY TITLE THAT WE PUBLISH, BUTTERWORTH-HEINEMANN
WILL PAY FOR BTCV TO PLANT AND CARE FOR A TREE.

Composition by Genesis Typesetting, Laser Quay, Rochester, Kent
Printed in Great Britain at the University Press, Cambridge

Contents

Preface to the third edition

Paediatric hepatology is benefiting greatly from developments in cellular and molecular biology. Advances particularly in inborn errors of metabolism, viral hepatitis and immunology have had an increasing impact on practice in the past 5 years. There is a better understanding of pathophysiological mechanisms. Effective vaccines have been produced for hepatitis A and B and there have been major breakthroughs in the biology of hepatitis C and E. Progress in radiology, endoscopy and laparoscopy have added exciting new modes of investigation and treatment procedures which are less invasive. The increased availability of liver transplantation has had a major impact on care in all forms of liver disease except self-limiting disorders. Liver transplantation has highlighted the need for even earlier diagnosis, better classification and for more information on prognosis.

The major objective of this new edition is to assist the clinician in earlier diagnosis and to highlight developments which allow better management of hepatobiliary disorders. Every chapter in this edition has been modified to include clinically relevant advances. The text highlights soluble problems for both clinical and laboratory research workers.

I owe a great debt to many colleagues at King's College Hospital, especially to Dr Giorgina Mieli-Vergani and Professor Diego Vergani, for guiding me through the intricacies of immunology of liver disorders and much else and to Mr E. R. Howard whose invaluable advice on surgical management now has a wider audience with the publication of his textbook. Dr John Karani and Dr Hylton Meire have kept me up to date with developments in diagnostic imaging and therapy and supplied many of the figures. I would also like to acknowledge the support I have had from Dr Colin Ball, Professor A. L. W. F. Eddleston, Miss Jane Ely, Dr Bernard Portmann, Mrs Jeanette Singer, Mr K. C. Tan and Dr Roger Williams.

Thanks are due also to Mr Pike and his staff at the photography department at King's College Hospital and to Dr Paul Cheeseman and Mr Alec Dionysiou who provided the line drawings. I am grateful to Romana Kebe for typing and collating the manuscripts.

My wife Ann has again provided understanding patient support which has made the completion of this text possible.

Alex P Mowat
1993

Preface to the second edition

Advances in paediatric hepatology in the last seven years extend from the application of sophisticated genetic engineering techniques in the diagnosis, prevention and management of metabolic disorders and viral infections, through to computer-assisted analysis of liver blood flow by ultrasonically guided Doppler probes. These advances have led to stricter categorization of liver disorders, improved understanding of their pathogenesis and better management. Every chapter in this edition has been modified to include clinically relevant developments in aetiology, prevention, disease mechanisms, diagnosis and management. Liver transplantation, now a therapeutic option, is covered in a new chapter in which the selection of patients, timing of liver transplantation, management and results are considered. The major objective is to assist the clinician in earlier diagnosis and more precise management of hepatobiliary disorders. The text may also stimulate and challenge both clinical and laboratory research workers by illustrating the rapid advances occurring over a whole range of liver disorders in childhood and the many problems still requiring a solution.

I am indebted to many colleagues at King's College Hospital for their support. Again I thank particularly Professor C. Eric Stroud, Dr Roger Wiliams, Dr Giorgina Mieli-Vergani, Mr E. R. Howard, Dr B. Portmann, Professor A. L. W. F. Eddleston and Dr H. Meire.

My thanks are also due to my son Neil who provided the new line drawings, to Mr Pile and his staff of the Photographic Department at King's College Hospital for the photographs and particularly to Mrs Pamela Golding who again typed the manuscript.

My wife Ann has again provided unstinting, patient support, without which compiling this text would have been impossible.

Alex P. Mowat

Preface to the first edition

This book aims to provide a comprehensive and up-to-date account of disorders of the liver and biliary system in childhood. The main justification for writing such a book at this time is the need to synthesize for the clinician the many important developments in diagnosis, categorization and treatment of liver disease in childhood which have occurred in the last two decades. The developments considered range through new knowledge of the mechanisms of physiological jaundice; the controversy of jaundice associated with breast feeding; surgery for extrahepatic biliary atresia; the role of hepatitis B virus infection in chronic liver disease; presymptomatic diagnosis of Wilson's disease; liver transplantation to surgical treatment of metabolic disorders such as glycogen storage disease. Throughout, important aspects in diagnosis and management are stressed from the viewpoint of the paediatrician. The value and limitations of investigative procedures, both old and new, are critically discussed.

The secondary aim is to summarize recent research developments and to indicate some of the outstanding clinical problems and areas in which research is urgently required. The book incorporates advances in knowledge of hepatocyte and bile duct cell structure and function derived from electronmicroscopic and biochemical studies, where these contribute to our understanding of the pathogenesis of liver disease.

Information gleaned from studies in genetic disorders which lead to liver damage have also been included since these give important insights both into liver function and mechanisms of liver damage. Such advances in knowledge are important to the clinician and clinical research worker trying to understand and modify the many metabolic disturbances which can occur secondarily to liver damage or bile duct obstruction.

Recent developments in the understanding of disordered immune mechanisms associated with liver disease suggest that these are important not only because of their role as diagnostic indicators but because of their putative role in pathogenesis. Evidence relating the outcome of liver disease to the interaction between the many cell types within the liver and the cells of the reticulo-endothelial system is also scrutinized.

This bok has been written primarily for clinicians, especially paediatricians, paediatric surgeons and gastroenterologists; but it is hoped that it will be of value also to pathologists, biochemists and laboratory research workers concerned with understanding aspects of hepatic function and elucidating pathogenic mechanisms.

I wish to acknowledge my indebtedness to all my many teachers, especially Dr G. A. Levvy, Professor Ross G. Mitchell and Dr Irwin M. Arias who gave me so much help in developing my interest in liver disease.

This work would not have been possible without the help and encouragement of many colleagues at King's College Hospital. I am particularly grateful to Professor C. Eric

Stroud, Dr Roger Williams, Dr Adrian L. W. F. Eddleston and Mr Edward R. Howard for their help in providing an academic environment in which to pursue clinical research in liver disease.

My thanks are due to the many past and present fellow students in the Department of Child Health and the Liver Unit for contributing to my continuing education by stimulating discussion.

Dr K. Cottrall, Dr D. I. Johnston, Dr V. C. Larcher, Mr D. J. Manthorpe, Dr G. Mieli, Dr A. Nicholson, Dr C. A. Porter, Dr B. I. Portmann, Dr H. T. Psacharopoulos, Dr A. L. Smith and Dr M. S. Tanner, co-workers in the last seven years, have contributed much information which has modified my understanding of conditions considered in this book.

Clinical photographs were the work of Mr Blewitt and his staff of the Photographic Department of King's College Hospital. Dr Meili, Dr Portmann and Dr W. G. P. Mair provided photomicrographs.

Dr Heather Nunnerley performed many of the radiographic procedures shown, and provided the radiographs.

I would like to thank the Editors of the *Archives of Disease in Childhood, Tohoku Journal of Experimental Medicine, Journal of Clinical Investigation* and Churchill Livingstone, Publishers, for permission to include illustrations and tables from their works.

Many colleagues have invited me to see patients under their care and advised me on their subsequent progress. These patients and their parents provided the stimulus which has seen this book to completion, assisted by the tactful, succinct and helpful guidance of Dr John Apley.

The complete manuscript was typed by Mrs Pamela Golding, while continuing her duties as secretary in the Department of Child Health, King's College Hospital. Without her the book would not have been completed.

I am greatly indebted to my wife and children for their patient support and understanding during the gestation of this book.

Alex P. Mowat

Chapter 1

Anatomy and physiology of the liver

Anatomy of the liver

The liver is a highly organized tissue with five different types of highly specialized and interacting cells. These are arranged in intimate contact with a complex but ordered system of channels carrying blood and bile. The liver lies in the right upper quadrant of the abdomen attached to the lower surface of the diaphragm. It accounts for one-twentieth of the body weight of the neonate and one-fiftieth of that of the adult. It receives 25–30% of the cardiac output. The structural organization of the liver and its vascular elements is designed to allow it to occupy a central place in metabolism while interposed as a guardian between the digestive tract (and spleen) and the rest of the body. An essential function of the liver is to maintain the concentration of macromolecules and solutes in hepatic vein blood and in bile within a very narrow concentration range irrespective of dietary intake or the metabolic demands of other organs. Substrates are rapidly taken into the liver cells, metabolized, stored and their products transferred as required into the blood and bile. Blood, bile and lymph-containing channels transport nutrients, metabolites, antigens, antibodies, hormones and drugs, to and from liver cells. The vascular arrangements ensure that hepatocytes, Kupffer cells and sinusoidal endothelial cells are in intimate contact with blood flowing through the liver. Electron microscopic examination of hepatocytes shows an equally complex arrangement of channels and transport mechanisms connecting plasma membranes and intracellular organelles. A knowledge of the microanatomical relationships necessary for normal liver function is essential in appreciating some of the pathophysiological events that follow liver damage. In this chapter the gross structure is described and emphasis is given to the structural arrangements which ensure that each hepatocyte is in intimate contact with the blood flowing through the liver, facilitating transport of materials into and out of the hepatocyte and, at the same time, facilitating secretion of bile.

Gross structure

The liver is a continuous, uniform organ adopting a shape enforced on it by body cavities, other intraperitoneal structures and vascular forces – the positive pressure from the portal vein and the hepatic artery and the often negative pressure in the hepatic veins. The conventional division into right and left lobes does not coincide with the intrahepatic branching of vessels and ducts. Some knowledge of the normal distribution of these structures is necessary to understand some of the pathological consequences of disease within the liver or in the portal or hepatic venous systems and in the planning of liver resections.

Portal vein branches

The portal vein, which is formed by the junction of the superior mesenteric vein and the splenic vein and carries 70–80% of the blood supply to the liver, is directed towards the right lobe as it approaches the portahepatis. It branches into a short right trunk and a longer left trunk. The intrahepatic branches are subject to minor variations but a 'typical' pattern can be described. The right branch gives rise to a lateral branch directed to segments 5 and 8 in the posterolateral part of the liver the right upper lobe, a large central branch supplying segments 6 and 7 in the anterolateral section of the right lobe and an inferior branch supplying the area to the right of the gall bladder. From the left trunk, superior, intermediate and inferior branches supply segments 2, 3 and 4 in the lateral aspects of the left lobe and branches run also to the quadrate (Figure 1.1). The caudate

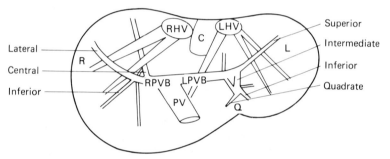

Figure 1.1 Diagrammatic representation of portal blood distribution to the right (R), left (L), quadrate (Q), and caudate (C) lobes of the liver, and the main right (RHV) and left (LHV) hepatic veins

receives blood from both veins. Otherwise anastomoses or overlap in territory between the branches of the right and left portal vein branches are unusual. Each terminal branch has a sharply defined territory, the smaller branches having the characteristic of 'end-arteries'. The portal vein 'territories' are shared by branches of the hepatic artery and tributaries of the hepatic duct which accompany the branches of the portal vein.

Hepatic artery

The hepatic artery and its intrahepatic branches are much less constant than the portal vein. In 55% of individuals the main hepatic artery arises as a single trunk from the coeliac artery but in the remainder two or three main arteries arise from the coeliac, superior mesenteric, gastroduodenal, left or right gastric arteries, or even directly from the aorta.

Within the liver the artery or its branches follow the appropriate branches of the portal vein. Sometimes two anastomosing arteries may accompany one vein, but the terminal branches are end-arteries supplying independently a circumscribed volume of liver. There are no intrahepatic communications between the right and left hepatic arteries.

Most of the hepatic artery blood flow goes initially to the bile ducts, stroma and gall bladder but a little may go to portal vein branches as they enter sinusoids. Around the bile ducts hepatic arterial blood enters peribiliary capillary plexuses which drain via interlobular branches of the portal vein to the sinusoids. The peribiliary capillary plexus facilitates reabsorption of substances, such as bile salts, from the bile ducts giving an intrahepatic cholehepatic circulation. In the presence of decreased portal blood flow hepatic arterial flow increases up to 100%. The factors controlling the relationship are undefined.

Hepatic vein tributaries

There are three main hepatic veins: the right hepatic vein drains the right upper lobe, the middle vein drains an area supplied by both the right and left portal veins, and the left vein drains the left lobe. The hepatic veins are relatively straight and follow a radial course to the inferior vena cava. The branches of the portal vein interdigitate between these vessels, the convexity of their course being directed to the diaphragm and to the anterior and lateral body walls. The hepatic vein tributaries have sharply defined areas of drainage which do not relate directly to the portal vein end-branch or hepatic end-artery territory, yet they do interdigitate with these to give uniform drainage of the liver. On both a microscopic and

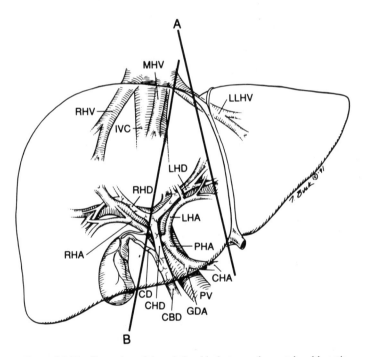

Figure 1.2 The illustration of the relationship between the portal and hepatic veins with liver surface markings used in reduction hepatectomy. Lines A and B indicate the planes of parenchymal transaction for the creation of a segment 2 and 3 graft (A) and a full left lobe graft (B). LLHV, left hepatic vein; MHV, middle hepatic vein; IVC, inferior vena cava; RHV, right hepatic vein; RHA, right hepatic artery; RHD, right hepatic duct; LHD, left hepatic duct; LHA, left hepatic artery; PHA, posterior hepatic artery; CD, cystic duct; CHD, common hepatic duct; CBD, common bile duct; GDA, gastroduodenal artery; CHA, common hepatic artery; PV, portal vein. (Reproduced with permission from Broelsch *et al.*, 1991.)

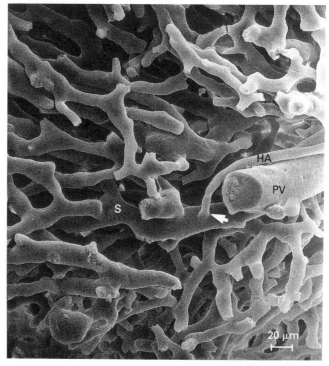

Figure 1.3 Arteriolosinusoidal anastomosis (arrow). At the terminal portal tract of a 4-week-old rat. HA, hepatic arteriole; PV, portal venule; S, sinusoid. (Reproduced with permission from Haratake *et al.*, 1991.)

a macroscopic scale, portal vein and hepatic veins run as nearly perpendicular to one another as is geometrically possible. The interrelationship of the main hepatic and portal vein branches define the division of the liver into eight segments which form the basis of modern liver surgery. (Figure 1.2). Other fairly constant hepatic veins drain the posterior cranial part of both lobes, the inferior part of the right lobe, and a number lead from the caudate lobe (segment 1) .

Microanatomical features

Portal tract

The portal tract, sometimes described as the portal *triad* because it contains, typically, terminal branches of the portal vein, hepatic artery and a bile ductule as its three most prominent structures; it also includes lymph vessels, nerves and an occasional mast cell and lymphocyte. It is surrounded by a sheath of connective tissue continuous with the external capsule of the liver. This connective tissue, referred to as the 'limiting plate', bounds the portal canal or tract.

From the portal tracts, portal venous blood and the hepatic artery branches pass through the limiting plate, through channels which are controlled by a sphincter. These channels discharge into a specialized network of capillaries termed 'sinusoids'.

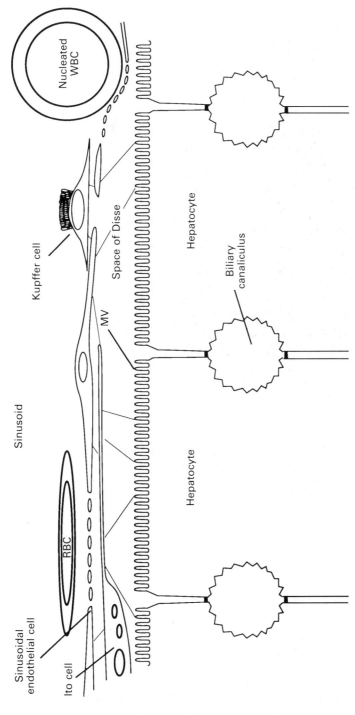

Figure 1.4 Diagrammatic representation of relationship of the functional unit formed by sinusoidal lining cells, space of Disse and hepatocyte microvillus (MV) membrane to facilitate rapid transfer between the hepatocyte and the sinusoidal lumen. Elliptical red cells pass freely along the sinusoid. The nucleated white blood cell (WBC) is compressing the sinusoidal lining cells and the space of Disse augmenting movement of fluids between space of Disse and sinusoidal lumen (endothelial massage). The fine lines in the space of Disse represent extracellular matrix (ECM) components. MV, microvillus on hepatocyte cell surface; WBC, white blood cell; RBC, red blood cell.

Sinusoids

Sinusoids are capillaries with a unique structure which both facilitates transfer of metabolites between hepatocytes and blood perfusing the liver and allows the liver to function as an efficient guardian between the gut and the rest of the body.

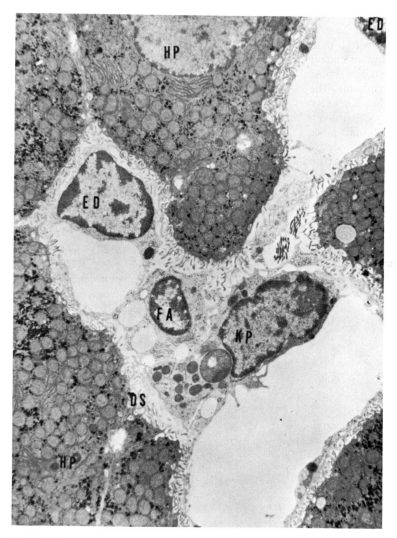

Figure 1.5 A survey picture of the sinusoid of rat liver fixed by perfusion. A Kupffer cell (KP); an endothelial cell (ED); a fat storage cell (FA); a hepatocyte (HP); the space of Disse (DS). The Kupffer cell has a small nucleo-cytoplasmic ratio, many cytoplasmic projections, ample cytoplasm containing many lysosomes with various size and density. An endothelial cell is characterized by a large nucleo-cytoplasmic ratio, the smooth cell surface, attenuated cytoplasmic processes forming the large part of the sinusoidal wall and well developed vacuolar apparatus. There is a paucity in lysosomes ($\times$ 6800, reduced to nine-tenths in reproduction). From Ogawa *et al.* (1973), reproduced by courtesy of the Editor of the *Tohoku Journal of Experimental Medicine*

Three types of highly specialized cells, which play a critical role in maintaining homeostasis, line the sinusoids. The *sinusoidal endothelial cells*, which account for 3% of liver cells, are large flat cells with fine processes which form the barrier that gives the sinusoids vascular integrity. These cells do not appear to adhere to one another but overlap loosely. They have in their cytoplasm fenestrae of approximately 1000Å occurring in small patches called sieve plates. The fenestra provide channels between the plasma and the space of Disse through which fluid, metabolites and chylomicron remnants devoid of triglyceride can readily move. Their diameter is changed by endogenous and exogenous factors. Numerous pinocytotic vesicles reflect the role of these cells in receptor-mediated phagocytosis of endogenous and exogenous macromolecules. They are important in the turnover and catabolism of many glycoproteins, lipoproteins and mucopolysaccharides present in plasma. They synthesize important mediators such as prostaglandin E_2 and prostacyclin. The second type of cell usually given the eponym *Kupffer cell* and comprising 2% of liver cells, are anchored to the sinusoidal aspect of endothelial cells by fine cytoplasmic process. Their functions include phagocytosis of particulate matter, catabolism of endotoxin, lipids and glycoproteins including many enzymes, antigen processing and secretion of mediators and cytotoxic agents. The Kupffer cells are also thought to have the ability to bulge into the lumen of the sinusoid and perhaps control sinusoidal blood flow. A third type of perisinusoidal cell, on the non-luminal side of the endothelial cells, is the *Ito cell*, also called 'fat-storing cell' or stellate cell, reflecting two of its functions: vitamin A storage and metabolism and its ability to send out prolonged cytoplasmic projections which may control the diameter of sinusoids. During fibrogenesis these cells become myofibroblasts and secrete massive amounts of extracellular matrix components. Pit cells have features of large lymphocytes with 'natural killer' activity which may play a role in defence against viruses and tumour cells.

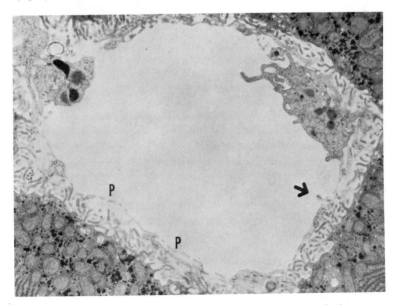

Figure 1.6 The transverse section of the sinusoid. There are many pores in the attenuated process of the endothelial cell (P). The size of the pores is about 0.1 μm. A microvillus of the hepatocyte penetrates the sinusoidal wall through the pore (arrow) (× 10 200, reduced to seven-tenths in reproduction). From Ogawa *et al.* (1973) reproduced by courtesy of the Editor of the *Tohoku Journal of Experimental Medicine*

Between these endothelial cells and the hepatocytes in health there is no basement membrane but a large extravascular space, the space of *Disse*, extending to the tight junction between adjacent hepatocytes. The space of Disse contains very scanty amounts of extracellular matrix components. The lumina of the sinusoids are less than the diameter of circulating cells, particularly if nucleated. As cells move along the sinusoids fluid is forced into and out of the space of Disse, enhancing transfer to and from the intravascular and the microvilli of the hepatocyte membrane which project into the space of Disse. Excess fluid in this space drains to lymphatics within the portal triads (Figures 1.2 to 1.5). The polyhedral *hepatocytes* are in a maze-like arrangement of sheets around which the

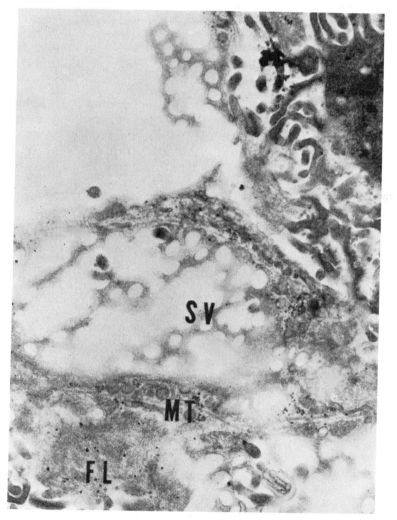

Figure 1.7 The tangential section of the attenuated process of the endothelial cell. The pores are round or oval in shape creating the sieve plate-like structure (SV). Fine filaments (FL) and microtubules (MT) can be seen in the cytoplasm around the pores (× 20 900, reduced to nine-tenths in reproduction). From Ogawa *et al.* (1973), reproduced by courtesy of the Editor of the *Tohoku Journal of Experimental Medicine*

sinusoids form a continuous three-dimensional network. The liver cell plates are two cells thick in the first 2 years of life gradually changing to plates one cell thick by 6 years.

Extracellular matrices components

Extracellular matrices components are insoluble structures initially considered as a scaffold holding cells in place but are now known to incorporate adhesive proteins which interact with specific cell surface receptors. They consist of five distinct classes of macromolecules: collagens, elastins, glycoproteins, proteoglycans and hyaluronic acid. They form a weblike structure to which cells adhere. Components of these macromolecules interact with specific cell surface receptors which connect via cytoskeletal elements to the nucleus and thus modify the phenotypic expression of the cell. The interaction is inhibited by circulating proteoglycans at physiological concentrations. Extracellular matrix/cell interaction also has an important role in cell position, locomotion, growth, differentiation and regeneration. Dramatic quantitative and qualitative changes occur in cirrhosis and during the development of malignant change.

The hepatic acinus and hepatocyte heterogeneity

The functional unit of the liver is an acinus, a three-dimensional mass of parenchyma dependent upon blood supply through a single portal tract. Blood exits the acinus by two or more hepatic veins. These hepatic venules, called 'central veins' are at the periphery of the acinus. In this concept parenchymal cells are arranged in concentric zones around the portal tracts. Zone 1, the nearest, receives blood with a high content of oxygen, insulin and glucagon, has a high metabolic activity and is the last to undergo necrosis and the first to show signs of regeneration after injury. It contains more Kupffer cells than other zones. Zone 3 nearest the terminal hepatic veins receives blood last and is described as being in the micro-circulatory periphery of the acinus. This perivenular area is formed by the most peripheral portions of Zone 3 of several adjacent acini. In injury to this zone the damaged area frequently has the outline of a starfish. Sinusoids are narrow and tortuous in Zone 1 becoming larger and straighter in Zone 3. There are striking differences between the morphology, biochemistry and function of hepatocytes in Zones 1 and 3, with a continuous and gradual transition in characteristics in the intervening 20 to 25 hepatocytes along the acinus. Sequential modification of both blood and bile occurs as they traverse the acinus. Hepatocyte heterogeneity is essential to ensure that the concentration of solutes in the hepatic venules and bile is within closely defined limits.

Hepatic development

Much of our current knowledge of the development of the liver and its functions has been derived from studies in animals or very abnormal situations in the human fetus. Because of the great variability between species in fetal growth rates, relative maturity at different stages in gestation, particularly at birth, and in postnatal feeding habits, extrapolation of these findings to the intact human fetus may lead to erroneous conclusions.

The liver appears in the third week of gestation as an invagination of the foregut into the mesoderm of the septum transversum. At 4 weeks' gestation the endodermal derived hepatic diverticulum has a cranial bud from which the hepatocytes are derived and a caudal one from which bile ducts are formed. Cords of epithelial cells grow to the right and left from the cranial bud, and rapidly proliferate between endothelium lined spaces which connect with the vitelline veins. Intrahepatic bile ducts, thought to be derived from hepatocyte precursors surrounding portal vein branches, become evident at 8 weeks' gestation. A double-layered ductal plate in the form of a sheath is formed around portal vein branches. The ductal plate is progressively remodelled to form ever smaller segments of bile duct as gestation proceeds. Interlobular bile ducts are seen at 10 weeks' gestation with bile secretion commencing at 12 weeks. Even in the third trimester intralobular bile ducts are sparse and at birth may be difficult to identify by light microscopy. Arrest of this remodelling offers an explanation for the vascular and bile duct changes seen in congenital disorders of the intrahepatic bile ducts. The liver lobes are of equal size until 3 months' gestation after which the right lobe predominates.

The caudal bud becomes the cystic duct and gall bladder. The original diverticulum elongates to become the hepatic and common bile ducts. Initially the gall bladder and bile ducts are hollow but at 5 weeks they are solid because of epithelial proliferation. Recanalization starts around 7 weeks and is complete by 14 weeks. The ventral pancreas develops in close proximity to the hepatic diverticulum and shares a common exit into the duodenum. Congenital anomalies involving the gall bladder, biliary and pancreatic ducts are, understandably, relatively common with a frequency of 10%. The mesoderm forms the marrow elements, endothelial cells, Kupffer cells, connective tissue matrix and blood vessels. All branches of the portal and hepatic veins can be identified by the 10 mm stage. By late gestation the ultrastructural features of hepatocytes are very similar to those in the adult. Until 2 years of age the majority of the hepatocyte plates are two cells thick limiting entry and egress of substrates. It is not until the age of 5 or 6 years that all plates are one cell thick. Umbilical venous blood from the placenta is largely deviated from the liver via the ductus venosus to the inferior vena cava. The remainder of the umbilical vein blood passes via the portal vein through the liver, rejoining the circulation via the hepatic veins. At this stage, the right and left hepatic lobes are of equal size, but the portal venous drainage to the left lobe is less satisfactory than that to the right, causing a relative retardation of growth of the left lobe before birth. The ductus venosus probably closes soon after birth. By 10–20 days of age closure is complete.

A further complexity is the gradual development of hepatocyte heterogeneity and differences in metabolic function across the acinar zones. The factors controlling the development and maintenance of this complex, highly organized structure are the subject of much current research. It seems likely that all of the cells within the liver interact with one another. They also interact with components of the extracellular matrix via specific receptors on cell surfaces. These adhesive proteins of the extracellular matrix not only control cell migration but also metabolic activity within hepatocytes. A host of growth factors and specific growth factor receptors have been identified in recent years. Of those purified the majority are tyrosine kinases whose activity is determined by the degree of phosphorylation. These stimulate or inhibit the growth of many tissues. In the fine tuning of hepatocyte growth a hepatotropin, a number of hepatopoietins and a hepatic proliferation inhibitor, as yet poorly characterised, may be crucial.

Haemopoietic cells are still prominent in the liver at birth but clear by 6 weeks of age unless hyperactive because of haemolysis.

Physiology of the liver

Hepatocellular functions: developmental and pathophysiological aspects

The liver plays a major role in metabolism, maintaining within narrow limits the supply of carbohydrates, proteins, lipids and macromolecules to other tissues, in spite of wide variations in dietary intake and in metabolic demands. The liver is involved in the chemical transformation of many endogenous and exogenous substances, thereby changing their metabolic, therapeutic or toxic effects and facilitating biliary excretion of many substances. By bile formation it contributes to digestion and absorption. It serves as a store for carbohydrates in the form of glycogen, and also for the fat-soluble vitamins, A, D, E and K and vitamin B_{12}.

During much of childhood the liver has considerable reserve capacity for these functions. In the neonatal period and first 2 years of life there is a temporary inefficiency in some its roles, particularly in infants born prematurely.

In fetal life many enzymes have negligible activity, possibly because many of the functions of the liver are at this time performed by the placenta and maternal tissues. It is thought that changes in the function of the liver in the perinatal period occur in association with intrahepatic and extrahepatic vascular changes, together with extensively studied, but only partially understood, changes in enzymatic activity. These may be mediated by postnatal falls in plasma insulin and increase in glucagon. Many of the enzymatic studies on which current knowledge is based have been carried out in experimental animals, often using artificial substrates for the enzyme.

Each of the main physiological roles of the liver are considered briefly below, together with changes during development and in disease. For further details Chapter 16 should be consulted together with major textbooks (Arias et al., 1988; Scriver et al., 1989; McIntyre et al., 1991).

Carbohydrate metabolism

Monosaccharides, glucose, galactose and fructose absorbed from the intestinal tract are avidly taken up by the liver, where they may be utilized for immediately required energy, being incorporated in the citric acid cycle, or they may be used to form glycogen. During fasting hepatic glycogen is an invaluable source of carbohydrate, releasing glucose to other tissues and preventing hypoglycaemia. Gluconeogenesis in the liver increases with prolonged fasting utilizing amino acids released from peripheral tissues. Muscle glycogen does not release glucose into the general circulation.

Large amounts of glycogen appear in the liver towards the end of gestation. Glycogen is rapidly mobilized immediately following birth; hypoglycaemia may occur at this stage. It is thought that this arises because of ineffective gluconeogenesis which does not replenish hepatic glycogen. Liver glycogen stores are lower in the premature or light-for-gestational age infant.

Hypoglycaemia occurs in inborn errors of carbohydrate, amino acid and lipid metabolism, fulminant hepatic failure, Reye's syndrome and with poisoning by drugs such as ethanol or hypoglycin.

Lipids: bile salts

The liver has a key role in the synthesis, catabolism and biliary excretion of lipids, lipoproteins, phospholipids, sphingolipids, cholesterol-derived steroids and enzymes involved in their metabolism. Neutral fats absorbed from the small intestine are oxidized within the liver into glycerol and free fatty acids. Fatty acids may be further oxidized to acetyl coenzyme A (CoA) which enters Kreb's tricarboxylic acid cycle. Glycerol may be utilized to form other triglycerides or degraded via acetyl CoA. Hepatic fat is usually triglyceride synthesized from fatty acids and glycerol-3-phosphate. There is continuous recycling of fatty acids between the liver and adipose tissue. Hepatic uptake increases with serum fatty acid concentrations. The liver has a limited ability to oxidize fatty acids and to secrete triglyceride as very low density lipoproteins. Fat accumulation in the liver may thus occur because of increased lipolysis in adipose tissue or from hepatic derangement limiting fatty acid oxidation or triglyceride secretion.

Cholesterol is synthesized in the liver, intestinal mucosa, adrenal cortex and arterial walls. It is excreted in the bile as a neutral steroid. As well as providing the basic structure for steroid hormones, cholesterol is the precursor of bile salts. These are synthesized only within the liver. The liver also has a key role in the uptake, reabsorption and conjugation of free bile acids arriving in the portal blood. These are rapidly conjugated with glycine or taurine, prior to biliary secretion (See Chapter 2).

In the newborn infant serum bile acid and cholesterol concentrations are lower than in older children or in adults. Bile acid synthesis is reduced. The bile acid pool, when corrected for surface area, is less in the neonate than in the adult. Bile acid secretion is low although there is no defect in bile acid transport. Malabsorption of fats results. These physiological defects are not seen in infants who have been born to mothers who have received dexamethasone to prevent hyaline membrane disease. Presumably this agent induces metabolic pathways involved in bile acid formation.

All forms of hepatocellular injury and cholestasis cause mild hypertriglyceridaemia, decreased serum cholesteryl ester, a reduced alpha-lipoprotein concentration and an increased beta-lipoprotein concentration. With cholestasis there is also a striking rise in free cholesterol and unusual lipoproteins, particularly lipoprotein-X and a deficiency of cholesterol acyltransferase (LCAT).

Protein and amino acid metabolism

The liver, with muscle, plays a key role in amino acid metabolism. Amino acids absorbed from the intestine are rapidly taken up by the liver. There they are utilized in protein synthesis, gluconeogenesis or ketogenesis following deamination or transamination. Ammonia produced by the deamination of amino acids is rapidly converted to urea.

Most of the proteins in plasma, other than the immunoglobulins, are synthesized by the rough endoplasmic reticulum of the hepatocytes. Quantitatively, albumin is the most important of these, but haptoglobin, transferrin, caeruloplasmin, C reactive protein, alpha-1 antitrypsin, alpha-2 globulin, ferritin and alpha- and beta-lipoprotein are formed in the liver.

The other important proteins are those involved in clotting mechanisms. Fibrinogen, prothrombin and Factors V, VII, IX, X and, to some extent, Factor VIII, are formed within the liver. Factors II, VII, IX and X are dependent on the presence of vitamin K for their synthesis. Inhibitors of the coagulation system, notably anti-thrombin III and components of the fibrinolytic system, for example, plasminogen, are also synthesized within hepatocytes. The liver avidly binds desialylated glycoproteins clearing them from the circulation.

Protein synthesis is very active in fetal life and in the newborn period. The main serum protein in fetal life is alpha-fetoprotein. It first appears in the serum at 6 weeks' gestation, rising to a peak concentration of 300 mg/dl at 13 weeks' gestation and then declining linearly to around 7 mg/dl in cord blood. By the age of 6 weeks the concentration has fallen to less than 25 µg/litre. Albumin synthesis starts at approximately 3 to 4 months' gestation, the serum concentration is at the adult value by birth. Low levels are commonly found in prematurely born infants. Proteins involved in coagulation are frequently of low concentration around the time of delivery but increase to normal levels within a few days. Caeruloplasmin is low at birth and reaches its highest concentration at about the age of

3 months, thereafter falling slowly to the adult level by the age of 2 years. There is thus no uniformity in the time course of changes in homeostasis of different proteins.

Although amino acids, except cystine, are in higher concentrations in fetal blood than in the adult, the enzymes involved in metabolism or degradation of amino acids are at low activity around the time of birth. The elevated phenylalanine levels frequently found in premature infants are attributed to a deficiency of enzymes involved in this degradation. Premature infants given a high protein intake may be unable to metabolize amino acids and have dangerously elevated serum concentrations as a result. If liver function is impaired significantly serum concentrations of amino acids increase, except branched chain amino acids which are preferentially taken up by muscle. Protein synthesis decreases as shown clinically by low concentrations of clotting factors produced by the liver and by low serum albumin concentrations, although fluid retention may contribute to the latter. The role of the liver in acidbase homeostasis is controversial. Alkalosis in advanced liver disease may be due to impaired urea synthesis as well as potassium depletion or hyperaldosteronism. During hepatic regeneration alpha-fetoprotein production increases (see Chapter 8). Alpha-fetoprotein production is prolonged and increased in neonatal obstructive liver diseases; it is also produced by 70–90% of hepatocellular tumours.

Drug, toxin and xenobiotic metabolism

The metabolism of drugs, toxins and xenobiotics within the liver occurs in two stages in most instances. The first step (phase I) is a biochemical transformation resulting in oxidation, reduction, hydrolysis, hydration or isomerization. This is followed by conjugation (glucuronidation, glycosylation, sulphation, methylation, acetylation, amino-acid, glutathione or fatty acid condensation), which renders the compound more water-soluble, making it more readily excreted in the urine or bile. Continuous administration of drugs such as phenobarbitone, phenytoin or rifampicin, which are metabolized by the endoplasmic reticulum, has the effect of increasing the concentration and activity of enzymes involved in drug metabolism. This process known as 'enzyme induction', is non-specific, that is one drug may induce changes in the metabolism of other drugs or endogenous substances such as steroids. The outcome may or may not be to the patient's advantage; adverse effects include e.g. patients treated with phenobarbitone having increased vitamin D and cyclosporin requirements.

In the first 2–4 weeks of life, drug metabolism is frequently very different from that in the adult because of differences in the binding of drugs by serum proteins, inefficient renal function, and differences in hepatic metabolism. The metabolic handicaps in drug handling in the newborn are very similar to those found in bilirubin excretion. Phase 2 reactions are generally normal in early infancy but it is 3 months of age before Phase 1 drug metabolizing enzyme activity levels are similar to those in adult life. As a result, both the pharmacological action of drugs and their half-life are often very different in the newborn period. It is generally necessary to give low doses less frequently. In childhood it has been estimated that hepatic metabolism of drugs such as theophylline is twofold higher than in adults. In hepatic insufficiency the effects on drug metabolism are complex and depend on the degree of biotransformation in other tissues, changes in binding protein concentrations in addition to changes in liver function. In general the pharmacological half-life is prolonged.

Vitamins   The liver has a critical role in the uptake, storage, metabolism and transport of both water-soluble and fat-soluble vitamins, frequently being the main organ of synthesis of specific transport proteins. Hepatocytes and Ito cells are involved in vitamin A metabolism. Thiamine, riboflavin, niacin, vitamin B_{12}, B_6, folic acid, biotin and pantothenic acid are metabolized in the liver and are essential for other aspects of hepatic metabolism. The liver produces essential active metabolites of vitamins D and E. Vitamin K is essential for the synthesis of clotting factors II, VII, IX, X and proteins C and S. Normal bile production is essential for absorption of fat-soluble vitamins. In hepatic insufficiency the main effects are deficiency of fat soluble vitamins, but other tissues suffer from deficiency of metabolically active vitamin products.

Hormones

The liver has an important role in the metabolism of glucocorticoids, mineralocorticoids, thyroxine, parathyroid hormone, insulin, glucagon, growth hormone, oestrogens, aldosterone and gut hormones. The main step is usually production of an inactive metabolite which is then conjugated to either glucuronic acid or sulphate which can then be excreted by the kidney. Many of the binding proteins are synthesized in the liver as is somatomedin. The liver is a major target organ for many hormones, frequently producing secondary messengers which are essential for the full effects of a particular hormone. Feedback control mechanisms minimize the effects of liver disease on most hormonal derangements in childhood.

Reticulo-endothelial function

In fetal life, the liver is an important site of haematopoiesis, activity being maximal at 7 months' gestation. Within 6 weeks of birth haemopoiesis is normally confined to the bone marrow, but in the presence of haemolytic anaemia, or where the bone marrow space has been destroyed, the reticulo-endothelial cells of the liver are again found to be involved in haem formation.

Kupffer cells are phagocytic and have an important function in removing a variety of bacterial products, such as endotoxin, and other antigens which have been absorbed into the portal blood. They produce many cytokines with antiviral effects and others including leukotrienes which influence metabolism in hepatocytes and Ito cells. The Kupffer cells may have an important role in conjunction with the rest of the reticulo-endothelial system in producing antibodies. The source of secretory IgA in human bile is unclear. In other species it can be secreted from hepatocytes or from plasma cells in the biliary system (NouriAria and Eddleston, 1991).

Hepatic ultrastructure and function

Electron microscopy coupled with advances in histochemistry at a subcellular level, has permitted exciting advances in the correlation of structure and function within the hepatocytes. Histochemical studies, although they have been used to demonstrate only a few enzymes, are important, particularly if quantified by microdensitometry, since they have provided a correlation between cell morphology and the results of biochemical studies which have exploited classic cell fractionation techniques.

These histochemical studies allow speculation about function of the structures seen with the electron microscope. The hepatocyte is permeated by a continuous complex tubular network, the plasma membrane, with all intracellular organelles except mitochondria.

The major structures within the hepatocytes – organelles – will be described and their function considered.

Plasma membrane The plasma membrane of the hepatocyte is a complex and active tissue, possibly conferring on the liver cell many of its unique properties of selective hepatic uptake of chemicals and their biliary excretion. The sinusoidal aspects of the cell are bounded by long, often tortuous villi, which stain actively with such enzymes as alkaline phosphatase and nucleosidase-monophosphatase. In the cytoplasm immediately adjacent to the membrane are numerous vesicles which participate in the transport of proteins, lipids and macromolecules into the hepatocyte. The membrane contains highly specialized areas which facilitate absorption and secretion by endocytosis. It can occur in the fluid phase, by adsorption to specific membrane sites or be receptor mediated. In this last mode the receptor–substrate complex is internalized and remains segregated from the cytoplasm within vesicles. The receptor may be metabolized, returned to the plasma membrane or excreted in bile. The microfilament system is involved in the process of endocytosis and the internal direction of vesicles to the organelle in which they are further metabolized or to the biliary pole of the hepatocyte. Cholesterol, albumin, fibrinogen and other proteins are secreted into the circulation via the plasma membrane by a similar series of processes.

The bile canalicular surface is the other main area of specialization on the hepatocyte cell membrane. It has slender villi up to 0.5 mm in length which are actively involved in bile secretion. The bile canaliculi are formed by such specialized areas of cell membrane on opposing liver cells. Microfilaments surround the canaliculus, protrude into the microvilli, and may exert rhythmic contractions of the canaliculus to enhance bile flow. The third area of specialization of the plasma membrane is the so-called 'junctional' complex, a reinforced adherent area of plasma membrane bounding the bile canaliculi and effectively separating the lumen of the canaliculi from the sinusoids. The lateral or intrahepatic plasma membranes are relatively simple, being interrupted with occasional interdigitations linking adjacent cells. They do have microvilli.

Endoplasmic reticulum Endoplasmic reticulum is a complex system of membranous cisterna traversing the cytoplasm and closely associated, if not continuous with, all other organelles except the mitochondria. It is composed of proteins, phospholipids and RNA. Its functions are thought to include synthesis and transport of proteins, lipids and mucopolysaccharides and metabolism of many xenobiotics. Two types are recognized: a smooth endoplasmic reticulum, and a rough endoplasmic reticulum which has attached to it 12×10^6 ribosomes per hepatocyte.

Nucleus The nucleus is the principal site for the regulation of hereditary characteristics. The nuclear envelope consists of an outer ribosome-studded membrane and an inner smooth membrane. The membranes fuse in parts called 'membrane pores'. Continuity between the outer nuclear membrane and the endoplasmic reticulum has been reported in many cell types.

A nuclear cytoplasmic pathway has been demonstrated in some types of cells. The nucleus has many fibrillar deoxyribonucleic acid and granular components containing ribonucleic acid precursors. It has an important role in ribosomal ribonucleic acid biosynthesis. Euchromatin, representing active parts of the genome, or complete gene complement, is seen as dense fibres in isolated chromatin fractions. Mitotic figures are very rare (1/20 000).

Mitochondria The main function of these organelles is in oxidative phosphorylation and in the storage of energy as adenosine triphosphate. Mitochondria are closely related to the endoplasmic reticulum but are most dense in the perinuclear and sub-sinusoidal zones.

They have a characteristic appearance, being delineated by a smooth outer membrane which is separated by a small space from the inner membrane. The inner membrane is convoluted and on projections into the matrix has prominent, fine club-shaped particles. Each base part is thought to represent an electron transport system, while the head of the club represents ATPase coupling factors. Within the matrix, granules containing calcium and phosphorus may be seen. The mitochondria also contain both deoxyribonucleic acid and ribonucleic acid. They thus have a complete mechanism for the transport of genetic material, although the exact relationship of this mechanism to the nuclear genetic material is unclear.

Ultrastructural histochemical techniques show that the enzymes cytochrome, B5 and monoamine oxidases are localized to the outer layers of the mitochondrial membrane, while enzymes of the respiratory chain are on the inner membrane. The inner membrane also contains a range of substrate specific transport mechanisms for glutamate alpha-ketoglutarate, carnitine and fatty acid derivatives. The matrix is a concentrated solution of enzymes involved in tricarboxylic acid and fatty acid metabolism and urea synthesis.

Mitochondria are sensitive indicators of cell damage. Swelling, bizarre shape and the development of crystal-like material in the matrix have been described in a variety of hepatic disorders.

Golgi apparatus   The Golgi apparatus is a complex arrangement of vesicles and saccules, often stacked in a parallel fashion near the bile canaliculi. Adjacent to the Golgi apparatus is a distinct system of smooth membrane tubules from which lysosomes may arise (GERL – Golgi-endoplasmic reticulum-lysosomes). The Golgi apparatus is involved in the addition of carbohydrate moieties to polysaccharides, glycoproteins and glycolipid proteins. It may be involved in the coupling of lipids with protein and in their 'packaging' prior to secretion from the hepatocytes.

Lysosomes   Lysosomes are a morphologically heterogeneous group of organelles found throughout the hepatocyte. They contain more than 30 acid hydrolysases which are capable of degrading a wide range of biological compounds if activated. The relationship to other intracellular compartments is unclear. They may contain other organelles in various states of degeneration, haemosiderin granules or ferritin particles and lipofuscin. Whether they function entirely as intracellular scavengers has not been resolved.

Peroxisomes   These are small spherical or ovoid structures 0.1–1.5 μm in diameter. They have no specific intracellular distribution and how they communicate with other intracellular organelles is uncertain. Their functions include respiration, gluconeogenesis, lipid metabolism, thermogenesis and purine catabolism. They contain two essential enzymes involved in the glycerol ether bond formation required for the production of plasmalogens. They also contribute to bile acid synthesis (see Zellweger's syndrome).

Microtubules   Microtubules are smooth membrane tubules found throughout the hepatocyte. They are less prominent in the liver cells than in many other cells. The main role is thought to be in intracellular transport, but this has yet to be fully defined.

Clinical assessment of liver size and texture

Inspection   Where hepatomegaly is massive, or where there are large nodules on the surface of the liver, this may be evident on inspection.

Palpation and percussion   The extent of downward displacement of the liver is determined most easily by palpation just lateral to the right rectus muscle in the midclavicular line. Serial measurement of the extension down from the right costal margin is helpful in monitoring disease. In the newborn the liver edge is 3–4 cm below the right costal margin but by 4 months of age it has usually receded to 2 cm below the costal margin. In older children it is rarely more than 1 cm below the costal margin, except in deep inspiration. It may be normally palpable in the mid-line 3 or 4 cm below the base of the xiphisternum.

If the liver is palpable at a lower level, one cannot immediately conclude that the liver is enlarged until the position of the upper border has been determined by light percussion. It should be at the level of the fifth or sixth rib in the right mid-axillary line, at about the seventh intercostal space in the mid-axillary line, and at the ninth rib posteriorly. The left lobe extends from the mid-line out as far as the left mid-clavicular line. Increase in lung volume displaces downwards the upper limits of hepatic dullness.

Auscultation   Auscultation is of value in detecting increased hepatic blood flow in vascular lesions such as tumours and haemangiomata.

Auscultation may be used to assess the position of the lower border of the liver by placing a stethoscope on the xiphisternum and scratching the abdomen lightly in a transverse direction, advancing the line of the scratch cephalad in the right mid-clavicular line. If the edge of the liver is below the costal margin a change in intensity and quality of the auscultated sound is noted as the edge is crossed. In general, this technique has little to add to palpation, but it may be helpful when the liver is large but soft, for example, in glycogen storage disease. In a recent study the extent of liver enlargement determined by auscultation corresponded more accurately than palpation with the liver size as determined by scanning techniques. An alternative method is to determine the 'liver span', the distance in the mid-clavicular line between the upper limit of hepatic dullness and the palpated or percussed edge of the liver. Average values are 5 cm at 2 months of age, 7 cm at 3 years and 9 cm at 12 years. Where the latter technique has been compared with radioisotope scans, considerable discrepancies have been found.

Very large livers are associated with storage disorders, disorders of the reticulo-endothelial system, such as leukaemia, gross fatty change, malignant disease and congestive cardiac failure. Rapid changes in size occur in congestive cardiac failure and in bile duct obstruction. A reduction in the size of the liver occurs in acute liver failure and in cirrhosis except when due to biliary lesions. Reidel's lobe is an anatomical variation consisting of a downward tongue-like projection from the right lobe of the liver which may extend to the right iliac crest. The liver may be central or left sided in biliary atresia-polysplenia syndrome.

Some information on the nature of the liver disease may be inferred from the consistency of the edge of the liver and from its surface. The normal edge is soft, fairly sharp, and is not tender. Livers swollen by infection, infiltration or congestion are firm, have somewhat rounded edges, smooth surfaces and are tender if the swelling is acute. As fibrosis increases the liver becomes harder. In cirrhosis the liver is hard and has an irregular surface and edge. The liver is pulsatile in tricuspid incompetence.

Spleen

In health the spleen is not palpable except in the first few weeks of life when it may be palpated from 1 to 2 cm below the left costal margin. It is very commonly palpably enlarged during generalized infections. It is best detected by gentle palpation starting from the right iliac fossa and moving towards the left costal margin. The spleen is a very superficial organ, and the edge is very distinct. The splenic notch is very rarely palpable in health. On percussion the dullness extends up beyond the costal margin. Spleen size should be recorded as the distance in its long axis from the costal margin to the tip. Splenomegaly may reflect portal pressure as well as infiltration, abnormal storage of metabolites or occur in response to infection. Ultrasonic scanning is valuable in detecting and monitoring the degree of splenomegaly, particularly in the presence of ascites.

Bibliography and References

Arias, I. M., Jakoby, W. P., Popper, H, Schachter, D. and Shafritz, D. A. (eds) (1987) *The Liver – Biology and Pathobiology*, 2nd edn. Raven Press, New York

Arias, I. M., Jakoby, W. B., Popper, H., Schachter, D. and Shafritz, D. A. (eds) (1988) *The Liver – Biology and Pathobiology*. 2nd edn, Raven Press, New York

Ashkenazi, S., Mimouri, F., Merlob, P., Litmanovitz, I. and Reisner, M. (1984) Site of liver edge in full-term healthy infants. *Am. J. Dis. Child.*, **138**, 377

Broelsch, C. E., Whitington, P. F. and Emond, J. C. (1991) Liver transplantation in children from living related donors. *Annals of Surgery*, **214**: 428–39

Desmet, V. J. (1992) Congenital diseases of intrahepatic bile ducts: variations on the theme 'Ductal Plate Malformation'. *Hepatology*, **16**: 1069–1083

Drews, U. (1991) Embryology of the liver. In *Hepatobiliary Surgery in Childhood* (eds Schweizer, P., Schier, F.), Schattauer, Stuttgart, pp.3–10

Fuller, G. N., Hargreaves, M. R., King, D. M. (1988) Scratch test of clinical examination of liver. *Lancet*, **i**: 181

Gumucio, J. J. (1989) Hepatocyte heterogeneity: the coming of age. From the description of a biological curiosity to the partial understanding of its physiological meaning and regulation. *Hepatology*, **9**, 154–160.

Haratake, J., Hisaoka, M., Furuta, A., Horie, A. and Yamamoto, O. (1991) A scanning electron microscopic study of postnatal development of rat peribiliary plexus. *Hepatology*, **14**: 1196–1200

McIntyre, N., Benhamou, J. P., Bricher, J., Rizzetto, and Rodes J. (eds) (1991) *Oxford Textbook of Clinical Hepatology*, Oxford Medical Publications, Oxford

Mowat, A. P. (1976) Development of liver function. In *Topics in Paediatric Gastroenterology* (ed J. A. Dodge), Pitman Medical, London, p.51

Naveh. Y. and Berant. M. (1984) Assessment of liver size in normal infants and children. *J. Pediatr. Gastroenterol. Nutr.*, **3**: 346

Nouri-Aria, K. T. and Eddleston, A. L. W. F. (1991) Immunological functions of the liver. In *Oxford Textbook of Clinical Hepatology*. (eds N. McIntyre, J. P. Benhamou, J. Bricher, Rizzetto and J. Rodes) Oxford Medical Publications, Oxford, pp.97–101

Ogawa, K., Minase, T., Enomolo, K. and Gnoe, T. (1973) Ultrastructure of fenestrated cells in the sinusoidal wall of rat liver after perfusion fixation. *Tohuky J. Exp. Med.*, **110**: 89

Peters, R. L. (1983) Early development of the liver. A review. In *Paediatric Liver Disease* (eds M. M. Fischer and C. C. Roy) Plenum Press, New York, p.1

Reif, S., Sykes, D., Rossi, T. and Weiser, M. M. (1992) Changes in transcripts of Basement Components during rat liver development: Increase in laminin messenger RNAs in the neonatal period. *Hepatology*, **15**: 310–315.

Rieff, M. I. and Osborn, L. M. (1983) Clinical estimation of liver size in newborn infants. *Pediatrics*, **71**, 46

Reubner, B. H., Blankenberg, T. A., Burrows, D. A., Soo Hoo, W. and Lund, J. K. (1990) Development and transformation of the ductal plate in the developing human liver. *Paediatr. Pathol.*, **10**, 55–68

Scriver, C. R., Beaudet, A. L., Sly, W. S. and Valle, D. (eds) (1989) *The Metabolic Basis of Inherited Disorders*, 6th edn. McGraw-Hill, New York

Sokal, E., Trivedi, P., Portmann, B. and Mowat, A. P. (1989) Developmental changes in the intra-acinar distribution of succinate dehydrogenase, glutamate dehydrogenase, glucose 6 phosphatase and NADPH dehydrogenase in rat liver. *J. Ped. Gastroenterol. Nutrition*, **8**, 522–527

Suchy, F. J., Bucuvalas, J. C. and Novak, D. A. (1987) Determinants of bile formation during development: ontogeny of hepatic bile acid metabolism and transport. *Sem. Liver Dis.*, **7**, 77–84

Taylor, I. M. (1983) Developmental aspects of the hepatic circulation. In *Paediatric Liver Disease* (eds M. M. Fischer and C. C. Roy), Plenum Press, New York, p.17

Traynor, O., Castaing, D. and Bismuth, H. (1988) Peroperative ultrasonography in the surgery of hepatic tumours. *Br. J. Surg.*, **75**, 197–202

Chapter 2

Anatomy and physiology of the biliary tract

Anatomy and physiology

The biliary tract extends from the bile canalicular membrane in the hepatocyte through a system of ductules, ducts and the gall bladder to the sphincter of Oddi where it joins the duodenum. Bile formation starts in the hepatocyte but the whole biliary system is lined by cells which play an important part in the production and modification of bile. The surface area of these bile duct and gall bladder lining cells is increased by the presence of microvilli. Its role in secretion and absorption of bile is emphasized by its profuse blood supply.

Anatomy and ultrastructure

The biliary system starts in the *bile canaliculi*, which are channels of uniform diameter between two or three adjoining hepatocytes. The walls of bile canaliculi are specialized segments of the hepatocyte cell wall bearing regularly shaped cylindrical microvilli which jut into the lumen of the canaliculi. Along the margin of the grooves which form the bile canaliculi the hepatocytes are attached to one another by junctional complexes. These include gap junctions which permit electrical communication between liver cells, desmosomes which act as fastening bodies, and so-called 'tight junctions' which form continuous bands along the entire length of the canalicular network. The bile canaliculi are surrounded by specialized pericanalicular cytoplasm which contains microtubules, vesicles, lysosomal-like structures and, frequently, a Golgi apparatus. Within the pericanalicular cytoplasm there is a rich network of actin microfilaments which also extend into the microvilli. These microfilaments maintain the shape of the hepatocyte including the microvilli and contribute to the structural integrity of the canaliculus. They also have a contractile function which requires the integrity of the Ca^{2+}-calmodulin and actin-myosin systems to promote bile flow in the canalicular network within the hepatocyte plate towards the portal tract.

Bile leaves via channels lined by two spindle-shaped cells (canal of Hering) which drain into fine cholangioles at the periphery of the portal tracts. They have a diameter less than that of a liver cell and are lined by cuboidal epithelial cells. They drain to interlobular bile ductules lined by cells which are smaller than hepatocytes, have a clear cytoplasm, fewer mitochondria, but have up to 70 widely spaced microvilli on their epithelial surface. These ductules join ducts of ever-increasing calibre which form plexuses around portal vein branches as they carry bile towards the portahepatis, forming septal, then segmental ducts which drain into the major right and left hepatic ducts before emerging from the right and

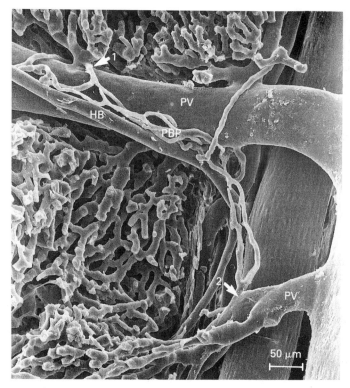

Figure 2.1 Anastomosis between peribiliary plexus (PBP) and inlet venule (1) and between peribiliary plexus and portal vein branch (2) in a preterminal portal tract of a 4-week-old rat. (Reproduced with permission from Harate *et al.*, 1991)

left lobes of the liver at the portahepatis to form the common hepatic duct (Figure 2.1). The lining cells of these larger ducts become more cylindrical but still bear many microvilli.

All of the intrahepatic biliary epithelium is surrounded by a dense capillary network derived from tributaries of the hepatic artery and draining via terminal branches of the portal vein into the sinusoids. Another feature of these major tributaries of the common hepatic duct are two diametrically opposed rows of glands which produce both serous and mucous secretions. These glands lie outside the ducts but open into them. Simpler, smaller, but less frequent glands are seen along the common bile duct. The common bile duct has a columnar epithelium with prominent microvilli. The mucosa is often arranged in longitudinal oblique folds or rugae with a highly vascular lamina propria. A few thin smooth muscle fibres are found in the connective tissues surrounding the duct.

The common hepatic duct is joined by the cystic duct from the gall bladder to form the common bile duct, which terminates at the choledocho-duodenal junction uniting with the main pancreatic duct in a *complex ampulla* which opens on to a papilla on the mediodorsal aspect of the second part of the duodenum. A sphincter is found at the lower end of the common bile duct with another within the ampulla and its papilla. The ampulla has a complex arrangement of valve-like structures with smooth muscle and mucus-producing glands which may assist in the mixing of bile and pancreatic juices. The usual gross

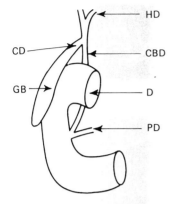

Figure 2.2 Diagrammatic representation of a normal extrahepatic biliary tree showing the hepatic duct (HD), common bile duct (CBD), gall bladder (GB), cystic duct (CD), duodenum (D), and pancreatic duct (PD)

anatomy of the extrahepatic biliary system is shown in Figure 2.2 but many variations in size, position, orientation and site of confluence occur.

The *gall bladder* is a pear-shaped highly vascular well enervated bag, the broad end of which is directed anteriorly towards the abdominal wall. The fasting volume in adults ranges from 10 to 50 ml. The body extends into a narrow neck continuing into the cystic duct which may have a sphinteric action. The mucosa of the gall bladder is lined by columnar epithelium bearing long, fine microvilli. The surface area is markedly increased in area by highly vascular rugae or interconnecting ridges. These mucosal folds extend into the cystic duct.

The wall of the gall bladder consists of muscular fibres without definite layers except in the neck and fundus where the muscle is particularly prominent. The muscle is embedded in elastic connective tissue. The gall bladder receives its rich blood supply from the tortuous cystic artery, usually a branch of the hepatic artery. The gall bladder stores and concentrates bile and secretes glycoproteins. The gall bladder contracts to 25 to 50% of its fasting volume with a t_2 of 15 minutes in response to acid food in the duodenum while the sphincter of Oddi relaxes reciprocally under the influence of cholecystokinin and neural control.

Physiology of bile formation

Bile is formed in the bile canaliculi, modified in the bile ducts, concentrated in the gall bladder and ultimately is mixed with food in the intestines. There, certain organic acids, particularly bile salts, are reabsorbed, enter the circulation and return to the liver where they are avidly taken up by hepatocytes to undergo further enterohepatic circulation. Bile salts are believed to provide the main driving force in bile formation.

Bile is a complex solution of cholesterol (90–20 mg/dl; 2.4–8.5 mmol/litre), phospholipids in the form of phosphatidyl choline (1.4–8.0 g/litre), conjugated bile salts (3–45 mmol/litre), protein (0.3–3.0 g/dl) and electrolytes. The bile salts promote the secretion of lipids and stabilize these in bile. The osmolality of bile is that of plasma since cholesterol, phospholipid and bile salts are aggregated to form mixed micelles. The proteins include immunoglobulin IgA at a concentration 10 times that of plasma. The concentration of electrolytes reflects that in plasma except that the concentration of bicarbonate is higher.

Bile secretion is a complex process involving at least four steps: (a) uptake or synthesis of substances by the liver or bile duct cells; (b) metabolic transformation of these

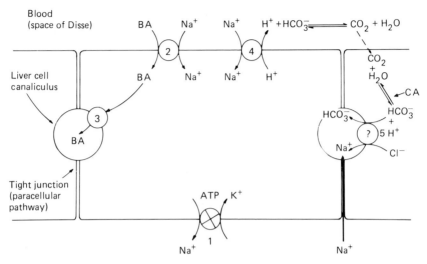

Figure 2.3 Diagrammatic representation of major bile acid (BA) transport systems considered to be involved in hepatic uptake and biliary secretion. The evidence for these transport systems is based largely on studies using membrane vessicles. (1) represents Na^+, K^+–ATPase; (2) bile acid–Na^+ co-transport system; (3) canalicular carrier for bile acids; (4) Na^+/H^+ antiport system. This may be linked via carbonic anhydrase (CA) to a Cl^-–HCO_3^- exchanger(s). The paracellular pathway may carry H_2O as well as NA^+

principally by the endoplasmic reticulum and Golgi on route to the bile; (c) transcytotic microtubular-dependent movement of vesicles (formed at the basolateral membrane or within hepatocytes) to the bile canaliculi; and (d) excretion of water, organic and inorganic material into the bile canaliculi. In addition, paracellular secretion of electrolytes, water and inert solutes occurs via the junctional complex (Figure 2.3).

The transcytotic microtubular-dependent vesicular pathway accounts for only 10% of bile flow but is the principal mechanism for the biliary secretion of proteins, ligands, lipids and inert non-electrolytes. Intracellular regulation of bile secretion appears to be mediated via cAMP and protein kinase A which are stimulatory, protein kinase C which is usually inhibitory and cytosolic Ca^{2+} which may have contrasting effects on different components of secretion.

Biliary lipid secretion is bile salt dependent, requires intact microtubular function and is presumed to be vesicular rather than derived from specialized parts of the bile canalicular membrane. Proteins such as IgA, which are concentrated in bile, are taken up by a receptor protein on the sinusoidal membrane and rapidly endocytosed. The receptor protein is recycled to the sinusoidal membrane and the IgA transported across the hepatocyte and exocytosed into bile bound to a fragment of its receptor at the bile canaliculus. Other proteins are metabolized or degraded before secretion by up to six different postulated pathways.

Great difficulties exist in performing quantitative studies of biliary secretion, particularly in humans, but qualitative studies determining the constituents of bile and their concentrations have been possible. Collections usually involve having a T tube in the common bile duct, which implies that the circumstances studied are more likely to be pathological than physiological; or by duodenal intubation, in which substantial amounts of bile may be lost. Endoscopic cannulation of the ampulla of Vater and the common bile duct may give additional information and obviate the problem of loss of bile but has too many complications to be used as a physiological investigation. Unfortunately, there are substantial differences from species to species in bile constituents and in bile flow. Thus, the results of animal studies cannot be applied uncritically to humans. Nevertheless, by using techniques comparable to those used in determining glomerular filtration rate, in which the biliary clearance of inert solutes such as erythritol is determined, and by the use of methods validated *in vitro* and *in vivo* in the experimental animal, a tentative assessment of bile flow and the factors controlling it in humans may be made.

Bile acid-dependent secretion of bile

A linear relationship exists between the excretion of bile acid, bile flow and electrolyte output in bile in humans and many other species. Factors controlling bile acid metabolism are thus important in consideration of the control of bile flow. Between 30 and 60% of canalicular bile flow is estimated to be bile salt-dependent.

The secretion of bile salts are the main driving force in bile formation. They are excreted in bile in concentrations which are approximately 5000 times greater than that in serum – an enormous concentration gradient. Canalicular water flow is thought to be a passive osmotic response to the transport of bile salts. The pathways involved in bile salt uptake and secretion and their integration with electrolyte and water movement are given in Figure 2.3.

Bile acids reabsorbed from the intestine are very efficiently removed from the portal blood by hepatocytes, between 60 and 80% being cleared in a single passage. *De novo* synthesis of bile salts from cholesterol occurs in the liver. Before secretion, bile salts are conjugated with the amino acids glycine or taurine. Within the hepatocyte they are bound to ligandin Y (glutathione S-transferase), endoplasmic reticulum and a high affinity site on the Golgi apparatus. The latter may be involved in a vesicular pathway of bile salt

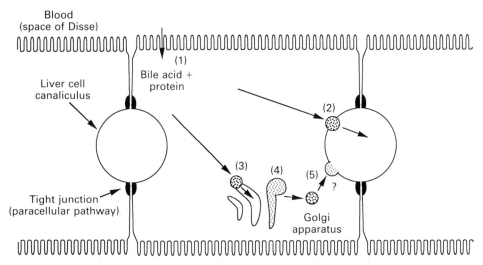

Figure 2.4 Bile acid transport through the hepatocyte. After active uptake by the hepatocyte bile acids are bound to cytosolic proteins such as glutathione S-transferases of the Y family. Bile acids may then pass via microtubules to be secreted by canalicular carriers (2). Another pathway involves uptake and internalization with a specific carrier into the Golgi apparatus (3–4), transport in Golgi derived vesicles (5) and secretion by exocytosis. (Redrawn from Erlinger, 1992.)

secretion by exocytosis. The other mode of secretion is via a carrier-mediated active transport system. Only a small amount of the total bile salts excreted at any one time is newly synthesized, the remainder having already undergone repeated cholehepatic and enterohepatic circulation. They will have been concentrated, stored in the gall bladder to be released in high concentration into the duodenum when food is taken and reabsorbed largely in the ileum (Figure 2.4).

Digestion and enterohepatic circulation of bile salts   In the upper small intestine bile salts play a crucial role in digestion and absorption of lipids. The exact mechanism of their action in this regard is still not clear but they do aid in the formation of micelles and accelerate the uptake of both fatty acid and monoglyceride by the small bowel mucosa. They activate pancreatic lipase and may have a role in the release of enterokinase and enteric hormones. They are also necessary for the absorption of fat-soluble vitamins A, D, E and K, as well as calcium. Bile salts undergo passive reabsorption throughout the small bowel but pass into the ileum where they are absorbed by an active transport system ideally adapted for taurine and glycine conjugates of bile acids and also efficient at absorbing unconjugated bile acids.

This whole process is so efficient that the total bile salt pool (2–4 g in the adult) may be excreted and reabsorbed twice with every meal with only 3% of the total pool being lost in the faeces every 24 hours.

Cholesterol and phospholipid metabolism and bile salts   The liver is a key organ in the regulation of cholesterol balance, compensating for changes in dietary intake. It synthesizes and secretes various lipoprotein particles which transport sterols. It clears from the circulation both chylomicrons which have given up apolipoproteins and triglycerides to peripheral tissue but still carry cholesterol and lipoproteins carrying cholesterol from other tissues. It secretes cholesterol, steroid hormones and other lipids in bile. The movement of cholesterol into bile occurs simultaneously with phospholipids and bile salts but the exact physicochemical form in which they are secreted is unclear.

The metabolism of bile salts and cholesterol is closely related in a variety of ways as follows:

(1) The excretion of bile salts formed from cholesterol probably accounts for 40% of its turnover.
(2) Absorbed bile salts exert a negative feedback control on their own synthesis (that is, the more absorbed, the less new bile salts are formed) and thus influence cholesterol degradation.
(3) Cholesterol synthesis decreases with increased dietary intake but bile salts also control the synthesis of cholesterol both in the liver and in the intestine.
(4) Bile salts promote the secretion of insoluble cholesterol and maintain it in micellar solution in bile.
(5) Bile acids may stimulate lecithin (phosphatidyl-choline) synthesis.

Bile acid-independent component of bile flow

Factors controlling bile acid-independent bile production by hepatocytes are poorly understood. It accounts for 30–60% of canalicular bile flow in different species. It is reduced by agents which inhibit the enzyme sodium potassium ATPase and is thus thought to be produced by active sodium transport across the bile canaliculi. In experimental animals enzyme inducers such as phenobarbitone and hydrocortisone increase this component of bile flow. Agents such as glycogen, thyroid hormone and theophylline which increase cyclic AMP, also increase this component of bile flow. It may be mediated via a chloride bicarbonate-exchanger or carrier mediated glutathione conjugates.

Specific pathways of secretion into bile

At least three further distinct and independent pathways of hepatocyte secretion into bile have been identified for the following classes of substances: (a) a bile acid transporter; (b) a separate multiple organic anion transporter; and (c) and organic cation transporter – the multidrug resistance gene product – which may be responsible for the secretion of drugs and other organic cations. The driving forces for such secretion includes ATP and Ca^{2+}– ATPase with bicarbonate mediating SO_4^{2-} excretion which promotes excretion of dicarboxylic acids.

In general, compounds excreted in the bile in concentrations much higher than in plasma increase bile flow, others such as bilirubin do not, while yet others, such as lithocholic acid, bromsulphthalein and radio-opaque dyes, may be cholestatic, that is, they may reduce the bile flow.

Role of bile ducts

Studies using isolated segments of bile ducts and *in vivo* experiments, confirm that bile ducts modify canalicular bile by reabsorption and secretion. In humans 40% of basal bile flow has been estimated to come from bile duct epithelium. Secretin released by vagal stimulation from acid in the duodenum produces a bicarbonate enriched bile with a rise in pH and a fall in bile salt concentration. Cholecystokinin and gastrin in some species have similar effects. Bile ducts can reabsorb water, electrolytes, amino acids, glucose and at least some bile salts such as ursodeoxycholate. Prior to reabsorption bile ducts are protonated liberating bicarbonate which is excreted in the bile.

Role of the gall bladder

In the fasting state bile produced in the liver (estimate 600 ml/day in the adult) is diverted into the gall bladder, the sphincter of Oddi being closed. In the gall bladder there is active reabsorption of sodium bicarbonate and water by means of a neutral anion-cation pump which causes a 10-fold increase in the concentration of non-absorbable organic compounds.

Within 30 minutes of eating, there is a sharp increase in bile acid concentration of the duodenum due to contraction of the gall bladder and relaxation of, and perhaps propulsive actions by, the sphincter of Oddi. If the gall bladder is removed, is non-functioning owing to disease, or is inert as in coeliac disease, the sharp rise in duodenal concentration of bile does not occur and enteric absorption of fats may be impaired.

Cholestasis: impaired bile formation and secretion

Cholestasis, literally a standing still of bile, may be defined as impaired biliary secretion. To the pathophysiologist it means a measured reduction in bile flow or a reduction in the concentration of a major bile constituent. To the clinician cholestasis means the demonstrable accumulation in the blood of substances normally excreted in the bile (bilirubin, bile salts and cholesterol) giving jaundice with yellow bilirubin-containing

Table 2.1 Cellular mechanisms in impaired bile formation

Site of lesion	Suspected mechanism	Examples of cuases
Changes in basal lateral hepatocyte membrane	Inhibition of Na, K–ATPase	Ethinyl oestradiol
Altered intracellular transport	Disturbed microfilament or microtubular function	Chlorpromazine, colchicine
	Specific abnormalities of bile salt transport or metabolism	Genetic
Intracellular secretory	Pertubation of secretory processes	Intracellular calcium binding by bile salts
	Inhibition of Golgi function	Genetic (Alagille's syndrome)
Peri-canalicular	Inhibition of canalicular contractions	Phalloidin
Canalicular membrane	Inhibition of metabolic processes associated with dilated canaliculi with few microvilli	Chlorpromazine
Tight junction	Loss of intracanalicular water giving super-concentrated bile	Oestrogens

urine, pale stools, pruritus and xanthelasma. It may be demonstrated semiquantitatively by the delayed appearance in the gut of radiopharmaceuticals avidly taken up and secreted by the liver. To the pathologist cholestasis means visible bile in liver tissue within hepatocytes or biliary channels. Such cholestasis occurs with bile duct obstruction and with the general perturbation of hepatic perfusion and function as occurs in acute and chronic hepatitis or cirrhosis. Examples of more specific factors which may be associated with cholestasis are given in Table 2.1 to illustrate the multiplicity of process required for bile formation.

References

Arias, I. M., Jakoby, W. P., Popper, H., Schachter, D. and Shafritz, D. A. (eds) (1987) *The Liver Biology and Pathobiology*, 2nd edn. Raven Press, New York

Balistreri, W. F. (1983) Immaturity of hepatic excretory function and the ontogeny of bile acid metabolism. *J. Paediatr. Gastroenterol. Nutr.*, **2**, S207–14

Boyer, J. L. (1986) Mechanisms of bile formation and organic anion transport. In *Membrane Physiology*, 2nd edn (eds T. E. Andriole, J. F. Hoffman and D. Fenestil), Plenum Press, New York, p.274

Boyer, J. L., Graf, J. and Gautam, A. (1988) Mechanisms of bile secretion: insight from the isolated rat hepatocyte couplet. *Sem. Liver. Dis.*, **8**, 308–16

Elias, E. and Murphy, G. (eds) (1986) Bile in health and disease. In *Proceedings of the 6th BSG/SK&F International Workshop, 1985*. Smith, Kline and French, Welwyn Garden City

Erlinger, S. (1992) Bile secretion *Br. Med. Bull.*, **48**, 860–76

Frimmer, M. and Ziegler, K. (1988) The transport of bile acids in liver cells. *Biochim. Biophys. Acta*, **947**, 75–99

Gautam, A., Ng, O. C., Strazzabosco, M., Boyer, J. L. (1989) Quantitative assessment of canalicular bile formation in isolated hepatocyte couplets using microscopic optical planimetry. *J. Clin. Invest.*, **83**, 565–573

Haratake, J., Hisaoka, M., Furuta, A., Horie, A. and Yamamoto, O. (1991) A scanning electron microscopic study of postnatal development of rat peribiliary plexus. *Hepatology*, **14**, 1196–1200.

McIntyre, N., Benhamou, J.-P., Bircher, J., Rizzetto, M. and Rodes, J. (eds) (1991) *Oxford Textbook of Clinical Hepatology*. Sections 1.2, 2.3, 2.5, 2.10. Oxford University Press, Oxford
Nathanson, M. H. and Boyer, J. L. (1991) Mechanisms and regulation of bile secretion. *Hepatology*, **14**, 551–566
Watanabe, S., Miyazaki, A., Hirose, M. *et al.* (1991) Myosin in hepatocytes is essential for bile canalicular contraction. *Liver*, **11**, 185–189

Chapter 3

Unconjugated hyperbilirubinaemia

Jaundice

Jaundice, a yellow discoloration of sclera, skin and other tissues caused by the accumulation of bilirubin, is an important sign of disease or functional disorder affecting the hepatic, biliary or haematological systems. It appears in children and in adults when the serum bilirubin concentration exceeds 2 mg/dl (34 µmol/litre), but in neonates it is rarely noticeable below a concentration of 5 mg/dl (85 µmol/litre). Except in the newborn, the total serum bilirubin is less than 1.5 mg/dl (25 µmol/litre).

At all ages investigation of the causes of jaundice is simplified if it is classified into unconjugated or conjugated hyperbilirubinaemia. *Conjugated bilirubin* has been made water soluble by the enzymatic addition of glucuronide in the hepatocyte as a necessary step prior to its excretion in the bile. If the process of biliary excretion is impaired for any reason bilirubin glucuronide passes into the serum and is excreted in the urine. There its presence is confirmed easily by test strips impregnated with a diazo reagent. They detect as little as 2 µmol of bilirubin per litre. They are an underused, sensitive and highly specific test of liver dysfunction. Instead clinicians overrely on the routine laboratory estimation of direct bilirubin which underestimates serum bilirubin glucuronide concentrations at normal serum bilirubin concentrations, overestimates them at total serum bilirubin concentrations of less than 70 to 80 µmol/litre and underestimates them at higher levels. With automated methods routine laboratory measurement of total serum bilirubin concentration, by the intensity of colour produced by the action of diazotized sulphonic acid in the presence of an accelerator such as methanol, is standardized and reproducible. In contrast, direct bilirubin measurement, in which the same reaction takes placed with no accelerator, is not standardised and influenced by factors which may be poorly controlled. Classification of jaundice into direct and indirect may be misleading if interpreted without urinanalysis and/or standard laboratory biochemical tests for the detection of liver disease (usually termed 'liver function tests' although they do not test liver function *per se*). Accurate measurement of bilirubin mono- and diconjugates is possible with alkaline methanolysis and high performance liquid chromatography. These show that less than 5% of bilirubin is conjugated in health. Such methods allow distinction of Gilbert's syndrome from jaundice due to haemolysis. In the former less than 2% will be conjugated. Diazo testing even in a good laboratory will not detect less than 0.5 mg/dl (7 µmol/litre: approximately 33%) in the direct reacting form.

Unconjugated hyperbilirubinaemia is characterized clinically by jaundice without bile in the urine. In unconjugated hyperbilirubinaemia the total serum bilirubin is raised with less than 15% bilirubin reported to be in the direct reacting form (See above). It may be physiological in the newborn. It is frequently due to haematological causes; rarely, it is due to genetic or familial functional disorders considered in this chapter. Very high concentrations of unconjugated bilirubin cause brain damage.

Conjugated hyperbilirubinaemia is characterized clinically by jaundice with bile in the urine. The stools may be pale brown or even chalky white in colour. The total serum bilirubin is raised and more than 15% of the bilirubin is in the direct reacting form (See above). It is always indicative of significant hepatobiliary disease.

Bilirubin metabolism

Bilirubin is an orange organic anion with a molecular weight of 584, exclusively derived from haem or haemoglobin in senescent red blood cells, from extravasated red blood cells, from premature destruction of haemoglobin haem in developing red cells or from other tissue haem proteins such as the enzyme cytochrome P450. It is produced largely in the reticulo-endothelial system of the spleen, liver and bone marrow. Haem is first converted to biliverdin by the rate-limiting microsomal enzyme haemoxygenase, which produces equimolar amounts of carbon monoxide and biliverdin. Biliverdin is changed to bilirubin by the action of the abundant cytoplasmic biliverdin reductase enzyme. Bilirubin has a limited aqueous solubility at physiological pH. It is carried from the reticulo-endothelial system to the liver in the circulation firmly bound to serum albumin. Within the liver an ill-understood but very efficient mechanism dissociates bilirubin from albumin and the bilirubin passes into the hepatocyte. What determines hepatic selectivity of bilirubin uptake is not clear, nor is the process of uptake understood; recent research, however, has shown that this process requires no energy but has many experimental *in vitro* features consistent with a carrier-mediated membrane transport system.

Within the hepatocyte bilirubin is transported to the endoplasmic reticulum, possibly being carried by cytoplasmic proteins with a high affinity for bilirubin, such as ligandin (glutathione S-transferase B) or Z protein (fatty acid binding protein). In the endoplasmic reticulum an enzymatic process converts bilirubin to a water-soluble form, largely bilirubin diglucuronide but as recent studies have shown also to the monoglucuronide and possibly also forming conjugates with glucose, xylose and sulphate. In humans it would seem that diglucuronide is the major conjugate. The exact enzymatic process involved in these conversions is probably complex, and as yet the enzymes involved have not been purified or characterized. A surprising new finding that bilirubin monoglucuronide is formed in the endoplasmic reticulum but is subsequently converted to bilirubin diglucuronide and bilirubin by an enzyme in the liver cell membrane has been challenged in recent studies. The bilirubin conjugates are excreted into the biliary system by an energy-dependent process. The bilirubin is then carried in the bile to the bowel where it is converted to stercobilin and excreted in the stool. There is little or no enteric reabsorption.

Kernicterus

Kernicterus is a disorder in which unconjugated bilirubin is deposited in parts of the brain causing death or permanent neurological damage, typically nerve deafness, choreoathetosis, cerebral palsy and mental retardation. In full term infants with haemolytic anaemia serum bilirubin concentrations of greater than 20 mg/dl (340 μmol/litre) are associated with a significant risk of kernicterus. Acidosis, asphyxia, hypo-albuminaemia and prematurity may cause kernicterus to occur at serum bilirubin concentrations as low as 8 mg/dl (136 μmol/litre). Bilirubin can also cause a transient encephalopathy with acute changes in behaviour and in neurophysiological responses. Whether severe neonatal hyperbilirubinaemia can cause a lesser degree of permanent learning difficulty is contentious. In a recent study it was shown that serum bilirubin values above 20 mg/dl (340 μmol/litre) in full term male subjects was associated with lower IQ score at 17 years, an association not seen in female subjects. The pathogenesis of bilirubin encephalopathy is not fully understood. Unconjugated bilirubin can diffuse into the brain if the serum concentration of unconjugated bilirubin exceeds the capacity of the serum proteins, particularly albumin, to bind bilirubin. It is not possible to measure unbound bilirubin in serum. Estimation of the reserve capacity of serum proteins to bind bilirubin has not proved to be a more precise indication of the risk of kernicterus than serum bilirubin concentration itself. Although a wide range of endogenous anions such as haematin, bile acids and fatty acids, and many drugs compete *in vitro* with bilirubin for albumin binding only, sulphonamides and maternal salicylates have been shown to reduce binding and provoke kernicterus. The role of free fatty acids is controversial. The duration of exposure to high serum bilirubin levels, acidosis, alteration in the 'bloodbrain' barrier and pre-existing brain damage have all been postulated to be important contributory factors.

Genetic abnormalities in bilirubin metabolism

Crigler–Najjar syndrome (Type 1)

In 1952, Crigler and Najjar described a syndrome of severe persistent unconjugated hyperbilirubinaemia, without haemolysis or evidence of hepatic disease, usually complicated by the early onset of kernicterus and, frequently, death in the first year of life. Since then over 100 cases have been described. With the improved treatment of jaundice in the newborn period patients now survive into adult life but remain at risk of kernicterus. The condition is inherited in an autosomal recessive fashion. It occurs in all races. There is complete absence of activity of the enzyme bilirubin uridine diphosphate glucuronyl transferase (bilirubin UDPGTase) in liver. A number of genetic mutations have been found in association with this disorder but their exact effect on the enzyme glycoprotein is uncertain. In one patient a point mutation in exon 3 of the human bilirubin UDPGTase gene complex, in which a C is replaced by a T, produced a truncated and inactive enzyme. Heterozygotes are phenotypically normal with normal serum bilirubin but may have impaired glucuronidation of other substrates.

Clinical features

Jaundice appears within a few hours of birth, bilirubin rapidly rising to values greater than 20 mg/dl (340 μmol/litre), uncontrolled by phototherapy and requiring treatment by repeated exchange transfusion. At the end of the first week of life the serum bilirubin may stabilize at levels between 15 and 45 mg/dl (250 and 750 μmol/litre) but with fasting or intercurrent infection exacerbations to much higher levels occur increasing the risk of kernicterus. Kernicterus usually develops in the perinatal period or in infancy but in a few instances the onset is delayed until the late teens. Investigations fail to show haemolysis or other factors aggravating jaundice in the neonatal period. There may be a history of parental consanguinity or of similar severe icterus in other family members. The urine contains no bilirubin but may contain yellow photobilirubin derivatives.

Diagnosis

A provisional diagnosis may be made on the basis of the clinical features in the absence of other causes of hyperbilirubinaemia. Liver function tests, serum bile salt concentration and oral cholecystograms are normal. Confirmation requires percutaneous liver biopsy. There is no histological abnormality except for scattered bile plugs in bile canaliculi and bile ductules. These may represent bilirubin photoconjugates which have precipitated after biliary secretion. Bilirubin UDPGTase activity is absent.

Treatment

The object is to maintain the serum bilirubin to a level at which brain damage will not occur. Since jaundice becomes more severe during intercurrent infections the aim should be to reduce the serum bilirubin to values of less than 250 μmol/litre. Phototherapy for periods of up to 15 hours a day is the mainstay of treatment. For exacerbations continuous phototherapy, exchange transfusion or plasmapheresis may be required. In early infancy one or two standard neonatal phototherapy units usually provide sufficient photo energy, but as the infant grows more powerful specially designed light sources are likely to be required. After 4 years of age, phototherapy gradually becomes less effective. Oral cholestyramine by binding bilirubin in the gut may diminish the requirement. Liver transplantation should be considered since it is at present the only long-term means of preventing kernicterus.

Crigler–Najjar (Type 2)

This variant of the Crigler–Najjar syndrome is characterized by a less severe non-haemolytic unconjugated hyperbilirubinaemia with a serum bilirubin concentration of between 5 and 20 mg/dl (85–340 μmol/litre) which falls by at least 30% when enzyme-inducing agents such as phenobarbitone are given. The disorder is thought to be inherited in an autosomal dominant fashion with variable penetrance, but in some families inheritance may be autosomal recessive (Labrune et al., 1989). There is defective but not absent UDPGTase activity. Some conjugated bilirubin may be found in the bile, 50% in the form of bilirubin monoglucuronide.

Clinical features

Jaundice may start in the first year of life but may be delayed until childhood or even the fourth decade; its severity varies from time to time. A family history of similar jaundice may be obtained. Hyperbilirubinaemia in relatives may be shown chemically. Brain damage is infrequent.

Diagnosis

A provisional diagnosis may be made if there is no other evidence of liver disease and there is a positive family history of unconjugated hyperbilirubinaemia. Confirmation requires the demonstration of normal hepatic pathology, virtually absent activity of UDPGTase, increased bilirubin monoglucuronide in serum and bile and a reduction of serum bilirubin concentration with enzyme-inducing agents, e.g. phenobarbitone.

Treatment

The bilirubin falls to levels ranging from normal to 5 mg/dl (35 μmol/litre) in 2 to 4 weeks when enzyme-inducing agents such as phenobarbitone are given in a dose of 5–10 mg/kg body weight each evening. Since exacerbation may cause kernicterus they require similar treatment to Type 1 Crigler–Najjar syndrome.

Gilbert's syndrome

Definition

Mild, chronic, variable, unconjugated hyperbilirubinaemia with serum bilirubin levels of around 2–5 mg/dl (34–85 μmol/litre) without significant haemolysis or abnormality of liver function tests are the characteristic features of this condition. Serum bilirubin concentrations are at the high end of a skew distribution curve of bilirubin values in healthy populations, suggesting that this is a term applied to subjects with the highest serum bilirubin concentration in the population rather than a disease state. It is likely that this is a heterogeneous condition with differing pathogenic mechanisms contributing in individual patients. Mechanisms demonstrated include: slightly reduced red blood cell survival in 50% of cases, impaired hepatic uptake of bilirubin, deficient UDPGTase activity *in vitro* or a mild excretory defect.

The prevalence has been quoted to be as high as 6% but this is dependent on the value chosen as the upper limit of normal. Family studies suggest an autosomal dominant inheritance with incomplete expression but this is contentious.

Clinical features

There is a mild fluctuating jaundice. It may be accompanied by unexplained vague symptoms such as upper abdominal discomfort, lethargy and general malaise. Intercurrent infection, exertion and fasting, particularly if lipid is withdrawn from the diet, aggravates the jaundice but no more so than in other hyperbilirubinaemic states. Intravenous nicotinic acid in a dose of 50 mg in the adult also causes a sharp increase in serum bilirubin levels. Such an injection and fasting have been used clinically to support the diagnosis. Males are more commonly affected than females. The age of onset is difficult to determine but most cases come to light at around the age of 10 years but there is frequently much delay in diagnosis. Low levels of cholylglycine with normal chenodeoxycholic acid levels support the diagnosis.

Diagnosis

Diagnosis should be restricted to patients who have no history of liver disease, who show no abnormality on clinical examination, except icterus, who have normal haematological studies and liver function tests including normal serum bile acids but do have a persistent documented mild hyperbilirubinaemia. The liver histology is normal, but biopsy is unnecessary. The main conditions to be considered in differential diagnosis are compensated haemolytic states, the post-viral hepatitis syndrome, shunt hyperbilirubinaemia and Crigler–Najjar syndrome Type 2.

Treatment

The disorder is benign. If the jaundice is distressing the patient it may be cleared by the administration of phenobarbitone in a dose of 6–10 mg/kg of body weight given each evening in gradually increasing doses. Surprisingly, this therapy often causes diminution of other symptoms.

Neonatal unconjugated hyperbilirubinaemia

Of all the liver disorders, jaundice due to unconjugated hyperbilirubinaemia in the newborn infant is by far the most frequent, being evident in half of all neonates. Marked hyperbilirubinaemia can cause brain damage. The appearance of jaundice has two beneficial effects, namely, the earlier diagnosis of disorders such as septicaemia haemolysis or galactosaemia which cause jaundice and which require specific treatment; measures are taken to prevent kernicterus (irreversible brain damage due to staining of the brain by bilirubin). A great deal of research effort has gone into factors controlling the production and excretion of bilirubin. Unfortunately, in the study of neonatal jaundice much research has been done on experimental animals which do not suffer from physiological jaundice. Frequently, substances more easily measured than bilirubin have been used in *in vitro* work. Extrapolation of the results of such work to bilirubin metabolism in the newborn infant has caused a great deal of confusion.

Since, in most circumstances, bilirubin does neither harm nor good, the results of such studies may be of more importance for the information they provide about the metabolism of other organic anions, of greater physiological or pharmacological importance, which share the same metabolic pathways as bilirubin.

Physiological jaundice of the newborn

Physiological jaundice of the newborn is a transient benign icterus which occurs during the first week of life in otherwise healthy newborn infants. In full-term infants jaundice appears after the age of 24 hours and serum bilirubin rises to a mean maximum level of 6 mg/dl (100 μmol/litre) on the second to fourth days of life returning to normal by the seventh day. In breast-fed babies values are higher with the 95 percentile for bottle-fed infants being 11.6 mg/dl (195 μmol/litre) but 14.5 mg/dl (245 μmol/litre) in breast-fed infants. In premature infants levels of between 12–15 mg/dl (200–240 μmol/litre) are commonly reached on the fifth to seventh days of life and return to normal by the 14th day.

Pathogenesis

It is now considered likely that there is no single cause of physiological jaundice in the neonate but that it results from the complex interaction of factors which cause: (a) increased bilirubin production; (b) impaired hepatic uptake, conjugation and excretion of bilirubin; and (c) enteric reabsorption of bilirubin. In the individual infant all the factors influencing bilirubin metabolism can rarely be rigorously investigated. Statistical associations between the parameters that can reasonably be measured only point at aspects which require further study. Much of the laboratory research into this condition has been done with experimental animals which do not have physiological jaundice adding to interpretative difficulties when the results are applied to human.

Studies of possibly greater significance in understanding the condition in humans are those performed in the Rhesus monkey which does have a physiological jaundice, albeit a biphasic one. The serum bilirubin increases from less than 1 mg/dl (17 μmol/litre) to 4.5 mg/dl (76 μmol/litre) in the first 24 hours of life (phase 1), falling to 2 mg/dl (42 μmol/litre) on the second, third and fourth day (phase 2) returning to 0.1 mg/dl (less than 2 μmol/litre) on the fifth day. By infusion studies on this animal it has been shown that bilirubin formation is at five times the adult values in the first 18 days of life, activity of the enzyme bilirubin UDPGTase is almost zero at birth but very rapidly reaches high levels in the first 24 hours, attaining adult levels by the third day. Hepatic uptake which is at only 30% of the adult value at birth rises more slowly, reaching adult levels only on the fifth day. It is thus considered that the rapid rise of bilirubin in phase 1 is due to deficient bilirubin conjugation, but that the impaired hepatic uptake may be a major factor in phase 2. The cause of the impaired hepatic uptake has still to be identified but the virtual absence of ligandin within the hepatocyte at birth but reaching adult levels during the first week of life may possibly be related. By cannulating the bile duct and interrupting the passage of bile into the bowel it has been shown that absorption of bilirubin from the bowel adds considerably to the load of bilirubin which has to be excreted in this age group.

In the *human infant* there is good evidence of increased bilirubin production from reduced red blood cell survival shown experimentally both by the use of radioactively labelled glycine incorporated in haemoglobin and also from studies of the production of carbon monoxide, released from haem. Both techniques give the red blood cell life of approximately 90 days in the newborn compared with 120 days in the adult. There is, in addition, increased bilirubin production from non-haemoglobin sources giving a total bilirubin production of approximately 8.5 ± 2.3 mg/kg of body weight per day (145 ± 39 μmol/kg per day) in infants compared with 3.6 mg/kg of body weight per day (75 μmol/kg per day) in the adult.

Lower ligandin levels have been demonstrated in human neonatal livers. The role of the possible deficient activity of the enzyme bilirubin UDPGTase is yet to be established. In an early study of this enzyme activity done on human biopsy material the time course of development was totally different from that seen in physiological jaundice, adult levels not being reached until the 70th day. It should be noted, however, that methylumbelliferone was used as a substrate rather than bilirubin. There is at present no direct evidence to implicate ineffective hepatic perfusion or diminished transport across the hepatocellular membranes as a factor in physiological jaundice. Intestinal absorption of unconjugated bilirubin derived from hydrolysis of bilirubin glucuronide by beta-glucuronidase is increased. If there is constipation this can be particularly important since the gut at birth contains an average 360 μmol of bilirubin (more than 300 mg).

Pathological neonatal unconjugated hyperbilirubinaemia

Pathological neonatal unconjugated hyperbilirubinaemia indicates that a disease process or processes may be present aggravating or accentuating the mechanisms causing physiological neonatal unconjugated hyperbilirubinaemia. Any degree of jaundice in the first 24 hours of life is pathological. In full-term bottle-fed infants bilirubin concentrations should not exceed 12 mg/dl (200 μmol/litre) on the second to fourth day and should have returned to normal by the eighth day. In breast-fed infants values should not exceed 15 mg/dl (255 μmol/litre) but may remain elevated beyond 2 weeks of age. In prematurely born infants the peak concentration may not occur until the fifth to seventh day but should be less than 15 mg/dl (255 μmol/litre) and return to normal by the 14th day. Any deviation from this pattern is abnormal and is indicative of possible underlying disease. An infant with such jaundice must be urgently investigated to identify treatable conditions such as septicaemia or galactosaemia and to institute measures to prevent kernicterus.

Causes of pathological neonatal jaundice

The many factors which may contribute to hyperbilirubinaemia in the newborn are listed in Tables 3.1, 3.2 and 3.3. It would be inappropriate in a textbook such as this to consider these in detail. The conditions listed in Table 3.1 require active treatment, and priority in assessment and investigation must be to exclude these. Those listed in Table 3.2 are important to appreciate since they may save the child much unnecessary investigation. The conditions listed in Table 3.3 are some of those in which a statistical correlation has been shown although the mechanism of action is far from clear.

Table 3.1 Causes of neonatal unconjugated hyperbilirubinaemia which require urgent identification and treatment

Infection
Haemolytic disorders, e.g. blood group incompatibility, defects of red cell membranes, red blood cell enzyme deficiencies, ingestion of haemolytic agents
Increased red blood cell mass, e.g. placental transfusion, twin-to-twin transfusion, infant of diabetic mother, late clamping of the cord
Hypoxia
Hypoglycaemia
Hypothyroidism
Dehydration
Galactosaemia
Fructosaemia
Administration of drugs competing with bilirubin for hepatic excretion
Meconium retention
High intestinal obstruction

Table 3.2 Established associations with neonatal hyperbilirubinaemia

Prematurity	Excessive bruising
Infant of diabetic mother	Down's syndrome
Breast milk jaundice of late onset	Transient familial neonatal hyperbilirubinaemia
Gilbert's syndrome	

Table 3.3 Factors possibly implicated in aggravating physiological jaundice

Male sex – summer birth	Progesterone therapy
Previous use of oral contraceptives with breast feeding	Breast feeding
Prolonged labour	Antepartum haemorrhage
Family history of hyperbilirubinaemia	Vitamin E deficiency
Previous use of oral contraceptives	

Table 3.4 Maternally administered drugs and serum bilirubin concentrations in the newborn infant

Drugs causing a reduction in serum bilirubin concentration	Drugs causing an increase in serum bilirubin concentration	Drugs having no effect on serum bilirubin concentration
Narcotic agents	Diazepam	Phenothiazine derivatives
Barbiturates	Oxytocin	General anaesthetics
Aspirin		Local anaesthetics
Chloral hydrate		Sulphadimidine
Reserpine		Ampicillin
Sodium phenytoin		Penicillin
Alcohol		

Drugs administered during pregnancy, in labour or in the neonatal period may also affect bilirubin metabolism. Most important are those causing depressed respiration with hypoxia and its sequelae. Table 3.4 lists the effects on serum bilirubin concentration in the newborn infant of drugs given to the mother. It is important to appreciate, however, that these effects are often minimal and of no clinical significance; they are included to illustrate how difficult it is in this field to associate a particular event with subsequent bilirubin metabolism.

When many risk factors are present then there is a high probability of jaundice and provided the infant is otherwise healthy it is likely to be unrewarding to undertake a battery of laboratory investigations to find a pathological cause. On the other hand more modest elevation of serum bilirubin in an infant with few or no risk factors might require investigation (Maisels and Gifford, 1986).

Breast milk jaundice

During the first week of life jaundice may be observed more commonly in breast-fed infants than in bottle-fed infants. In a study of serum bilirubin concentrations in 2416 infants breast feeding was associated with a serum bilirubin concentration of more than 12.9 mg/litre 3.7 times more frequently than bottle feeding. A possible compounding factor is the frequency of breast feeding: infants fed more than 8 times per 24 hours had lower bilirubin concentrations than those fed less frequently (DeCarvallo et al., 1982). The distribution of jaundice in healthy breast-fed infants may be bimodal. The serum bilirubin concentration in the majority, both in the first week and subsequently, is similar to that of the formula-fed infant. The minority have higher serum bilirubin values in the first week of life; these remained abnormally elevated at day 21 with a mean level of 70 μmol/litre (4 mg/dl) (Kivlahan and James, 1984). It is estimated that such early hyperbilirubinaemia associated with breastfeeding may be followed by mild prolonged hyperbilirubinemia in between 25% and 40% of infants (Kivlahan and James, 1984). There may be an overlap between such jaundice and the socalled breast-milk jaundice syndrome.

The reasons for this are not clear but possibly result from the combination of handicaps in bilirubin handling causing physiological jaundice, aggravated by low calorie intake, steroids in breast milk, possibly in inhibition of bilirubin excretion by fatty acids in breast milk and contentiously by some action of prostaglandins. In most instances jaundice disappears within 2 weeks of birth.

A rarer form of jaundice associated with breast feeding is that in which the serum bilirubin concentration rises to between 15 and 20 mg/dl (255–360 μmol/litre) in the second or third week of life in infants who are otherwise entirely well. Such jaundice may persist for as long as 4 months. If breast feeding is discontinued, however, the jaundice will resolve spontaneously within 6 days and, surprisingly, may not recur if breast feeding is recommenced. An incidence of 2.5% has been reported (Maisels *et al.*, 1988).

The aetiology of the syndrome is not known. Seventy-five per cent of siblings of affected infants are similarly affected. Breast milk from the mothers of affected infants can be shown to competitively inhibit bilirubin and chenodeoxycholate glucuronide formation *in vitro*. Among the putative mechanism is the presence in the mother's milk of $3\alpha_1 20\beta$-pregnanediol, an isomer of a natural steroid found in breast milk. It has been found in a few instances in breast milk of mothers of affected infants. When given to two infants it did cause a rise in serum bilirubin. It is not found in every case, however. Free fatty acids, powerful inhibitors of bilirubin conjugation *in vitro*, have been implicated but refuted by further studies. Enteric bilirubin reabsorption in adult rats is inhibited by normal human and cow's milk, but is not inhibited by milk from mothers whose infants have breast milk jaundice suggesting that such milk may allow increased enteric reabsorption of bilirubin. Recent studies have suggested that the high beta-glucuronidase activity in breast milk may be an important factor in the neonatal hyperbilirubinaemia of breast-fed babies (Gourley and Arend, 1986, Shinzawa *et al.*, 1988). A mild degree of liver dysfunction, immaturity or cholestasis may contribute. In a study of 58 such infants Tazawa *et al.* (1991) found in one-third elevated levels of serum alkaline phosphatase, gamma-glutamyl transpeptidase or total bile salts. On stopping breast feeding for 3 days the rate of fall of the bilirubin was slower in those with high serum bile salt concentrations.

Clinical aspects

As has already been stated, these children are entirely well. It is important, however, to consider hypothyroidism in differential diagnosis. Kernicterus has not been reported to complicate this condition but it is my practice to recommend that breast feeding be stopped for a period of 24–48 hours if the serum bilirubin levels are greater than 17 mg/dl (290 μmol/litre). If the jaundice is less than this the mother should be encouraged to continue breast feeding.

Transient familial hyperbilirubinaemia

Infants with this condition develop jaundice with serum bilirubin values peaking at 9–65 mg/dl (153–1100 μmol/litre) in the first few days of life which persists into the second or third week. The mothers are apparently healthy but all their children develop jaundice which may be complicated by kernicterus or death. Jaundice is thought to be caused by an unidentified inhibitor of bilirubin glucuronide formation which can be recovered from the serum of the mothers and of their infants.

Control of hyperbilirubinaemia

Identification and specific treatment of the causes of hyperbilirubinaemia in Table 3.1, minimizing the effects listed in Table 3.2, and the prevention of kernicterus are the objectives in management. Prevention by good antenatal care, followed by an atraumatic delivery of a mature infant and an appropriate environment in the newborn period with an

Table 3.5 Laboratory investigations in unconjugated hyperbilirubinaemia in the newborn

Serial determination of total and direct serum bilirubin
Haemoglobin and reticulocyte determination
Red blood cell morphology
Blood group of mother and child
Direct Coomb's test in saline and albumin on infant's red blood cells
Maternal antibodies and haemolysins
Urine microscopy and culture
Urine analysis for reproducing substances
Blood culture and other appropriate bacteriological investigations
Specific enzyme test for abnormality of red blood cells
Serum thyroxine and thyroid stimulating hormone concentration

adequate intake of both fluid and calories, is paramount. It would be inappropriate to consider in detail all that is implied by the above.

Laboratory investigations required for diagnosis and treatment are listed in Table 3.5. Some comments on the relative place of exchange transfusions, phototherapy and phenobarbitone – the major specific measures in controlling hyperbilirubinaemia – are appropriate.

Exchange transfusion

The most rapid and effective method of controlling hyperbilirubinaemia is an exchange transfusion in which twice the calculated blood volume is progressively replaced by compatible whole blood less than 48 hours old. In infants with haemolytic disorders immediate exchange transfusion is indicated when the serum bilirubin level exceeds 20 mg/dl (340 μmol/litre) if full term. In premature infants there are no established criteria but it would seem prudent to intervene at levels of 15 mg/dl (250 μmol/litre) in premature infants, in infants of 1.5 to 2.0 kg or as low as 10 mg/dl (170 μmol/litre) at weights of 1.0 kg. Sepsis, acidosis, hypotension, hypothermia, hypoalbuminaemia or hypoglycaemia may prompt transfusion at lower levels.

Phototherapy

In the last three decades phototherapy has become established as an effective and widely used means of controlling unconjugated hyperbilirubinaemia in infancy. In spite of its many potentially adverse acute pathophysiological effects it has proved remarkably free from adverse long-term sequelae. Hyperbilirubinaemia may be prevented and controlled by exposing the jaundiced infant to lamps which produce radiation in the range of 450–460 nm with a minimum irradiance flux of 4 μW/m². While narrow-band blue lights with peak emission near 450–460 nm (the peak absorption spectrum of bilirubin-albumin complex) are, in theory, ideal, the optimum spectrum *in vivo* may be on the long wavelength side of the absorption band, from 480 to 510 nm because skin transmittance is greatest at these wavelengths (Eggert *et al.*, 1988; McDonagh and Lightner, 1988; Romagnoli *et al.*, 1988). The major photochemical effect is the production of stereoisomers of bilirubin. Photobilirubin produced in nanoseconds by rotation of the terminal pyrrole ring of bilirubin through 180°, moves out of the skin over 1–3 hours and is then rapidly excreted in bile without conjugation. Shielding the liver in Gunn rats decreases the efficiency of phototherapy suggesting a direct hepatic effect. *In vitro* the photochemical derivatives of bilirubin are less toxic to microsomal functions than bilirubin. Phototherapy is commonly introduced at around 250 μmol/litre (15 mg/dl) in term infants but at lower levels in prematures, empirically when the serum bilirubin concentration in μmol/litre is one-tenth of the birth weight in grams (e.g. at 110 μmol/litre in an infant of birth weight 1100 g). Phototherapy for 1 hour every 4 hours is probably as effective as continuous phototherapy.

Side-effects   A number of side-effects have been recognized as complications of phototherapy. The most important is an increase by 2–3-fold in the insensible water loss which may lead to dehydration and thereby aggravate hyperbilirubinaemia. It is important, therefore, to supply an increased water intake. Loose stools may occur due to lactose malabsorption. A low lactose feed may help. It is important to protect the eyes because of the possibility of retinal damage. Phototherapy increases platelet turnover; it increases concentrations of follicular stimulating hormone and luteinizing hormone.

To date no permanent abnormality has been detected in human infants treated with phototherapy but because of the immense biological effects of light on the neuro-endocrine system it would seem prudent to limit the use of phototherapy to infants who have been shown to require it. Although it has been postulated that neonatal hyperbilirubinaemia may cause a continuum of brain damage from kernicterus to minor intellectual impairment, this has never been confirmed. It is important not to use phototherapy until diagnostic studies to identify the cause of jaundice have been undertaken. Phototherapy is the only means of controlling hyperbilirubinaemia in Crigler–Najjar Type 1.

Phototherapy is contraindicated in infants with liver disease as evidenced by a conjugated hyperbilirubinaemia. It causes acute haemolysis and an unusual bronzing of the skin. Copper retention and abnormal porphyrin metabolism have been implicated (Rubaltelli *et al.*, 1983).

Phenobarbitone

Carefully controlled studies have shown that phenobarbitone, particularly if given to the mother for some days before delivery of the infant, is effective in both premature and full-term infants in controlling neonatal hyperbilirubinaemia even when caused by haemolysis. The mode of action of phenobarbitone in humans has not been determined. Animal studies suggest that the drug stimulates hepatic uptake, conjugation and excretion of bilirubin as well as increasing the bile salt-dependent component of bile flow. Since the effect of phenobarbitone on reducing serum bilirubin is not apparent until 48 hours after commencing therapy, it is of little value in the treatment of established hyper-bilirubinaemia. It should be remembered that phenobarbitone has been shown to influence many other metabolic systems including hormones, clotting factors, vitamins and drugs in addition to changing the intercellular ratios of reduced and oxidized forms of NAD(H) and NADP(H). Routine use of phenobarbitone in the management of hyperbilirubinaemia is therefore to be discouraged.

It has to be recognized, however, that many infants are born in conditions where optimum highly technical perinatal care is not possible. In these circumstances the small risk of complications with relatively simple measures, particularly phototherapy, may be discounted if they give an increased chance of survival without brain damage.

Tin protoporphyrin

A new and potentially useful mode of treatment of neonatal jaundice, parenteral tin protoporphyrin (Kappas *et al.*, 1988), a haemoxygenase inhibitor, ameliorated the severity of hyperbilirubinaemia in full-term infants with direct Coombs positive ABO incompatibility and decreased the requirement for phototherapy. Although no significant side-effects were recorded it should be noted that the combination of phototherapy and tin protoporphyrin, in concentrations similar to those used in infants, produced a high mortality in 7-day-old rats (Keino *et al.*, 1990).

Jaundice in later infancy and childhood

Unconjugated hyperbilirubinaemia with normal coloured stools and urine is likely to be due to haemolytic disorders, pyloric stenosis, Gilbert's disease, primary shunt hyperbilirubinaemia or Crigler–Najjar syndrome. Biochemically it is characterized by an elevated unconjugated bilirubin usually to levels of less than 6 mg/dl (100 µmol/litre). The serum conjugated bilirubin, alkaline phosphatase transaminase, albumin and globulin will be normal. In haemolytic disorders the serum haptoglobulins will be diminished. The total haemoglobin is low with a reticulocyte count greater than 2% of the total red cell count: frequently it is as high as 20%. Unconjugated hyperbilirubinaemia may also complicate hypersplenism and portal hypertension due to portal vein obstruction

If anaemia is severe this may cause hepatocellular dysfunction with an elevation in the conjugated bilirubin. This may also occur if haemolytic anaemia is due to infection, or complicating the haemolytic uraemic syndrome. It may be found also in haemolytic anaemia complicating Wilson's disease.

Bibliography and References

Alonso, E. M., Whitington, P. F., Whitington, S. H., Rivard, W. A. and Given, G. (1991) Enterohepatic circulation of nonconjugated bilirubin in rats fed with human milk. *J. Pediatr.*, **118**, 425–430

Auerbach, K. G. and Gartner, L. M. (1987) Breastfeeding and human milk: their association with Jaundice in the neonate. *Clin. Perinatol.*, **14**, 89–107

Blankaert, N. and Heirwegh, K. P. M. (1986) Analysis and preparation of bilirubins and biliverdins. In *Bile Pigments and Jaundice. Molecular, Metabolic and Medical Aspects* (ed. J. D. Ostrow). Marcel Dekker, New York, ch 3, pp.31–80

Bongers-Schokking, J. J., Colon, E. J., Hoogland, R. A., Van Den Brande, J. L. V. and De Groot, C. J. (1990) Somatosensory evoked potentials in neonatal jaundice. *Acta Paediat. Scand.*, **79**, 148–155

Bosma, P. J., Chowdhury, N. R., Goldhoorn, B. G., Hofker, M. H., Elferink, R. P. J. O, Jansen, P. L. M. and Chowdhury, J. R. (1992) Sequence of exons and the flanking regions of human bilirubin-UDP-Glucuronyl transferase gene complex and identification of a genetic mutation in a patient with Crigler-Najjar syndrome, type 1. *Hepatology*, **15**, 941–947

Buchan, B. C. (1979) Pathogenesis of neonatal hyperbilirubinaemia after induction of labour with oxytocin. *Br. Med. J.*, **2**, 1255

Clarke, D. J., Keen, J. N. and Burchell, B. (1992) Isolation and characterisation of a new hepatic bilirubin UDP-glucuronosyltransferase. *FEBS Letters*, **299**, 183–186

Crigler, J. F. and Najjar, V. A. (1952) Congenital familial nonhemolytic jaundice with kernicterus. *Pediatrics*, **10**: 169

deCarvalho, M., Klaus, M. H. and Merkatz, R. B. (1982) Frequency of breast-feeding and serum bilirubin concentration. *Am J. Dis. Child.*, **136**: 747–48

Eggert, P., Stick. C. and Swalve, S (1988) On the efficacy of various irradiation regimens in phototherapy of neonatal jaundice *Eur. J. Pediatr.*, **147**, 525–528

Fevery, J. and Blanckaert, N. (1991) Bilirubin metabolism. In *Oxford Textbook of Clinical Hepatology* (eds N. McIntyre, J. P. Benhamou, J. Bricher, Rizzetto and Rodes J.). Oxford Medical Publications, Oxford, pp.107–115

Galbraith, R. A., Drummond, G. S. and Kappas, A. (1992) Suppression of bilirubin production in the Crigler–Najjar Type I syndrome: studies with the heme oxygenase inhibitor tin-mesoporphyrin, *Pediatrics*, **89**, 175–182

Gentle, S., Orzas, M. and Persico, M. *et al.* (1985) Comparison of nicotinic acid and caloric restriction induced hyperbilirubinaemia in the diagnosis of Gilbert's syndrome. *J. Hepatol.*, **1**, 537

Gollan, J. L. (1988) Pathobiology of bilirubin and jaundice. In: *Seminars on Living Disease* (ed. P. D. Berk). Thieme Medical Publishers, New York, pp.1–199

Gourley, G. R. and Arend. R. A. (1986) Beta glucuronidase and hyperbilirubinaemia in breast-fed and formula-fed babies. *Lancet*, **ii**, 644

Hansen, T. W. R., Bratlid, D. and Walaas, S. I. (1988) Bilirubin decreases phosphorylation of synapsin I, a synaptic vesicle-associated neuronal phosphoprotein, in intact synaptosomes from rat cerebral cortex. *Pediatr. Res.*, **23**, 219–223

Jansen, P. L. M., Mulder, G. J., Burchell, B. and Bock, K. W. (1992) New developments in glucuronidation research: report of a workshop on 'Glucuronidation, its role in health and disease', *Hepatology*, **15**, 532–544

Kappas, A., Drummond, G. S., Manola, T., Petmezaki, S. and Valaes, T. Sn-protoporphyrin use in the management of hyperbilirubinemia in term newborns with direct Coombs-positive ABO incompatibility. *Pediatrics*, **81**, 485–497

Keino, H., Nagae, H., Mimura, S., Watanabe, K. and Kashiwamata, S. (1990) Dangerous effects of tin-protoporphyrin plus phototherpy on neonatal rats. *Eur. J. Pediatr.*, **149**, 278–279

Kivlahan, C. and James, E. J. P. (1984) The natural history of neonatal jaundice. *Pediatrics*, **74**: 363–70

Labrune, P., Myara, A., Hennion, C., Gout, J. P., Trivin, F. and Odievre, M.(1989) Crigler-Najjar type II disease inheritance: a family study. *J. Inher. Metab. Dis.*, **12**, 302–306

Labrune, P., Myara, A., Huguet, P., Folliot, A., Vial, M., Trivin, F. and Odievre, M. (1992) Bilirubin uridine diphosphate glucuronosyl transferase hepatic activity in jaundice associated with congenital hypothyroidism, *J. Pediatr. Gastroent. and Nutr.*, **14**, 79–82

Lee, K. and Gartner, L. M. (1986) Fetal bilirubin metabolism and neonatal Jaundice. In *Bile Pigments and Jaundice Molecular, Metabolic and Medical Aspects* (ed. J. D. Ostrow). Marcel Dekker, New York, ch 15, pp.373–394

Lemaitre. B., Toubas, P. L., Suillo, T. M., Drew. N. C. and Relier, J. P. (1977) Changes of serum gonadotrophin concentrations in premature infants submitted to phototherapy. *Biology of the Neonate*, **32**, 113

Levine, R. L. (1988) Neonatal jaundice. *Acta Paediatr. Scand.*, **77**, 177–182

Mcdonagh, A. F. and Lightner, D. A. (1988) Phototherapy and the photobiology of bilirubin. *Sem. Liver Dis.*, **8**, 272–283

Mair, B. and Klempner, L. B. (1987) Abnormally high values in Direct Bilirubin in the Serum of Newborns as measured with the DuPont aca Analyser. *Amer. J. Clin. Path.*, **87**, 642–644

Maisels, M. J., Gifford, K., Antle, C. E. and Leib, G. R. (1988) Jaundice in the healthy newborn infant: a new approach to an old problem. *Pediatrics*, **81**, 505–511

Maisels, M. J. and Gifford, K. (1986) Normal serum bilirubin levels in the newborn and the effect of breastfeeding. *Pediatrics*, **78**, 837–843

Mowat, A. P. (1982) Familial inherited abnormalities: Hepatic disorders. *Clin. Gastroenterol.*, **11**, 171

Olsson, R., Bliding, A., Jagenburg, R., Lapidus, L., Larsson, B., Svardsudd, K. and Wittboldt, S. (1988) Gilbert's Syndrome – Does it exist? *Acta Med. Scand.*, **224**, 485–490

Ostrea, E. M., Ongtengco, E. A., Tolia, V. A. and Apostol. E. (1988) The Occurrence and Significance of the Bilirubin Species, Including Delta Bilirubin, In Jaundiced Infants. *J. Pediati Gastroenterol. Nutr.*, **7**, 511–516

Ostrow, J.D. (ed.) (1986) *Bile Pigments and Jaundice. Molecular, Metabolic and Medical Aspects.* Marcel Dekker, New York

Perlman, M. and Frank, J. W. (1988) Bilirubin beyond the blood-brain barrier. *Pediatrics*, **81**, 304–315

Pett, S. and Mowat, A. P. (1987) Crigler-Najjar Syndrome Types I and II. Clinical experience – King's College Hospital 1972–1987. Phenobarbitone, phototherapy and liver transplantation. *Mol. Aspects Med.*, **9**, 473–482

Plastino, R., Buchner, D. M. and Wagner, E. H. (1990) Impact of Eligibility Criteria on Phototherapy Program Size and Cost. *Pediatrics*, **85**, 796–800

Ritter, J. K., Chen, F., Sheen, Y. Y., Tran, H. M., Kimuras, S., Yeatman, M. T. and Owens, I. S. (1992) A novel complex locus UGT1 encodes human bilirubin, phenol and other UDP-Glucuronosyltransferase isozymes with identical carboxyl termini. *J. Biol. Chem.*, **20**, 947–950

Roda, A., Roda, E., Sama. C. *et al.* (1982) Serum primary bile acids in Gilbert's syndrome. *Gastroenterology*, **82**, 77

Romagnoli, C., Marrocco, G., de Carolis MP, Zecca, E. and Tortorolo, G. (1988) Phototherapy for hyperbilirubinaemia in preterm infants: green versus blue or white light. *J. Pediatr.*, **112**, 476–478

Rosenthal, P., Blanckaert, N., Kabra, P. M and Thaler, M. M. (1986) Formation of bilirubin conjugates in human newborns. *Paediatr. Res.*, **20**, 947–950

Rubaltelli, F. F., Jori, G. and Reddi, E. (1983) Bronze baby syndrome. A new porphyrin-related disorder. *Pediatr. Res.*, **17**, 327

Scheidt, P. C., Bryla, D. A., Nelson, K. B., HIrtz, D. G. and Hoffman, H. J. (1990) Phototherapy for neonatal Hyperbilirubinaemia: six-year follow-up of the National Institute of Child Health and Human Development Clinical Trial. *Pediatrics*, **85**, 455–463

Shinzawa, T., Mura, T. and Shiraki, K. (1988) Inhibition of rat liver UDP-glucuronyltransferase isozymes toward bile acid by breast milk causing prolonged jaundice. *Yonago Acta Medica*, **31**: 39–52

Tazawa, Y., Abukawa, D., Watabe, M., Nakagawa, M. and Yamadw, M. (1991) Abnormal results of biochemical liver function tests in Breast fed infants with prolonged indirect hyprbilirubinaemia. *Eur. J .Pediatr.*, **150**, 310–313

Ullrich, D., Fevery, J., Sieg, A., Tischler, T. and Bircher, J. (1991) The influence of gestational age on bilirubin conjugation in newborns. *Eur. J. Clin. Invest.*, **21**, 83–89

Vohr, B. R., Karp, D., O'Dea, C. *et al.* (1990) Behavioral changes correlated with brain-stem auditory evoked responses in term infants with moderate hyperbilirubinaemia. *J. Paediatr.*, **117**, 288–291

Wooster, R., Sutherland, L., Ebner, T., Clarke, D., Da Cruz e Silva, O. and Burchell, B. (1991) Cloning and stable expression of a new member of the human liver phenol/bilirubin: UDP-glucuronosyl-transferase cDNA family. *Biochem J.*, **278**, 465–469.

Chapter 4

Hepatitis and cholestasis in infancy: intrahepatic disorders

Conjugated bilirubin is produced by the enzymatic addition of glucuronide to bilirubin in the endoplasmic reticulum of the hepatocyte. It is water soluble and in health is efficiently excreted in bile. In hepatobiliary disorders conjugated bilirubin passes back into serum and is excreted in the urine. Conjugated hyperbilirubinaemia is, therefore, always pathological in contra-distinction to unconjugated hyperbilirubinaemia which may be physiological in the first 2 weeks of life (Chapter 3). It must be suspected in any jaundiced infant in whom *the urine is never colourless* but yellow at all times. One of the main reasons for delay in recognition of conjugated hyperbilirubinaemia is that the *urine is very rarely dark yellow or brown*, even in infants with complete bile duct obstruction, in the first months of life as it would be in an older child or adult. The urinary volume is relatively high in infancy reducing the intensity of the colour. Conjugated hyperbilirubinaemia is confirmed when the urine gives a positive reaction for bilirubin with test strips impregnated with a diazo reagent or by a raised direct bilirubin (see Chapter 3).

Conjugated hyperbilirubinaemia is a most important and specific sign of underlying liver or biliary disease. In infants it is relatively sensitive. It should allow the early identification of a clinical syndrome, hepatitis of infancy, due usually to intrahepatic

Table 4.1 Disorders associated with conjugated hyperbilirubinaemia in infancy

Intrahepatic disorders

Infective
Inherited disorders
    Inborn errors of metabolism
    Genetic disorders
    Familial disorders
Chromosomal anomalies
Endocrine abnormalities
Vascular abnormalities
Intravenous nutrition
Drugs
Severe haemolytic disease
Chronic hypoxia and circulatory abnormalities
Idiopathic

disease, less commonly to lesions of the intra- or extrahepatic biliary tree. It occurs in approximately one in 500 infants. However mild the icterus, it always indicates significant hepatobiliary disease which requires urgent investigation to identify disorders for which specific medical or surgical treatment, if instituted early, can prevent permanent damage to the liver, brain and other organs. Whatever the cause it may be complicated by life-threatening spontaneous bleeding due to vitamin K malabsorption unless parenteral vitamin K is given. In addition it allows the early identification of associated genetically determined disorders. Even if no specific treatment is available precise diagnosis will determine the prognosis of the individual case and the risk of recurrence in subsequent pregnancies. The associated clinical features and degree of abnormality shown by standard biochemical tests of liver damage ('liver function tests') are rarely helpful in differential diagnosis. The disorders associated with the syndrome are legion (see Table 4.1). Very rarely, conjugated hyperbilirubinaemia may be caused by a specific genetically determined abnormality in the excretion of bilirubin glucuronide without other derangement of liver function.

Hepatitis syndrome of infancy

Clinical and laboratory features

Hepatitis syndrome of infancy is characterized by clinical and laboratory features of liver dysfunction, particularly conjugated hyperbilirubinaemia. The term 'hepatitis' indicates an inflammation of the liver. The cause in this age group is not necessarily infective. The vast majority of patients present with jaundice usually continuous with physiological jaundice, but a small number present at between 5 and 8 weeks of life and some even later in infancy. Because of the high urinary output in infants the *urine is always yellow – never dark brown* as it would be in adults with conjugated hyperbilirubinaemia *nor colourless* as it is frequently in the healthy infant or in the infant with an unconjugated hyperbilirubinaemia. In many instances the stools have reduced yellow or green pigment. If cholestasis is severe the stools are white, cream-coloured or brown with no yellow or green pigment. Less commonly, infants may present with other evidence of liver dysfunction such as a bleeding diathesis, hypoglycaemia or fluid retention. Most commonly the bleeding diathesis is due to vitamin K deficiency associated with fat malabsorption which may also cause slow weight gain. Hepatomegaly is usual. Palpable splenomegaly occurs in 40–60% of cases.

Standard biochemical tests of liver function although unhelpful in differential diagnosis are of value in following progression of disease and assessing its severity. Serum aspartate aminotransferase, alkaline phosphatase and usually gamma-glutamyl transpeptidase are elevated to values between 1.5 and six times normal. Serum albumin is usually in the normal range at presentation but may be low if liver disease is severe or if there is marked fluid retention. The prothrombin time may be prolonged and usually corrects to normal with intravenous vitamin K unless acute failure is present. Serum lipids and cholesterol are normal in the first 4 months of life but increase thereafter, particularly in patients with bile duct hypoplasia syndromes. Hypoglycaemia suggests a metabolic or endocrine disorder (See below).

Pathological features

The gross pathological findings are an enlarged green liver with splenomegaly. In patients with intrahepatic disease the extrahepatic bile ducts are frequently very thin because of reduced bile flow. It may be difficult to demonstrate a patent lumen in the proximal extrahepatic or major intrahepatic bile ducts by endoscopic cholangiography or even with operative cholangiography. Intraoperative cholangiography using methylene blue may be helpful. In this age group intrahepatic bile duct dilatation is most unusual except in association with choledochal cysts and in the rarer entity, Caroli's syndrome, occurring with or without congenital hepatic fibrosis. It may occur with distal intrinsic or extrinsic obstruction of the common bile duct. The likelihood of progression to chronic disease varies with the site of major pathological change (Table 4.2).

On histological examination there is conspicuous cholestasis with bile staining within the hepatocytes and occasionally within bile canaliculi and in bile ductules. Hepatocytes show, in many instances, a variable degree of multinucleated giant cell transformation. This occurs both in patients with intrahepatic disease and in extrahepatic bile duct obstruction as in biliary atresia. The term 'giant cell hepatitis' therefore has little to recommend it since it does not exclude major bile duct disease.

Table 4.2 Pathological categories

Pathological category	Associated factors	Prognosis
Bile duct hypoplasia	Syndrome	100% chronic liver disease but progressive in only 10–20%
Extrahepatic bile duct obstruction		Chronic liver disease unless surgically corrected
Progressive intrahepatic cholestasis	Consanguinity	100% cirrhosis
	Positive family history	100% cirrhosis

Hepatocellular necrosis as indicated by eosinophilic necrosis is inconspicuous with haematoxylin and eosin staining but is reflected by crowding of reticulin fibres with appropriate stains. Throughout the hepatic parenchyma and in the portal tracts there is a diffuse, often mild, infiltrate with lymphocytes or polymorphs. Clumps of haemopoietic cells are often conspicuous, particularly in the first 6 weeks of life. Increased iron staining, both in hepatocytes and in Kupffer cells, occurs in association with infective, genetic and idiopathic hepatitis.

The portal tracts are often widened with cellular infiltration, conspicuous bile ductular proliferation and increased fibrosis. These changes occur to varying extents in patients with disorders affecting primarily the hepatic parenchyma, but occur with oedema in all portal tracts in patients with disorders of the major intrahepatic and/or extrahepatic ducts.

Pathobiological considerations

The infant seems more prone than the older child or adult to develop liver dysfunction as evidenced by conjugated hyperbilirubinaemia. It occurs more commonly than in older children or adults with infections such as septicaemia, urinary tract infection, with total parenteral nutrition and in some patients with alpha-1 antitrypsin deficiency, cystic fibrosis or Niemann–Pick disease Type C. In this latter group of patients the subsequent clearing of jaundice while clinical evidence of liver disease persists, suggests that reduced bilirubin clearance, reflecting an age-related inefficiency of hepatic excretory function, is a major component of such jaundice in infancy. The best evidence for such inefficiency

Table 4.3 Possible aetiological factors in cryptogenic hepatobiliary disease in infancy

Causes	Timing	Mechanisms	Examples
Genetic	Antenatal – / + or –	Infections	Bacterial toxins Unidentified viruses
and/or	Perinatal – + or –	Toxins	Drugs in pregnancy or labour, sedatives, antihistamines, milk additives, DDT in maternal fat stores, intravenous fat
			Immunological incompatibility between infant and mother
Environmental		Immunological factors	Absorption of polypeptides Transient immunodeficiency Abnormalities of cell-mediated immunity
	Postnatal –	+ or –	
		Perinatal handicaps	Transiently depressed enzymatic activity Impaired hepatic perfusion during postnatal vascular changes Excessive demand due to haemolysis especially in severe haemolytic disease Perinatal hypoxia Decreased gut hormone production Bile salt retention Atypical bile salt formation

in hepatic excretion in the human infant is the pattern of change of serum primary bile salt concentrations. These rise in the first week of life in a similar fashion to unconjugated bilirubin. They fall gradually after 6 to 9 months of age but remain elevated for 3–6 years with adult values of serum cholylglycine concentration being found only in children of 3–4 years of age and of chenodeoxycholic acid found at ages 6–10 years. Infants also show an exaggerated rise in serum bile acid concentration after meals. There is, in addition, reduced bile salt concentration in the bowel lumen, particularly in the premature infant (Table 4.3).

Since numerous studies indicate a direct relationship between bile acid excretion and bile secretion, these observations, together with studies in experimental animals, have given rise to the concept of *physiological cholestasis* in which there is increased susceptibility to jaundice in response to noxious agents. An anatomical factor which may contribute to the cholestasis is the arrangement of hepatocytes in plates two cells thick in the first 5 years of life, rather than as single cell plates as occurs in later life. The rate of maturation of transport mechanisms and enzymatic activities involved in both bile salt and bile salt-independent components of bile formation and secretion, as yet undetermined in humans, are also likely to be of major importance.

The cellular response to hepatic injury in this age group has three distinctive features.

Giant cell transformation   The exact nature of giant cell transformation of hepatocytes to multinucleated large cells with pale cytoplasm and many variable stained nuclei is still a

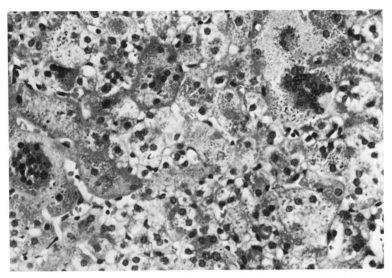

Figure 4.1 Hepatitis in infancy. Hepatic parenchyma showing great variability of hepatocyte size with many giant cells. Two multinucleated cells are seen. The normal lobular pattern cannot be distinguished. There is slight cellular infiltrate. (Percutaneous liver biopsy; haematoxylin and esosin; × 250, reduced to seven-eighths in reproduction)

mystery (see Figure 4.1) but is usually attributed to fusion rather than incomplete division of hepatocytes. It appears to be a non-specific response to injury, particularly in intrauterine life or in the first 24 months of extrauterine life. It can occur in adults with drug-induced or non-A,B,C hepatitis. In the experimental animal it has been shown that endotoxin from *Escherichia coli* can produce such changes. They are seen also with galactosamine-induced hepatitis.

Viral infection may be associated with the nuclei dispersed around the periphery of the hepatocyte rather than clumped in the centre as seen in idiopathic disease. While the increased number of nuclei suggest a regenerative process the electron microscopic appearance suggests degeneration. When serial biopsies have been done it has been concluded that these cells have a relatively short life span. They may represent a reversion to or an arrest at a more primitive level of functioning since the degree of elevation of serum alpha-fetoprotein found in infants has been related to the degree of giant cell change seen on liver biopsy. Both phenomena, however, may represent an unrelated response to injury.

Bile ductular proliferation The second distinct pathological change is ductular proliferation within and at the margin of portal tracts. This is seen particularly in bile duct obstruction but occurs also in infants with genetic deficiency of serum protein alpha-1 antitrypsin, cystic fibrosis, endocrine deficiencies and idiopathic disease. Experimentally bile duct ligation, hepatocellular injury caused, for example, by aflatoxin and by infusions of abnormal bile salts, can all produce such bile duct proliferation. These distorted, angulated bile ductules may arise by cholangiocyte proliferation, be derived from hepatocytes by direct transformation, from perilobular cells which are incompletely differentiated into hepatocytes or cholangiocytes or from a persistence of the primitive duct plate.

Fibroblastic activity and extracellular matrix components   Around these abnormal bile ductules there is marked fibroblastic activity. Liver biopsies from such patients show increased activity of the enzyme prolyl hydroxylase, a rate-limiting enzyme in collagen formation. Serum concentrations of markers of connective tissue formation, components of Types III and V collagen and of laminin, are increased irrespective of the nature of the underlying liver disease. What determines whether connective tissue accumulation will be progressive or reversible is as yet uncertain.

The development and progression of liver disease in this age group is clearly dependent on the interaction between the many cell types within the liver. Injury primarily to hepatocytes, sinusoidal endothelial cells, Kupffer or Ito cells or to bile duct epithelial cells will disturb the functioning of the other types of cells. Equally important is the interaction of these liver and biliary cells and components of the extracellular matrix via integrins with the migratory cells of the reticulo-endothelial system, particularly polymorphonuclear leucocytes, lymphocytes, eosinophils and macrophages. It is important therefore that research into causes of liver disease in this age group include factors affecting all cells within the liver and not be limited to hepatocytotrophic viruses or to hepatocyte toxins.

Management and differential diagnosis

A full clinical evaluation is essential. The age, occupation, ethnic origin, degree of consanguinity and illnesses of both parents must be noted together with the state of health, birth order and age of other siblings and the presence or absence of liver disease in other family members. A careful history of the pregnancy, noting illnesses, contact with infectious disease, drug therapy, blood transfusions or blood group incompatibility must be noted, together with the gestation and details of perinatal condition and perinatal events. Parental consanguinity or a family history of liver disease in other family members should raise the suspicion of a genetic cause for the problem. Complications of prematurity, particularly infection, hypoxia and disorders preventing oral nutrition and requiring total intravenous alimentation may be followed by cholestasis. Up to 40% of those with hepatocellular disease are born prematurely or with birth weights of less than 2.5 kg but 10% of those with biliary atresia are also born prematurely with 5% being light-for-gestational age. The mode of onset of the hepatic features, particularly when the urine first became other than colourless, changes in stool colour, pattern of feeding, feed composition and weight gain may give a clue to the underlying disorder. Clinical examination should include documentation of the weight, length, head circumference, chest circumference, abdominal girth, midarm circumference, triceps and subscapular skinfold thickness as well as liver size, consistency and spleen size and presence or absence of ascites and abdominal masses (Figure 4.2). Serial measurements are particularly valuable in monitoring the course of the disorder. Careful clinical examination of the remainder of the child with specific attention to the cardiovascular system, eyes, face, skin and genitalia may reveal features listed in Table 4.4 which suggest a particular diagnosis. Ophthalmic examination including slit-lamp examination for embryotoxon is essential.

Stool colour   It is essential that the doctor sees a specimen of stool and notes its colour. In our unit we organize that a sample of every stool is collected in a plastic transparent container, and placed in a black plastic bag for examination during ward rounds. If the stool contains green or yellow pigment cholestasis is incomplete and biliary atresia is excluded *at that time*.

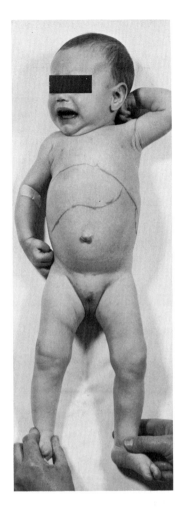

Figure 4.2 Child aged 6 months with alpha-1 antitrypsin phenotype PiZ. There is marked hepatomegaly, splenomegaly, and an everted umbilicus. The child demonstrated marked pruritus. Jaundice had been present since the third day of life. By the age of 3 weeks the stools were acholic and the urine dark. There was marked hepatomegaly, splenomegaly but no ascites. Laboratory investigations showed features of severe cholestasis with Rose Bengal faecal excretion of <5% in 72 hours. Jaundice persisted until the age of $5\frac{1}{2}$ months. Routine tests of liver function remained abnormal. By the age of 11 months ascites was evident and there was marked failure to thrive. The infant died of cirrhosis at the age of 17 months

Table 4.4 Disorders which may be suspected from clinical findings

Disorders	Abnormal physical signs
Generalized viral infections	Skin lesions, purpura, choroidoretinitis, myocarditis, etc.
Galactosaemia, hypoparathyroidism	Cataracts
Trisomy 21, 18 or 13	Multiple congenital anomalies
Choledochal cyst	Cystic mass below the liver
Spontaneous perforation of the bile ducts	Ascites and bile-stained herniae
Biliary hypoplasia	Systolic murmur, abnormal facies, embryotoxon
Hepatic or biliary haemangioma	Cutaneous haemangiomata
Extrahepatic biliary atresia	Situs inversus
Septo-optic dysplasia	Optic nerve hypoplasia and/or micropenis

Immediate investigations (Table 4.5)

On identifying conjugated hyperbilirubinaemia it is immediately necessary to exclude treatable infections such as septicaemia, urinary tract infection, toxoplasmosis, syphilis, listeriosis, tuberculosis and malaria, and to consider the dietary treatable metabolic disorders, galactosaemia and fructosaemia. Equally urgent is the detection of severe prolongation of the prothrombin time so that spontaneous haemorrhage, particularly intracranial, may be prevented by intravenous vitamin K and, if necessary, fresh frozen plasma. Hypoglycaemia or abnormal serum sodium concentrations may indicate endocrinopathy.

Initial investigations must therefore include urine culture, urinanalysis for non-glucose reducing substances, particularly if a patient has had galactose in the preceding 4 hours, a full blood count and a prothrombin time. Blood sugar and electrolytes are also required. If fever or other features of infection are present blood and ascitic fluid should be taken for culture and wide spectrum antibiotic treatment started. It is important to appreciate that even if septicaemia is confirmed there may be serious underlying liver or biliary disease which requires subsequent definition. Similarly the finding of non-glucose reducing substances in the urine does not necessarily indicate galactosaemia since galactosuria can occur in some normal infants and is present in up to 50% of infants in our unit with hepatic or biliary disease. Nevertheless a galactose-free, fructose-free diet should be instituted until these disorders have been definitely excluded.

Urgent consideration must then be given to excluding the surgically correctable disorders, extrahepatic biliary atresia (p.79), spontaneous perforation of the bile duct (p.419), and choledochal cyst (p.414) and rare causes of bile duct obstruction. Skilled ultrasonography of the biliary tract is required in all cases to detect biliary dilatation, a finding confirming a lesion requiring assessment by an experienced surgeon. It is equally important to consider the endocrine disorders associated with this syndrome which have to be excluded on the basis of the clinical and appropriate laboratory investigations. Familial erythrophagocytic reticulosis is another potentially treatable condition which must be excluded.

Because such a large percentage of cases will have cryptogenic disease a percutaneous liver biopsy to determine whether the disorder is primarily biliary or hepatocellular (See Chapter 5) should be performed at an early stage particularly if there is complete cholestasis. It may reveal abnormal storage in hepatocytes or Kupffer cells, indicating that a metabolic disorder may be present. It indicates the severity of liver disease and likely prognosis. It is essential that some of the material obtained is frozen at −70°C so that it can be used for subsequent biochemical analysis if the liver histology or vacuolation of peripheral blood leucocytes indicate that a metabolic disorder is likely.

If there is complete cholestasis there is equal urgency in identifying alpha-1 antitrypsin deficiency (PIZZ, protese inhibitor phenotype 22) by phenotyping and cystic fibrosis by immunoreactive trypsin levels and/or sweat sodium concentration. The clinical, laboratory and pathological features of liver disease with these disorders are frequently indistinguishable from biliary atresia. The prognosis is much worse than that of idiopathic hepatitis of infancy. Because of the high frequency of the carrier state for these disorders in our community they must be excluded in all infants with hepatitis syndrome.

The next priority is to exclude systematically genetic/metabolic disorders and viral infections not indicated by the history or physical findings. Identification of abnormalities of bile salt formation is particularly important since treatment with oral primary bile salts may reverse liver damage. Niemann–Pick Type 3 is second in frequency only to alpha-1 antitrypsin deficiency as a genetic factor associated with hepatitis in infancy. It is now our

Table 4.5 Serial investigation of infants with conjugated hyperbilirubinaemia

Investigations to be initiated immediately
  Prothrombin time
  Bacterial culture of blood and urine
  Urine microscopy, 'Dipstick' analysis and Clinitest analysis for non-glucose reducing substances
  Peripheral blood count including reticulocyte count if anaemia is present
  Blood group, saving serum for cross-matching
  Blood sugar and urea or creatinine
  Serum sodium, potassium, bicarbonate and calcium

If acutely ill, save as much urine and serum as possible at –70°C for subsequent biochemical analysis
Diagnostic paracentesis of abdomen if appropriate.

Investigations to be initiated as soon as normal laboratory service is available
  Standard biochemical test of liver function including total and direct bilirubin and gamma-glutamyl
    transpeptidase
  Serum cholesterol
  Alpha-1 antitrypsin phenotype
  Red blood cell galactose-1 phosphate uridyl transferase
  Sweat electrolyte determination
  Immunoreactive trypsin
  Serum and urinary amino acids
  Urinary succinyl acetone and delta-aminolaevulinic acid
  Serum thyroxine; TSH; cortisol (9:00 am)
  Viral culture of urine
  WR or VDRL
  HbsAg
  Antibody tests for toxoplasmosis, cytomegalovirus, herpes simplex, rubella, hepatitis C virus and HIV
  Ultrasound of abdomen to identify focal hepatic lesion or dilated ducts. If either are present refer to
    specialist centre
  X-ray chest to exclude cardiac lesion; long bones for evidence of rickets or intrauterine infection; vertebral
    bodies for failure of fusion
  Ophthalmic examination for embryotoxon, optic nerve hypoplasia, choroidoretinitis

If stools acholic, contact specialist centre to plan transfer to exclude biliary atresia

Specialist centre

If no contraindication percutaneous liver biopsy: tissue for histological, electron microscopic and enzymatic
  studies: viral and bacterial culture

Laparotomy
  If above genetic disorders and endocrine deficiencies are excluded, stools lack green or yellow pigment
    and biopsy is compatible with biliary atresia: laparotomy, operative cholangiography or definitive
    surgery by an experienced paediatric hepatobiliary surgeon.
  If biopsy equivocal and stool colour not convincingly green or yellow ^{99m}Tc-tagged
    methylbromo-iminodiacetic acid biliary excretion scan after 3 days of phenobarbitone may be useful if
    it demonstrates bile duct patency
  If biliary atresia a possibility but laparotomy can be deferred: endoscopic cholangiography

If no cause identified and cholestasis incomplete:
  Bone marrow aspirate for storage disorders
  White blood cell lysosomal enzyme concentration
  Mass spectroscopy of urine to exclude defects of fatty acid metabolism. May need to be repeated on a
    fasting sample
  Blood lactate and pyruvate
  Very long chain fatty acids
  Serum tetrasialotransferrin
  Urinary bile acid identification by gas chromatography: mass spectrometry
  Fibroblast culture for enzyme studies

practice to perform bone marrow aspiration before considering any case as idiopathic or cryptogenic.

The remaining disorders must also be excluded systematically if there is a family history of liver disease in infancy or of consanguinity. In these circumstances it is essential to establish fibroblast culture and to preserve liver biopsy tissue frozen at −70°C for subsequent biochemical studies. Enzymatic studies in peripheral blood lymphocytes may be appropriate in some cases. If there is no such family history and liver histology indicates hepatocellular disease without disturbance of liver architecture or features of metabolic abnormalities, and no associated abnormality has been discovered except prematurity or infections, further investigations to identify associated abnormalities should be postponed until it is clear that a chronic disorder is present. Follow-up at 6, 12 and 24 months will detect this.

Details of intrahepatic disorders causing conjugated hyperbilirubinaemia in infancy or a hepatitis syndrome are considered elsewhere in this chapter, extrahepatic disorders in Chapter 5, Alpha^{-1} antitrypsin deficiency in Chapter 18 and metabolic disorders in Chapter 15. Liver disorders associated with genetic disorders without a known biochemical basis are considered elsewhere, e.g. cystic fibrosis (p.349), autosomal recessive polycystic disease of the kidneys (p.303) and haemophagocytic lymphohistiocytosis (p.295).

Management of consequences of prolonged cholestasis

Retention by the liver of substances normally excreted in the bile, decreased delivery of bile salts to the proximal intestine with low intraluminal bile acid concentrations and malabsorption of fats and fat-soluble vitamins, and hepatocellular dysfunction, are the mechanisms underlying the main clinical consequences of cholestasis (Table 4.6).

Nutritional Supplements   Infants with cholestasis frequently fail to grow and gain weight at normal rates. A major contributory factor is malabsorption of fats and fat soluble

Table 4.6 Pathophysiological consequences of prolonged cholestasis

Abnormality	Effect	Management
Failure of biliary excretion		
Bilirubin	Jaundice	Cholestyramine: 4–16 g/day
Bile salts	Pruritus	Phenobarbitone: 5–10 mg/kg/day
Cholesterol	Xanthelasma	IR phototherapy
		Terfenadine: 1–3 mg/kg/bd
Decreased bile salts in intestine		
Malabsorption of long-chain triglycerides	Poor growth	
Vitamin D	Osteoporosis	
	Rickets and osteomalacia	
Vitamin K	Bleeding diathesis	
Vitamin A	Night blindness	See text
Vitamin E	Haemolytic anaemia	
	Neuromuscular degeneration	
Hepatocellular dysfunction	Cirrhosis	That of underlying disorder
	Portal hypertension	
	Liver failure	
	Susceptibility to infection	

vitamins caused by reduced bile salt concentration in the gut lumen and portal hypertension. In addition there may be reduced calorie intake caused by anorexia or early satiety from gastric compression from enlarged viscera and ascites. Liver disease may cause malutilization of nutrients as shown by high serum amino acid levels. There may be increased energy requirements in part due to the hyperdynamic circulation. Intercurrent infections add to the problems.

To promote increase calorie absorption formulas with a high proportion of medium chain triglycerides are used since medium chain fats (MCF) are less dependent on bile salts for absorption.

Calorie intake may be further increased by the addition of glucose polymers or combined fat/carbohydrate supplements. It is important to ensure that 2–3% of calorie intake is in the form of polyunsaturated long chain fats to prevent essential fatty acid deficiency. Essential amino acid intake must be sufficient for growth. With calorie intakes of up to 200 kcal/day it is possible to increase rates of weight gain and increase skinfold thickness. It may be necessary to used continuous overnight nasogastric feeding to achieve such intakes. In some instances linear growth rates will increase but this is unusual unless there is concomitant improvement in the underlying liver disease.

To what extent high serum amino acid concentrations, the decreased ratio of branched chain to aromatic acids or high blood ammonia levels contribute to developmental delay (see below) is unknown. Supplements of branched chain amino acids which are preferentially metabolized in muscle have also been used to increase calorie utilization but it is unclear whether they have any advantages over carbohydrate sources. Whether MCFs are adequately metabolized in advanced liver disease is uncertain.

Fat-soluble vitamin deficiencies must be prevented. Hypoprothrombinaemia due to vitamin K deficiency is an immediate and constant risk. It may be prevented by oral vitamin K_1 (phytomenadione) 1 mg/day. While jaundice persists the prothrombin time should be checked at 4-weekly intervals, and vitamin K_1 given intravenously if prolonged. Vitamin D deficiency is the next to become manifest. Vitamin D requirements are increased by dark skin colour, severe malabsorption, enzyme-inducing drugs such as phenobarbitone or rifampicin and rapid growth rates and decreased by exposure to sunlight. Oral supplements of 400 IU daily in infants fed on milk preparations fortified with vitamins and 1200 IU daily in breast-fed infants usually suffices to prevent rickets if jaundice lasts for less than 3 months. If jaundice persists for longer, 40 000 IU intramuscularly at 4-weekly intervals should be given to white infants but in dark-skinned patients the dose is increased 2 to 3-fold. Serum phosphate and calcium concentrations should be checked at 4-weekly intervals to determine whether supplements are needed and, with an X-ray of wrists at 8-weekly intervals, to monitor control of rickets. Despite normal calcium absorption and normal serum concentrations of the hepatic metabolite of vitamin D, 25-hydroxy-cholecalciferol, osteoporosis with reduced bone mass and an increase risk of pathological fractures is a frequent and unexplained complication of cholestasis which has persisted for periods usually longer than 1 year.

In the past 10 years it has become clear that in infants and children with liver disease, particularly if jaundiced, failure to absorb sufficient vitamin E causes a progressive neuromuscular disorder. Initially this causes loss of tendon reflexes and hypotonia but it progresses to give paralysis of gaze, ataxia, decreased vibratory sensation and proprioception. It may cause changes in the central nervous system. Vitamin E deficiency is rarely clinically manifest before 18 months of age and may be absent after jaundice lasting 15 years. Neurological abnormalities have been found in a proportion of patients when the vitamin E concentration is less than 9 µmol/litre (0.4 mg/dl) or the vitamin E/total lipid ratio (mg vitamin E/g of lipid) is less than 0.6. Pathological evidence of deficiency may be seen as early as 5 months of age and biochemical deficiency as early as 2 months of age. The mechanism of neurological damage is not clear. Whether vitamin E levels must be maintained above those levels at which neurological damage can occur to prevent subclinical damage is at present unknown. Our practice is to give all jaundiced infants 15 mg vitamin E (α-tocopherol acetate) orally and to monitor vitamin E/lipid ratios at 2-monthly intervals from 2 months of age. If mild biochemical deficiency is detected, oral vitamin E is increased to as much as 200 mg/kg/day to maintain a normal vitamin E/lipid ratio. If the ratio is less than 0.2 oral therapy is ineffective and a parenteral vitamin E preparation (Roche) is given in a dose of up to 10 mg/kg (but not more than 200 mg) at 2-weekly intervals for a 3-month period and thereafter vitamin E requirements are reassessed based on serum concentrations.

If cholestasis is severe or prolonged, serum vitamin A levels are low. Night blindness and skin thickening are rarely observed in children of less than 8 years of age but retinal degenerative changes in children with both vitamin E and vitamin A deficiency have been noted earlier. Two of 24 children aged 2 months to 6 years and 24 of 106 of unspecified age had punctate keratopathy. Hepatic levels of vitamin A may be low when serum levels are normal. There are no established biochemical parameters with which to monitor therapy. Our practice is to supplement the diet of all infants with oral vitamin A in a dose of 2500 IU daily. If biochemical evidence of vitamin A deficiency is seen (Plasma retinol < 20 μg/dl (0.7 mol/litre), oral supplements should be increased 10-fold. If levels remain low a water miscible preparation in a dose of 50 000 IU intramuscularly at monthly intervals prevents features of vitamin A deficiency without causing high liver concentrations (Amedee-Manesme et al., 1988). Too much vitamin A can cause hepatotoxicity

Neurodevelopmental problems   The advent of portoenterostomy for biliary atresia and liver transplantation for end-stage liver disease in infancy and childhood has stimulated studies of neurodevelopmental problems associated with liver disorders which previously caused death in early childhood. In the majority malnutrition and cholestasis with malabsorption of fat and fat soluble vitamins is a compounding factor which may contribute to neurodevelopmental problems (Stewart et al., 1987, 1988). Subsequent studies of children requiring liver transplantation identified low IQ in nine of 21 in whom the liver disease had started in the first year of life compared with two of 15 with liver disease of later onset. The children with intellectual impairment had a longer duration of disease, poorer nutritional status, smaller head and mid-arm circumference and lower serum vitamin E concentration. Whether vitamin E supplements or a high calorie diet would optimize development in such children is still to be proved (Stewart et al., 1988). Following liver transplant the relationship between early onset of liver disease and delayed intellectual function persists (Stewart et al., 1991). In a study of 28 such patients compared with 18 patients with cystic fibrosis matched to control for effects of growth retardation, chronicity of illness, age of onset and socioeconomic status significant differences were seen. The liver transplant recipients had lower mean nonverbal intelligence scores, poorer academic achievement and scored less satisfactorily in tests of learning and memory, abstraction, concept formation, visual spatial function and motor function. Whether more intensive nutritional intervention early in life or better educational facilities following liver transplantation would reverse this remains to be seen.

Control of pruritus

To enhance biliary excretion and to control pruritus a number of agents may be tried. Cholestyramine is effective in controlling pruritus in most patients provided enough is ingested. The rationale underlying its use is that it binds bile salts in the intestinal lumen. It is also claimed that by interrupting the enterohepatic circulation it may stimulate *de novo* bile acid synthesis and thus bile salt-dependent bile flow but since the serum bile salt concentration is high in almost every case, any beneficial effect it may have on liver function may have other mechanisms. The side-effects which may cause difficulties are malabsorption of fat-soluble vitamins and drugs, folic acid deficiency, constipation and acidosis. It should be given with food and not at the same time as drug or vitamin supplements. Ursodeoxycholic acid (UDCA), a relatively hydrophilic bile acid, has been shown in recent studies to be an effective antipruritic agent when given in a dose of 15 to 45 mg/kg/24 hours. It may aggravate pruritus in the first weeks of therapy. It has a choleretic action thought to be due to increased bicarbonate release by bile duct epithelial cells as UDCA is reabsorbed to undergo a cholehepatic recirculation. Its use in a variety of liver disorders such as cystic fibrosis produces improvement in liver function tests attributed to a cytoprotective action. It is not universally effective. Improvement was observed in only five of 17 children in our service with chronic liver disease and pruritus not controlled by cholestyramine. One patient had an unexplained deterioration in liver function when the dose was increased from 15 to 30 mg/kg/day which resolved when the drug was withdrawn.

Phenobarbitone may be given to stimulate bile salt-independent bile flow. Oral administration of 5–10 mg/kg may decrease jaundice and, less commonly, control pruritus. Whether its action on metabolism, as a non-specific enzyme-inducer, operates for the patients' wellbeing or conversely is a matter for speculation. The same stricture applies to rifampicin which in a dose of 10 mg/kg/day alleviates pruritus which has not been controlled by cholestyramine. Furthermore this drug has well recognized hepatic side-effects (Chapter 14). It has been postulated that the antimicrobial action of this drug may limit the production of toxic secondary bile salts in the colon. It may limit hepatic uptake of bile salts.

Phototherapy with infrared or ultraviolet irradiation lessens pruritus if given in suberythematous doses for 3–10 minutes daily. Terfenadine is an antihistamine with mild antipruritic effects.

Genetically determined metabolic disorders

Liver dysfunction and structural changes due to genetically determined metabolic disorders listed in Table 4.7 may present with a hepatitis syndrome in infancy. (Further details are given in Chapters 15 and 18.) *Galactosaemia*, fructosaemia and tyrosinaemia must be identified as early as possible in every case since specific dietary and drug treatments are essential. Galactosaemia and fructosaemia may be suspected clinically from the characteristic onset of symptoms after ingesting the monosaccharide. The urine may contain a non-glucose reducing substance identified with a positive test using Clinitest tablets or Benedict's solutions. If the glucose oxidase test is negative it provides some corroboration of the diagnosis; however, up to one-half of patients with other forms of hepatobiliary disease in infancy have galactosuria because hepatic metabolism of galactose is impaired. A further problem is that urine testing may only be positive if the offending monosaccharide has been ingested shortly before the time of testing. In some patients galactosuria does not occur. In up to one-third of patients with galactosaemia the presentation is with an overwhelming, septicaemia-like illness in the first 48 hours of life.

Table 4.7 Metabolic disorders associated with the neonatal hepatitis syndrome

Disorder	Screening investigation	Definitive investigation	Associated clinical features
Galactosaemia	Non-glucose reducing substance may be found in the urine when galactose is ingested (not invariably)	Decreased concentration of RBC Galactose-1-phosphate uridyl transferase	Onset at birth with vomiting, failure to thrive, haemorrhagic diathesis, septicaemia, and later cirrhosis, mental retardation and cataracts
Fructosaemia	Fructosuria may be present when fructose is ingested	Decreased or absent hepatic fructose-1-phosphatase	Onset after introduction of sucrose-supplemented milk. Vomiting, hypoglycaemia, haemorrhagic diathesis, hepatomegaly, pallor, failure to thrive, anorexia, glycosuria, hyperaminoaciduria
Phosphoenolpyruvate carboxykinase (PEPCK) deficiency	Hypoglycaemia, raised lactate or pyruvate	PEPCK deficiency in skin fibroblasts	Hypotonia, delayed development, hepatic steatosis with fibrosis and liver failure. Cot death
Tyrosinaemia	Positive ferric chloride test, positive Phenistix. High serum concentrations of tyrosine phenylanine	Increased urinary succinyl-acetone	Onset at 1–4 weeks of age with failure to thrive, hepatocellular failure, bleeding diathesis, renal tubular dysfunction, and vitamin D resistant rickets
Alpha-1 antitrypsin deficiency	Protein inhibitor phenotype		
Cystic fibrosis	Albumin in meconium, elevated immunoreactive trypsin in serum	Sweat sodium chloride greater than 70 mmol/litre	Meconium ileus, failure to thrive, malabsorption, anaemia, oedema, respiratory tract infection
Niemann–Pick disease	Sphingomyelin accumulation in bone marrow	Sphingomyelinase deficient in leucocytes, lymph nodes or liver biopsy	Hepatosplenomegaly, progressive dementia, blindness
Niemann–Pick type II (C) (Neurovisceral storage disease with ophthalmoplegia)		Defective cholesterol esterification in cultures fibroblasts	Hepatosplenomegaly, progressive dementia presenting with incoordination and supranuclear ophthalmoplegia after 6 years of age

Gaucher's disease	Cells in marrow	Deficient glucosyl ceramide beta-glucosidase in leucocytes, bone marrow or liver biopsy	Splenomegaly, hepatomegaly, lymph node enlargement, pulmonary infiltration and central nervous system involvement
Wolman's disease		Deficiency of acid esterase in leucocytes or liver biopsy	Vomiting, diarrhoea, failure to thrive, abdominal distension, hepatosplenomegaly, steatorrhoea, adrenal calcification, developmental delay
Defects in bile acid synthesis	Positive Lifschutz test	Very low or undetectable primary bile acids, increased 7-hydroxycholesterol derivatives in urine	
Zellweger's syndrome	High serum iron with saturation iron-binding capacity, increased urinary or serum pipecholic acid, decreased plasmalogens	Absence of peroxisomes on electron microscopy of liver biopsy. Increased di- and tri-hydroxy-coprostanic acid and very long chain fatty acids in serum	Low birth weight, prominent forehead, with open metopic suture, sagittal suture synostosis, congenital cataracts, hypertelorism, high-arch palate, severe developmental delay and failure to thrive, cirrhosis, cysts of kidney, stippled cartilage in diaphysis and patella
Dubin–Johnson syndrome	Bromsulphophthalein sodium clearance reduced with rebound increase in concentration at 120 minutes	Pigment in the liver on biopsy (may not be evident until the age of 4 years)	Positive family history
Trihydroxycoprostatic acidaemia (THCA)	Very low serum cholic acid	Defect of specific THCA hydroxylating enzyme	Persistent cholestasis. Biliary hypoplasia progressing to cirrhosis and death by the age of 3 years

Fructosaemic patients may not have fructosuria even when challenged with a fructose load. If the onset is clearly related to fructose intake a presumptive diagnosis is warranted while awaiting results of definitive investigations. In *tyrosinaemia* the prothrombin ratio is increased and the albumin concentration is usually low. Diagnosis is established in nearly every case by the finding of succinyl acetone in urine in concentrations 20 to 100 times normal. Rarely deficiency of fumarylacetoacetate hydrolyase in tissue is required to establish the diagnosis. Dietary and drug therapy dramatically improves liver function and delays consideration of liver transplantation.

If there is complete cholestasis there is equal urgency in identifying alpha-1 antitrypsin deficiency (PIZZ) by phenotyping, and cystic fibrosis as already emphasized. As discussed above it is important to identify the other disorders because of the implications for genetic counselling and prognosis. This should always include Niemann–Pick Type 3. The remaining disorders must be excluded if there is a family history of liver disease in infancy or of consanguinity. In these circumstances it is essential to establish fibroblast culture and to preserve liver biopsy tissue frozen at –70°C for subsequent biochemical studies.

Enzymatic studies in peripheral blood lymphocytes may be appropriate in some cases. More commonly observed liver disorders associated with genetic disorders without a known biochemical basis are considered elsewhere, e.g. cystic fibrosis (p.349), Zellweger's syndrome (p.284), autosomal recessive polycystic disease of the kidneys (p.303), haemophagocytic lymphohistiocytosis (p.295).

Familial syndromes with as yet uncharacterized biochemical basis

Liver diseases with cholestatic features have been described in a number of distinct familial syndromes. In the majority the occurrence is compatible with an autosomal recessive inheritance. The underlying metabolic defect(s) is (are) unknown.

Syndromic biliary hypoplasia

See intrahepatic biliary hypoplasia.

Cholestasis with lymphoedema

Obstructive jaundice in infancy followed by recurrent episodes of jaundice throughout childhood and in adult life and *lymphoedema* has been reported in a group of patients with common ancestry in south west Norway. A similar disease has been described in families in Italy, North America and Australia. Liver biopsy in infancy shows hepatitis with giant cell transformation, whereas in adults the main abnormalities are intracanalicular cholestasis (Aagenaes, 1974). Towards puberty these patients develop oedema of the legs with hypoplasia of the lymph vessels in the limbs. Cirrhosis may develop in adolescence (Henriksen *et al.*, 1981). It has been suggested that deficiency of the intrahepatic lymphatics may contribute to the cholestasis.

Benign recurrent cholestasis

This is characterized by multiple episodes of cholestasis with jaundice and pruritus, with complete clinical, functional and morphological recovery during remissions. During attacks liver biopsies show prominent centrilobular cholestasis with minimal hepato-cellular necrosis and a mild inflammatory cell reaction in the portal tracts. The age of onset may be from early infancy through to adult life. Episodes typically start with anorexia and malaise followed by intense pruritus. Jaundice if it occurs start 13 weeks later. There may weight loss, steatorrhoea and mild abdominal pain. The liver may be slightly enlarged and tender. Episodes last for a few days to 24 months. Males and females are equally affected. A family history of the disease or of cholestasis of pregnancy is obtained in 50% of cases suggesting an autosomal recessive mode of inheritance. Cholestyramine given prophylactically may reduce the number of exacerbations. Corticosteroids may terminate relapses.

Progressive intrahepatic cholestasis

Progressive intrahepatic cholestasis is a heterogeneous assortment of familial disorders of unknown cause which progress to cirrhosis and death, usually in the first or second decades. Most reported cases are without distinguishing pathological or biochemical criteria. The presenting feature may be jaundice in the neonatal period or jaundice, pruritus or malabsorption appearing later in infancy. Some families present with a syndrome which initially seems similar to benign recurrent cholestasis. Pruritus is frequently severe. Diarrhoea, steatorrhoea and failure to thrive are often prominent features. Remission is never complete. Rarely clinical features clear but liver function tests remain abnormal. Exacerbations lasting a few days to 20 months occur, often provoked by infection. Families with high sweat sodium concentrations but without other features of cystic fibrosis have been identified. Kayser-Fleischer rings have been noted in those with long-standing cholestasis. Inspissated bile, gall-stones, large gall bladder, pancreatitis and myocarditis have all been described. Hepatomegaly persists with increasing intrahepatic fibrosis proceeding usually to biliary-type cirrhosis but in some patients, particularly of Arab descent, with features of chronic aggressive hepatitis. Splenomegaly, portal hypertension and bleeding from varices ensues. Hepatoma may develop (Ugarte and Gonzalez-Crussi, 1981).

A number of distinct subgroups have been described within specific families or racial groups.

Cholestasis with actin and microfilament accumulation in North American Indian children

Prominent pericanalicular microfilament accumulation with much actin surrounding dilated bile canaliculi and well preserved microvilli, are characteristic features of a disorder described in 14 North American Indian children. Jaundice in the neonatal period progressing to cirrhosis by 2 years of age was the usual presentation, but some presented with features of cirrhosis without prior jaundice. Pruritus, heart murmurs, recurrent skin and ear infections, severe epistaxis and a characteristic leash of small blood vessels on the cheeks, are prominent clinical features (Weber *et al.*, 1981).

Fatal familial cholestatic syndrome in Greenland Eskimo children

Persistent jaundice starting in the first 3 months of life, pruritus, malabsorption and its complications, thrombocytosis and low serum cholesterol concentrations were distinctive features of this autosomal recessively inherited syndrome. Eight of 16 died of infection and bleeding between 6 weeks and 3 years with the oldest survivor being 30 months. The ultrastructural features were unremarkable but even at postmortem examination there was no cirrhosis although there was portal-portal fibrosis.

Byler disease   Severe familial idiopathic cholestasis proceeding to cirrhosis with early death, often in the first decade was described in eight members of the Byler family and in other Amish families (Clayton *et al.*, 1969). The longest life span recorded is 18 years (Jones *et al.*, 1976).

Three further categories have been identified recently, two on the basis of unusual biochemical findings of uncertain pathogenic significance and one by distinctive changes in the major intrahepatic bile ducts.

Maggiore and coworkers (1987) reported a subgroup characterized by normal gamma-glutamyl transpeptidase concentrations in serum which is most unusual in infants with any other form of hepatobiliary disease. These infants had clear clinical and pathological evidence of progressive hepatic fibrosis with the emergence of complications of cirrhosis in the first decade. Other biochemical test of liver damage were abnormal.

Strumm *et al.* (1990) more recently have demonstrated impaired apolipoprotein A-1 synthesis in hepatocytes with very low serum levels as a distinctive feature in 18 patients with this disorder.

Sclerosing cholangitis of neonatal onset   Amedee-Manesme *et al.* (1989) described eight children, three of whom had consanguineous parents with jaundice in the first 36 months of life with the cholangiographic features of sclerosing cholangitis. Although jaundice cleared other liver function tests remained abnormal and cirrhosis with portal hypertension was established by 9 years of age. The same findings were observed in two siblings of consanguineous patents, with the elder being performed successfully at 6 years of age (Baker *et al.*, 1993).

Iron storage disorders

These usually lethal disorders are characterized by a four- and sevenfold increase in iron in the liver, pancreas, heart, endocrine and exocrine glands and in skin (see Chapter 15). Haemosiderosis, both hepatocellular and reticulo-endothelial, is found in leprechaunism. In this disorder the liver also contains multiple small nodules composed of large, pale foamy hepatocytes with large quantities of glycogen and little fat. Some cases show intrahepatic cholestasis and bile duct proliferation. Others have no hepatic abnormality (Ordway and Stout, 1973).

Hepatosteatosis

A number of families have been described with conjugated hyperbilirubinaemia, sometimes kernicterus, a bleeding disorder and marked fatty infiltration in the liver as well as other organs and viscera, leading to death in the neonatal period. In some families males only are affected. In one case serum lipids and fatty acids were markedly increased. With modern investigations these should be found to have specific inborn errors of metabolism (see Chapter 15).

Rare associations

Liver disease presenting in infancy has been associated with mild de Jeune's syndrome and also with renal tubular insufficiency and multiple congenital anomalies (see chapter 16).

Chromosomal abnormalities

In trisomy 13 and 18, between 20% and 30% of patients have hepatitis. The presence of such trisomies may be suspected clinically from the marked physical abnormalities and can be confirmed by analysis of the chromosomal karyotype. The hepatitis may contribute to failure to thrive. Hepatitis may be slightly more common in infants with Down's syndrome and there is often the suggestion that it occurs more frequently in female phenotypes with Turner's syndrome, but it is difficult to be certain whether there is indeed an increased incidence in these two conditions.

Endocrine disorders associated with hepatitis syndromes

An awareness that hepatitis syndromes may be associated with underlying endocrinopathy is essential if these are to be rapidly identified and specific treatment given before complications develop. Furthermore, liver disease frequently will not resolve until the endocrinopathy is treated. Full consideration of these disorders and their treatment is outside the scope of this text but associated clinical features which should raise clinical suspicion and appropriate diagnostic investigations are given in Table 4.8. Hypothyroidism is classically associated with an unconjugated hyperbilirubinaemia. Its presence in hepatitis syndromes may merely change what would have been an anicteric cryptogenic hepatitis into an icteric one which is recognized. Hypothyroidism is so common that it must be excluded in every instance.

Septo-optic dysplasia is an extremely variable neuro-optical malformation characterized by three major clinical manifestations: anterior midline prosencephalic developmental defects such as absence of the septum pellucidum or corpus callosum, bilateral or unilateral optic nerve hypoplasia, and varying degrees of hypopituitarism. Liver disease in infancy was first associated with septo-optic dysplasia in 1975 in an infant with hypopituitarism. Studies in our unit in the past 5 years suggest that presentation with conjugated hyperbilirubinaemia may be more frequent than previously appreciated (Roberts-Harry et al., 1990). We have identified nine cases of septo-optic dysplasia and two possible cases identified in a 6-year period. Features which should promote consideration of the diagnosis are prolonged second stage of labour, severe hypoglycaemia

Table 4.8 Endocrine disorders associated with hepatitis syndrome of infancy

Disorder	Diagnostic investigations	Associated features
Hypopituitarism	Low HGH, ACTH, TSH and T_4, FSH and LH	Hypoglycaemia, micro-genitalia, micro-ophthalmia, absent septum pellucidum
Diabetes insipidus	Fixed urinary osmolality on water deprivation increasing with $10\,\mu g$ of DDAVP	High serum sodium
Hypoadrenalism	Low plasma cortisol levels after ACTH	Hypoglycaemia, hypotension, low serum sodium
Hypothyroidism	High TSH, low T_4	Cretinism, goitre
Hypoparathyroidism	Low serum parathormone concentrations	Low calcium, DiGeorge syndrome

in the immediate postnatal period, unconjugated hyperbilirubinaemia starting in the first 24 hours of liver sometimes requiring exchange transfusion and high or low serum sodium concentrations. In typical cases the optic nerve head is small occupying only a proportion of the disc area and being surrounded by a pale or pigmented halo or crescent between the optic head and the pigmented retinal epithelium. It may be so minor that it can only be diagnosed by comparing the width of the disc with the disc macular distance. The anomaly may be unilateral or bilateral, mild or severe. There may be impairment of visual acuity. Only 30% of patients had all three major components of the syndrome (Morishima and Aranoff, 1986).

Liver disease associated with hypopituitarism usually presents with jaundice dating from the neonatal period persisting for up to 6 months, associated with abnormal biochemical test of liver function which return to normal within 12–24 months. Liver biopsies are characterized by cholestasis with dilated bile canaliculi, and focal areas of hepatocellular necrosis. There may be features of bile duct obstruction or bile duct hypoplasia. None of our patients have developed chronic liver disease. Two reported cases had cirrhosis or portal hypertension.

Infections associated with hepatitis in infancy

A wide range of agents causing generalized infection of the neonate produce hepatitis as a major or minor component of the illness. The hepatitis may range in severity from fulminant liver failure to elevation of transaminases without clinical features of liver disease. Bacterial infections such as *Escherichia coli* septicaemia and infection with *Listeria*, toxoplasmosis, cytomegalovirus, rubella, Reo type III virus and hepatitis B virus, have all been associated with extrahepatic biliary atresia as well as hepatitis. In addition, septicaemia may complicate liver disease primarily due to a metabolic abnormality such as galactosaemia. Cytomegalovirus may frequently be found in the urine of infants who are well. Considerable care, therefore, is necessary before the neonatal hepatitis syndrome can, in an individual patient, be attributed to any of these alleged pathogens, unless the hepatitis is associated with the severe extrahepatic clinical manifestations listed in Table 4.9

In clinical management it is essential to exclude treatable bacterial infection, listeriosis, toxoplasmosis malaria and infection with *Treponema pallidum* since specific anti-microbial therapy for these is available. For viral infections, no effective treatment has as yet been devised other than acyclovir for herpes simplex. Note that infants developing hepatitis B are particularly likely to have a fulminant course if born to mothers who are are HBsAg and anti-HBe positive. Chronic liver disease is unusual in the absence of an underlying metabolic cause except with hepatitis B virus infection (Chapter 6) and rare instance of cytomegalovirus infection.

Liver disease associated with total parenteral nutrition

Intravenous nutrition using solutions of amino acids, carbohydrates and lipids with added electrolytes, trace elements and vitamins is an essential part of modern paediatric care. It is used for augmenting nutrition in low birth weight, premature infants. It may be the only mode of nutrition in severe and/or extensive small gut disorders. Liver disease may be caused by a combination of catheter-related complications, metabolic effects of the nutrients, lack of gut stimulation in the absence of oral intake and effects of the underlying

Table 4.9 Infections associated with hepatitis syndrome of infancy

Infecting agents	Screening investigations	Definitive investigations	Principal extrahepatic manifestations
Cytomegalovirus	CF antibody in serum	Isolation from urine and liver with demonstration of virus in liver by IF	Small for dates; microcephaly; meningoencephalitis; intracranial calcification; neonatal thrombocytopenic purpura; splenomegaly; retinitis, deafness
Rubella virus	CF and HAI antibodies in serum	Specific IgM antibody, virus isolation from nasopharynx and liver	Small for dates; cataracts, retinitis; congenital heart defects; microphthalmia, buphthalmos and corneal oedema; myocarditis; neonatal thrombocytopenic purpura; splenomegaly; osteopathy; lymphadenopathy
Hepatitis A		IgM anti-HAV	Usually asymptomatic in infancy
Hepatitis B virus	HBs antigen in mother	HBs antigen in infant	None described
Non-A, B, C hepatitis	None	Absence of HBsAg and anti HAV and HCV	Non-A, B, C hepatitis in mother
Herpes simplex virus	Perinatal herpes in mother	Isolation and demonstration of virus from superficial lesions and liver	Splenomegaly; heart failure, pneumonitis; skin vesicles; meningoencephalitis
Coxsackie A9, B Echo virus 9, 11, 14, 19 Adenovirus Human herpes virus 6,	Isolation from respiratory tract and faeces	Isolation from liver	Myocarditis; meningoencephalitis; pneumonitis
Reo virus Type III Epstein-Barr virus	Paul–Bunnell test	CF antibody in serum Indirect immunofluorescent antibody IgM antibody to EG virus	
Varicella zoster virus	Demonstration of virus from superficial lesions	Demonstration of virus in the liver	Disseminated infection as in herpes simplex: skin lesions more obvious
Psittacosis		IgM antibody to psittacosis	
Bacterial infection		Blood culture, urine culture, CSF	Anaemia; any other system may be involved
Listeria		Isolation of organisms from blood culture, CSF or liver	Septicaemia; meningitis; pneumonitis; purpura
Treponema pallidum	VDRL or TPI, particularly in mother	Demonstration of Treponema by dark ground illumination	Rhinitis; skin rash; bone lesions; anaemia; lymph-adenopathy; meningoencephalitis
Toxoplasma gondii	CF antibody in serum	Rising antibody titre in infant; specific IgM antibody; isolation of organisms from liver and CSF; visualization of organism from liver and CSF	Microcephaly; macrocephaly; meningoencephalitis; intracranial calcification; choreoretinitis; thrombocytopenia; purpura
Malaria		Plasmodium in blood film	Splenomegaly
Tuberculosis	Chest X-ray	Tuberculosis in gastric aspirate	Respiratory distress

CF = Complement fixing; HAI = Haem. agglutination inhibition; IF = Immunofluorescence microscopy; EM = Electron microscopy; CSF = Cerebrospinal fluid

disease. The prevalence increase with increasing prematurity and the duration of parenteral nutrition. The disorder remits gradually if intravenous feeding can be stopped but progresses to cirrhosis if it has to be maintained. Progression may be arrested if some oral feeding is possible.

Pathology

Cholestasis, hepatocellular damage, lobular disarray and mild to moderate degrees of multinucleated giant cell transformation with hyperplasia of the Kupffer cells are the main features. Cholestasis is both canalicular and hepatocellular being more severe towards the central portions of the lobule. There are no bile plugs in the portal tracts. Hepatocytes show rarefaction and vesiculation of the cytoplasm. They may contain moderate accumulations of glycogen, haemosiderin and lipofuscin. There is frequently a mild, inflammatory cell infiltrate in the portal tracts and parenchyma. The hyperplastic Kupffer cells contain PAS-positive pigments, lipofuscin and bile pigment. The portal tracts are widened and show increased fibrosis.

Ultrastructural studies show giant mitochondria of various sizes and shapes and damaged endoplasmic reticulum. There are increased collagen fibres in the space of Disse. From these develop a fine pericellular fibrosis which progresses to cirrhosis. This may be complicated by carcinoma. Bile canaliculi may be massively dilated, devoid of microvilli and plugged with bile. Acute acalculous cholecystitis, biliary sludge and cholelithiasis may develop.

Pathogenesis

The aetiology is unknown. The frequency increases with decreasing gestational age, the duration of intravenous nutrition and the persistent absence of any oral intake. The majority of infants have been exposed to other factors which themselves may impair liver function and cause cholestasis. These include sepsis, hypoxia, blood transfusion, intra-abdominal surgery and drugs. Shock with poor peripheral perfusion associated with severe infection or hyaline membrane disease may be the critical factor in the premature infant without intra-abdominal disease (Dosi *et al.*, 1985).

The main components of the intravenously administered solutions – carbohydrates, lipids and amino acids – are all equally suspect as possible contributory factors, since they produce abnormal biochemical tests of liver function or pathological changes in the liver in humans or experimental animals. Amino acid solutions may cause hyperammonaemia, metabolic acidosis and hyperaminoacidaemia. They may have a direct effect on bile salt-independent bile flow. Solutions deficient in taurine may limit bile salt excretion. Total or relative lack of essential nutrients and trace elements have also been implicated. The other possible contributory factor is the absence of the normal intestinal stimuli to bile formation which occurs when the infant is not fed. Production of gut hormones which stimulate bile secretion may be limited. The rate of recycling of the bile acid pool is reduced and thus a stimulus to bile formation is removed. The observation that the frequency of cholestasis increases with the duration of fasting may merely reflect how ill these babies are rather than indicate any aetiological importance.

Clinical features and laboratory findings

The first clinical indication of hepatic involvement is usually the appearance of a conjugated hyperbilirubinaemia. Conjugated hyperbilirubinaemia, abnormal biochemical tests of liver function and hepatomegaly develop after periods of intravenous nutrition lasting from 10–180 days, the onset being earlier in premature ill infants. The incidence is typically around 15% in those of less than 32 weeks' gestation, 5% in those of between 32 and 36 weeks and 1.5% after 36 weeks' gestation. Hepatomegaly and splenomegaly may be noted. The stools are rarely acholic unless there is complicating biliary obstruction. If intravenous feeding is maintained, hepatomegaly becomes progressively more marked and the liver harder. Features of cirrhosis may develop. Fifteen of 16 infants with massive bowel resection requiring intravenous nutrition for periods ranging from 8–21 months developed liver disease with three deaths and three survivors having end-stage liver disease.

Usually prior to the onset of jaundice elevation of aspartate aminotransferase, gamma-glutamyl transpeptidase or alkaline phosphatase may be detected. Serum bile acid concentration may rise. Values are usually within two or three times the upper limit of normal. The blood ammonia may be as high as three times normal. The serum bilirubin concentration ranges from 34 μmol/litre to levels greater than 300 μmol/litre (2–9 mg/dl), returning to normal within 7–100 days of discontinuing intravenous nutrition.

Treatment and prognosis

The essentials of treatment are to replace intravenous feeding with as much oral feeding as possible, to exclude other cause of cholestasis including biliary obstruction by sludge and stones and vitamin supplements. Percutaneous, endoscopic or laparoscopic cholangiography may be therapeutic as well as diagnostic if there is secondary bile duct obstruction. When intravenous nutrition is withdrawn the jaundice settles and liver function tests improve, returning to normality usually within 5 months. Liver biopsy changes may persist for up to a year. If intravenous feeding has to be continued progressive liver disease with cirrhosis is the inevitable sequela, particularly if no oral feeding is possible. It is recommended therefore that intravenous feeding should be curtailed as much as possible if jaundice or other features of hepatocellular injury appear. Tests of liver function should be carried out regularly while intravenous feeding is in progress.

Circulation disturbances – anaemia and hypoxia associated with cholestasis

The combination of circulatory changes with hypoxia may result in glycogen depletion, fatty metamorphosis, hyaline degeneration, infarction and necrosis. In babies dying of uncomplicated hyaline membrane disease, foci of cellular degeneration and necrosis may be associated with fibrin thrombi in the sinusoids. Cholestasis associated with total parenteral nutrition is more common in uninfected premature infants who have had hyaline membrane disease and shock. Fatty change in hepatocellular necrosis is also reported in congenital heart disorders where left heart function is impaired. It seems possible that similar mechanisms contribute to cholestasis occurring during the recovery phase of erythroblastosis. The hepatic complications associated with hypoxia are in general reversible if the primary cause is removed.

Drugs, environmental toxins and iatrogenic disorders

There is a similar paucity of reports of drug-induced liver injury in infancy as in older children (see p.151); nevertheless there are sufficient to emphasize that the infant is no less susceptible than other age groups and may, indeed, be at particular risk because of age-related metabolic changes. Neither the placenta nor breast offer much protection from xenobiotics. Maternal alcohol ingestion has been associated with intrahepatic pathology in the fetal alcohol syndrome and more contentiously with biliary atresia (Donigan and Werlin, 1981). The neonate is likely to receive one, two or three drugs at delivery and if intensive care is required, a further three or four, as well as the hazards of parenteral nutrition. A proprietary intravenous vitamin E supplement containing polysorbate has been implicated in causing a progressive intralobular cholestasis with inflammation of hepatic venules and extensive sinusoidal veno-occlusion by fibrosis in premature infants. A particular hazard in the premature nursery is the umbilical vein catheter which rather than having its tip in the inferior vena cava passes into a portal vein branch causing thrombosis and hepatic necrosis.

Recently reported examples of drug-induced hepatic problems include frusemide as a suggested cause of gall stones (Mowat, 1986) and erythromycin estolate causing complete cholestasis in an infant of six weeks (Krowchuk and Seashore, 1979). Chloramphenicol may cause grey syndrome in neonates and an increased incidence of bone marrow depression and hepatitis in infants and older children. Chloral hydrate has recently been implicated as a cause of liver damage in infancy. Could the unusual self-limiting hepatitis with pneumonitis, haemolytic anaemia, fat-soluble vitamin deficiency and relative failure to thrive reported by Godel and Hart (1984) in infants of less than 3 months of age living in coastal areas of Arctic Canada be caused by an environmental toxin?

Post-haemolytic cholestasis (inspissated bile syndrome)

Transient conjugated hyperbilirubinaemia occurs during the recovery phase in erythro-blastosis in which it appears that the bilirubin is conjugated more rapidly than it can be excreted. Liver function tests are, however, normal. When the unconjugated hyper-bilirubinaemia has been protracted and severe, or if there has been marked anaemia at birth, the urine may contain bile and the stools become acholic. Laboratory investigations show typical features of the hepatitis syndrome in infancy. The liver biopsy shows hepatocellular necrosis and giant cell transformation. There may be both hepatocellular and canalicular cholestasis. There is little increased fibrosis, or changes in the portal tracts. Prognosis is good.

Cholestasis in the ill premature infant

The premature infant requiring intensive care may be exposed to a series of episodes of illness which adversely affect liver function, already compromised by prematurity. All of the disorders considered above may contribute, particularly hypoxia, infections, surgical procedures preventing oral feeding and parenteral nutrition. Drugs, blood and blood products may cause hepatitis. In addition all of the disorders considered in this and the following chapter have to be considered. Prematurity does not exclude biliary atresia, choledochal cyst or alpha-1 antitrypsin deficiency. The principles of investigation and management of the term infant apply except that these infants frequently have had blood transfusions which makes investigation for serological markers of infection and tests for some inherited disorders difficult to interpret. Finding the parents are heterozygotes for the PIZZ state or galactosaemia may be the only way to make an early diagnosis.

Idiopathic or cryptogenic hepatitis (hepatocellular jaundice) of infancy (Figure 4.3)

Despite an increasing range of specific disorders associated with liver disease in infancy, between 60% and 80% of cases in most series have either extrahepatic biliary atresia or idiopathic or cryptogenic liver disease. The percentage in which no cause can be found in any series is determined by the genetic composition of the community, environmental factors, referral patterns, the investigation facilities available at the time of the study and the rigidity of criteria for an aetiological diagnosis (see Tables 4.10 and 4.11). Some of those currently labelled 'cryptogenic' no doubt have an as yet unidentified metabolic or infectious disorder. Long-term follow-up for such infants may allow a more precise diagnosis in a few when new features appear, e.g. central nervous system involvement in storage disorders. In others the birth of a second affected sibling reinforces the possibility of an unrecognized genetic disorder.

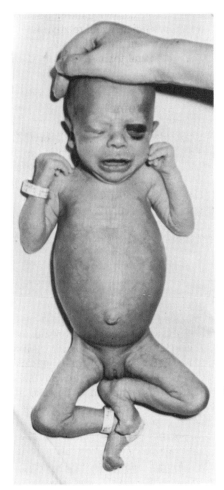

Figure 4.3 Infant aged 2 weeks with conjugated hyperbilirubinaemia, purpura and abdominal distension due to ascites. The birth weight was 2.3 kg at 39 weeks' gestation. No cause for the liver disease was identified. Steroids were started at 5 days after birth because of persistent purpura with thrombocytopenia, the platelet count being less than 10 000 and the prothrombin time prolonged by 110 seconds. The bleeding diathesis settled over the course of 2 weeks. Steroids were continued when liver function tests remained abnormal and a percutaneous liver biopsy showed features consistent with chronic aggressive hepatitis. Steroids were eventually stopped at the age of 2 years when liver function tests had been normal for 12 months. A liver biopsy at 5 years of age showed slight hepatic fibrosis. There was no clinical or biochemical evidence of liver disease. Although the outcome was satisfactory in this case, there is no evidence that steroids affect the course of hepatocellular disease in this age group

Table 4.10 Causes of obstructive jaundice in infancy; the influence of environmental factors and diagnostic facilities on the apparent cause in three areas

Cause	King's College Hospital, London, England (1970–1976)	Royal Children's Hospital, Melbourne, Australia[1]	Verwoerd Hospital, Pretoria, S. Africa[2]
Extrahepatic biliary atresia	62	55	21
Idiopathic hepatitis	91	88	52
Alpha-1 antitrypsin deficiency	35	8	0
Galactosaemia	2	6	0
Cystic fibrosis	2	2	0
Rubella	2	3	0
Cytomegalovirus	3	13	0
Hepatitis B$_s$ Ag	2	1	0
Syphilis	0	1	28
Toxoplasmosis	1	2	0
Blood group incompatibility	4	6	6
Veno-occlusive disease	0	0	8
Miscellaneous	0	0	13

[1] Danks et al. (1977)
[2] Pretorius and Roode (1974)

Table 4.11 Relative frequency of causes of conjugated hyperbilirubinaemia (Paediatric Liver Service, KCH)

Disorder	Referred cases	Epidemiological study
Extrahepatic biliary atresia	337	11
Choledochal cyst	34	1
Spontaneous perforation of the bile ducts	6	0
Idiopathic hepatitis of infancy	331	29
Alpha-1 antitrypsin deficiency (PIZZ)	189	7
Other associated disorders	94	6
Alagille's syndrome	41	0
	1032	54

Clinical features

The presentation is with a hepatitis syndrome, hypoglycaemia, malabsorption, failure to thrive, liver failure with bleeding tendency (Chapter 8) or, rarely, cirrhosis and ascites (see p. 13), mimicking all disorders in this chapter and Chapter 5.

Infants with idiopathic disease are frequently of low birth weight, born following abnormal pregnancies and come to medical attention because of prematurity or low birth weight as well as because of hepatocellular disease. Jaundice frequently starts in the first 2 weeks of life but the onset may be up to 6 months of age. Jaundice may last anything from 2 weeks to 6 months. In an epidemiological study of cases in south-east England, half were sufficiently severe to give acholic stools.

Diagnosis and management

The diagnosis requires demonstration of bile duct patency usually by seeing that the stools are green, excluding rarer biliary disorders on the basis of the ultrasound, liver biopsy and in some instances cholangiogram findings and the systematic exclusion of disorders considered elsewhere in this chapter. The management is that of cholestasis and/or acute liver failure.

Prognosis

In the epidemiological study referred to above two died of liver disease in the first 6 months of life. In five of 27 survivors, biochemical tests of liver function were abnormal up to 10 years of age. All patients were asymptomatic. Biopsies in four of these patients at ages between 5 and 12 years were normal except in one patient who had mild fibrosis. The fifth, one of two children with an affected sibling in the series, had cirrhosis (Dick and Mowat, 1985). This patient has now developed features of Niemann–Pick Type II (C). Deutsch *et al.* (1985) gave a much poorer prognosis with 25 deaths from liver disease in 73 patients but with only three of 40 survivors aged between 6 and 17 years having chronic liver disease. Henriksen *et al.* (1981) also gave a poor prognosis with 15 of 27 dying and four of seven survivors studied having biochemical evidence of continuing liver disease. Chang *et al.* (1987) reported six deaths in the first 11 months, one at 4 years, two surviving with cirrhosis with the remaining 45 having made a complete hepatic recovery. In eight jaundice persisted for more than 6 months. Half had evidence of cytomegalovirus infection. In contrast, Odievre *et al.* (1981) reported only four deaths in 64 infants with 85% of the survivors making a good recovery. A similarly favourable prognosis was reported from Japan. The majority of these reports emphasize the poor prognosis in patients with familial occurrence of similar disease. It appears that those infants who have stools that are acholic for a long time, hard livers and histological features suggesting bile duct obstruction have the worse prognosis. Laparotomy and/or operative cholangiography aggravate the disorder. Since laparotomy findings may be misleading in up to 20% of cases with the danger of removal of narrow but patent bile ducts, laparotomy is best avoided.

Intrahepatic biliary hypoplasia

This disorder is characterized by an absence or reduction in the number of bile ductules seen in portal tracts within the liver substance. The diagnosis requires that within interlobular portal tracts normal sized branches of the portal vein and hepatic artery can be identified, but the bile ductules are absent or disproportionately small and the cuboidal epithelial cell lining them may be dysmorphic. The term has been used synonymously with biliary dysgenesis, hepatic ductular hypoplasia, paucity of the intralobular bile ducts and intrahepatic biliary atresia. Such hypoplasia may occur in association with specific genetic disorders such as alpha-1 antitrypsin deficiency or impaired cholic acid synthesis, in chromosomal abnormalities such as Down's syndrome and, rarely, with intrauterine infections such as rubella and cytomegalovirus. It has also been reported with hepatitis B. This section will consider only two forms: the rare syndromic variety occurring in association with a range of characteristic extrahepatic abnormalities (syndromic biliary hypoplasia) and an isolated abnormality (non-syndromic biliary hypoplasia).

Syndromic paucity of the interlobular bile ducts (Alagille's syndrome, syndromic biliary hypoplasia, arteriohepatic dysplasia)

In this disorder biliary hypoplasia is associated with a range of cardiovascular, skeletal, facial and ocular anomalies detailed below. The estimated incidence is one per 100 000 live births.

Aetiology

The aetiology is unknown. The occurrence of familial cases, identified both vertically and horizontally, suggest a genetic aetiology in such families. The majority of observations of familial cases are compatible with an autosomal dominant disorder of variable expression and reduced penetrance. However, the studies of Mueller *et al.* (1984) suggest that in some affected sibships the mode of inheritance is autosomal recessive. Sixteen cases with partial deletion of chromosome 20 have been reported (Desmaze *et al.*, 1992). The majority of cases are sporadic. For these an active teratogen such as rubella infection could account for anomalies in many systems.

The pathogenesis of the paucity of the bile ducts is intriguing. In the 20% of infants who have bile ducts present in their early biopsies a destructive, inflammatory process is suggested as a possible mechanism. An alternative is simple atrophy as a consequence of reduced bile production secondary to a defect in hepatocellular excretion.

The ultrastructural findings of bile canaliculi that are not dilated and have normal microvilli together with the lack of prominence of the Golgi apparatus – features which are prominent in other forms of cholestasis of infancy – has led to the suggestion that a reduced bile flow may result from a secretory block proximal to the Golgi apparatus or in the pericanalicular cytoplasm. A further possible mechanism is excessive clearance of embryonic duct remnants, as opposed to ineffective clearance in genetic disorders complicated by congenital hepatic fibrosis (Desmet, 1992).

Pathology

Typical histological features are shown in Figure 4.4. The portal tracts may be so inconspicuous that the biopsy may be interpreted as normal by inexperienced observers. In up to 20% of cases liver biopsies in the first 1–2 years of life contain easily identifiable interlobular bile ducts and ductules with up to 10% showing bile duct reduplication.

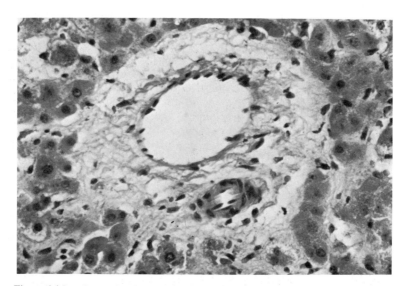

Figure 4.4 Portal tract showing a portal vein branch and, below, a small branch of the hepatic artery. No bile ductules can be seen. The spaces within the portal tract may be lymphatic channels. There is no increased fibrosis or cellular infiltrate. (Percutaneous liver biopsy; haematoxylin and eosin: × 320, reduced to seven-eighths in reproduction)

Repeat biopsies 4–10 months later show typical histological findings. In the jaundiced patient there is conspicuous bile retention in the hepatocytes but bile plugs are usually absent. There may be distension of hepatocytes, focal giant cell transformation and mild lobular disarray. Periportal or central lobular fibrosis is usually absent but in up to 20% of cases may be mild or moderate in infancy. Up to 15% go on to develop a biliary cirrhosis by the second decade. Ultrastructural examination shows marked intercellular bile pigment in vesicles in the GERL (Golgi-endoplasmic reticulum-lysosomes). The bile canaliculi are lined with normal microvilli, a feature unique to this form of cholestasis. The extrahepatic bile ducts are structurally normal but may be so narrow in the severely cholestatic patient that a lumen cannot be demonstrated even by operative cholangiography. Methylene blue injected into the biliary system may demonstrate patency.

Clinical features

Chronic cholestasis dominates the clinical picture in the vast majority but in up to 10% cyanotic heart disease is the main problem. Very rarely pruritus with abnormal biochemical tests of liver function may be the only manifestation. The sex incidence is equal. The family history is positive in 15% of cases; 20% are prematurely born or light for gestational age.

Hepatic features   The first feature to appear is conjugated hyperbilirubinaemia usually dating from the neonatal period, followed by pruritus occasionally starting at 2 months of age but rare before 5 months and finally in severe cases, xanthelasma, rare before 16 months but usually present at 2 years of age. Up to 90% present with a hepatitis syndrome often complicated by spontaneous bleeding caused by vitamin K malabsorption. Cholestasis is frequently so severe that the stools are acholic.

The remainder are anicteric but present with pruritus or failure to thrive. Of 27 patients studied in our unit 24 were jaundiced, 19 including four anicteric patients developed pruritus, while eight had xanthelasma (Figure 4.5). Throughout the first decade an

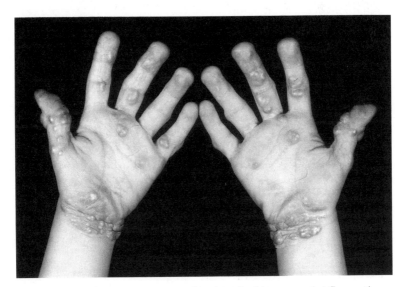

Figure 4.5 Xanthalesma, most pronounced at sites of mild trauma and at flexures, in a 6-year-old boy with Alagille's syndrome.

enlarged firm or hard liver is palpable in nearly all cases with splenomegaly present in up to 50%. There are few reports on long-term prognosis but it seems that in the majority of patients features of cholestasis gradually remit. Jaundice cleared in eight of the above patients at ages ranging from 3 months to 7 years, pruritus has lessened in the first decade in four and cleared in one, but only one has cleared the xanthelasma. In a review of 45 patients 14% have developed cirrhosis at a mean age of 12 years but nine anicteric patients aged 18 to 35 years were non-cirrhotic although biochemical tests of liver function were abnormal (Perrault, 1981). In a series of 80 patients of whom 21 died, in only four were the deaths attributed to liver disease the remainder dying of heart disease or infection (Alagille *et al.*, 1987). Chronic malabsorption of fat occasionally contributed to by exocrine pancreatic insufficiency, in addition to lack of intraluminal bile salts, is universal. Supplements of fat-soluble vitamins are essential. Severe growth retardation may, in part, be due to malabsorption.

Laboratory features   Aspartate aminotransferase and alkaline phosphatase concentrations are invariably raised at values ranging up to 10 times the upper limit of normal with gamma-glutamyl transpeptidase raised in the majority with concentrations ranging from three times to 30 times the upper limit of normal. These tests usually remain abnormal after jaundice clears. Eighty per cent have elevated serum cholesterol and triglyceride values ranging up to three times the upper limit of normal for age. Serum albumin and prothrombin time (after vitamin X) are normal except in decompensated cirrhosis.

Extrahepatic features   The frequency of the characteristic extrahepatic features on which a diagnosis is based is given in Table 4.12. The most characteristic cardiovascular anomaly is peripheral pulmonary artery stenosis. An important diagnostic feature is the distinctive facial appearance of a prominent forehead with deeply set moderately widely separated eyes, a saddle-shaped or straight nose which in profile is in the same plane as the forehead, and a small pointed chin. It should be noted that the specificity of this facial appearance has been challenged by the observations of Sokol *et al.* (1983) who considered that the facies are a feature of any form of persistent intrahepatic cholestatic liver disorder occurring in early childhood.

Another helpful diagnostic feature is the presence of vertebral anomalies, particularly failure of fusion of the bodies, giving rise to the so-called 'butterfly vertebrae'.

Table 4.12 Frequency of extrahepatic features in syndromic biliary hypoplasia

Extrahepatic features	Frequency (%)
Skeletal anomalies	50
Posterior embryotoxon	70
Abnormal facies	73
Cardiac anomalies	95
Benign anomalies	50
Symptomatic and fully investigated	
Isolated peripheral pulmonary artery stenosis	50
Peripheral pulmonary artery stenosis + other lesion	40
Other defects	10

Renal, neural and endocrine anomalies have also been described together with delayed mental and sexual development.

Embryotoxon, an accumulation of material on the inner aspects of the cornea near its junction with the iris, can only be demonstrated on slit-lamp examination of the eyes. Unfortunately it is present in up to 15% of the normal population. Nevertheless these features, particularly if all are present, do allow a firm diagnosis in the presence of typical pathological features. In the infants with complete cholestasis and persisting bile ducts and bile duct reduplication, differentiation from biliary atresia may be possible by endoscopic cholangiography.

Treatment

The treatment is that of chronic cholestasis. If diarrhoea is present, pancreatic exocrine insufficiency should be excluded. Pancreatic supplements may increase the rate of weight gain. Liver transplantation may be required for complications of cirrhosis and rarely for complications of cholestasis. There are no satisfactory means of limiting the hypercholesterolaemia.

Non-syndromic biliary hypoplasia (without associated developmental anomalies)

This is an extremely rare disorder of unknown aetiology. It has been a feature of cryptogenic intrahepatic cholestasis in siblings (Jubero *et al.*, 1966; Gray and Saunders, 1966; Sharp *et al.*, 1967; Ballow *et al.*, 1973) suggesting It may have a genetic basis. The main pathological difference from the syndromic variety is much more marked fibrosis which progresses rapidly to a biliary cirrhosis. There may be prominent giant cell transformation. The disorder usually starts with cholestasis in infancy followed by pruritus. The majority of cases progress rapidly to liver failure with death by 3 years of age.

Bibliography and references

General

Adcock, E. W. and Lester, R. (eds) (1984) Neonatal cholestasis: Causes, syndromes and therapy. *Report of the 87th Ross Conference on Paediatric Research.* Ross Laboratories, Columbus, Ohio

Amedee-Manesme, O., Mourey, M. S., Couturier, M., Alvarez, F., Hanck, A. and Bernard, O. (1988) Short- and long-term vitamin A treatment in children with cholestasis. *Am. J. Clin. Nutr.*, **47**, 690–693

Balistreri, W. F. (1985) Neonatal cholestasis. *J. Pediatr.*, **106**, 171

Balistreri, W. F., A-Kader, H. H., Ryckman, F. C., Heubi, J. E., Setchel, K. D. R. and the UDCA study group (1992) Ursodeoxycholic acid in paediatric patients with chronic cholestasis. In *Paediatric Cholestasis. Novel Approaches to Treatment* (eds M. J. Lentze, J. Reichen). Kluwer Academic Publishers, London p. 333

Becker, M., Von Bergmann, X., Rotthause, H. W. and Leiss, O. (1984) Biliary lipid metabolism in children with chronic intrahepatic cholestasis. *Eur. J. Pediatr.*, **143**, 35

Blanckaert, N. and Heirwegh, K. P. M. (1986) Analysis and preparation of bilirubins and biliverdins. In *Bile Pigments and Jaundice, Molecular, Metabolic and Medical Aspects* (ed. J. D. Ostrow). Marcel Dekker, New York, ch 3, pp. 31–80

Chang, M. H., Hsu, H. C., Lee, C. Y., Wang, T. R. and Kao, C. L. (1987) Neonatal Hepatitis: a follow up study. *Journal of Pediatric Gastroenterology and Nutrition*, **6**: 203–7

Charlton, C. P. J., Buchanan, E., Holden, C. E., Preece, M. A., Green, A., Booth, I. W., and Tarlow, M. J. (1992) Intensive enteral feeding in advanced cirrhosis: reversal of malnutrition without precipitation of hepatic encephalopathy. *Arch. Dis. Childh.*, **67**, 603–607.

Danks, D. M., Campbell, P. E., Smith, A. L. and Rogers, J. (1977) Studies of the aetiology of neonatal hepatitis and biliary atresia. *Arch. Dis. Childh.*, **52**, 360

Desmet, V. J. (1992) Congenital disease of intrahepatic bile ducts: variations on the theme 'ductal plate malformation', *Hepatology*, **16**, 1069–1083.

Deutsch, J., Smith, A. L., Danks, D. M. and Campbell, P. E. (1985) Long-term prognosis for babies with neonatal liver disease. *Arch. Dis. Childh.*, **60**, 447

Dick, M. C. And Mowat, A. P. (1985) Hepatitis syndrome in infancy – an epidemiological survey with 10-year follow-up. *Arch. Dis. Childh.*, **60**, 512

Ekelund, H. (1991) Late haemorrhagic disease of the newborn in Sweden, 1987–98. *Acta Paediatr.*, **80**, 966–969

El Tumi, M. A., Clark, M. D., Barrett, J. J. and Mowat, A. P. (1987) A ten minute radiopharmaceutical test in suspected biliary atresia. *Arch. Dis. Childh.*, **62**, 180–184

Fitzgerald, J. F. (1988) Cholestatic disorders in infancy. *Pediatr. Clin. of N. Am.*, **35**, 357–373.

Henriksen, M. T., Drablos, T. A. and Aagenaes, O. (1981) Cholestatic jaundice in infancy. The importance of familial and genetic factors in aetiology and prognosis. *Arch. Dis. Childh.*, **56**, 622

Howard, E. R. and Mowat, A. P. (1983) Hepatobiliary disorders in infancy: hepatitis; extrahepatic biliary atresia; intrahepatic biliary hypoplasia. In *Recent Advances in Hepatology*, Volume 1 (eds H. C. Thomas, and R. N. M. McSween). Churchill Livingstone, Edinburgh, p.153

Lukaszkiewicz, J., Ryzko, J., Socha, J. and Lorenc, R. S. (1989) Endogenous, cutaneous vitamin D synthesis stimulation as an effective way of improving the vitamin D status in children with hepatobiliary malfunctions. *Digestion*, **42**, 158–162

McNinch, A. W. and Tripp, J. H. (1991) Haemorrhagic disease of the newborn in the British Isles: a two year prospective study. *Br. Med .J.*, **303**, 1105–1108

Maggiore, G., Bernard, O., Riely, C. A., Hadchouel, M., Lemonnier, A. and Alagille, D. (1987) Normal serum gamma-glutamyl-transpeptidase activity identifies groups of infants with idiopathic cholestasis with poor prognosis. *Journal of Pediatrics*, **III**: 251–52

Mair, B. and Klempner, L. B. (1987) Abnormally high values in Direct Bilirubin in the Serum of Newborns as measured with the DuPont aca Analyser. *Am. J. Clin. Path.*, **87**, 642–644.

Montgomery, C. X. And Reubner, D. X. (1976) Neonatal hepatocellular giant cell transformation. A review. *In Perspectives in Paediatric Hepatology*, Volume 3 (eds. H. S. Rossenberg and R. P. Bolandi), p. 85. Chicago Year Book Publishers

Odievre, M., Hadchouel, M., Landrieu, P., Alagille, D. and Elliott, N. (1981) Long-term prognosis for infants with intrahepatic cholestasis and patent extrahepatic biliary tract. *Arch. Dis. Childh.*, **56**, 373

Ostrea, E. M., Ongtengco, E. A., Tolia, V. A. and Apostol, E. (1988) The Occurrence and Significance of the Bilirubin Species, Including Delta Bilirubin, In Jaundiced Infants. *J. Pediatr. Gastroent. Nutr.*, **7**, 511–516

Pretorius, P. J. and Roode, H. (1974) Obstructive jaundice in early infancy. *S. Afr. Med. J.*, **48**, 811

Robbins, C. and Holzman, I. R. (1992) Diffuse hepatic infarction with complete recovery in a neonate. *J. Pediatr.*, **120**, 786–788

Rosenthal, P., Blanckaert, N., Kabra, P. M. and Thaler, M. M. (1986) Formation of Bilirubin Conjugates in Human Newborns. *Paediatr. Res.*, **20**, 947–950

Rushton, D. I. (1981) Fetal and neonatal liver disease. *Dia. Histopathol.*, **4**, 17

Sokol, R. (1992) Vitamin deficiency and replacement in childhood cholestasis. In *Paediatric Cholestasis. Novel Approaches to Treatment* (eds M. J. Lentze, J. Reichen). Kluwer Academic Publishers, London, p.289

Sokol, R. J., Guggenheim, M. A. Iannaccone, S. T. *et al.* (1985) Improved neurologic function after long-term correction of vitamin E deficiency in children with chronic cholestasis. *New Engl. J. Med.*, **313**, 1580

Sokol, R. J., Guggenheim, M. A. and Heubi, J. E. *et al.* (1985) Frequency and clinical progression of vitamin E deficiency neurological disorder in children with prolonged neonatal cholestasis. *Am. J. Dis. Child.*, **139**, 1211

Sutor, A. H., Dagres, N. and Neiderhoff, H. (1992) Vitamin-K-mangelblutungen bei sauglingen. *Hamostaseologie*, **12**, 116–126

Trivedi, P., Mieli-Vergani, G. and Mowat, A. P. (1992) Cholestasis in infancy and children. An overview. In *Paediatric Cholestasis. Novel Approaches to Treatment* (eds M. J. Lentze, J. Reichen). Kluwer Academic Publishers, London, p.129

Wilkinson, M. L., Mieli-Vergani, G., Ball, C., Portmann, B. and Mowat, A. P. (1991) Endoscopic retrograde cholangiopancreatography (ERCP) in infantile cholestasis. *Arch. Dis. Child.*, **66**, 121–123

Endocrine disorders

Kaufman, F. R., Costin, G., Thomas, D. W., Sinatra, F. R., Roe, T. F. and Neustein, H. B. (1984) Neonatal cholestasis and hypopituitarism. *Arch. Dis. Childh.*, **59**, 787

Morishima, S. M. and Aranoff, S. D. (1986) Syndrome of septo-optic/pituitary dysplasia: the clinical spectrum. *Brain and Development*, **8**: 233–39

Roberts-Harry, J., Green, S. H. and Willshaw, H. E. (1990) Optic nerve hypoplasia: associations and management. *Archives of Disease in Childhood*, **65**: 103–6

Salisbury, D. M., Leonard, J. F., Dezateau, C. A. and Savage, M. O. (1984) Micropenis: An important early sign of congenital hypopituitarism. *Br. Med. J.*, **288**, 621

Infections associated with conjugated hyperbilirubinaemia

Abzug, M. J. and Levin, M. J. (1991) Neonatal adenovirus infection: four patients and review of the literature. *Pediatrics*, **87**, 890–896

Alford, C. A., Stagno, S., Pass, R. F. and Britt, W. J. (1990) Congenital and perinatal CMV infections. *Rev. Infect. Dis.*, **12**, S745–S753

Benador, N., Mannhardt, W., Schranz, D. *et al.* (1990) Three cases of neonatal herpes simplex virus infection presenting as fulminant hepatitis. *Eur. J. Pediatr.*, **149**, 555–559

Berge, P., Stagno, S., Federer, W. *et al.* (1990) Impact of asymptomatic congenital cytomegalovirus infection on size at birth and gestational duration. *Pediatr. Infects. Dis. J.*, **9**, 170–175

Boppana, S.B., Pass, R. F., Britt, W., Stagno, S. and Alford, C. A. (1992) Symptomatic congenital cytomegalovirus infection: neonatal morbidity and mortality. *Pediatr. Infect. Dis. J.*, **11**, 93–99

Brown, W. R., Sokol, R. J., Levin, M. J., Silverman, A., Tamaru, T., Lilly, J. R., Hall, R. J. and Cheney, M. (1988) Lack of correlation between infection with reovirus 3 and extrahepatic biliary atresia or neonatal hepatitis. *J. Pediatr.*, **113**, 670–676

Chen-Chih, J. S., Keene, L. and Nagey, D. (1990) Hepatic fibrosis in congenital cytomegalovirus infection: with fetal ascites and pulmonary hypoplasia. *Pediatr. Pathol.*, **10**, 641–646

Davenport, M. (1986) Neonatal malaria and obstructive jaundice. *Arch. Dis. Childh.*, **61**, 515

Ghishan, F. X., Greene, H. L., Halter, S., Barnard, J. A. and Moran, J. B. (1984) Non-cirrhotic portal hypertension in congenital cytomegalovirus infection. *Hepatology*, **4**, 684

Glaser, J. H., Balistreri, W. F. and Moreki, R. (1984) Role of the Reo virus Type III in persistent infantile cholestasis. *Pediatr.*, **105**, 912

Grathwohl, J., Ndumbe, P., Leke, R., Uy, A., Gerlich, W. H. and Repp, R. (1992) *Perinatale hepatitis-B-virus-ubertragung*, **140**, 366–368.

Griffiths, P. D., Baboonian, C., Rutter, D. and Peckham, C. (1991) Congenital and maternal cytomegalovirus infections in a London population. *Brit. J. Obstet. and Gynaecol.*, **98** 135–140

Hsu, H. C., Chang, M. H., Lee, C. Y. and Chen, D. S. (1988) Fulminant hepatitis in infants in Taiwan: strong association with hepatitis Be antigen-negative but antibody-positive maternal hepatitis B surface antigen carriage. *J. Gastroenterol. Hepatol.*, **3**, 17

Kahn, E., Greco, A., Daum, F. *et al.* (1991) Hepatic pathology in Pediatric Acquired Immunodeficiency Syndrome. *Human Pathol.*, **22**,1111–1119

Kiyosawa, K., Sodeyama, T., Tanaka, E. *et al.* (1991) Intrafamilial transmission of hepatitis C virus in Japan. *J. Med. Virol.*, **33**, 114–116

Kosai, K., Kage, M. and Kojiro, M. (1991) Clinicopathological study of liver involvement in cytomegalovirus infection in infant autopsy case. *J. Gastroenterol. Hepatol.*, **6**, 603–608

Kuss, J. T., Fischbach, M., Stephan, M., Juckert, F. and Levy, J. (1979) Bronze-baby syndrome and cholestatic icterus following neonatal listeriosis. *Ann. Pediatr.*, **26**, 493

Levy, I., Shoshat, M., Levy, Y., Alpert, G. and Nitzhan, M. (1989) Recurrent ascites in an infant with perinatally acquired cytomegalovirus infection. *Eur. J. Pediatr.*, **148**, 531–532

Lurie, M., Elmalach, I., Schuger, L. and Weintraub, Z. (1987) Liver findings in infantile cytomegalovirus infection: similarity to extrahepatic biliary obstruction. *Histopathology*, **11**, 1171–1180

Luyer, B. Le, Menager, V., Le Roux, P. *et al.* (1990) Infection néonatale á ctytomégalovirus á évolution hépatique fibrogéne. *Arch. Franç. de Pediatr.*, **47**, 361–364

Mannhardt, W. and Schumacher, R. (1991) Progressive calcifications of lung and liver in neonatal herpes simplex virus infection. *Pediatr. Radiol.*, **21**, 236–237

Morecki, R. and Glaser, J. (1989) Reovirus 3 and neonatal biliary disease: discussion of divergent results. *Hepatology*, **10**, 515–517

Mowat, A. P. (1980) Viral hepatitis in infancy and childhood. *Clin. Gastroenterol*, **9**, 191

Novati, R., Thiers, V., Monforte, A. D. *et al.* (1992) Mother-to-child transmission of hepatitis C virus detected by polymerase chain reaction. *J. Infect. Dis.*, **165**, 720–723

Numzaki, Y., Oshima, T. and Tanaka, A. *et al.* (1980) Demonstration of IgG EA and IgM MA antibodies in CMV infection of healthy infants and those with liver disease. *Pediatr.*, **97**, 545

Peckham, C. S. (1991) Cytomegalovirus infection: congenital and neonatal disease. *Scand. J. Infect. Dis. (suppl)*, **80**, 82–87

Raga, I., Chrystal, V. and Coovadia, H. M. (1984) Usefulness of clinical features and liver biopsy diagnosis of disseminated herpes simplex infection. *Arch. Dis. Childh.*, **59**, 820

Remington, I. S. and Desmonts, G. (1976) Toxoplasmosis. In *Infectious Diseases of the Fetus and Newborn Infant* (eds J. S. Remington and J. O. Klein). Saunders, Philadelphia, p.191

Rosenblum, L. S., Villarino, M. E., Nainan, O. V. *et al.* (1991) Hepatitis A outbreak in a neonatal intensive care unit: risk factors for transmission and evidence of prolonged viral excretion among preterm infants. *J. Infect. Dis.*, **164**, 476–482

Rushton, T. I. (1981) Fetal and neonatal liver disease. *Diag. Histopathol.*, **4**, 17

Shiraki, K., Yohihara, N., Sakuri, M., Eto, T. and Kawana, T. (1980) Acute hepatitis B in infants born to carrier mothers with the antibody to hepatitis B e antigen. *J. Pediatr.*, **97**, 768–770

Sinatra, F. R., Shah, P., Weissman, J. Y., Thomas, D. W., Merritt, R. J. and Tong, M. J. (1982) Perinatal transmitted acute icteric hepatitis B in infants born to hepatitis B surface antigen-positive and anti-hepatitis B e-positive carrier mothers. *Pediatrics*, **70**, 557–559

Spencer, J. A. D. (1987) Perinatal listeriosis. *Br. Med. J.*, **295**, 349

Talsma, M., Vegting, M. and Hess, I. (1984) Generalised coxsackie A infection in a neonate presenting with pericarditis. *Br. Heart J.*, **52**, 683

Terazawa, S., Kojima, M., Yamanaka, T. *et al.* (1991) Hepatitis B virus mutants with precore-region defects in two babies with fulminant hepatitis and their mothers positive for antibody to hepatitis B e antigen. *Pediatr. Res.*, **29**, 59

Thaler, M. M., Park, C. K., Landers, D. V. *et al.* (1991) Vertical transmission of hepatitis C virus. *Lancet*, **338**, 17–18

Vanclaire, J., Cornu, C. H. and Sokol, E. M. (1991) Fulminant hepatitis B in an infant born to a hepatitis Be antibody positive, DNA negative carrier. *Arch. Dis. in Childh.*, **66**, 983–985

Liver disease associated with total parenteral nutrition

Cooper, A., Floyd, T. F., Ross, A. J., Bishop, H. C., Templeton, J. M. and Zeigler, M. N. (1984) Morbidity and mortality of short-bowel syndrome acquired in infancy. An update. *J. Pediatr. Surg.*, **16**, 711

Dosi, P. C., Raut. A. J. and Bhaktharaj, P. *et al.* (1985) Perinatal factors underlying neonatal cholestasis. *Pediatr*, **106**, 471

Patterson, K., Kapur, S. and Chandra, R. (1985) Hepatocellular carcinoma in a non-cirrhotic infant after prolonged parenteral nutrition. *Pediatr.*, **106**, 797

Whittington, P. F. (1985) Cholestasis associated with total parenteral nutrition in infants. *Hepatology*, **5**, 693

Whittington, P. F., Farrell, M. K, Balistreri, W. F. (1986) Parenteral Nutrition and hepatobiliary dysfunction. *Clin. Perinatol.*, **13**, 197–212

Whittington, P. F. and Merritt, R. J. (1986) Cholestasis associated with total parenteral nutrition. *J. Paediatr. Gastroenterol. Nutr.*, **5**, 922

Whittington, P. F., Brown, M. R., Thunberg, B. J., Golub, L., Maniscalco, W. M., Cox, C. and Shapiro, D. L. (1989) Decreased cholestasis with enteral instead of intravenous protein in the very low-birth-weight infant. *J. Pediatr. Gastroenterol .Nutr.*, **9**, 217

Whittington, P. F., Balistreri, W. F., Bucuvalas, J. C., Farrell, M. K. and Buve, K. E. (1992) Total parenteral nutrition-associated cholestasis: factors responsible for the decreasing incidence. In *Paediatric Cholestasis. Novel approaches to treatment* (eds M. J. Lentze and J. Reichen). Kluwer Academic Publishers, London, p.191

Zahavi, I., Shaifer, E. A. and Gall, D. G. (1985) Total parenteral nutrition-associated cholestasis: acute studies in the infant and adult rabbits. *J. Pediatr. Gastroenterol. Nutr.*, **4**, 622

Circulation disturbances, anaemia and hypoxia associated with cholestasis

Raju, T. N. K. and Javed, D. F. S. (1981) Fetal intrahepatic cholestasis secondary to ABO haemolytic disease. *J. Natl. Med. Assoc.*, **73**, 747

Rushton, D. I. (1981) Fetal and neonatal liver disease. *Diag. Histopathol.*, **4**, 17

Drugs, environmental toxins and iatrogenic disorders

Bove, K. E., Kosmeatos, N., Wedig, K. E. *et al.* (1985) Vasculopathic hepatotoxicity associated with E-Ferol syndrome in low-birthweight infants. *J. Am. Med. Assoc.*, **254**, 2422

Donigan, T. H. and Werlin, J. (1981) Extrahepatic biliary atresia and renal anomalies in fetal alcohol syndrome. *Am. J. Dis. Child.*, **135**, 1067

Godel, J. C. and Hart, A. G. (1984) Northern Infants Syndrome: a deficiency state? *Can. Med. Assoc. J.*, **131**, 199

Krowchuk, D. and Seashore, J. H. (1979) Complete biliary obstruction due to erythromycin estolate administration in an infant. *Pediatrics*, **64**, 956

Mowat, A. P. (1986) Paediatric liver disease. In *Liver Annual*, Volume 5 (eds I. M. Arias, M. Frenkel. and I. H. P. Wilson). Elsevier, Amsterdam, p.328

Mowat, A. P., Lambert, G. H., Muraskas, J., Anderson, C. L. and Myers, T. F. (1990) Direct hyperbilirubinaemia associated with chloral hydrate administration in the newborn. *Pediatrics*, **86**, 77–281 (A rare example of drug induced liver damage in the neonate)

Familial syndromes

Aagenaes, O. (1974) Hereditary recurrent cholestasis with lymphoedema. Two new families. *Acta Paediatr. Scand.*, **63**, 465

Amedee-Manesme, O., Bernard, O., Brunelle, F. *et al.* (1987) Sclerosing cholangitis with neonatal onset. *J. Pediatr.*, **111**, 225–229

Baker, A., Portmann, B., Westaby, D., Wilkinson, S., Karani, J., Mowat, A. P. (1993) Neonatal sclerosisng cholangitis in 2 siblings: a category of progressive intrahepatic cholestasis. *J. Paediatr. Gastroenterol. Nutr.*, (in press)

Ballow, M., Margolis, C. Z., Schachtel, B. and Hsia, Y. E. (1973) Progressive familial intrahepatic cholestasis. *Pediatrics*, **51**, 998

Chobert, M. N., Bernard, O., Bulle, F., Lemonnier, A., Guellaen, G. and Alagille, D. (1989) High hepatic gamma-glutamyltransferase (gamma-GT) activity with normal serum gamma-GT in children with progressive idiopathic cholestasis. *J. Hepatol.*, **8**, 225

Clayton, R. I., Iber, E. L., Ruebner, B. H. and Mckusick, V. A. (1969) Byler disease. Fatal familial intrahepatic cholestasis in an Amish kindred. *Am. J. Dis. Child.*, **117**, 112

Endo, T., Uchida, K., Amuro, Y. *et al.* (1979) Bile acid metabolism in benign recurrent intrahepatic cholestasis. *Gastroenterology*, **76**, 1002

Goldfisgher, S., Grotsky, H. W., Chang, C. A. *et al.* (1981) Idiopathic neonatal iron storage involving liver, pancreas, heart, and endocrine and exocrine glands. *Hepatology*, **1**, 58

Henriksen, N. T., Drablos, P. A. and Aagenaes, O. (1981) Cholestatic jaundice in infancy. The importance of familial and genetic factors in aetiology and prognosis. *Arch. Dis. Childh.*, **56**, 622

Hillemeier, A. C., Henn, I. and Reily, C. A. *et al.* (1982) Meconium peritonitis and increased sweat chloride determinations in a case of familial progressive intrahepatic cholestasis. *Pediatrics*, **69**, 325

Hudgins, L., Rosengren, S., Treem, W., Hyams, J. (1992) Early cirrhosis in survivors with Jeune thoracic dystrophy, *J. Pediatr.*, **120**, 754–756.

Imal, U., Watanabe, T., Kondo, Y. *et al.* (1981) Caroli's Disease: its diagnosis with non-invasive methods. *Br. J. Radiol.*, **54**, 526

Jones, E. A., Rabin, L., Buckeley, C. H., Webster, G. K. and Owens, D. (1976) Progressive intrahepatic cholestasis of infancy and childhood. A clinico-pathological study of patient surviving to age of 18 years. *Gastroenterology*, **71**, 675

Kaplinsky, C., Sternlieb, I., Javitt, N. and Rotem, Y. (1980) Familial cholestatic cirrhosis associated with Kayser-Fleischer rings. *Pediatrics*, **65**, 782

Linarelli, L. G., Williams, C. N. and Phillips, M. I. (1972) Byler's disease. Fatal intrahepatic cholestasis. *J. Pediatr.*, **81**, 484

Lloyd-still, J. D. (1981) Familial cholestasis with elevated sweat electrolyte concentrations. *J. Pediatr.*, **99**, 580

Mikati, M. A., Baraket, A. Y., Sulh, H. B. and Der Kaloustian, V. M. (1984) Renal tubular insufficiency, cholestatic jaundice breast versus bottle feeding. *J. Am. Med. Assoc.*, **253**, 2679

Mulberg, A. E., Arora, S., Grand, R. J. and Vinton, N. (1992) Sclerosing cholangitis in children with immune deficiency: Expanding the spectrum of neonatal cholestatic liver disease. *Hepatology*, **16**, 192a

Neilson, I M., Ornvold, K., Jacobsen, B. B. and Ranek, L. (1986) Fatal familial cholestatic syndrome in Greenland Eskimo children. *Acta Paediatr. Scand*, **75**, 1010

Odievre, M., Gautier, M., Hadchouel, M. and Alagille, D. (1973) Severe familial intrahepatic cholestasis. *Arch. Dis. Childh.*, **48**, 806

Ordway, N. I. C. and Stout, L. C. (1973) Intrauterine growth retardation, jaundice and hypoglycaemia in a neonate. *J. Pediatr.*, **83**, 867

Rotthauwe, H. W., Becker, S. T. and Ch.Bosch, M. (1981) Progressive intrahepatic cholestasis. *Monatsschr. Kinderheilkd.*, **129**, 515

Strum, E., Brudelski, M., Bojanowski, M. *et al.* (1990) Progressive intrahepatic cholestasis; a defect in apolipoprotein A-1 synthesis. *Hepatology*, **12**, 984

Summerfield, J. A., Scott. I., Berman, M. *et al.* (1980) Benign recurrent intrahepatic cholestasis. Studies of bilirubin kinetics, bile acids and cholangiography. *Gut*, **21**, 154

Ugarte, N. and Gonzalez-crussi, F. (1981) Hepatoma in siblings with progressive familial cholestatic cirrhosis of childhood. *Am. J. Clin. Pathol.*, **76**, 172

Vs. R., Wolf-peeters, C., Desmet, V., Eggermont, E. and Van Acker, K. (1975) Progressive intra hepatic cholestasis (Byler's disease): case report. *Gut*, **16**, 943

Weber, A. M., Tuchweber, B., Yousee, I. *et al.* (1981) Severe familial cholestasis in North American Indian children: a clinical model of microfilament dysfunction? *Gastroenterology*, **81**, 653

Whitington, P. F., Treese, D. K., Alonso, E. M., Fishbein, M. H. and Emond, J. C. (1992) Progressive Familial intrahepatic cholestasis. In *Paediatric Cholestasis. Novel Approaches to Treatment* (eds M. J. Lentze, J. Reichen). Kluwer Academic Publishers, London, p.165

Whitington, P. F. and Whitington, G. L. (1988) Partial external diversion of bile for the treatment of intractable pruritus associated with intrahepatic cholestasis. *Gastroenterol.*, **95**, 130–136

Syndromic biliary hypoplasia

Alagille, D. (1985) Management of paucity of interlobular bile ducts. *J. Hepatol.*, **1**, 561

Alagille, D., Estrada, A., Hadchouel, M., Gautier, M., Odievre, M. and Dommergues, J. P. (1987) Syndromic paucity of interlobular bile ducts (Alagille syndrome or arteriohepatic dysplasia): Review of 80 cases. *J. Pediatr.*, **110**, 195–200

Chong, S. K. F., Lindridge, J., Moniz, C. and Mowat, A. P. (1989) Exocrine pancreatic function in syndromic paucity of interlobular bile ducts. *J. Pediatr. Gastroenterol. Nut.*, **9**, 445–449

Deprettere, A., Portmann, B. and Mowat, A. P. (1987) Syndromic paucity of the intrahepatic bile ducts: diagnostic difficulties, severe morbidity throughout childhood. *J. Pediatr. Gastroenterol. Nutr.*, **6**, 865–871

Desmaze, C., Deleuze, J. F., Dutrillaux, A. M., Thomas, G., Hadchouel, M. and Aurias, A. (1992) Screening for microdeletions of chromosome 20 in patients with Alagille syndrome. *J. Med. Genet.*, **29**: 233–35

Kahn, E. and Daum, E. (1984) Arteriohepatic dysplasia (Alagille's syndrome): a common cause of conjugated hyperbilirubinaemia. *Ann. Clin. Lab. Sci.*, **14**, 480

Kocoshis, S. A., Cottrell, C. M., O'Connor, W. N. *et al.* (1981) Congenital heart disease, butterfly vertebrae and extrahepatic biliary atresia: a variant of arteriohepatic dysplasia? *J. Pediatr.*, **99**, 436

Mueller, R. F., Pagon, R. A., Pepin, M. G. *et al.* (1984) Arterio-hepatic dysplasia: phenotypic features and family studies. *Clin. Genet.*, **25**, 323

Perrault, J. (1981) Paucity of interlobular bile ducts. *Dig. Dis. Sci.*, **26**, 481

Shulman, S. A., Hyems, J. S. and Gunte, R. (1984) Arterio-hepatic dysplasia (Alagille's syndrome): extreme variability amongst affected family members. *Am. J. Med. Genet.*, **19**, 325

Sokol, R. J., Heubi, O. E. and Balistreri, W. F. (1983) Intrahepatic cholestasis facies: is it specific for Alagille's syndrome? *J. Pediatr.*, **103**, 203

Stewart, S. M., Uauy, R., Waller, D. A. *et al.* (1987) Mental and motordevelopment correlates in patients with end-stage biliary atresia awaiting liver transplantation. *Pediatrics*, **79**: 882–88

Stewart, S. M., Uauy, R., Kennard, B. D., Waller, D. A., Benser, M. and Andrews, W. S. (1988) Mental development and growth in children with chronic liver disease of early and late onset. *Pediatrics*, **82**: 167–172

Valencia-Mayoral, P., Weber, J., Kutz, E. *et al.* (1984) A possible defect in the bile secretory apparatus in arteriohepatic dysplasia (Alagille's syndrome). *Hepatology*, **4**, 691

Non-syndromic biliary hypoplasia

Alagille, D. (1985) Management of paucity of interlobular bile ducts. *J. Hepatol.*, **1**, 561

Ballow, M., Maroolis, C. Z., Schachtel, B. and Hsia, Y. E. (1973) Progressive familial intrahepatic cholestasis. *Pediatrics*, **51**, 998

Gray, O. P. and Saunders, R. (1966) Familial intrahepatic cholestatic jaundice in infancy. *Arch. Dis. Childh.* **41**, 320

Jubero, R. C., Holand-Moritz, R. M. and Henry, K. S. (1966) Familial intrahepatic cholestasis with mental and growth retardation. *Pediatrics*, **38**, 819

Perrault, J. (1981) Paucity of inter-lobular bile ducts. *Dig. Dis. Sci.*, **26**, 481

Sharp, H. L., Carey, J. B., White, J. G. and Krivit, W. (1967) Cholestyramine therapy in patients with a paucity of intrahepatic bile ducts. *J. Pediatr.*, **71**, 723.

Chapter 5

Extrahepatic biliary atresia and other disorders of the extrahepatic bile ducts presenting in infancy

Disorders of the extrahepatic biliary tree causing jaundice or liver disease in infancy are amenable to surgical treatment. They present in a manner which may be indistinguishable clinically from the infective, metabolic, endocrine and other forms of hepatobiliary disease reviewed in Chapter 4. In this chapter extrahepatic biliary atresia and rarer disorders of the extrahepatic bile ducts will be discussed. Choledochal cyst is discussed on p.414, spontaneous perforation of the bile ducts on p.419.

Introduction

Extrahepatic biliary atresia, a disorder unique to infancy, affects one in 14000 liveborn infants. It is the most frequent single life-threatening hepatic disorder in early childhood in Europe, North America and Japan. Mortality can be reduced dramatically by early portoenterostomy followed, when necessary by liver transplantation. In the past two decades it has become clear that the mortality and morbidity can be considerably reduced by the radical operation hepatic portoenterostomy. If this is performed by 8 weeks of age the jaundice clears in 70–90% of infants, arresting the progression of liver disease and giving an 87% chance of survival with a good quality of life through to 15 years of age (Ohi *et al.*, 1990). Operation by 45 days of age may give even better results. This has to be contrasted with a mean survival of 11 months in the untreated infant who faces a miserable death with pruritus adding to the problems caused by cirrhosis and malabsorption. Unfortunately in many areas infants with biliary atresia are identified later, when successful operation is less likely or are referred to surgeons with little experience of this unusual operation. For infants in whom portoenterostomy has failed, or produced only palliation of the disease process, liver transplantation, performed electively gives a good quality of life and 5 year survival rates of over 80% (de Ville, de Goyet and Otte, 1992).

Definitions

Extrahepatic biliary atresia is characterized by complete inability to excrete bile associated with obstruction, destruction or absence of the extrahepatic bile ducts anywhere between the duodenum and the first or second order of branches of the right and left hepatic ducts. The extent and site of the atretic bile duct are extremely variable. To allow comparison of series from different units a standard classification of biliary atresia was produced by the Japanese Society of Paediatric Surgeons in 1976 (Howard, 1991).

Three main types are defined on the basis of the site of the atresia determined by the macroscopic appearances at laparotomy:

Type 1: Atresia of the common bile duct with patent proximal ducts
Type 2: Atresia involving the hepatic duct but with patent proximal ducts
Type 3: Atresia involving the right and left hepatic ducts at the portahepatis

Types 1 and 2, corresponding to those previously described as surgically correctable, should be treated by hepaticojejunostomy if the ducts contain bile. Types 1 and 2 accounted for only 12% in a series of 643 cases (Ohi *et al.*, 1987). Further subdivisions of this classification attempt to define the condition of the distal common bile duct and the hepatic duct radicals at the portahepatis. Only Type 1a is of clinical significance in that the gall bladder lumen is in continuity with the duodenum via the distal common bile duct and can thus be used as a biliary conduit (*see* p.87).

The term *extrahepatic biliary hypoplasia* refers to the cholangiographic demonstration of a patent but narrow biliary tree. The contrast usually flows freely from the gall bladder into the duodenum and with difficulty may be made to extend up into the liver parenchyma. This is found in jaundiced infants with intrahepatic disease.

The term *intrahepatic biliary atresia* is a misnomer which should be replaced by paucity of the intrahepatic bile ducts or intrahepatic bile duct hypoplasia (Chapter 4, p.69).

Pathology and pathogenesis

Pathological study of tissues removed from the portahepatis and of the proximal extrahepatic bile ducts suggests that biliary atresia in the vast majority of infants results from a sclerosing, inflammatory lesion initiated in ductular tissues. It may start in fetal life, around the time of birth or early in postnatal life. In the majority of infants with biliary atresia the unconjugated physiological jaundice merges into the conjugated hyperbilirubinaemia of biliary atresia making the exact time of onset uncertain. Stool contains no yellow or green pigment once meconium is passed and the urine is never colourless but persistently yellow because of its bilirubin content from day 4 onwards. In up to 30% of infants stools, initially pigmented, become acholic during the first 3 months of life. In rare cases there is cholangiographic evidence that the bile ducts were patent. The degree of duct involvement is very variable in its extent as is the intensity of inflammation. Histological sections may show degeneration of bile duct epithelial cells with a marked inflammatory cell response and fibrosis in the periductular tissues and luminal obliteration. In some instances there is complete destruction of bile duct tissues with only the persistence of biliary mucus-producing glands suggesting that bile ducts were present previously. Occasionally even these are absent and there is only fibrous tissue. Some segments of bile ducts may remain and dilate in the form of non-communicating cysts which may be mistaken for choledochal cysts or Type 1 atresia.

Irrespective of the time of onset of atresia, in nearly all patients the bile ducts within the liver extending to the portahepatis are patent until some weeks after birth. The main intralobular bile ducts are thereafter progressively destroyed by a pathological process which seems similar to that affecting the extrahepatic ducts.

Within the liver substance there is widening of the portal tracts with oedema, inflammatory cell infiltrate and increased activity of fibroblasts leading to the deposition of fibrous tissue. Around the periphery of the portal tracts and sometimes within the fibrotic inflammatory tissue there are numerous channels, lined with bile duct cells, which may be angulated and distorted giving the appearance of almost aimless proliferation. Some ducts contain bile plugs. Within the hepatic parenchyma there is inflammatory cell infiltrate and frequently giant cell proliferation. Cholestasis is prominent.

Without surgical drainage there is increasing fibrosis with a gradual decrease in the number of bile ducts. In cases that survive beyond the age of 12 months the histological appearance may be similar to that of bile duct paucity. Biliary cirrhosis may be established as early as 6 weeks of age but there is considerable case-to-case variation in the rapidity with which this develops. Hepatocellular carcinoma may complicate the cirrhosis. Even at 8 weeks of age portal hypertension is almost universal. Whether the intrahepatic changes in biliary atresia occur in response to whatever causes the extrahepatic lesion or arise secondarily to the bile duct obstruction (e.g. mediated by leukotrienes) is unresolved.

Even with successful bile drainage with the serum bilirubin falling to normal following surgery severe fibrosis and features of biliary cirrhosis will affect parts of the liver from which bile drainage is not effective. Livers resected at transplantation in such patients frequently shows cirrhotic changes in the capsule of the liver with central areas macroscopically and histologically normal. In such instances the patient's prognosis is dependent on whether there are sufficient unaffected segments to maintain good liver function and on whether the haemodynamic changes in the liver lead to increasing portal hypertension.

Aetiology

The aetiology of biliary atresia is unknown. The present evidence suggests that four distinct aetiopathological groups should be considered. Numerical and structural anomalies of chromosomes are identified in 1–2% (Silveira *et al.*, 1991a): 20–25% have significant abnormalities in other organs, such as absence of the inferior vena cava or situs inversus, splenic malformation syndrome, absence of portal vein, ventricular septal defects or intestinal malrotation, abnormalities which may have resulted from insults during organogenesis at 3–4, 5–7, 6–8 and 10 weeks respectively. The splenic malformation syndrome comprising poly- or asplenia with a preduodenal portal vein, intestinal malrotation and/or abdominal situs inversus, occurring in from 5–29% of reported series are an intriguing subset. The finding of biliary atresia (two) and biliary stenosis (one) in three newborn who alone had low gamma-glutamyl transpeptidase values among 10 000 amniotic fluid samples taken before 18 weeks' gestation also points to an early event leading to atresia. What the postulated teratogenic insult may be is undetermined. The third category (2–5%) have intestinal atresias or cardiovascular anomalies which could have been caused by disruptive events occurring after organogenesis is completed. A possible mechanism of damage is ischaemia (Gautier, 1979). It is not clear whether these events prevent bile duct formation or predispose to damage late in gestation, at birth or postnatally as presumably occurs in the major fourth group, who have no associated congenital abnormalities. The finding of bile duct remnants in excised tissue in over 95% of cases provides confirmation that in these cases biliary atresia does not occur from a failure of development, migration or canalization of the extrahepatic biliary tree. Possible initiating mechanisms include immune-mediated damage (Kawai *et al.*, 1980; Hadchouel *et al.*, 1981) or pancreatic enzymes encroaching on the biliary system via a long common pancreatic bile duct channel (Miyano *et al.*,

1979). Perinatal viral infections with such agents as Reo virus have been suspected as possible contributory factors but if they are it can only be in association with other reproductive, environmental or genetic factors. Increased maternal and paternal ages and a decrease in the number of firstborn infants have been reported in a number of studies together with an increased incidence of abortions in previous pregnancies and illnesses in pregnancies (Silveira *et al.*, 1992). An increased incidence of maternal diabetes mellitus has been associated with splenic malformation syndrome (Davenport *et al.*, 1991). One possible genetic factor determining susceptibility to infection may be the HLA status. HLA B12 occurs more commonly in those patients with biliary atresia without anomalies than in those with. This observation provides further support for the hypothesis that biliary atresia is an aetiologically heterogeneous disorder. There is no other evidence of a genetic basis. Only 17 familial instances have been recorded. The majority of these reports have not included histological findings in the resected bile ducts and may thus represent cases of extrahepatic bile duct hypoplasia associated with severe genetically-determined intrahepatic disease. Of 22 twins pairs, including five monozygotic twins, all were discordant for the disorder, except one reported in abstract form (Silveira *et al.*, 1991b).

Clinical features in the first 3 months of life (Figure 5.1)

Biliary atresia presents with prolongation of jaundice beyond the usual duration of physiological jaundice. It must thus be considered in any infant jaundiced beyond 14 days of age. The degree of jaundice is frequently slight with total serum bilirubin values as low

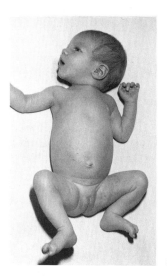
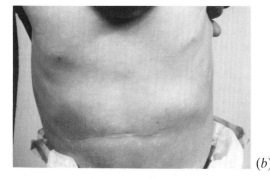

(*a*)   (*b*)

Figure 5.1 The clinical presentation of biliary atresia, 1985. (*a*) Infant aged 24 days with Type 3 biliary atresia. Jaundice was mild (serum bilirubin 120 mmol/litre) and the liver edge palpable only 3 cm below the costal margin but the urine was yellow and the stool contained no yellow or green pigment. There were no other abnormal clinical signs. (*b*) Close up of the abdomen 1 year following portoenterostomy. There are no clinical features of liver disease and growth and development are normal. Sadly, few cases are identified at this age and have more advanced liver damage before referral

as 100 μmol/litre (6 mg/dl). It is a conjugated jaundice with bilirubin in the urine which is light yellow in colour. This usually dates from birth. The urine is rarely dark in spite of the conjugated hyperbilirubinaemia, presumably because of the large urinary output occurring normally at this age. When biliary atresia is established the stool contains no trace of yellow or green pigment. This usually dates from birth but in up to 30% of infants with biliary atresia histories are obtained of pigmented stools persisting for some weeks after birth. There may be no other abnormal signs.

In many babies this mild jaundice is disregarded by parents and discounted as physiological or breast-milk jaundice by their medical advisers. It is often the development of complications such as spontaneous bleeding due to vitamin K malabsorption or failure to thrive which prompts referral for further investigation. To facilitate earlier diagnosis of hepatobiliary disorders including biliary atresia and to prevent complications, it is essential that any infant jaundiced after 14 days of age should have urinalysis for bilirubinuria and a direct serum bilirubin measured. If positive immediate assessment by a paediatrician is essential.

The range of birth weights of infants with biliary atresia is the same as other infants. The incidence of biliary atresia in prematurely born or light-for-gestational age infants is probably similar to that in term infants. Postnatal weight gain is usually normal for at least 6 weeks.

The liver progressively enlarges. By 2 months of age the edge will be more than 3 cm below the costal margin and its consistency increased. The spleen may be palpable. At this age it is unusual to find ascites or subcutaneous portosystemic shunts or other cutaneous features of chronic liver disease. If ascites is present spontaneous perforation of bile ducts should be suspected. Careful examination for a cystic mass between the liver and duodenum, for significant congenital heart disease and for situs inversus is essential. The clinical assessment is completed by viewing stool specimens. If these are stored before inspection they should be in a black plastic bag to exclude light. If the stool has no yellow or green pigment the most likely diagnosis is biliary atresia. It must be confirmed or excluded as rapidly as possible.

Early biochemical features

The serum bilirubin on presentation at the age of 2–8 weeks is commonly in the region of 136–204 μmol/litre (8–12 mg/100 ml) with between 50% and 70% of the bilirubin conjugated. Rarely, the total bilirubin may be as low as 90 μmol/litre (5.5 mg/dl) with only 51 μmol/litre conjugated (3 mg/dl), but in over 90% of cases, more than 68 μmol/litre (4 mg/100 ml) of the serum bilirubin will be conjugated in the first 10 weeks of life. Note that day-to-day fluctuations in serum bilirubin level of more than 51 μmol/litre are common. The bilirubin rarely rises progressively.

The serum aspartate aminotransferase and other tests of hepatocellular integrity are always abnormal, the vast majority of cases having serum levels at between two and 10 times normal, but rarely high values are obtained. The serum alkaline phosphatase level is also usually elevated but in only 50% of cases does the value exceed 230 IU/litre. The gamma-glutamyl transpeptidase is commonly elevated to values more than 10 times normal, but is occasionally normal. The serum albumin is normal, and the cholesterol may be at the upper limit of normal. Between 5 and 10% of cases would have prothrombin times prolonged to over 3 minutes which corrects to normal within 6 hours of giving intramuscular vitamin K. Anaemia is unusual.

Late clinical features

The child who survives beyond 4–6 months of life with biliary atresia suffers progressively from the effects of cirrhosis and fat malabsorption. The rate of development of these features is variable. All structures, tissue fluids and secretions, including tears, become jaundiced, the child eventually developing a greenish hue. Intestinal secretions pigment the previously acholic stools. The abdomen becomes markedly distended because of hepatomegaly, splenomegaly and ascites. In contrast, the remainder of the body becomes emaciated with lack of subcutaneous fat, muscle bulk and bone structure. Growth is retarded and motor development slowed. Unless vitamin D supplements are given, rickets develops. Pruritus adds to the child's misery. Hypersplenism and alimentary blood loss due to portal hypertension cause anaemia with all its consequences. There is increasing fluid retention which with diaphragmatic elevation and pulmonary oedema causes respiratory distress. Death, due to alimentary bleeding, chronic hepatic failure, systemic bacterial infection or bronchopneumonia, usually occurs by the age of 2 years but some infants die within 8 months, while a few survive to the age of 3 years. With partial bile drainage survival to 5 to 8 years and exceptionally to 13 or 14 years may occur.

Diagnostic investigations

The first consideration is to exclude treatable infectious, metabolic or endocrine causes of conjugated hyperbilirubinaemia (see Chapter 4) and to make sure that the prothrombin time is normal. Significant bacterial infection may complicate any form of hepatobiliary disease. If jaundice does not clear with specific treatment further investigation is essential. Choledochal cysts or cysts in an otherwise atretic biliary tree are identified by ultrasonography. If there is significant ascites (in the first 2 months of life) spontaneous perforation of the bile ducts should be suspected. The diagnosis is confirmed by aspirating bile-containing ascitic fluid or by the appearance of technetium-labelled iminodiacetic acid derivatives in the ascitic fluid. All three conditions require early surgical correction.

Other known causes of conjugated hyperbilirubinaemia with acholic stools, particularly alpha-1 antitrypsin deficiency (PIZZ), cystic fibrosis or septo-optic dysplasia must be excluded by appropriate investigations.

Indications for laparotomy in suspected biliary atresia

Laparotomy is ultimately required to confirm the diagnosis and to allow its surgical correction. Since laparotomy in patients with hepatitis will almost certainly cause some temporary deterioration in liver function (due to drug effects, changes in blood flow through the liver caused by intermittent positive pressure respiration, loss of fluid and blood) and may even cause an increased incidence of cirrhosis in the long term, it must be avoided as a primary investigation. Laparotomy should only be undertaken by an experienced surgeon who can assess changes in the portahepatis and proceed to porto-enterostomy or hepaticojejunostomy (McClement et al., 1985) Even with operative cholangiography, extrahepatic ducts (hypoplastic because of severe intrahepatic cholestasis) may be incorrectly considered atretic leading to a destructive unnecessary operation.

Laparotomy is indicated in any infant with persistent conjugated hyperbilirubinaemia and acholic stools in whom: (a) genetic, familial, metabolic, endocrine and infectious causes have been excluded; (b) the liver biopsy findings are compatible with extrahepatic biliary atresia; and (c) bile duct patency is not demonstrated with radiopharmaceuticals, duodenal aspirate or cholangiography.

Percutaneous liver biopsy (Figure 5.2)

There are no unique histological features which distinguish extrahepatic biliary atresia from infantile hepatitis. Nevertheless, the histopathologist with experience of liver biopsies in this age group can provide invaluable assistance in determining whether the cholestasis is due to a bile duct obstruction in which there is involvement of all portal tracts, or a disorder of hepatocytes. Bile accumulation within hepatocytes, giant cell transformation, haemosiderin deposition, disorganization of tubercular pattern in the hepatic lobule, and increased haemopoietic activity occur in both disorders. The main histological abnormalities of diagnostic importance are given in Table 5.1. It is important

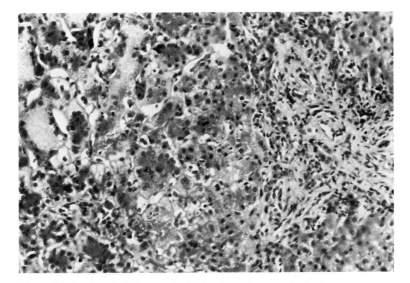

Figure 5.2 Extrahepatic biliary atresia. Widened portal tract with bile duct reduplication, increased fibrosis and cellular infiltrate in an infant aged 7 weeks with extrahepatic biliary atresia. Note that there is extensive giant cell transformation in the hepatic parenchyma ($\times$ 320, reduced to seven-eighths in reproduction)

Table 5.1 Histological features of diagnostic value on percutaneous liver biopsy

Bile tract disorders	Hepatocellular disease
Enlarged portal tract	Collection of mononuclear cells in the hepatic lobules
Numerous bile ducts	Fatty changes in the hepatocytes
Distorted elongated and angulated bile ductules	Uneven staining of hepatocytes
Increased fibrosis in portal tracts	
Lymphoedema of portal tracts	
Infiltration of portal tract with inflammatory cells	

that the biopsy should contain four or five portal tracts for a diagnosis to be attempted, since in hepatitis individual portal tracts may show features similar to those of atresia but portal tract involvement is not uniform.

Even with an experienced histopathologist bile duct obstruction can be confirmed or excluded in only 77% (Manolaki *et al.*, 1983).

Radiopharmaceutical tests

With over 20% of biopsies giving equivocal or misleading results radiopharmaceuticals have an important role in deciding whether cholestasis is complete or partial in which case laparotomy is unnecessary. Radionucleotide demonstration of bile duct patency using technetium-99m-tagged iminodiacetic acid derivatives (IDA) such as methylbromo IDA (MBr IDA), which have good hepatic uptake and limited renal excretion, have replaced earlier unhelpful IDA preparations such as *p*-butyl IDA (Manolaki *et al.*, 1983) and the [131]I Rose Bengal faecal excretion test (Dick and Mowat, 1986). Discrimination from intrahepatic cholestasis is enhanced if the infants are pretreated with phenobarbitone (5 mg/kg for at least 3 days). Repeated imaging up to 24 hours after intravenous injection may be required to demonstrate isotope in the gut. Equally effective discrimination may be achieved by computer analysis of distribution between the liver and heart within 10 minutes of intravenous injection. These radionucleotide studies are only of value in excluding atresia (El Tumi *et al.*, 1987).

Duodenal aspirate positive for bilirubin

This test is reliable in excluding atresia but it may be necessary to repeat it on a number of occasions (Shiraki *et al.*, 1987). Whether it is more informative than the stool colour is unclear.

Endoscopic cholangiography

Syndromic intrahepatic bile duct hypoplasia or bile duct paucity can be a difficult differential diagnosis since up to 25% of cases have no histological features of this condition in liver biopsies in the first 6 months of life. The biopsy features are those of bile duct obstruction. Even if there are distinctive syndromic features endoscopic or operative cholangiographic confirmation of bile duct patency may be necessary if the stools are not pigmented and there is no biliary excretion of radiopharmaceuticals.

Surgery

Preoperatively the infant continues on phenobarbitone in a dose of 5 mg/kg, vitamin K 1 mg/day. Before surgery oral neomycin 50 mg/kg in six divided doses and metronidazole 20 mg/kg/day are given for 24 hours with 10% dextrose for 48 hours.

Operative procedures

The abdomen is opened using a transverse laparotomy approach, sectioning both recti muscles, well above the level of the umbilicus at the same horizontal level as the portahepatis. The liver is usually found to be uniformly enlarged but occasionally one lobe may be more enlarged than the other. Even in early cases it feels firm on palpation, but in late cases cirrhosis will have developed. Ascites is rare. There may be features of portal hypertension.

Most commonly the gall bladder is small and firm and may be partially hidden by hypertrophy of surrounding parenchyma. In these circumstances, it is usually impossible to inject radio-opaque material through the gall bladder. In approximately 25% of cases the gall bladder, although small, will contain approximately 1 ml of colourless material, and in these circumstances it may be possible to show a lumen in the gall bladder and common duct, but the common hepatic duct is unlikely to be visualized. Further dissection is undertaken towards the portahepatis, examining particularly tissues in front of the right branch of the hepatic artery. Atretic or absent bile ducts will usually be found.

Hepaticojejunostomy

In individual series between 4 and 35% of cases have a patent segment of extrahepatic bile duct extending into the portahepatis. In these it is possible to fashion an anastomosis between the bile duct and a retrocolic Roux-en-Y loop of jejunum but only a minority drain bile satisfactorily (Figure 5.3). Successful surgery is rare after the age of 4 months.

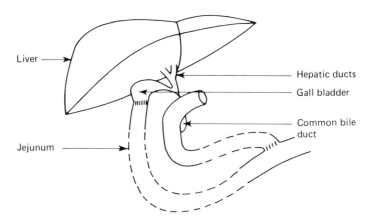

Figure 5.3 Diagrammatic representation of surgically correctable extrahepatic biliary atresia (Type 1A). The distal common bile duct is atretic but the common hepatic duct and main hepatic ducts are patent and are in continuity with the gall bladder via the cystic duct. A cholecyst-jejunostomy with a Roux-en-Y loop should give satisfactory bile drainage without cholangitis. Unfortunately, long-term cure is exceptional

Ascending cholangitis or lymphangitis is a frequent complication. Cirrhosis gradually develops in most cases and prolonged cure is exceptional, although one patient has been reported well at the age of 12 years and another moderately well at the age of 25 years (Berenson *et al.*, 1974).

Hepatic portoenterostomy ('Japanese' operation or Kasai procedure)

Where no patent extrahepatic bile duct remains, because the pathological process extends to the porta hepatitis, hepatic portoenterostomy is performed. In this operation an anastomosis is fashioned between the area of the porta hepatis and the bowel. Bile duct

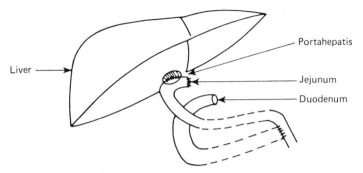

Figure 5.4 Hepatic portoenterostomy for an extrahepatic biliary atresia involving the main right and left hepatic ducts and the common hepatic duct (Type 3). These have been removed and the area of the portahepatis bared. A side opening in the Roux-en-Y loop of the jejunum is anastomosed to the edge of the bared area. Bile is thought to flow from the intrahepatic bile ducts into the bowel but in some patients it is suspected that lymphatic drainage into the bowel may occur

remnants or fibrous tissue in front of the right branch of the hepatic artery are carefully dissected free giving a cone of tissue with its base at the portahepatis above the bifurcation of the portal vein. This cone of tissue is then cut flush with the liver surface exposing an area, which extends laterally to where vessels enter the liver, through which bile may drain via residual bile channels. A side opening in a retrocolic jejunal Roux-en-Y loop, at least 40 cm in length is carefully anastomosed around the bare area of the portahepatis, making no attempt to link bile ductules to bowel mucosa (Figure 5.4).

To prevent ascending cholangitis caused by reflux of intestinal contents and bowel organisms to the hilar anastomosis a large number of modifications have been developed. Most include exteriorization of the Roux-en-Y loop with cutaneous bile drainage. The internal loop may be made more complex in a number of ways. There is no evidence that the frequency of cholangitis is thereby reduced (Ohi, 1991). These procedures have their own complications. Severe fluid and electrolyte losses, which may be fatal, may occur from stoma. Any bile which drains must be re-fed to the patient to facilitate fat absorption. Catastrophic bleeding may occur from varices at the mucocutaneous junctions of stoma. Such modifications should no longer be performed.

Portocholecystostomy

If the gall bladder and distal bile duct are patent it may be possible to anastomose the gall bladder to the portahepatis and provide bile drainage without the risk of direct contamination of portahepatis by bowel organisms but kinking of the mobilized gall bladder or ducts or progression of the atretic process in the extrahepatic biliary system may lead to obstruction with bile leaks and cholelithiasis (Ohi *et al.*, 1987).

To minimize attack rates of cholangitis in the first month after surgery it is our practice to give intravenous gentamicin and cefoxitin for 7 days and oral cephradine from days 8–28. Prophylactic co-trimoxazole (Septrin, Wellcome) given in a randomized control trial did not decrease the attack rate subsequently.

To promote bile flow phenobarbitone, dehydrocholic acid, ursodeoxycholic acid, glucagon and prostaglandin E all have their advocates but their efficacy has not been tested in controlled clinical trials. With the same aim and to prevent bile duct obstruction by scar formation many Japanese surgeons gave prednisolone in the second week after surgery. We give phenobarbitone and are evaluating prednisolone in a randomized study in those infants who have surgery between 8 and 12 weeks of age.

Oral fat soluble vitamin supplements vitamin K 1 mg daily, Ketovite tablets 3 daily, Ketovite liquid 5 ml daily are given to all infants. Maximum bile flow may not be achieved for up to one year following surgery and even then bile constituent concentration may not be normal (Howard and Mowat, 1984). During this period, dietary supplements with medium-chain triglycerides and glucose polymers may be necessary to achieve normal weight gain and growth. Vitamin D, 30 000 units, is given intramuscularly every 4 weeks until the jaundice clears. The dose of vitamin D must be monitored by the response of the patient's serum calcium, phosphate (if low, give additional phosphate) and the radiological appearances on wrist X-ray. If jaundice persists beyond 5 months of age it is essential to maintain the serum vitamin E concentration within the normal range by oral or parenteral vitamin supplements (*see* also Chapter 4, p.52).

Results

Short-term

Most centres with considerable experience emphasize the importance of early surgery, reporting good bile drainage with a return of the serum bilirubin to normal in 80–90% of those operated on before 60 days of age falling to 30–60% between 61 and 70 days and to 25–50% between 71 and 90 days and 20–35% in those operated up to 6 months of age. Exceptionally, later surgery may be effective (Mieli-Vergani et al., 1989). Centres with less experience have less satisfactory results (McClement et al., 1985). The success rate may be influenced by the presence or absence of other anomalies particularly if they are themselves life-threatening (Davenport et al., 1991). Cholangitis reduced the 5-year survival rate from 91% to 54% in one study (Houwen et al., 1989).

Although the serum bilirubin often falls to normal within 6 months of surgery, the aspartate aminotransferase concentration remains elevated through the first decade. The alkaline phosphatase follows a similar course. The gamma-glutamyl transpeptidase concentration frequently rises for 1 to 2 years even following successful surgery and gradually falls in the first decade. The serum albumin may be low for 1–2 months after surgery but thereafter returns to normal unless hepatic decompensation occurs. When bile drainage is not sufficient to clear jaundice liver function deteriorates and 80% of the infants die before their third birthday unless liver transplantation is performed.

Long-term results (Figure 5.5)

Although after portoenterostomy many patients have evidence of persisting disease, with pessimistic reports on liver histology (Gautier et al., 1984) recent studies from Japan, Europe and North America have emphasized that long-term survival with normal growth and development and a good quality of life is possible for an appreciable percentage (Chiba et al., 1992). In Kasai's unit the percentage of cases surviving 10 or more years climbed from 10% in those operated on in 1953–67 to 54% in the 1973–79 series. Early surgery is important if more are to benefit. In another study from Japan 73% of those operated on by 60 days are alive at 10 years in contrast to only eight of 71 (11%) operated on after 90 days and none operated on after 121 days (Ohi et al., 1990). Of 48 patients

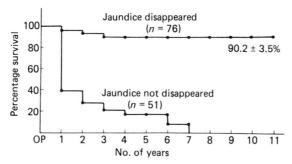

Figure 5.5 Survival curve of patients after corrective surgery for biliary atresia at the Tohoku University Hospital, Sendai, Japan from 1971 through 1983. Reprinted from *World J. Surg.* with permission

over 10 years of age 10 had splenomegaly. Among 37 who were leading normal lives were six who had had problems related to portal hypertension. Eleven had ongoing liver problems. Four who had cholangitis were mildly jaundiced, while 40% still had mildly raised transaminases. A 25-year-old woman had a child although menstrual problems may be more common than normal (Nakano *et al.*, 1990). Of 325 survivors over 10 years of age approximately 50% were entirely well but 30% had problems with cirrhosis or portal hypertension (Akiyama *et al.*, 1989). The oldest patient in these series is over 34 years old. Gottrand and coworkers (1991) report similar results from Paris. A 5-year survival rate without transplantation of 60% has been reported from London (Howard, 1991) and Denver (Lilly *et al.*, 1989). Survival with a good quality of life in spite of underlying cirrhosis has been described at 37 years (Figure 5.6).

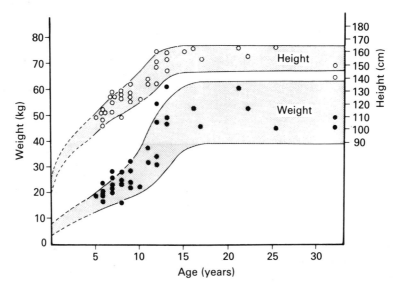

Figure 5.6 Growth in long-term female survivors following portoenterostomy. (Reproduced with permission from Ohi *et al.*, 1990.)

Complications

Cholangitis with or without bacteraemia

The most frequent, serious early postoperative complication is bacterial cholangitis. This diagnosis strictly requires recovery of organisms from portal tracts or the demonstration of acute inflammation in portal tracts. In practice it is usually defined as a febrile illness with deteriorating liver function and a polymorphonuclear neutrophil response in the peripheral blood. In most series the incidence of this complication is up to 50% but an incidence of 100% has been reported (Howard and Mowat, 1984). Although often described as an ascending bacterial cholangitis, the mode of infection may be luminal, lymphatic or venous. Clinically it is characterized by fever, the recurrence or aggravation of jaundice and frequently features of septicaemia. The stool pigment or bile flow is reduced. There may be increased abdominal distension with hepatic tenderness and peritonitis. The serum bilirubin rises, standard biochemical tests of liver function deteriorate.

E. coli, Klebsiella, Pseudomonas, Staphylococcus, Streptococcus pneumoniae, Enterobacter, Streptococcus faecalis, Haemophilus influenzae, Bacteroides fragilis, Clostridia perfringens and Candida may be isolated in blood cultures and/or liver biopsy cultures. Episodes occur most commonly in the first month after surgery but remain frequent in the first 2 years. Each attack causes acute and often chronic deterioration in liver function. This is particularly so with attacks occurring in the first months after surgery. Cholangitis may be difficult to distinguish from generalized viral infection in which a similar exacerbation of jaundice with deterioration of liver function may occur and indeed cholangitis may coincide with such viral infection.

On suspicion of the diagnosis, once blood culture, ascitic aspirate or liver biopsy have been taken, treatment should commence with intravenous broad spectrum antibiotics. Gentamicin and cefoxitin are currently our initial choice of antibiotics but these are modified in the light of the patient's response and bacteriological studies.

The incidence of cholangitis was not reduced by prophylactic Septrin as assessed in a controlled clinical trial. Twenty-four attacks, eight with septicaemia, occurred in 29 patients receiving Septrin as opposed to 26 attacks, six with septicaemia, occurring in the 37 patients receiving no Septrin.

In patients with recurrent attacks, intrahepatic bile duct dilatation, intrahepatic cysts or partial obstruction to the jejunal loop should be excluded by ultrasonography, biliary excretion scintiscans or percutaneous cholangiography with a view to surgical correction. Note that cysts not causing obstruction should be allowed to resolve spontaneously (Werlin et al., 1985).

Portal hypertension

Portal hypertension is present in almost all cases at the time of initial surgery even if it is performed by 8 weeks of age. It frequently resolves spontaneously in many in whom the serum bilirubin returns to normal, particularly if no attacks of cholangitis occur (Houwen et al., 1989). The incidence of varices on barium studies ranges from 20–50%. Varices are detected at endoscopy in 30–70% of those more than 3 years of age (Ohi 1991; Davenport et al., 1991). Bleeding from portal hypertension is much rarer, occurring in approximately 25% of those known to have varices. All patients with biliary atresia should nevertheless be advised not to consume salicylate-containing medicines. If bleeding occurs or if the varices are large and bleeding is anticipated, endoscopic sclerotherapy is the current treatment of choice. Portosystemic surgical shunts should be avoided since portal hypertension may stabilize and regress and also because the surgery involved makes subsequent liver transplantation (if it becomes necessary) more difficult. There have been no systematic studies of the use of propranolol in this disorder.

Destruction of intrahepatic ducts and progressive intrahepatic fibrosis

In approximately 10% of cases in whom the serum bilirubin returns to normal, intrahepatic cholangiopathy continues, jaundice recurs, intrahepatic bile ducts are destroyed and progressive biliary cirrhosis develops. The factors causing this are poorly understood but current evidence suggests that 'cholangitis is a major contributory factor'. Assessing the extent and significance of intrahepatic fibrosis in patients with surgically corrected biliary atresia is difficult, even with laparotomy and open liver biopsy. The distribution of fibrosis may not be homogeneous. Focal severe fibrosis may not indicate cirrhosis; on the other hand, narrow fibrotic septa may surround cirrhotic nodules; cirrhotic changes may be present in parts of the liver while large areas have normal architecture (Kimura *et al.*, 1980).

Pulmonary complications.

We have seen a number of well grown children and adolescents with mild icterus and an otherwise well compensated cirrhosis develop progressive cyanosis due to hepato-pulmonary syndrome. A 10-year-old boy leading a very active life after an apparently successful Kasai operation died suddenly from unsuspected pulmonary hypertension (Moscoso *et al.*, 1991).

Malabsorption

(see Chapter 4)

Liver transplantation

For the child in whom the serum bilirubin does not return to normal after portoenterostomy liver transplantation is only mode of management. Irrespective of the age and body weight it should be undertaken as soon as growth arrest occurs despite full nutritional support or when life-threatening complications of cirrhosis develop. Although anatomical abnormalities add to the complexity of surgery they are now rarely contraindications (see Chapter 22). Modifications to portoenterostomy and re-explorations of the porta hepatis should be avoided since they add to the difficulties of transplantation. Liver transplantation requires many more resources than portoenterostomy. The patient requires lifelong immunosuppression with close supervision for both medical and surgical complication and the longer-term prognosis is unknown. Although an important mode of management for end-stage liver disease the role of liver transplantation in biliary atresia is secondary to that of portoenterostomy except in infants who at presentation already have decompensated cirrhosis.

Emotional support for parents and families

In view of the very uncertain prognosis of biliary atresia early in its course, with the spectrum of early death or consideration of the advisability of liver transplantation if portoenterostomy fails, together with all of the complications, it is not surprising that the parents of infants with biliary atresia find the disorder causes much personal stress. To the problems of the disorder itself must be added the strains of travel to distant hospitals, sometimes causing family separation and difficulties with employment. Parents find it helpful to receive full information about biliary atresia in general and about their own child

Table 5.2 Disorders of the extrahepatic bile ducts causing hepatobiliary disease in infancy

Extrahepatic biliary atresia
Choledochal cyst
Spontaneous perforation of the bile ducts
Inspissated plugs in the biliary system associated with haemolytic disorders, cystic fibrosis and total parenteral nutrition
Gall-stones
Malignant nodes
Peritoneal bands
Tumours of the duodenum and/or pancreas
Haemangioendotheliomata
Inflammatory infiltrate
Duplication of the intestine
Radiotherapy
Ectopic gastric mucosa in bile ducts
Toxoplasmosis

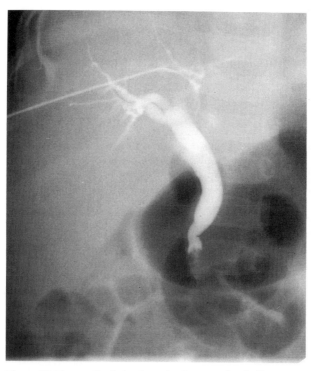

Figure 5.7 Fine needle cholangiography demonstrating fusiform dilatation of the common bile duct with an intralumenal filling defect at the level of the ampulla, typical of inspissated bile.

in particular. Written information is particularly appreciated. Careful follow-up with close attention to details of management is essential whether the patient is progressing towards a full healthy and independent adult life or is a potential liver transplant recipient.

Rare surgical causes of bile duct obstruction

These are given in Table 5.2. There may be clinical features of the associated disorders (Howard and Heaton, 1991). The stools contain no bile pigment if bile flow is completely obstructed. Diagnosis may be suspected by finding a dilated proximal bile duct (Figure 5.7) on ultrasonography with luminal or extrinsic abnormalities depending on the cause. Percutaneous or endoscopic cholangiography confirms the anatomical abnormality and may be effective in clearing inspissated material from the biliary tree. If the stricture is post-traumatic surgical balloon dilatation in conjunction with cholangiography may be possible. Liver biopsy is best avoided because of the risk of bile leaks. Usually laparotomy is required to confirm cause. Cholecystostomy with a saline flush, sphincteroplasty, cholecystectomy or a surgical bypass procedure may be required, depending on the cause of the obstruction.

Bibliography and references

Alagille, D., Laurent, J. and Roy C. C. (1989) Is there still a place for the Kasai procedure in the treatment of extrahepatic biliary atresia? *J. Pediatr. Gastroenterol. Nutr.*, **9**, 405–408

Anonymous (1989) Long term survival in biliary atresia. *Lancet* **2**, 597–598

Berenson, M. M., Garde, A. R. and Moody, F. G. (1974) Twenty-five year survival after surgery for complete extrahepatic biliary atresia. *Gastroenterology*, **66**, 260

Brown, W. R., Sokol, R J., Levin, M. J. *et al.* (1988) Lack of correlation between infection with reovirus 3 and extrahepatic biliary atresia or neonatal hepatitis. *J. Pediatr.*, **113**, 670–676

Chiba, T., Ohi, R., Nio, M. and Ibrahim, M. (1992) Late complications in long term survivors of biliary atresia. *European Journal of Pediatric Surgery*, **2**: 22–25

Daum, F. and Fischer, S. E. (1983) *Extrahepatic Biliary Atresia.* Marcel Dekker, New York

Davenport, M., Savage, M., Mowat, A. P. and Howard, E. R. (1991) The biliary atresia-splenic malformation syndrome. *Proceedings of the 5th International Sendai Symposium on Biliry Atresia*, p. 11–14

de Ville de Goyet, J. and Otte, J. B. (1992) Place of liver transplantation in biliary atresia. In *Paediatric Cholestasis. Novel Approaches to Treatment* (eds M. J. Lentze, J. Reichen) Kluwer Academic Publishers, London, p.265

Dick, M. and Mowat, A. P. (1986) Biliary scintigraphy with DISIDA. A simpler way of showing bile duct patency in suspected biliary atresia. *Arch. Dis. Childh.*, **61**, 191

El Tumi, M. A., Clarke, M. B., Barrett, J. J. and Mowat, A. P. (1987) Ten minute radiopharmaceutical test in biliary atresia. *Arch. Dis. Child.*, **62**, 180–181

Gautier, F., Laurent,J., Bernard, O. and Valayer, J. (1991) Improvement of results after Kasai operation. The need for early diagnosis and surgery. *5th international symposium on biliary atresia. Professional Postgraduate Services*, Japan, p.139–147

Gautier, M. (1979) Extrahepatic biliary atresia: aetiological hypothesis based on a study of 130 bile duct specimens. *Arch. Fr. Pediatr.* **36** (suppl.), 3–18

Gautier, M., Vallayer, J., Odievre, M. and Alagille, D. (1984) Histological liver evaluation 5 years after surgery for extrahepatic biliary atresia: A study of 20 cases. *J. Pediatr. Surg.*, **19**, 263

Gottrand, F., Bernard, O., Hadchouel, M., Pariente, D., Gauthier, F. and Alagille, D. (1991) Late cholangitis after sucessful surgical repair of biliary atresia. *Am. J. Dis. Child* , **145**, 213–215.

Hadchouel, M., Hogan, R. N. and Odievre, M. (1981) Immunoglobulin deposits in the biliary remnants in extrahepatic biliary atresia. *Histopathology*, **5**, 217

Hayes, D. M. and Kimura, K. (1980) *Biliary Atresia. The Japanese Experience.* Harvard University Press, Cambridge, MA and London

Houwen, R. H. J., Zwiersta, R. P., Severijnen, R. S. V. M. *et al.* (1989) Prognosis of extrahepatic biliary atresia. *Arch. Dis. Childh.* **64**, 214–218.

Howard, E. R., Davenport, M. and Mowat, A. P. (1991) Portoenterostomy in the eighties: The King's College Hospital Experience. *Proceedings of the 5th International Sendai Symposium on Biliary Atresia*, p.111–115

Howard, E. R. (1989) Biliary atresia. In *Maingot's Abdominal Operations,* 9th edition (eds) C. Schwartz, H. Ellis). Appleton-Lange, East Norwalk, CT, pp.1355–1364

Howard, E. R. (1992). Biliary atresia – complications and results of nontransplant surgery. In *Paediatric Cholestasis. Novel approaches to treatment* (Eds M. J. Lentze, J. Reichen). Kluwer Academic Publishers, London, p.273

Howard, E. R. (1991) Biliary atresia: aetiology, management and complications. *Surgery of Liver disease in Children* (ed. E. R. Howard). Butterworth-Heinemann, Oxford, pp. 39–59

Howard, E. R. and Mowat, A. P. (1977) Extrahepatic biliary atresia. Recent developments in management. *Arch. Dis. Childh.,* **52**, 825–827

Howard, E. R. and Mowat, A. P. (1984) Hepatobiliary disorders in infancy: Hepatitis; extrahepatic biliary atresia; intrahepatic biliary hypoplasia. In *Recent Advances in Hepatology,* (Thomas, H. C. and McSween, R. N. M., eds), p.153. Churchill Livingstone, London

Hussain, M., Howard, E. R., Mieli-Vergani, G. and Mowat, A. P. (1991) Jaundice at 14 days of age: exclude biliary atresia. *Arch. Dis. Childh.,* **66**, 1177–1179

Karrer, F. M., Lilly, J. R., Stewart, B. A. and Hall, R. J. (1990) Biliary atresia registry, 1976 to 1989. *J. Pediatr. Surgery,* **25**, 1076–1081

Kasai, M. and Suzuki, S. (1959) A new operation for 'non-correctable' biliary atresia: hepatic portoenterostomy. *Shujitsu,* **13**, 733

Kasai, M., Ohi, R., Chiba, T. and Hayashi, Y. (1988) A patient with biliary atresia who died 28 years after hepatic portojejeunostomy. *J. Pediatr. Surg.,* **23**, 431–434

Kawai, K., Kitagawa, H., Higshimori, T. *et al.* (1980) Experimental chronic non-suppurative destructive cholangitis in rabbits following immunization with bile duct antigen. *Gastroenterol. Jpn.,* **15**: 337

Kimura, S., Tomomatsu, T., Joko, Y. and Togon, H. (1980) Studies on the postoperative changes in liver tissue of long-term survivors after successful surgery for biliary atresia. *Z. Kinderchir.,* **31**: 228

Laurent, J., Gauthier, F., Bernard, O. *et al.* (1990) Long-term outcome after surgery for biliary atresia. *Gastroenterology,* **99**, 1793–1797

Lilly, J. R., Karrer, F. M., Hall, R. J. *et al.* (1989) The surgery of biliary atresia. *Ann. Surg.,* **210**, 289–296

McClement, J., Howard, E. R. and Mowat, A. P. (1985) Results of surgical treatment for extrahepatic biliary atresia in United Kingdom 1980–82. *Br. Med. J.,* **290**, 345–347

Manolaki, A. G., Larcher, V. F., Mowat, A. P., Barratt, J. J., Portmann, B. and Howard, E. R. (1983) The pre-laparotomy diagnosis of extrahepatic biliary atresia. *Arch. Dis. Childh.,* **58**, 591

Markowitz, J., Daum, F., Kahn, E. I. *et al.* (1983) Arteriohepatic dysplasia 1. Pitfalls in diagnosis and management. *Hepatology,* **3**, 74–76.

Mieli-Vergani, G., Howard, E. R., Portmann, B. and Mowat, A. P. (1989) Late referral for biliary atresia – missed opportunities for effective surgery. *Lancet,* **i**, 421–423

Miyano, T., Suruga, K. and Suda, K. (1979) Abnormal choledocho-pancreatico-ductal junction related to the aetiology of infantile obstructive jaundice. *J. Pediatr. Surg.,* **14**, 16

Moscoso, G., Mieli-Vergani, G., Mowat, A. P. and Portmann, B. (1991) Sudden death caused by unsuspected pulmonary hypertension, 10 years after surgery for extrahepatic biliary atresia. *J. Ped. Gastroenterol. Nutr.,* **12**, 388–393.

Muller, F., Gauthier, F., Laurent, J., Schmitt, M. and Boue J. (1991) Amniotic fluid GGT and congenital extrahepatic biliary damage. *Lancet,* **337**, 232–233

Nakano, M., Saeki, M. and Hagane, K. (1990) Delayed puberty in girls having biliary atresia. *J. Pediatr. Surg.,* **25**, 808–811

Nelson, R. (1989) Managing Biliary Atresia. Referral before 6 weeks is vital. *Br. Med. J.,* **298**, 1471

Nietgen, G. W., Vacanti, J. P. and Perez-Atayde, A. (1992) Intrahepatic bile duct loss in biliary atresia despite portoenterostomy: a consequence of ongoing obstruction, *Gastroenterology,* **102**, 2126–2133

Nittono, H., Tokita, A., Hayashi, M. *et al* (1988) Ursodeoxycholic acid in biliary atresia. *Lancet,* **i**, 528

Ohi, R. (1991) Biliary atresia: modification of the original portoenterostomy operation. In *Surgery of Liver disease in Children* (ed. E. R. Howard). Butterworth-Heinemann, Oxford, pp. 60–71

Ohi, R. *et al.* (1987) The present status of surgical treatment for biliary atresia: report of the questionnaire for the main institutions in Japan. In *Biliary Atresia.* Ohi, R. (ed) pp.125–30. Professional Postgraduate Services, Tokyo

Ohi, R., Nio, M., Chiba, T., Endo, N., Goto, M. and Ibrahim, M. (1990) Long-term follow-up after surgery for patients with biliary atresia. *J. Ped. Surg.,* **25**, 442–445

Ohi, R., Hanamatsu, M., Mochizuki, I., Chiba, T. and Kasai, M. (1985) Progress in the treatment of biliary atresia. *World J. Surg.* **9**, 285–293

Ohkohchi, N., Chiba, T., Ohi, R. and Mori, S. (1989) Long-term follow-up study of patients with cholangitis after successful Kasai operation in biliary atresia: selection of recipients for liver transplantation. *J. Pediatr. Gastroenterol. Nutr.* **9**, 416–420

Schwartz, M. Z., Hall, R. J., Reubner, B., Lilly, J. R., Brogen, T. and Toyama, W. M. (1990) A genesis of the extrahepatic bile ducts: report of 5 cases. *J. Paediatric Surg.,* **25**, 805–807

Shimotake, T., Iwai, N., Yanogihara, J., Deguchi, E. and Onouchi, Z. (1992) Postoperative management of children with biliary atresia and heart failure. *Eur. J. Pediatr. Surg.,* **2**, 110–113.

Shiraki, K., Okada, T. and Tanimoto, K. (1987) Evaluation of various diagnostic methods in biliary atresia. In *Biliary Atresia* (ed. R. Ohi) Professional Postgraduate Services, Tokyo, pp. 85–94

Silveira, T. R., Salzano, F. M., Howard, E. R. and Mowat, A. P. (1991a) Extrahepatic biliary atresia and twinning. *Braz. J. Med. Biol. Res.,* **24**, 67–71.

Silveira, T. R., Salzano, F. M., Howard, E. R., Mowat, A. P. (1991b) Congenital structural abnormalities in biliary atresia: Evidence for etiopathogenic heterogeneity and therapeutic implications. *Acta. Paediatr. Scand.,* **80**

Silveira, T. R., Salzano, F. M., Howard, E. R. and Mowat, A. P. (1992) The relative importance of familial, reproductive and environmental factors in biliary atresia: etiological implications and effect on patient survival. *Braz. J. Med. Biol. Res.,* **25**, 673–681.

Silveira, T. R., Donaldson, P. T., Mieli-Vergani Salzano, F. M., Howard, E. R. and Mowat, A. P. (1993) Extrahepatic biliary atresia with and without associated congenital anomalies: relation with HLA CLASS I antigens and rhesus blood group. *J. Pediatr. Gastroenterol. Nutr.* (in press)

Sokal, E. M., Veyckemans, F., de Ville de Goyet, J. *et al.* (1990) Liver transplantation in children less than 1 year of age. *J. Pediatr.,* **117**, 205–210

Stewart, B. A., Hall, R. J. and Lilly, J. R. (1988) Liver transplantation and the Kasai operation in biliary atresia. *J. Pediatr. Surg.,* **23**, 623–626

Stringer, M. D., Howard, E. R. and Mowat, A. P. (1989) Endoscopic sclerotherapy in the management of esophageal varices in 61 children with biliary atresia. *J. Pediatr. Surg.,* **24**, 438–442

Ullrich, D., Rating, D., Schroter, W., Hanefeld, F. and Bircher, J. (1987) Treatment with ursodeoxycholic acid renders children with biliary atresia suitable for liver transplantation. *Lancet,* **ii**, 1324

Vasquez-Estevez, J. J., Stewart, B., Shikes, R. H., Hall, R. J. and Lilly, J. R. Biliary atresia: early determination of prognosis. *J. Pediatr. Surg.,* **24**, 48–51

Werlin, S. L., Sly, J. R., Slarshak, R. J., Glicklich, M. and Nathan, R. (1985) Intrahepatic biliary tract abnormalities in children with corrected entrahepatic biliary atresia. *J. Pediatr. Gastroenterol. Nutr.,* **4**: 537

Wilkinson, M. L., Mieli-Vergani, G., Ball, C., Portmann, B. and Mowat, A. P. (1991) Endoscopic Retrograde Cholangiopancreatography (ERCP) in Infantile Cholestasis. *Arch. Dis. Child.* **66**, 121–123

Rare surgical causes of bile duct obstruction

Howard, E. R. and Heaton, N. D. (1991) Benign extrahepatic bile duct obstruction. In *Surgery of Liver disease in Children* (ed. E. R. Howard). Butterworth-Heinemann, Oxford, pp. 94–101

Chapter 6

Viral infections of the liver

Hepatitis

The term hepatitis indicates an inflammation of the liver, usually associated with hepatocyte degeneration or necrosis. The cause may be infective, toxic, genetically determined, physical, ischaemic or cryptogenic. The course may be acute or chronic. Although it is usual to characterize the hepatitis by the aetiological factor, the wide range of clinical manifestations seen in any of the above types is determined by the severity of the alterations in hepatocyte function. At one end of the scale is an asymptomatic hepatitis in which hepatocellular necrosis is minimal and revealed only by elevation of serum enzymes such as aspartate aminotransferase, at the other end is fulminant hepatitis associated with massive hepatocellular necrosis, hepatic encephalopathy and spontaneous haemorrhage. Hepatitis in infancy is considered in Chapter 4.

Viral hepatitis

Although the contagious nature of acute hepatitis was noted by Hippocratic writers in the fourth century BC and epidemic hepatitis recorded in the fourth century AD, and a viral cause suggested as early as 1908, it was not until the late 1930s that the term 'infectious hepatitis' replaced 'catarrhal jaundice'. The responsible agent was identified as hepatitis A virus (HAV) in 1973. Hepatitis spread by vaccinia vaccine was reported in 1855 but it was not until 1943 that the term 'homologous serum jaundice' or 'serum hepatitis' was introduced implying that a serum factor spread the infection.

The demonstration in 1969 that Australia antigen, now called the 'hepatitis B surface antigen' (HbsAg), was associated with serum hepatitis led to the identification of hepatitis B virus (HBV) in 1970. In 1977 the Delta virus (HDV) which causes hepatitis only in conjunction with HBV was discovered. By 1975 it was already apparent that acute hepatitis may be caused by agents other than HAV or HBV or other identified viruses. An enterically transmitted virus now known as hepatitis E virus (HEV) was identified in 1987 and its viral DNA cloned in 1990. Hepatitis C virus (HCV) was cloned in 1989 and although still not visualized it is already known to be responsible for much but not all post-transfusion and chronic hepatitis previously labelled non-A, non-B hepatitis. Safe, highly immunogenic and protective vaccines for both hepatitis A and B are available. The term viral hepatitis, is by convention, limited to hepatitis caused by the above viruses which

Table 6.1 Viruses that may involve the liver

RNA viruses:	DNA viruses:
Picorna viruses (Enteroviruses) 　Hepatitis A virus 　Coxsackie viruses 　Echo viruses	Adenoviruses Hepadna viruses 　Hepatitis B virus
Toga viruses 　Yellow fever virus 　Rubella virus	Herpes viruses 　Cytomegalovirus 　Epstein–Barr virus 　Herpes simplex virus 　Varicella zoster virus
Arena viruses 　Junin virus 　Machupo virus 　Lassa virus 　Rift Valley fever virus	
Rhabdo viruses 　Marborg virus 　Ebola virus	
Reo viruses 　? perinatal or neonatal	
Paramyxo viruses 　Measles virus 　Mumps 　Hepatitis C	
Delta hepatitis (hepatitis B-dependent). 　Hepatitis E	

produce hepatitis as the major clinical manifestation. Viruses currently believed to involve the liver are listed in Table 6.1. This chapter will deal with viruses which have a high degree of hepatic trophism.

Acute viral hepatitis type A

Definition

This is an acute inflammation of the liver with varying degrees of hepatocellular necrosis caused by the enterically transmitted hepatitis A virus (HAV), a member of the picornavirus family. The hepatitis is usually benign but severity may increase with age. There are no long-term sequelae but the disease may be relapsing.

Aetiology and pathogenesis

Hepatitis A is a non-enveloped virus, 27 to 28 nm in diameter. Its genome consists of a single strand of RNA which codes for four capsid proteins, a viral polymerase and proteases. Only one serotype has been recognized. Although classified taxonomically as a picornavirus with the designation enterovirus Type 72, unlike others it is resistant to heat and is less cytolytic in cell culture.

The first evidence of viral infection is the detection of the virus in the liver with immunofluorescent antibody staining 1–2 weeks after infection. In experimental animals

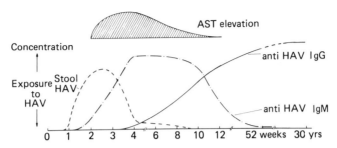

Figure 6.1 Diagrammatic representation of time course of changes in titre of viral excretion in stool, IgM and IgG antibody concentration and hepatitis following exposure to hepatitis A virus

this is associated with a rise in transaminases although there is no cytolysis. It is uncertain whether prior replication occurs in the alimentary tract. It has not been detected in intestinal mucosa of experimental animals. Within a few days the virus can be found in faeces and in bile. The virus has been detected in the blood before the onset of disease but the time of its appearance and duration of its presence is not well defined.

The virus is a very effective immune stimulus. An IgM antibody appears in serum 7–10 days after exposure, reaching peak concentrations after 20–40 days and thereafter rapidly declining to become undetectable by 60 days in the majority but occasionally persisting for as long as 1 year. IgG antibodies become detectable approximately 30 days after exposure, the titre rising over the course of the next month and persisting for up to 30 years (Figure 6.1). Faecal viral shedding as assessed by immunological tests of relatively low sensitivity is maximal 20–25 days after exposure and persists usually for up to 16 days after the onset of hepatitis. Excretion persist for 6 weeks in 10% of cases and longer in relapsing cases (Fagan *et al.*, 1990). Molecular hybridization and polymerase chain reaction techniques may show excretion prolonged for 3 to 4 months, as has recently been demonstrated in premature infants (Rosenblum *et al.*, 1991). Faecal IgA antibody to HAV is found 20 days after exposure and persists for up to 6 months. There is no chronic carrier state. It is thought that the virus is mildly cytopathic but that the major injury is due to cell-mediated immune responses.

Pathology

Liver cell damage or necrosis, regeneration, and inflammatory cell infiltrate in the hepatic parenchyma and portal tracts, with or without bile pigment retention, are the hallmarks of hepatitis. Liver damage occurs throughout the liver in all lobules, but to varying extents and is often most marked in the centrilobular areas. Damage may take the form of liver cell swelling with a granular cytoplasm (ballooning degeneration), shrinkage of liver cells (giving a deeply stained acidophilic cytoplasm), or loss of cells, best appreciated as an irregular collapse of the reticulum network. Such necrosis may be focal, affect groups of liver cells, or confluent. The inflammatory cell infiltrate, both in the parenchyma and portal tracts, is mainly of mononuclear cells but scanty polymorphonuclear neutrophil leucocytes are common. The inflammatory cell infiltrate of the portal tract may extend a little distance into the hepatic parenchyma. Kupffer cells become active macrophages replete with material from degraded cells.

The rate of progression of the pathological changes is very variable. After some weeks or months, features of acute hepatocyte injury regress; but the reticulo-endothelial cellular reaction persists, sometimes with increased portal tract changes which mimic large bile duct obstruction. Clumps of cells containing PAS-positive, acid-fast, ceroid pigment and stainable iron are characteristic of this stage. Such changes may persist for many months but healing is eventually complete.

Variations from this sequence of pathological changes may include the following:

(1) A period of persistent cholestasis.
(2) A period of improvement with a recurrence of cholestasis both proceeding to eventual complete recovery.
(3) A rapid progression to massive necrosis with hepatic encephalopathy.

As well as these intrahepatic changes, a generalized lymph gland enlargement, splenomegaly due to cellular infiltration and inflammatory lesions of the duodenum and kidney are commonly found. Myocarditis, pancreatitis, and aplastic anaemia are rare complications.

Epidemiology

In all age groups most infections are subclinical and anicteric. Data based on case reporting grossly underestimate disease incidence. The availability of serological markers for hepatitis A infection have confirmed earlier conclusions based on clinical observations and rare volunteer studies. The main source of infection is virus shed in the faeces late in the incubation period and within 2 weeks of onset of hepatitis. The faecal/oral route is the usual mode of spread. Transmission is by close personal contact or by contaminated food or water. In areas of the world where overcrowding, poor sanitation and sewage-contaminated drinking water is the norm, HAV infection is acquired very early in infancy. The mean age of exposure increases as standards of sanitation and hygiene improve.

In parts of western Europe and Scandinavia few children have been infected in the past two decades, antibodies to type A hepatitis being found in less than 20% of young adults. In areas of intermediate incidence the highest infection rates occur in nurseries, schools, military institutions and prisons. The secondary attack rate is high in children in households with an index case and can be high in neonatal intensive care units. Sewage-contaminated clams, mussels and oysters have been incriminated in some outbreaks. Blood or blood products taken during the viraemic stage are infrequent modes of infection. Infection in late pregnancy has not been shown to affect the newborn infant.

Clinical features

The incubation period is from 21 to 40 days. The severity of disease may vary from an asymptomatic subclinical infection to rapidly fatal hepatitis. In children aged 2–16 years in Thailand totally unapparent infections were three times more common than symptomatic ones. The proportion of infected children developing icteric hepatitis in a recent epidemic in a UK city ranged from 1 in 43 of those under 5 to 1 in 4.7 of 8 to 10-year-olds (Stuart et al., 1992). In an epidemic in Greenland the frequency of apparent hepatitis increase from less than 1% in children of under 1 year to 24% in 15-year-olds. One outbreak in children in China produced an attack rate of 22% with a mean age in symptomatic patients of 5.9 years and 4.5 in those with subclinical disease. In subjects over 8 years of age 20% were jaundiced and 34% had no abnormality in liver function tests (Feinstone *et al.*, 1991).

Symptomatic infection has two phases. The *pre-icteric* phase is characterized by anorexia, nausea, vomiting, lassitude and sometimes intermittent dull abdominal pain felt in the epigastrium or right hypochondrium. There may be fever and headache, particularly in older children.

In young infants the stool may be loose and failure to gain weight is common. Clinical examination may reveal tender hepatomegaly, also splenomegaly and lymph gland enlargement. It is suspected that in many affected children no features allowing a clinical diagnosis of hepatitis develop and the disease regresses at this stage.

When bilirubinuria, pale or clay coloured stools (30%) and scleral icterus appears at the *icteric phase* there is often a regression of all symptoms and a return of appetite, particularly in young children. In older children, as in adults, there is commonly an exacerbation of the original symptoms with, in some cases, depression and pruritus. The liver is usually enlarged and tender, and the spleen is palpable in 20–30% of cases. Jaundice may persist for only a few days but usually fades in the second week. Rarely it may persist for months. Complete recovery is the rule.

Laboratory findings

Serum transaminase levels are elevated from 3 to 4 days before the onset of jaundice, returning to normal typically in 2–3 months. In one series of hospitalized children 25% still had elevated transaminases at 6 months and 5% at 9 months. The serum bilirubin level rises when the transaminase concentration is already at its peak, which is usually somewhere between 400 and 800 IU/litre, but occasionally will exceed 1000 IU/litre. Serum alkaline phosphatase levels are rarely more than 50% of the normal value. Further elevation may occur in association with marked cholestasis but should raise the suspicion of extrahepatic bile duct disease. A prolonged prothrombin time should raise suspicion of severe liver cell necrosis or chronic underlying disease.

The *diagnosis* is based on these clinical and laboratory findings confirmed by detecting IgM antibodies to HAV. Clinical features of chronic liver disease or low serum albumin, prolonged prothrombin time and high immunoglobulin suggest coincidental underlying liver disease which may require urgent identification and treatment (see Chapter 13 on Chronic hepatitis). A mild leucocytosis may be found in the incubation period often to be followed by leucopenia and lymphopaenia, often with a few atypical lymphocytes. Haemolysis may occur in patients with glucose-6-phosphate dehydrogenase deficiency and other genetic haemolytic disorders but should raise suspicion of co-existing Wilson's disease.

Complications

The most serious complication is *fulminant hepatic failure* which occurred in 0.5% of jaundiced cases in one epidemic but rates of 0.1–0.35% are reported in hospitalized cases. The clinician should be alerted to the possibility of this developing by a number of clinical features such as persisting anorexia, progressively deepening jaundice, reappearance of the initial symptoms and, particularly, a reduction in liver size to less than normal or the development of ascites. Neuropsychiatric changes taking the form of irrational or aggressive behaviour or progressive encephalopathy are a sinister development. Laboratory investigations suggesting fulminant hepatic failure include prolongation of the prothrombin time, a falling serum albumin, hypoglycaemia, raised serum ammonia or respiratory alkalosis. Subacute hepatic necrosis, chronic hepatitis or cirrhosis has not been seen following serologically documented hepatitis A. After transaminases return to normal relapse may occur 15 to 90 days later (Chiriaco *et al.*, 1986) with transaminases of 200–2300 IU/litre, icterus, prolonged virus excretion and acute liver failure (Fagan, 1990). In one study 6% of icteric cases had a biochemical relapse (Sjorgen *et al.*, 1987).

Rare complications include bone marrow aplasia, or hypoplasia, pancreatitis, myocarditis, acute renal failure, cryoglobulinaemia, splenic rupture and Guillain-Barré syndrome. In two patients aged 14 years HAV infection was followed by autoimmune chronic active hepatitis (Vento et al 1991).

Management

There is no specific treatment: most patients are adequately cared for at home. It is important to describe modes of spread and to outline the probable course of the illness to parents so that they may be alerted to any atypical features heralding the onset of complications. The minimal investigations listed in Table 6.2 are necessary to determine the severity of the hepatitis and to exclude other aetiological causes.

Table 6.2 Minimal investigations necessary in sporadic acute hepatitis

Serum bilirubin, total and direct reacting	Full blood count, including reticulocyte count
Serum transaminase	Hepatitis B surface antigen
Serum alkaline phosphatase	Caeruloplasmin
Prothrombin time	Paul–Bunnell test
Serum albumin	Cytomegalovirus antibody
Serum immunoglobulins	IgM HAV antibody
Tissue autoantibodies	HCV antibody (2nd generation)

There is no evidence that diet and enforced, absolute or partial bed rest have any bearing on the rate of healing of the liver or that strenuous activity increases the duration of the illness. Many patients avoid fats since this intensifies nausea, but when this settles, fat should be taken normally; indeed, one study suggests that healing occurred more quickly when the fat intake was high. Anti-emetic drugs such as metoclopramide may be necessary, but it is important to limit the dosage of any drug metabolized by the liver otherwise side effects, such as dystonic reactions, may appear. Corticosteroids may reduce the duration of cholestasis but generally have no place in management.

Prevention

With the high incidence of asymptomatic cases and with maximum infectivity preceding the onset of recognized disease, an essential step in prevention is safe disposal of faeces and the provision of drinking water uncontaminated by faecal pathogens. Person-to-person spread may be minimized by scrupulous hand washing after defaecation and before handling food. The virus is inactivated by boiling for more than 5 minutes, by irradiation, formalin and chlorine in a concentration of 1 mg/litre if exposed for 30 minutes.

Active immunization is now possible using highly immunogenic, safe, well tolerated vaccines containing formaldehyde-inactivated attenuated virus. A single intramuscular dose is protective in more than 94% of recipients within 21 days (Werzberger *et al.*, 1992) and probably prevents unapparent infection (Innis *et al.*, 1992). Currently booster doses are recommended at 1 and 12 months but the duration of protection is not known. It could be life-long.

The role of passive immunization is now very limited. Human normal immunoglobulin (HNIg) contains sufficient antibodies to HAV to give passive protection for 3 months at a dose of 0.06 to 0.12 ml/kg (or 250 mg under 10 years of age; 500 mg if older). Whether this dose would control infection in closed communities and in the home better than active immunization or whether active and passive immunization at different site would be advantageous is unknown. Active immunization is preferable for travellers to endemic areas.

Viral hepatitis type B

Viral hepatitis type B is caused by the hepatitis B virus (HBV), a double-stranded DNA virus of the Hepadnavirus family which has unique biological properties (Hollinger *et al.*, 1991). Unlike hepatitis A virus the host immunological response may be ineffective leading to chronic infection. After years or decades this infective carrier state with pauci-symptomatic or asymptomatic chronic liver disease can resolve but it may progress to cirrhosis and/or liver cancer. It has been estimated recently that there are between 300 and 400 million HBV carriers in the world and that HBV causes 250 000 deaths per annum. The host, viral or environmental factors causing the variable immune and cytopathological effects are subjects of intensive research but remain to be fully elucidated. The recently discovered mutants of HBV contribute to the variability of outcome.

Aetiology

The hepatitis B virus

Hepatitis B virus is a 42 nm spherical DNA-containing virus. It has an inner nucleocapsid core 27 nm in diameter termed the hepatitis B core (HBc) which is a potent immunogen. It surrounds the viral genome and reverse transcriptase. The core produces a truncated core protein termed the hepatitis Be antigen (HBeAg), with a different antigenicity, which is found as a soluble protein in the blood during massive viraemia. HBc/e may suppress induction of beta-interferon by the virus. The outer lipoprotein coat has equimolecular amounts of three proteins, S, pre-S_1 and pre-S_2, the latter two being polypeptide extensions on the amino end of S. Pre-S_2 is a 55 amino acid extension with pre-S_1 having a further 119 amino acids added to pre-S_2. The virus has four functional genes; the S gene which encodes HBsAg has three start codons for pre-S_1, pre-S_2 and S proteins; the C region encodes HBc, the P gene viral polymerase and the X gene a small protein of which may regulate viral replication.

In the past 4 years a number of genetic variants of HBV have been identified. Using recombinant DNA and molecular hybridization techniques HBV DNA has been found integrated into chromosomes of liver cells of infected patients (Zuckermann, 1990). The virus appears to replicate only in liver but is found in other organs. Three different morphological forms of HBsAg may be detected in the sera of patients acutely or chronically infected: intact virus particles. Spherical 22 nm HBsAg particles and filamentous HBsAg with a diameter of 22 nm (Figure 6.2). In most sera the ratio of 22 nm HBsAg particles to intact virus particles exceeds 1000:1. The respective antibodies to the major products of HBV are anti-HBc, anti-HBe and anti-HBs.

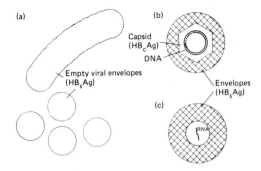

Figure 6.2 (*a*) 22 nm spherical particles and filaments carrying HB$_s$Ag. (*b*) a schematic representation of hepatitis B virus with its envelope carrying HB$_s$Ag and a capsid carrying HB$_c$Ag and containing the circular DNA molecule. (c) the Delta agent with the HB$_s$Ag envelope and its RNA-containing core.

Four major virus-determined subtypes of hepatitis B surface antigen, termed adw, adr, ayw and ayr, are useful markers in epidemiological studies but are identical in their clinical effects (Table 6.3). A virulent 'a' mutant, which is not neutralized by antiHBe, has been described.

Three additional indicators of HBV infection provide useful pathophysiological information but are not routinely available: HBV-specific DNA polymerase (which also indicates continuing viral replication), HBV DNA hybridization and the polymerase chain

Table 6.3 Significance of serological markers of viral hepatitis

Marker	Significance
Hepatitis A:	
IgM HAV Ab	Acute hepatitis (may be positive for up to 1 year).
IgG HAV Ab	Immunity to hepatitis A due to past infection, active immunization or passive immunization.
Hepatitis B:	
HBsAg	Acute or chronic hepatitis B infection
IgM HBcAb	High titre: > 600 acute hepatitis Low titre: chronic infection
IgG HBcAb	Past exposure to hepatitis B, or continuing hepatitis B infection (if HBsAb is positive)
HBsAb	Immunity to hepatitis B, post-infective or with active or passive immunization
HBeAg	Highly infectious state in acute or chronic infection
HBeAb	Less infective state in the HBsAb positive patient except with HBe minus variant
HBV-specific DNA polymerase	A more sensitive and specific indicator of persisting viral infection
HBV DNA by direct DNA hybridization	An even more sensitive indicator of viral replication detecting 10^5 genomes/ml.
Polymerase chain reation for HBV genome	Ultrasensitive technique detecting 10 genomes/ml
Delta agent	Acute or chronic infection with delta
IgM delta antibody	Continuing delta infection
IgG delta antibody	Past delta infection

reaction (PCR) for HBV specific oligonucleotides. This technique has allowed the detection of HBV DNA in sera in which even antiHBc is absent. Its main value has been in the identification of new variants of HBV. The technique is so sensitive that stringent precautions are necessary to prevent contamination.

Mutants   A worrying development is the emergence of virulent hepatitis B virus mutants which evoke unusual and ineffective immune responses. This first came to light in 44 of 1590 recipients of hepatitis B vaccine who developed evidence of hepatitis B surface antigen (HBsAg) replication in spite of adequate concentrations of antibody to HBsAg. Studies of virus isolated from a mother and child showed that a stable mutation had occurred causing a single amino acid substitution in hepatitis B surface antigen which was such that antibodies provoked by the vaccine could not bind to the modified virus (Carman *et al.*, 1990). At least three further variants have been described including one in the precore region which produces a virus incapable of encoding the e antigen and producing severe and even fulminant hepatitis B (Kosaka *et al.*, 1991). Mutants developing in HBsAg positive mothers with HBeAb have caused fulminant hepatitis in their infants (Terazawa *et al.*, 1991).

Serological response in HBV infection (Table 6.3)

Serological response is *variable both in the timing and intensity.* The viral components may be present so transiently that they are never detected or may persist in high concentrations for up to 30 years in carriers. IgM anti-HBc antibodies appear as the first evidence of disease and IgG anti-HBc antibodies persist for decades and are thus the best marker of disease prevalence. An exception was 10% of infected Taiwanese infants who did not develop anti-HBc on 5-year follow-up (Lee *et al.*, 1989). Antibodies to HBe and HBs appear weeks, months or years later as hepatitis resolves. They may never appear in the chronic carrier. Commonly, there is a time interval during which the viral antigen disappears from the serum and its antibody (other than anti-HBc) is undetectable.

Acute hepatitis (Figure 6.3)

In uncomplicated acute hepatitis HBV as HBV DNA or DNA polymerase, HBsAg and, more transiently, HBeAg are found in the serum usually 1–2 weeks after parenteral exposure and 6–8 weeks after oral exposure but occasionally as late as 7 months. Approximately 4 weeks after the first detection of antigens the patient becomes symptomatic or a rise in serum transaminase is detected. By then the first antibody to appear, anti-HBc IgM, is present in a very high concentration and will remain detectable for up to a year. HBe antigen disappears followed 2 or 3 weeks later by HBsAg. During this period anti-HBc may be the only serological evidence of HBV infection. Anti-HBe then appears apparently signalling the end of active viral replication. Finally, anti-HBs is detected indicating recovery and protection from reinfection. Years later anti-HBe, anti-HBsAb and finally anti-HBc become undetectable.

HBV carriers

The carrier state is characterized by persistence of HBsAg in the circulation for more than 6 months. It occurs in two forms. In the first the co-existence in the serum of HBeAg, HBV-DNA polymerase or HBV DNA indicates continuing viral replication. High titres of anti-HBc suggest persisting liver damage. After years of the carrier state an immune

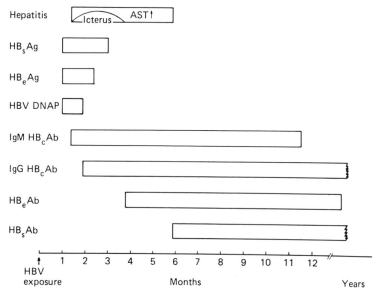

Figure 6.3 Diagrammatic representation of the sequential appearance and disappearance of hepatitis B antigens and antibodies in uncomplicated acute hepatitis with transient HB$_s$ antigenaemia

response to HBV infected hepatocytes may develop with a rise in transaminases in 70% of cases. HBeAg and HBV DNA disappear from serum. Anti-HBe is detected after an interval. In spite of this 5–15% reactivate with all the serological features of acute infection and sometimes rapidly progressive disease. A proportion of such cases has been associated with the emergence of mutant HBV. In the majority the immune response is completed when anti-HBs appears sometimes years after clearing HBe. HBV may still be detected in serum by PCR up to 6 years later (Bortolotti *et al.*, 1992) but its pathobiological significance is unknown. In the second form the carrier has no infective virus in the circulation. The hepatocytes contain viral DNA capable of producing HBsAg but not intact virus. Note that immunosuppressed patients, e.g. in Down's syndrome, patients with HIV infection, those requiring renal dialysis, or receiving cytotoxic drugs, have aberrant responses to infection, e.g. HBV infection within the liver without serological markers (Lok *et al.*, 1991) and are prone to acute and chronic exacerbations.

HBV within the liver

Using immunofluorescent and immunoperoxidase techniques, HBc can be detected within the nucleus of the hepatocyte as granular deposits in patients with chronic hepatitis. Cytoplasmic HBsAg can be identified by its 'ground glass' appearance with haematoxylin and eosin or Masson's trichrome stain or as a homogeneous brown material with orcein staining. It is particularly prominent in 'healthy' carriers. With DNA-DNA hybridization techniques and DNA Southern blotting, both viral replication and integration of viral DNA into host chromosomal DNA can be demonstrated.

Hepatocellular damage in HBV infection

The mechanisms causing persistent viral infection and hepatocellular injury in HBV infection are poorly understood even in chronic disease. How the virus enters the hepatocyte is unclear. The viral genome becomes encoded with host DNA leading to the assembly of complete virons and viral proteins which may have a direct cytopathic effect with minimal inflammatory response. HBs, c and e antigens are expressed on the liver cell surface membrane exciting humoral and cellular immune responses. These involved the coordinated action of antigen presenting cells, B and T lymphocytes and efficient interferon production (Figure 6.4) *In vitro* studies indicate that hepatocyte cytolysis is induced by T lymphocytes acting against HBs, Hbe and HBc expressed on the cell surface (Keller *et al.*, 1990; Penna, 1992). Other *in vitro* studies show that

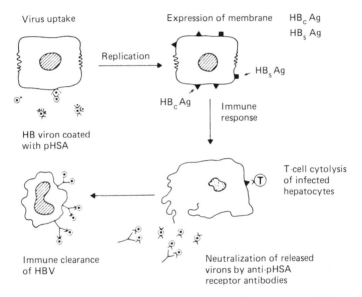

Figure 6.4 Schematic illustration of the sequence of events in acute HBV infection, from virus uptake through replication and liver cell damage to recovery. (pHSAA, polymerized human serum albumin.) Reproduced, with permission, from Mondelli and Eddleston (1984)

T cells activated by persistent HBV infection trigger a humoral response against hepatocyte membrane components which subsequently contribute to hepatocellular damage in an antibody-dependent non-T cell mediated cytotoxic reaction. Cells with integrated HBV genome without changes on their surface membranes are not subjected to these cytolytic attacks and persist with the potential for virus-associated oncogenesis (Figure 6.5).

Two other modes of liver injury are described. In acute hepatitis and fulminant hepatic failure the rapid appearance of antibodies to hepatitis B core and envelope proteins may lead to the development of immune complexes in the liver sinusoids with subsequent impairment of the microcirculation and ischaemic necrosis. T lymphocytes also produce soluble lymphokines which initiate in monocytes a coagulation protease

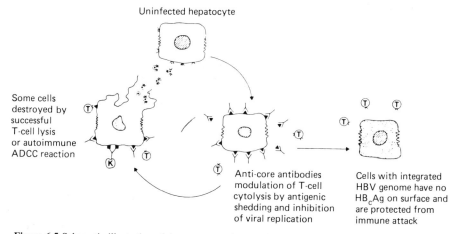

Uninfected hepatocyte

Some cells
destroyed by
successful
T-cell lysis
or autoimmune
ADCC reaction

Anti-core antibodies
modulation of T-cell
cytolysis by antigenic
shedding and inhibition
of viral replication

Cells with integrated
HBV genome have no
HB$_c$Ag on surface and
are protected from
immune attack

Figure 6.5 Schematic illustration of the sequence of events in chronic HBV infection, illustrating the circular path through viral replication, liver cell damage, and infection of other hepatocytes. The modulating effect of anti-core antibodies on this process is also shown, together with the protective effect of viral integration. Reproduced, with permission, from Mondelli and Eddleston (1984)

cascade. This causes platelet aggregation, fibrin deposition, local microthrombus formation and injury to vascular endothelium, as well as augmenting other cytotoxic mechanisms.

Severity of pathological change

A wide range of pathological changes may occur. These range from the healthy carrier state with no hepatocellular necrosis or cellular infiltrate through acute hepatitis to massive hepatocellular necrosis, various forms of chronic hepatitis, cirrhosis and hepatocellular carcinoma. Assessing the severity of liver disease is often difficult without liver biopsy. Asymptomatic subjects without clinical abnormality and with normal biochemical tests of liver function may have advanced liver disease. Coexistent Delta infection is usually associated with severe acute disease, chronic active hepatitis or cirrhosis (see below).

Epidemiology

Transmission of HBV occurs by the parenteral route but since *minute* quantities of blood are infective it may be blood-borne via unapparent fomites, e.g. sharp objects, toothbrushes, chewing gum or insect bites. In saliva and semen viral concentrations are 100 to 1000 times less than in blood but both have been shown to be infective in experimental studies. HBV has been detected in urine, tears, impetiginous lesions and breast milk but it is not known whether these are infective. Sources of infection in childhood are given in Table 6.4.

There is marked geographical variation in prevalence and in age at infection. In much of Asia and Africa where adult carrier rates are greater than 10% and, to a lesser extent, in Mediterranean countries and South America where 2–7% of adults are carriers, HBV infection is predominantly a disease acquired in early infancy and childhood. The higher the adult carrier rate, particularly carriers who are HBeAg positive, the higher the rate of

Table 6.4 Sources of hepatitis B infection in childhood

HBsAg positive mother	Infection acquired at delivery or postnatally transplacentally
HBsAg positive family member or other close contacts	Drug abusers, homosexuals, patients with renal failure, reticulosis, organ transplant, immigrant from areas of higher carrier rate Infection may be spread via formites, abrasions and possibly by arthropods
Blood products, particularly clotting factor concentrates prepared from paid donors	Haemophilic globulin, e.g. Factor VIII concentrated for haemophilia

acquisition in childhood. Close contact with an HBsAg, HBeAg positive mother or other family member is the main predisposing factor. In south-east Asia up to 30% become infected in the first year of life with evidence of infection appearing at 3 months of age. In the majority infection is acquired during delivery but the 5–10% vaccination failure rate may represent intrauterine infection or emergence of mutants. In contrast, in parts of Africa only 5% may be infected in the first year of life. These geographical differences in the rate of early infection are in part explained by the higher HBe Ag carrier rate in Chinese mothers (40% v 15%). HBV in food partially masticated by parents and passed into the mouths of infants during weaning may contribute to early infection in parts of Asia. After 1 year of age HBV infection can be detected in a gradually increasing percentage of children, so within some communities up to 90% are infected in the first decade. Infants born to HBeAg positive mothers have a 70–90% chance of HBV infection, in contrast to a risk of 10–40% if born to an HBeAg negative mother.

In north-west Europe and North America infection in infancy and childhood is very uncommon. When it does occur it is from an HBsAg positive parent from an area with a high carrier rate or in the setting of a family infection initiated by a visitor from an area of high prevalence or by a drug addict or homosexual. The routine screening of donor blood for HBsAg has largely eliminated therapeutic transfusion or injection of blood products as a mode of transmission. HBV infection did occur in up to 40% of institutionalized handicapped children, particularly those with Down's syndrome. It was more common in patients with leukaemia and other disorders with impaired immunity, particularly if much hospitalization was required or if multiple transfusions of blood products or coagulation factors were given. Patients with haemophilia receiving infusions of cryoprecipitate were at particularly high risk. Infection in adolescents and adults occurs by parenteral and sexual spread.

Clinical features

Acute infection

The incubation period is from 60–110 (mean 90) days but may range from 30–180 days. The serological response is described above and illustrated in Figure 6.3. Antibody to HBsAg can be detected during antigenaemia and before the hepatitis in 10–20% of patients who develop arthritis and rash associated with immune complex formation and during the hepatitis in a significant proportion of patients. In the majority, however, the anti-HBs can only be detected weeks or months after the disappearance of HBsAg.

Table 6.5 Expression of hepatitis B virus infection in childhood

Asymptomatic development of HBsAb
Acute hepatitis, asymptomatic, anicteric or icteric
Papular acrodermatitis
Acute hepatitis proceeding to chronic hepatitis or cirrhosis
Disorders associated with circulating immune complexes:
   glomerulonephritis, periarteritis, pericarditis, arthritis
Chronic hepatitis
Cirrhosis
Hepatocellular carcinoma
'Healthy' carrier state
Carrier state with immune disorders:
   Down's syndrome, malignant disease, renal failure, organ transplantation

Acute infection at its mildest produces an asymptomatic acquisition of HBsAb or an anicteric hepatitis (Table 6.5). An icteric hepatitis with the entire range of features occurring in HAV may develop. The rise in transaminases tends to be more gradual and prolonged with 20% still abnormal at 1 year (Chow et al., 1989). Fulminant hepatitis, with a mortality of 60–70% occurs in less than 1% of cases. It may occur in infants born to HBsAg positive carrier mothers who are HBeAg negative and anti-HBe positive, perhaps due to viral mutants. It may be due to hepatitis D infection (see hepatitis D).

A range of extrahepatic disorders are associated with HBV infection.

Papular acrodermatitis of childhood (Gianotti-Crosti syndrome)

In children HBV causes a specific flat erythematous non-pruritic papular eruption of the skin of the face and extremities, generalized lymph gland enlargement and hepatomegaly. The rash settles after 2–3 weeks. There is biochemical and pathological evidence of hepatitis which may be acute or chronic. Jaundice is rare.

HBV glomerulopathy

There appears to be an excess of acute and chronic HBV infection in patients with membranous or mesangioproliferative glomerulopathy (GN). HBeAg can be detected in the glomerular deposits. Whether the HBV causes the glomerulopathy or whether the antigens are trapped in abnormal glomeruli is unknown. An excess of HBV infection is not seen in other renal pathologies. The frequency of HBV GN correlates with the prevalence of HBV in that population. Where electron microscopy features are those of a secondary GN the renal lesion is indolent and remits with elimination of HBsAg from serum (Wrzolkowa et al., 1991). With other pathologies the outcome is not different from that in patients who are HBV negative. The spectrum of associated liver disease is wide.

Other extrahepatic manifestations

A serum sickness-like syndrome with fever, abdominal pain, vomiting, nodular, urticarial or pruritic rashes and arthritis, has been described during the prodromal period in children. Vasculitis, mononeuritis, Guillian-Barre' syndrome, pleural or pericardial effusions, and aplastic anaemia are rare complications.

Chronic HBV infection

In chronic carriers HBsAg is present in serum for longer than 6 months. It is not clear why certain patients progress to chronic infection while others clear HBV after acute infection. There is deficiency in interferon production in chronic HBV but this may be secondary to HBV infection. At all ages the reported carrier rate in males is greater than in females and more serious sequelae are more common. The carrier rate is greatest in those infected in early infancy or by 3 years of age. A persistent carrier state occurs in between 70 and 90% of acute infections in infancy and declines to between 6 and 10% of infections which occur after the sixth year of life. It may also be greater in subjects who have a relatively mild clinical hepatitis.

Many with chronic infection have no history of acute disease and are detected because of the finding of HBsAg in the blood on screening or during investigation of features of chronic hepatitis or cirrhosis (see Chapter 15). They may have non-specific features such as anorexia, lethargy or poor weight gain or features of liver disease such as abdominal distension, hepatomegaly, splenomegaly, palmar erythema, spider angiomata with or without abnormal biochemical tests of liver function. Chronic aggressive hepatitis and cirrhosis may be present even if there are no clinical signs and biochemical tests of liver function are normal. The severity of liver damage can only be assessed with further investigation, including ultrasonography, technetium colloid liver scans, percutaneous liver biopsy, laparoscopy and endoscopy.

Natural history of persistent hepatitis B infection: i.e. carriers

It is estimated that with sustained viral replication the life-time risk for death from hepatocellular carcinoma or cirrhosis is 40–50% for men and 15% for women. Data on the natural history of persistent HBV infection in childhood are sparse. Reported studies are usually cross-sectional rather than longitudinal. Infection for as long as 20 years has been documented. There is increasing evidence, however, that there is a tendency for the prevalence of infection to gradually decrease over many months or years.

Serological changes   The HBsAg titre falls slowly. In 2–40% of patients serum HBeAg disappears each year. HBsAg clears months or years later at a rate of 0.6 to 2% per year, and eventually HBsAb appears. The persistence of HBeAg was analysed in an outpatient study in Taipei, of 169 asymptomatic carriers and 59 symptomatic children, with a mean age of 4.8 years, followed for 3.4 years; 48 cleared HBeAg and 45 developed anti-HBe antibodies. The annual HBe clearance rate was less than 2% in the first 3 years of life but increased thereafter, being 35% in children of more than 6 years whose mothers were HBsAg negative and 14% in those whose mothers were HBsAg positive. Symptomatic children, particularly if the serum transaminases were elevated, had annual clearance rates as high as 42% as opposed to 14% in asymptomatic patients. In a study of 90 Spanish children of whom 61 were asymptomatic the clearance rate was 14% (Ruiz-Moreno *et al.*, 1989). In a prospective study of 420 carriers in Taiwan observed for 1–13 years, spontaneous loss of HBsAg occurred in only 10 (0.6%/year) (Hsu *et al.*, 1992).

Evolution of pathological changes   Patients presenting with features of acute hepatitis or with liver biopsy features of chronic persistent hepatitis have a good hepatic prognosis. A few of the latter will go on to chronic aggressive hepatitis. Chronic aggressive hepatitis or bridging necrosis is more frequently associated with cirrhosis. In a prospective study of 292 children (mean age, 5.6 years) with abnormal biochemical tests of liver function 3% had cirrhosis, 44% moderate chronic active hepatitis (CAH), 13% mild CAH, 5% chronic lobular hepatitis and 35% chronic persistent hepatitis (CPH) at presentation. During follow-up over a 1–10 year period (mean 4.0 ± 2.5 years) showed there was little propensity to change. Delta infection, blood transfusion and male sex were more common in those with cirrhosis (Bortolotti et al., 1988).

The evolution of chronic hepatitis B infection in children over 1 to 12 (mean 5) years has been clarified in two further papers from this group. The first comprised 27 children with antibody to hepatitis Be antigen. Severe hepatitis occurred in those with hepatitis B virus DNA in serum. This cleared and the alanine aminotransferase activity normalized within 4 years. In the 15 patients without HBV DNA disease biochemical remission occurred within 1 year in 10 and within 26 months in a further two. Only those two patients who were transfused at birth and two with hepatitis D had chronic liver disease. Of 76 HBeAg positive children aged 1–13 years 44 had CAH with two having cirrhosis. Over a mean period of observation of 5 years 30% remain HBeAg positive without biochemical and pathological improvement. In two with CPH initially, CAH developed; 70% seroconverted permanently to anti-HBe positive and cleared hepatitis B virus DNA from the serum, with permanent normalization of transaminase levels in 93% and improvement in histological features in 25 of 29 rebiopsied (Bortolotti et al., 1990); 9% developed anti-HBs. In a study of 90 children in Madrid of whom 79% had CAH initially the results were similar with an increased severity of histological change in eight of 17 who were still HBe positive and rebiopsied after a mean follow-up of 4 years. In five of seven who seroconverted liver histology had improved on repeat biopsy (Ruiz-Moreno et al., 1989).

In a study of almost 400 adults, many of whom were over 40 years of age, the 5-year survival for CPH, CAH, and CAH with cirrhosis was respectively 97%, 86% and 55%.

Hepatocellular carcinoma

Geographic areas with the highest incidence of hepatocellular carcinoma (HCC) are also the areas with the highest known frequency of chronic HBV infection. In middle-aged men in Taiwan and Japan the yearly incidence of hepatocellular carcinoma in HBsAg positive subjects is more than 200 times that of comparable HBsAg negative controls. Upwards of 60% have coincidental cirrhosis. HBV DNA has been found in the cellular DNA of tumours and tumour cell lines. Thus there is highly suggestive evidence that HBV is one factor causing hepatocellular carcinoma. The high incidence of HBV infection in mothers but not in fathers of patients with hepatocellular carcinoma and the low titre of HBsAg in such patients is compatible with prolonged infection derived from the mothers in the perinatal period or early infancy. Such studies imply a mean carrier duration of 35 years. The youngest reported case is less than 2 years. Every one of 51 consecutive children with HCC in Taiwan had detectable HBsAg either in the blood or in the liver tissue (Hsu, 1987) and seven of 11 cases of HCC in childhood in Germany had positive HBsAg serology. HBV does not have the properties of an oncogenic retrovirus. In Greenland and parts of Alaska where the carrier rate is as high as 20% hepatocellular carcinoma is rare, implying that genetic or other environmental factors, e.g. aflatoxins or other viruses, are required to cause the tumour.

Prevention

Immunization

Subjects at risk should be immunized using highly immunogenic efficacious and safe genetically engineered vaccines, derived from the S protein of HBs, which give protection with doses as low as 0.6 µg and with widely differing regimens. These vaccines are still relatively expensive but are being introduced to universal immunization regimens for infants in countries where the carrier rate is more than 1%. If the immediate risk of infection is high, as it is in an infant born to an HBsAg positive mother or after 'needle stick' or sexual exposure, vaccination (10 µg) should be combined with administration of hepatitis B immunoglobulin (HBIg age 0–4 years, 200 IU; 5–9 300; >9 500) given intramuscularly at a different site *as soon as possible and no later than 48 hours after exposure.*

If the risk of infection is particularly high a repeat dose may be given after 30 days and repeat doses of vaccine at 2 and 6 weeks rather than at 1 and 6 months as in the standard regimen. The efficacy of such management is not 100%. Mass hepatitis B vaccination in Taiwan had a protective efficacy of 85% with 11% of infants carrying hepatitis B surface antigen when a plasma derived vaccine in a dose of 5 µg at 1, 5, 9 and 52 weeks was used with, in addition, hepatitis B immunoglobulin given within 24 hours of birth to infants of mothers who were HBeAg positive. In a study of 235 infants of HBeAg carriers in Hong Kong 3 µg of vaccine at birth, 1, 2 and 6 months gave protection to only 65% but protection was achieved in 80% who also received HBIg at birth and 87% in those given additional doses at monthly intervals for 6 months. Three babies in this study were HBV carriers from birth. The 73 who developed transient and eight with chronic HBV infection, between 3 and 36 months of age, had relatively low antiHBs titres.

Although the best results in preventing perinatal infection have been achieved by combining passive and active immunization at birth, the cost of the specific immunoglobulin is prohibitive in many parts of the world. In areas of high endemicity where perinatal transmission plays the key role in maintaining chronic carriage of HBV, the only realistic hope for HBV control is the universal immunization of all newborns with HBV vaccine, without HBV specific immunoglobulin. Where infection is acquired later it will be more practical and economic to give three dose of the vaccine given in combination with other immunizations starting at 8 weeks of age. This compromise may give the best prospect of protection to the greatest number of children. In areas of very low or intermediate prevalence screening of all antenatal mothers is essential. Limiting screening to those who have had hepatitis during pregnancy, are known drug addicts or whose racial origins are from African, Far East, Middle East or Mediterranean areas, i.e. areas with a high carrier rate, will identify only a percentage of mothers who are infective. Active and passive immunization of newborns at risk with active immunization, in combination with other vaccines, of the rest of the population is essential in areas of intermediate prevalence. Booster doses before puberty are advised.

It is not yet clear how frequently revaccination is necessary. An antibody titre of > 1000 IU/litre will give protection for 5 years. A concentration of 10 IU/litre is believed to be the minimal effective titre. Vaccines of increase immunogenicity incorporating HBe, pre-S, s and mutant virus sequences are being developed.

General measures

All blood to be used for transfusion or plasma-derived products such as anti-haemophiliac globulin must be screened for hepatitis B by the most sensitive method available, and where positive rejected. Disposable needles, adequate sterilization of equipment and safe handling of all clinical specimens is essential.

All HBsAg positive subjects, but particularly those who are HBeAg positive, are potential sources of infection. HBV is present at high concentrations in blood and in infective concentrations in secretions such as saliva and in open sores. HBV persists for a long time in fomites such as toothbrushes. HBV appears to gain entrance via injured or infected skin or mucosa. It may possibly be acquired by ingestion. If infective subjects are identified and they and their attendants advised of the mode of infection, the risks of infection are smaller except within families or in nurseries. The wearing of plastic, disposable gloves when handling blood, secretions, urine or faeces is advisable. Thorough hand washing is also necessary. With such measures infection is rare, even in institutions for mentally retarded children. The risks of infection in ordinary schools is even less.

Treatment for HBV infection

Because chronic hepatitis B infection may be associated with the development of cirrhosis and/or hepatocellular carcinoma several antiviral treatments have been investigated with generally poor results in children, except in those in whom spontaneous clearance of the virus would have been expected. In a recent study (Ruiz-Moreno et al., 1992), recombinant alpha-2-beta-interferon (rα-IFN) given at the dose of 5 or 10 MU/m^2 three times a week was effective in inducing a serological, biochemical and histological remission of disease in approximately 50% of Spanish children treated. These children, however, had histologically active disease and high transaminases at the beginning of the study, suggesting that they were likely to clear the virus spontaneously. Treatment with IFN may have accelerated the natural course of the disease. rα-IFN inhibits intracellular viral replication and may prevent the entry of virus into host cells. It augments the primary antibody response to T cell-dependent antigens, increases the expression of cell surface HLA class I antigens and Fc receptors, and enhances both T cell mediated and natural killer cell cytotoxicity.

The results of a well conducted randomized study of carrier children aged between 2 and 17 years with no features indicative of a propensity to spontaneous cure suggests that a combination of prednisolone for 6 weeks followed by recombinant rα-IFN for 16 weeks may have a role; four of 31 treated in this fashion cleared HBV DNA, four becoming anti-HBe positive and one anti-HBs positive. In contrast 30 receiving placebo were unchanged while one of 29 treated with alpha-interferon alone seroconverted to anti-HBe, anti-HBs.

This study is noteworthy in that only one in the prednisolone interferon group and one in the control had elevated transaminases prior to instituting therapy, and thus spontaneous seroconversion would not be anticipated (Lai et al., 1991). A similar three armed study with steroid or placebo pretreatment followed by a 12-week course of human lymphoblastoid IFN (Wellferon) has just been completed in 118 children (mostly white). Preliminary results show that approximately 30% in both treatment groups became HBeAg negative compared with 17% in control patients (Mieli-Vergani, personal communication).

Prednisolone which decreases inflammatory activity in the liver and may improve well-being still has its advocates although randomized controlled trials in children (Vajro et al., 1985a) and adults indicated that it had an adverse effect on survival and increased the rate of viral replication. Note that both prednisolone withdrawal and rα-IFN treatment have produced fatal liver failure. Further controlled studies using different doses and duration of rα-IFN, carefully stratified for intensity of viral replication, disease activity and age at infection are nevertheless justified.

Sixty percent to 70% of patients who develop fulminant hepatic failure die, unless transplanted. With transplantation the mortality falls to 20–30%. The recipient has less risk of recurrence of HBV infection in the graft than those with chronic HBV infection, in whom HBIg seems to delay infection but does not eradicate it (O'Grady, 1992).

Viral hepatitis type C

In the last 5 years hepatitis C virus (HCV) has been shown to cause the majority of cases of post-transfusion non-A non-B hepatitis and much sporadic, community acquired non-A non-B hepatitis in many parts of the world. A remarkable amount of information has become available in a very short time particularly considering that the virus has still to be convincingly visualized. Given the problems of lack of sensitivity and specificity of the antibody tests used in many early studies of HCV, these should be interpreted with caution. A more precise picture of clinicopathological and epidemiological features should emerge over the next few years with the application of more specific 'second generation' antibody tests and polymerase chain reaction (PCR) techniques.

Aetiology

The hepatitis C virus

After 10 years of intensive effort Houghton and his colleagues (Choo et al., 1989) used an ingenious molecular cloning technique to identify the genome of an agent causing blood-borne non-A non-B hepatitis without isolating the agent. Since then a great deal of work has allowed the genetic location of its structural and non-structural proteins to be inferred. The virus, which has not yet been propagated in tissue culture or visualized, is a single-stranded RNA virus with characteristics intermediate between flaviviruses and pestiviruses. Considerable heterogeneity (22% difference in nucleotide sequencing) exists in different HCV isolates. Three distinct patterns of genetic heterogeneity have already been identified.

Diagnosis   To date the diagnosis of hepatitis C is largely based on methods which use the proteins produced by parts of the C genome in recombinant micro-organisms to detect antibodies found only in HCV infections. Assays of increasing sensitivity and specificity have been developed in the last 2 years. Initial assays detected antibodies to the viral product (C100-3 and C33c from the NS3 and NS4 genomic region) and were often negative until symptoms had been present for 6–12 weeks. False positive results did occur as, for example, that associated with hypergammaglobulinaemia in autoimmune chronic active hepatitis. A four-antigen recombinant immunoblot assay (4-RIBA) which detects anti-C100, anti-5-1-1, anti-C33c and anti-C22-3 simultaneously correlates well with the detection of hepatitis C RNA using nested PCR (see Figure 6.6). This combined assay identified about half of the cases of post-transfusion hepatitis in the first month of the illness compared with 20% using anti-5-1-1 and anti-C100-3 assay.

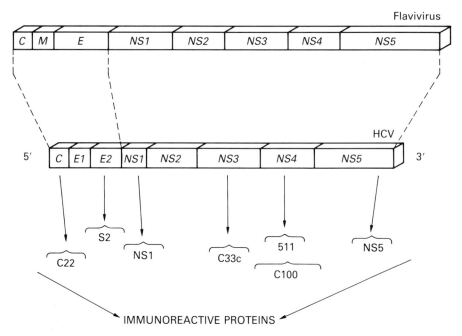

Figure 6.6 Relationship between flavivirus and hepatitis C virus genomes and the protein products used in serological testing for HCV infection. The C regions encode for nucleocapsid or core structural proteins, E regions for envelope structural proteins, NS regions for non-structural proteins of still undefined function. (Reproduced with permission from Alberti (1991)

Given the apparent genetic heterogeneity of HCV it will be crucial to choose appropriate genomic sequences which detect (by PCR techniques) all HCV variants but do not react with other viruses.

Pathology

Intense granular eosinophilic change in scattered hepatocytes, sinusoidal infiltrates of lymphocytes (cytotoxic T and NK) and macrophages, lymphoid aggregates in portal tracts and lymphocytic infiltration of the biliary epithelium are characteristic features although not specific. Chronic persistent or aggressive hepatitis, cirrhosis and hepatocellular carcinoma may develop.

Epidemiological features

At present it appears that the incubation period of hepatitis C is usually between 6 and 12 (range 2–26) weeks following blood transfusion but 4 weeks after the administration of infected coagulation factors. Intrafamilial transmission of HCV appears to be rare occurring in only 8% in a study of almost 200 family members of 107 index cases. Mother to infant transmission has been documented but seems to be much rarer than in hepatitis B infection. Hepatitis C infection appears to be relatively rare in children except in haemophiliacs where up to 90% are affected, and in patients who require many transfusions because of renal failure (20%: Jonas *et al.*, 1992) or leukaemia (25%: Locasciulli *et al.*, 1991).

Studies using first generation assays gave a seroprevalence for anti-HCV in Cameroon which rose from 6.6% in 4 to 6-year-olds to 17.5% for those aged 11 to 14 years (Ngatchu *et al.*, 1992) and was in 0.9% Saudi Arabian children aged 1 to 10 years (Al-Faleigh *et al.*, 1991). The use of clotting factor concentrates that were vapour or wet-heat treated prevented HCV infection in haemophiliacs (Blanchette *et al.*, 1991). In Taiwan, 14 of 144 (9.7%) children (mean age: 3 years, range: 1 month to 15 years) with chronic liver disease (Ding-Shinn *et al.*, 1991) and eight of 22 (36%) with non-A, non-B hepatitis were noted to have anti-HCV seroconversion (Shun-Chien *et al.*, 1991). HCV antibodies were found in 16 of 33 (48%) Italian children with chronic cryptogenic hepatitis (Bortolotti *et al.*, 1992). Between 1/1000 and 1/3000 blood donors in Scotland were HCV positive by PCR testing.

Clinical features

The acute disease is usually asymptomatic (Figure 6.7). There are no specific features which distinguish HCV from other forms of hepatitis except that the serum transaminases do fluctuate by up to 15-fold. Whether HCV causes fulminant non-A, non-B hepatitis is unclear. Chronicity occurs in one-third to three-quarters. Studies in adults suggest that about half of these go on to chronic aggressive hepatitis or cirrhosis. Nine of the 16 Italian children referred to above had a liver biopsy which showed chronic lobular/persistent hepatitis (five), chronic active hepatitis (three) and cirrhosis (one). In only one patient did the transaminase return to normal on follow-up from 1 to 14 (mean 5.4) years. None developed liver failure (Bortolotti *et al.*, 1992). In leukaemic children in long-term remission those who were persistently anti-HCV positive had the most severe histological changes on liver biopsy (Locasciulli *et al.*, 1991). The presence of HCV antibodies has

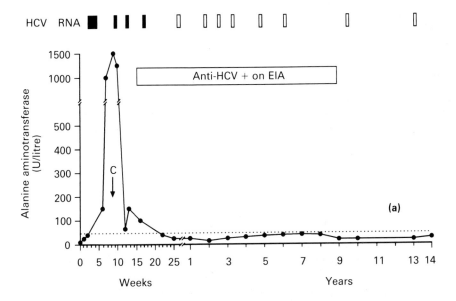

Figure 6.7 (*a*) Biochemical and biological course of acute HCV infection

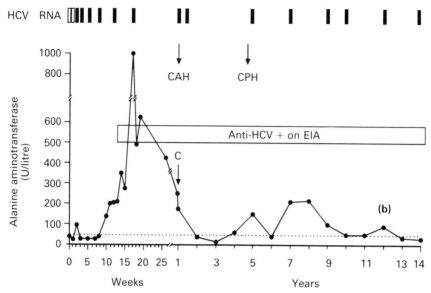

Figure 6.7 (*b*) Acute hepatitis progressing to chronic hepatitis in which serum samples were persistently positive for HCV for up to 14 years. There is a sustained antibody response

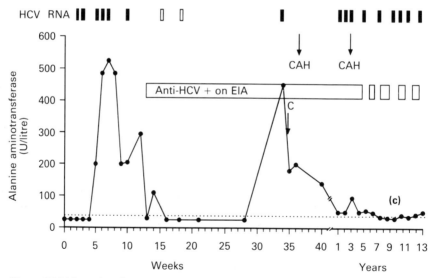

Figure 6.7 (*c*) Intermittently positive HCV RNA in serum with a fluctuating antibody pattern in a patient who progressed chronic active hepatitis 3 years after acute episode? These illustrate that the disappearance of HCV RNA appears to correlate with resolution of hepatitis C while antibody levels do not necessarily remain elevated in patients with chronic disease

●———●   alanine aminotransferase values
....   upper limit of normal solid bars indicate positive assay for HCV RNA by PCR, open bar negative assays.
CAH/CPH   biopsy showing chronic aggressive/persistent hepatitis
C   time of serum sampling of innoculum infective in chimpanzee (from Farci *et al.*, 1985, with permission)

been described in 80% of patients with liver kidney microsomal (LKM) antibody type II autoimmune chronic hepatitis (Lenzi *et al.*, 1990).

Recent reports however have shown that in patients with autoimmune chronic active hepatitis who are positive for anti-LKM antibody, antibodies to p450IID6 were present in 13 of 18 (72%) anti-HCV negative patients but in only 10 of 37 (27%) HCV-infected patients (Ma *et al.*, 1992). The possible role of viral infection in autoimmunity remains to be elucidated.

Prevention and Treatment

Screening of blood donors for anti-HCV and use of vapour-heated and wet heated clotting factor concentrates should decrease the risk of HCV transmission. Interferon therapy for 24–48 weeks in adults with pathologically active disease, reduces serum transaminase activity in about 50% of cases. In these HCV RNA activity disappears from the serum in 4 weeks. Doses have ranged from 0.25 to 10 MU, three times a week. Transaminases values usually revert to pretreatment levels when therapy is stopped. Alpha-lympho-blastoid interferon (3 MU/m^2 three times a week for 48 weeks) given to seven anti-HCV (+) children caused normalization of transaminase levels in six which persisted after 1 to 24 weeks of follow-up (mean: 11 weeks) (Iorio *et al.*, 1992). Similarly, 6 of 14 (43%) children with thalassemia major and chronic hepatitis C infection who were treated with recombinant alpha-interferon (3 MU/m^2 three times a week for 15 months) normalized alanine transaminase from 1 to 15 months from start of treatment with disappearance of HCV RNA in the serum (de Virgilis *et al.*, 1992).

Delta hepatitis

Delta hepatitis is caused by the hepatitis D virus HDV. It occurs only in conjunction with hepatitis B infection. Co-infection causes an acute hepatitis with a greater tendency to be fulminant (2–7%) than HBV alone. Superinfection also causes acute hepatitis and aggravates chronic HBV-related liver damage. Although first identified in 1977 it has been found in sera collected in 1947.

Hepatitis delta virus

This is a very small unclassified virus which is unique in that it requires HBV virus for replication and infectivity. The virus particle, 35–37 nm in diameter, consists of a borrowed HBsAg coat enclosing the HD protein and its single-stranded RNA genome. The variation in clinical expression may be due to genetic heterogeneity. Transmission is by horizontal direct parenteral inoculation or close body contact to subjects simultane-ously infected with HBV or already HBV carriers. It is directly pathogenic.

Epidemiology

Its distribution is worldwide but there is considerable geographical and local variation in prevalence. Peak areas include parts of eastern Europe where up to 60% of adult HBV-infected individuals are also delta-infected, northern South America, the Mediterranean Basin, the Middle East and parts of Africa. All age groups are susceptible. Perinatal infection is infrequent but infection in children, particularly males, can occur in circumstances where HBV spreads horizontally (Buitrago *et al.*, 1986). In the Amazon basin of Brazil, infection rate increases with age from 5% in children less than 10 years of age to 26% in those between 10 and 14 years and >40% in subjects more than 15 years of age (Bensabath *et al*., 1987). Serological evidence of HDV infection was demonstrated in 34 of 270 (12.5%) Italian children who were HBsAg carriers (Farci *et al*., 1985), but in only four of 247 (1.6%) Taiwanese children who had acute or chronic HBV infection (Hsu *et al*., 1988). In the Guangzhou area of China, six of 44 (13.6%) children had superinfection with the delta agent, an identical prevalence to adults (Chen *et al*., 1990).

Clinical and pathological features

Recent studies have shown considerable heterogeneity (Rizetto and Durazzo, 1991). Infection may be asymptomatic whereas initially HDV infection was considered to be consistently associated with clinical evidence of liver disease. *Co-infection* with HBV causes an acute hepatitis in which a biphasic rise in transaminase may occur, the second due to HBV. It may be fulminant in 2–7% but spontaneous recovery with no long-term sequelae is usual. *Superinfection* of HBV carriers causes an exacerbation of liver damage in between 50–90% of those infected (Benhamou, 1991). In the Amazon Basin, delta virus infection was demonstrated in 74% of fulminant hepatitis (Labrea hepatitis) and in 100% of chronic hepatitis B cases (Bensabath *et al*., 1987). Thirty-two of the 44 (73%) cases of fulminant hepatitis were in children less than 15 years of age, 31 of whom were males. In the same study, 44 delta virus-negative HBsAg carriers were followed-up for 1 to 5 years; among these, four males less than 10 years of age became superinfected with HDV and three developed fulminant hepatitis, fatal in two. Postmortem studies of patients with fulminant hepatitis showed eosinophilic necrosis and microvesicular steatosis of the liver. Asymptomatic carriers with minimal hepatitis prior to HDV infection may develop severe chronic hepatitis or cirrhosis; 15% progress to liver failure, a similar percentage eventually achieve remission while the remainder deteriorate over one or two decades. HBV replication is inhibited by HDV infection. Liver damage is most severe in those with active HBV replication. An association with hepatocellular carcinoma has not been demonstrated.

Laboratory detection

IgM antibodies to HDV infection are positive in 80–90% of cases; only transiently in co-infections but persistently in chronic infections. Total antibodies to HDV become positive by 1 month from onset of symptoms. Delta antigen is present in serum in high concentration late in the incubation period and briefly in 20% after onset of acute infections but is detectable only by HDV RNA dot hybridization in other circumstances. Note that HBsAg may be undetectable in a few patients with acute infections but IgM antiHBc is positive.

Treatment is unsatisfactory. Corticosteroids are unhelpful. Interferon reduces HDV RNA and transaminases but the effects are transient. Transplanted livers are reinfected in 80% of cases, hepatitis developing only when HBV markers are fully expressed. HBV vaccination should limit spread of HDV.

Viral hepatitis E

An epidemiological distinct form of non-A, non-B viral hepatitis principally spread by the faecal-oral route is caused by a single-stranded RNA virus, hepatitis E virus (HEV). It is

Table 6.6 Significance of serological investigation in apparent acute viral hepatitis

	1	2	3	4	5	6	7	8	9
Anti-HAV IgM	+	–	–	–	–	–	–	–	–
HBsAg	–	+	–	+	–	+	–	+	–
IgM anti-HBc	–	+	+	+	+	–	–	+	–
Anti-HDV	–	–	–	+	+	+	–	–	–
Anti-HCV	–	–	–	–	–	–	+	+	–
Anti-HEV	–	–	–	–	–	–	–	–	+

1, Acute HAV infection
2, Acute HBV infection or reactivation
3, Acute HBV with early seroconrversion
4, Acute HBV/HDV coinfection
5, Acute HDV infection with HBV suppression
6, Acute HDV infection in HBV carrier
7, Acute HCV infection
8, HBV/HCV coinfection
9, Acute HEV infection

a non-enveloped virus with characteristics of a calicivirus. The viral particle is 32–34 nm in diameter and appears in the stools of patients. Tests for genomic sequence and antibody detection have been developed but as yet have been used in only a small number of studies. Clinicopathological and epidemiological information is thus incomplete.

Pathology

The histological features are as in other forms of viral hepatitis except that ballooning of hepatocytes may be more prominent and the number of polymorphs may be increased disproportionately. Virus-like particles may be seen in bile ductular cells and sinusoidal lining cells. The pathogenesis of liver damage is unknown but it is believed that HEV has a direct cytopathic effect.

Epidemiology

The virus is spread by the faecal-oral route. Massive sewage contamination of drinking water is thought to have caused large epidemics in the subcontinent of India, Central and South-east Asia, the Middle East, parts of Africa, parts of North America, Mexico and the Soviet Union. Clinically evident attack rates are highest in young adults (2.95%) and only 1.4% in those under 14 years. Why children are not affected is unclear. The utilization of recently developed specific serological tests should clarify understanding. In a study of 39 children age 2–14 (mean 6) years with icteric hepatitis in the city of Khartoum 23 (59%) had IgM anti-HEV as had three of 39 age matched controls (Hyams et al., 1992). During the previous 6 months 15 of these cases had been in contact with a jaundiced patient. One hypothesis is that they have subclinical infection in childhood but that subsequent exposure to HEV leads to disease by an immune enhancement mechanism (Reyes et al., 1991). HEV is endemic in developing countries. Travellers are at risk.

Clinical features

The incubation period ranges from 3 to 9 (mean 9) weeks. The symptoms and signs are similar to those of hepatitis A. In the Khartoum study 30% had arthralgia. The illness is generally mild and of short duration. Biochemical results are also similar to those found in hepatitis A. Cases of fulminant hepatitis are reported, especially in pregnant women in whom the mortality rate is 10–20% and fetal complications are common (Tsega *et al.*, 1992). In Western countries the disease may affect people recently arrived from places where it is epidemic or endemic.

Diagnosis is confirmed by detecting genomic sequences in tissues or stool or by detection of antibodies to recombinant HEV antigens, investigations not yet routinely available. Prevention is by improving standards of hygiene. No treatment or prophylaxis are available.

Other viruses sometimes causing hepatitis as the main clinical manifestation

Infectious mononucleosis hepatitis

Infection with the human herpes virus IV (Epstein-Barr virus) leads to a generalized disturbance of the reticulo-endothelial system. The virus induces neoantigens on the surface of B lymphocytes. Reactive T-lymphocytes, the atypical mononuclear cells, produce cytolysis of infected cells. The incubation period is 30–40 days. In developing countries up to 80% are infected by 18 months of age; in affluent countries it is a disease of adolescence and adult life. Infection is usually asymptomatic in the first decade but between 25% and 50% of adolescents and adults get clinical disease. There is commonly enlargement of lymph nodes and pharyngeal lymphatic tissue plus splenomegaly (75%), palatal enanthema (50%), peri-orbital oedema (30%) and a variable exanthema. Pneumonitis and central nervous involvement with benign aseptic meningitis, encephalitis or infectious polyneuritis may also occur. The temperature may rise to 39°C and settle by lysis over a variable period averaging 6 days. In severe cases the temperature may rise to 40–41°C and remain at this level for more than 2 weeks. The virus may be recovered from the pharynx in 80–90% of patients, and may be excreted intermittently for years. It persists for life in lymphoid tissue and may reactivate periodically. Fatal X-linked lymphoproliferative disease (Duncan's syndrome) occurs in boys unable to mount a cytolytic T-cell response. In immunosuppressed patients including liver transplant recipients a fatal lymphoproliferative disorder may develop.

Hepatic features

Hepatic involvement with inflammation and necrosis as shown by raised serum transaminase levels occurs in over 90% of cases. Values may be more than 20 times normal. Histologically there is dense accumulation of large mononuclear cells in and around the portal tracts and within the hepatic parenchyma. The Kupffer cells are large and numerous. There are foci of liver cell necrosis but these are less diffuse than in viral hepatitis. Cholestasis is absent or slight. Recovery is associated with conspicuous mitotic activity in the hepatocytes, sometimes taking as long as 8 months to resolve.

The clinical course is often mild with minimal hepatic enlargement and tenderness, although occasionally this may be severe. Jaundice occurs in 5–15% of cases. It may proceed, follow or occur at the same time as lymph gland enlargement. The course may mimic chronic active hepatitis. Prolonged severe jaundice and even fatal hepatocellular necrosis have been recorded. A haemophagocytic syndrome may develop (Chen *et al.*, 1991).

Diagnosis

The diagnosis is made by a specific IgM antibody to Epstein-Barr virus (EBV), by finding atypical lymphocytes in the peripheral blood or by a positive heterophil antibody test (Paul-Bunnell test). EBV associated nuclear antigen (EBNA) is a marker of cells containing EB viral genome. Where hepatic features are prominent, cytomegalovirus infection and acute hepatitis types A and B are the main differential diagnosis.

Treatment

Most patients require no treatment. Ampicillin or amoxycillin must not be used since they produce an irritating drug rash. Contact sports should be avoided since there is a risk of splenic rupture. Acyclovir inhibits EBV *in vitro* and should be tried in high dose in severe cases although its efficacy is unproved. In severe cases, however, the administration of corticosteroids has a dramatic effect in reducing the size of the hypertrophied lymphoid tissue and should be used in instances of severe hepatitis.

Cytomegalovirus (human herpes virus, Type V)

Cytomegalovirus (CMV) like other herpes viruses is a DNA containing virus which may undergo latency and reactivation years after primary infection. It is transmitted by intimate contact or by blood products, being present in almost all secretions including breast milk and in circulating leucocytes. Perinatal infection occurs in 0.2 to 2.4% of all births (Berge *et al.*, 1990). Up to 5% are symptomatic in the neonatal period with encephalitis the most serious consequence (Peckham, 1991). Urinary and salivary excretion may continue for years. Later infection is usually asymptomatic. It may cause an infectious mononucleosis-like illness in healthy subjects and generalized infection in immunosuppressed patients.

Hepatic features

The characteristic pathological change, which may be observed in any affected tissue, is a multinucleated giant cell with large intranuclear inclusions. Such changes occur primarily in epithelial cells such as those lining the small bile ducts. Bile ductule proliferation and portal tract fibrosis may occur. There may be hepatocellular necrosis and inflammation. Rarely, fatal massive hepatic necrosis occurs. Rarely it is associated with cirrhosis. In transplant recipients it may contribute to chronic rejection.

Clinical features

In infants symptomatic infection is most commonly associated with generalized multisystem disorder acquired *in utero*. Petechiae, jaundice and hepatomegaly occurred in 70% in a recent study (Boppana *et al.*, 1992). Death occurs in 10% from pulmonary or brain involvement. In older children and adolescents symptoms resembling mild acute viral hepatitis or infectious mononucleosis may occur. The majority of patients have hepatomegaly with mildly abnormal biochemical tests of liver function. In those with jaundice, the features are those of a viral hepatitis with transaminases up to 20 times normal and jaundice persisting for up to 3 months. Often infection is asymptomatic or results in only a mild non-specific febrile illness.

Symptomatic disease is most commonly associated with the administration of immunosuppressive or cytotoxic drugs, or following major cardiovascular surgery with cardiopulmonary bypass techniques. In transplant recipients fever and elevated transaminases should raise suspicion of CMV hepatitis (Salt *et al.*, 1990).

Diagnosis of CMV infection is established by the isolation of the virus from the urine, blood or liver, or by antibody tests showing serum conversion and/or by the presence of IgM antibody to cytomegalovirus which can be detected before clinical features appear. It should be noted, however, that CMV may be provoked from latency by immunosuppressive drugs and debilitating illness. Some caution is necessary, therefore, in assuming an aetiological relationship between clinical features and the recovery of the virus from the urine or blood.

Prevention and treatment

An attenuated, live CMV vaccine is being developed (Alford *et al.*, 1990). Immunocompromised patients should only be given CMV negative blood or blood products. Cytomegalovirus-free recipients should receive organs only from donors who have no evidence of CMV infection. Three different prophylactic regimens are effective in 60–75% of liver transplant recipients: intravenous immunoglobulin (IgG: 0.5 mg/kg) at weekly intervals for 6 weeks and acyclovir for 3 months (Stratta *et al.*, 1991); acyclovir (800 mg four times daily for 3 months); ganciclovir (5 mg/kg twice daily for 1 week) followed by acyclovir (800 mg four times daily for 3 months) (Freise *et al.*, 1991).

Successful treatment of CMV disease following liver transplantation has been achieved in 60 of 84 (71%) patients after an initial course of Ganciclovir (5 mg/kg twice daily for 14 days) (Shaefer *et al.*, 1991).

Herpes simplex hepatitis

Herpetic hepatitis occurs particularly in infants with generalized herpetic disease and in children or adults who are immunosuppressed. It does occur in adults previously considered to be well.

Hepatic features

Hepatomegaly with tenderness, raised serum transaminases and a prolonged prothrombin time are the main manifestations. Fulminant hepatic failure is frequent in identified cases (Benador *et al.*, 1990). On liver biopsy, small punctate areas of haemorrhagic necrosis with a variable mononuclear reaction are seen (Brooks *et al.*, 1991). Cutaneous lesions are a useful diagnostic clue but are absent in 40% of affected neonates (Koskiniemi *et al.*, 1989). There may be typical intranuclear inclusion bodies. The diagnosis is established by virus isolation or identification using immunofluorescent or electron microscopic techniques.

Prevention and treatment

Immunosuppressed patients should avoid contact with overt herpetic lesions. Acyclovir in a dose of 10–20 mg/kg/day given in 8-hourly boluses and continued for a minimum of 5 days controls the infection.

Other common viral illnesses of childhood frequently causing anicteric hepatitis

All viruses probably affect the liver in common with other organs. Occasionally the patient may be frankly icteric. In the majority hepatic infection is detected only by a rise in serum transaminases, the patient having no hepatic symptoms. Rarely, the patient may develop fulminant hepatic failure. Virus-related hepatitis of this form is identified most commonly in patients who are immunosuppressed or patients who have underlying liver diseases. Common viruses implicated include measles, varicella, mumps, rubella, adenoviruses, ECHO and coxsackie virus. Neonates may be at particular risk of ECHO and adenovirus hepatitis. Note that features of hepatic involvement may appear before cutaneous lesions. Paramyxovirus-like particles have been associated with a severe giant cell hepatitis in childhood (Phillips *et al.*, 1991). Reovirus 3 has a contentious association with hepatobiliary disease in infancy.

Hepatic involvement in acquired immune deficiency syndrome   The human immunodeficiency virus type 1 (HIV-I) does not cause a specific liver lesion but it predisposes to focal infection which may be granulomatous; malignancy of any liver component; to chronic hepatotropic infection by hepatitis A, B or C, or non-specific changes due to cachexia. The cellular response to infection may be attenuated. Neonatal infection may be associated with giant cell hepatitis (Witzleben *et al.*, 1988). Hepatic pathological findings in children include: giant cell transformation, CMV inclusions, Kaposi sarcoma, chronic active hepatitis, lymphoplasmacytic infiltrate and granulomatous hepatitis secondary to fungal infection (Jonas *et al.*, 1989; Kahn *et al.*, 1991). A fibrosarcoma of the liver developed in an 8-year-old (Ninane *et al.*, 1985). Diagnosis is suspected from the clinical features, the immunological abnormalities and confirmed by specific antibody tests. Azidothymidine and treatment of opportunist infection may reverse temporarily some of the features.

Mosquito borne viral hepatitis

Yellow fever hepatitis

Hepatitis may occur as part of the generalized illness caused by the Group 4 arbovirus (*Flavivirus febricus*), a round 30–40 nm enveloped RNA virus. The infection is transmitted in enzootic areas in Africa and South America by the bite of the infected mosquito which acquires its infection from humans in the urban variety but from primates in the jungle variety. Infection is endemic but, rarely, epidemics may occur. The incubation period is 4–6 days. The disease varies in severity from a subclinical infection to a fatal illness: 5–10% of cases die.

Pathology

Within 24 hours of onset there is acidophilic necrosis of Kupffer cells followed a few days later by the characteristic hepatic lesion of a diffuse severe necrosis of hepatocytes in midzone of the hepatic lobule with little inflammatory change. Occasionally the hepatic necrosis may be diffuse. Some fatty change may occur in the hepatocytes. The connective tissue does not proliferate and no permanent scarring occurs if the patient recovers. Similar changes in the myocardium and renal tubules are equally important clinically.

Clinical aspects

Jaundice appears on the fourth to fifth day of an illness characterized by fever, prostration and headache. The liver is tender but not enlarged. Splenomegaly is unusual. In the malignant form a haemorrhagic diathesis occurs.

The diagnosis may be suspected on the basis of prolonged fever with a slowing of the pulse rate due to cardiac involvement, albuminuria, and hepatic features in the absence of hepatosplenomegaly. Leptospirosis is the main differential diagnosis. Confirmation may be made by antibody tests (complement fixation test and haemagglutination test) or virus isolation. Liver biopsy is contraindicated.

There is no specific treatment. Supportive care, correction of hypotension, and conservative management of renal failure may be required.

From the age of 6 months the disease may be prevented by vaccination which provides protection for at least 10 years. With currently available vaccine reactions are rare, but allergy to egg is a contraindication to their use.

Dengue haemorrhagic fever

This is a multisystem disorder caused by the dengue virus, a mosquito-borne member of the flavivirus group. India, South-East Asia, the West Pacific and Cuba are areas of high prevalence. The incubation period is 1–7 days. Children typically are affected. The illness is characterized by fever, myalgia, a bleeding diathesis and shock due to increased vascular permeability. Soft tender hepatomegaly and raised transaminase levels to levels 5–15 times normal are associated with mid-zonal necrosis, Kupffer cell hyperplasia and sinusoidal infiltration (Wang *et al.*, 1990). Rarely the presentation may be acute liver failure (George *et al.*, 1988). Diagnosis is confirmed by rising concentrations of antibodies to dengue antigen. Treatment is by fluid and colloid replacement for shock and blood and platelet infusions. Prevention is dependent on mosquito control. Some live attenuated vaccines are available and others are being assessed.

Enzootic 'exotic' hepatitis

The term 'exotic viruses' has been applied to some viral illnesses which affect animals as well as humans. Although exotic outside the area of distribution of hosts or vectors where they cause significant morbidity, because of air travel they may now occur anywhere. Nosocomial infection is a hazard.

Lassa fever is a multisystem disorder caused by an RNA containing arenavirus. Its host reservoir is a West African rat which excretes it in urine throughout life. Patients shed the virus for a month after infection. The disorder has been increasingly recognized in West Africa and in visitors returning from that area. After an incubation period of 3–17 days an infection which ranges from asymptomatic to lethal develops. Shock due to increased capillary permeability is a critical pathogenic mechanism. The liver is the major target organ. Diffuse hepatocellular necrosis, eosinophilic necrosis, prominent macrophages and increased mitotic activity are prominent histological features. Fetal and neonatal infections occur producing a 'swollen-baby syndrome' with oedema, ascites and a bleeding diathesis. A perinatal death rate of nearly 90% has been recorded (Price *et al.*, 1988). Diagnosis is established by virus isolation in specially equipped laboratories or by rising antibody levels which become apparent in the second week of the illness. Therapy with intravenous ribavirin 60 mg/kg/day starting within 6 days of onset of fever is effective if the transaminase levels and severity of viraemia are low (McCormick *et al.*, 1986).

Ebola virus infection and the rare *Marburg virus* disease are unusual viral infections in which the liver appears to be a major target organ. Species of monkeys in Sudan and Zaire are the putative hosts. Eosinophilic necrosis of hepatocytes with Kupffer cell hyperactivity are the main pathological findings. There may be confluent hepatic necrosis. Serum transaminases are raised, jaundice may occur.

Bunyaviridae are a large family of spherical enveloped RNA viruses a few species of which cause liver damage in humans. *Rift valley fever* is caused by a plebovirus found in domestic and wild animals and mosquitos in Africa and in Central and South America. After an incubation period of 3 to 6 days a generalized febrile illness with lymphadenopathy and petechiae develops. There may be widespread hepatic necrosis. Jaundice developing on the sixth day of the illness carries a poor prognosis. Vaccines for animal are available but not for humans! The *Crimean-Congo virus* which infects ticks and birds as well as animals causes a similar illness with even more purpura and a higher mortality. It is found in the Middle East and Pakistan as well as in Russia and Africa. There is as yet no specific treatment for any of these infections (Zuckerman and Ellis, 1991).

Bibliography and references

General

Balistreri, W. F. (1988) Viral hepatitis. *Pediatr. Clin. N. Amer.,* **35**, 637–69
Feinstone, S. and Gust, I. (1991) Hepatitis A. In *Oxford Textbook of Clinical Hepatology* (eds. N. McIntyre, J.-P. Benhamou, J. Bricher, Rizzetto and J. Rodes). Oxford Medical Publications, Oxford. pp.565–571
Hollinger, F. B., Lemon, S. M. and Margolis, H. S. (Eds) (1991) Viral Hepatitis and Liver Disease. Baltimore: Williams and Wilkins, 135–148.
Mieli-Vergani, G. Viral Hepatitis in Children (in press)
Zuckermann, A. (Ed.) (1990) Viral hepatitis. *British Medical Bulletin,* **46**, 300–684
Zuckermann, A. and Howard, H. C. (Eds) Viral hepatitis. (in press)

Hepatitis A

Amesty-Valbuena, A., Gonzalez-Pirela, Y. and Rivero, M. (1989) Seroepidemiologic study of hepatitis A virus among children of Maracaibo, Venenzuela. *Invest. Clin.,* **30**, 215–228
Azimi, P. H., Roberto, R. R. and Guralnick, J. *et al.* (1986) Transfusion acquired hepatitis A in a premature infant with secondary nosocomial spread in an intensive care nursery. *Am. J. Dis. Child.,* **140**, 23–27
Blaine-Hollinger, F., Andre, F. E. and Melnick, J. (Eds) (1992) Proceedings of the International Symposium on Active Immunization against Hepatitis A, Vienna, 27–29 January, *Vaccine,* **10**, 97–103
Boughton, C. R. (1991) Hepatitis A vaccine. *Med. J. of Aust.,* **155**, 508–509
Chin, K. P., Lok, A. S., Wong, L. S., Lai, C. L. and Wu, P. C. (1991) Current seroepidemiology of hepatitis A in Hong Kong. *J. Med. Virol.,* **34**, 191–193
Chiriaco, P., Guadalupi, C., Armigliato, M., Bortolotti, F. and Realdi, G. (1986) Polyphasic course of hepatitis A in children. *J. Infect. Dis.,* **153**, 378–379
Chow, C. B., Lau, T. T. Y., Leung, N. K. and Chang, W. K. (1989) Acute viral hepatitis: aetiology and evolution. *Arch. Dis. Childh.,* **64**, 211–213
Colepis, A. G., Locarnini, S. A., Lehmann, N. I. and Gust, I. D. (1980) Detection of hepatitis A virus in the faeces of patients with naturally acquired infections. *J. Infect. Dis.,* **141**, 151–156
Fagan, E. A., Yousef, G., Brham, J. *et al.* (1990) Persistence of hepatitis A virus in fulminant hepatitis and after liver transplantation. *J. Med. Virol.,* **30**, 131–136
Garcia-Puga, J. M., Toledano Cantero, E. and Ballesta Rodriguez, M. (1989) Outbreak of hepatitis A in day nursery: diagnosis and follow-up in a pediatric clinic. *Acta. Primaria,* **6**, 478–481, 484–485
Gordon, S. C., Reddy, R., Schiff, L. and Schiff, E. (1984) Prolonged intrahepatic cholestasis secondary to acute hepatitis A. *Ann. Intern. Med.,* **101**, 635–637
Gregory, P. B., Knauer, C. M., Kempson, R. L. and Miller, R. (1876) Steroid therapy in severe viral hepatitis A: a double blind, randomised trial of methyl-prednisolone versus placebo. *N. Engl. J. Med.* **294**, 681–687

Gust, I. D. and Feinstone, S. M. (1988) Epidemiology. In: *Hepatitis A*. CRC Press, Florida, pp.163–191

Gust, I. D. (1988) Prevention and control of hepatitis A. In *Viral Hepatitis and Liver Disease* (ed. A. J. Zuckerman). Alan R Liss, New York, 77–80

Hadler, S. C. and McFarland, L. (1986) Hepatitis in day care centers: epidemiology and prevention. *Rev. Infect. Dis.,* **8**, 548–557

Hermier, M., Descos, B., Collet, J. P., Philber, M., Pouillaude, J. P. and Pacros, J. P. (1985) Acute cholecystitis disclosing A virus hepatitis. *Arch. Fr. Ped., 42*, 525–529

Innis, B. L., Snitbhan, R., Kunasol, P. *et al.* (1992) Protection against hepatitis A by an inactivated vaccine (*Proceedings of the satellite symposium of the IX Asian-Pacific Congress of Gastroenterology and the VI Asian-Pacific Congress of Digestive Endoscopy*). Bangkok, Thailand, p 16

Innis, B. L., Snitbhan, R., Hoke, C. H., Munindhorn, W. and Laorakpongse, T. (1991) The declining transmission of hepatitis A in Thailand. *J. Infect. Dis., 163*, 989–995

Kurane, I., Binn, L. N., Bancroft, W. H. and Ennis, F. A. (1985) Human lymphocyte responses to hepatitis A virus-infected cells: interferon production and lysis of infected cells. *J. Immunol., 135*, 2140–2144

McNeill, M., Hoy, J. F., Richards, M. J. *et al.* (1984) Aetiology of fatal viral hepatitis in Melbourne, a retrospective study. *Med. J. Aust., 141*, 637–640

Najarian, R., Caput, D., Gee, W. *et al.* (1985) Primary structure and gene organisation of human hepatitis A virus. *Proc. Natl. Acad. Sci. USA, 82*, 2627–2631

Noble, R. C., Kane, M. A., Reeves, S. A. and Roeckel, I. (1984) Post-transfusion hepatitis A in a neonatal intensive care unit. *J. Amer. Med. Assoc., 252*, 2711–2715

O'Grady, J. G., Gimson, A. E. S., O'Brien, C. J., Pucknell, A., Hughes, R. and Williams, R. (1988) Controlled trial of charcoal haemoperfusion and prognostic indicators in fulminant hepatic failure. *Gastroenterology,* **94**, 1186–1192

Prince, A. M., Brotman, B., Richardson, L., White, T., Pollock, N. and Riddle, J. (1985) Incidence of hepatitis A virus (HAV) infection in rural Liberia. *J. Med. Virol., 15*, 421–428

Ramsay, C. N. and Upton P. A. (1989) Hepatitis A and frozen raspberries. *Lancet, 1*, 43–44

Robertson, B. H., Khanna, B., Naiman, O. V. and Margolis, H. S. (1991) Epidemiologic patterns of wild-type hepatitis A virus determined by genetic variation. *J. Infect. Dis., 163*, 286–292

Rosenblum, L. S., Villarino, M. E., Nainan, O. V. *et al.* (1991) Hepatitis A outbreak in a neonatal intensive care unit: risk factors for transmission and evidence of prolonged viral excretion among preterm infants. *J. Infect. Dis.* **164**, 476–482

Shimizu, H., Takebayashi, T., Goto, M. and Togashi, T. (1984) Studies on an outbreak of hepatitis A in an institution for the mentally retarded children. *Hokkaido Igaku Zasshi, 59*, 247–253

Sjogren, M. H., Hoke, C. H., Binn, L. N. *et al.* (1991) Immunogenicity of an inactivated hepatitis A vaccine. *Ann. Intern.Med., 114*, 470–471

Sjogren, M. H., Tanno, H., Fay, O. *et al.* (1987) Hepatitis A virus in stools during clinical relapse. *Ann. Intern. Med., 106*, 221–226

Song, Y. (1991) The investigation of anti-hepatitis A virus antibody rate in Guangzhou population. *Chung-Hua-Liu-Hsing-Ping-Hsueh-Tsa-Chih, 12*, 265–268

Stuart, J. M., Majeed, F. A., Cartwright, K. A. V., Room, R., Parry, J. V., Perry, K. R. and Begg, N. T. (1992) Salivary antibody testing in a school outbreak of hepatitis A. *Epidemiol. Infect., 109*, 161–6

Sun, Y. D., Zhang, Y. C., Ren, Y. H. and Meng, Z. D. (1988) Clinical/subclinical case ratio in hepatitis A. *Lancet,* **2**, 1082–83

Vallbracht, A., Gabriel, P., Maier, K. *et al.* (1986) Cell-mediated cytotoxicity in hepatitis A virus infection. *Hepatology, 6*, 1308–1314

Vento, S., Garofano, T., Di Perri, G., Dolci, L., Concia, E. and Bassetti, G. (1991) Identification of hepatitis A virus as a trigger for autoimmune chronic hepatitis type 1 in susceptible individuals. *Lancet, 337*, 1183–1187

Werzberger, A., Mensch, B., Kuter, B. *et al.* (1992) A controlled trial of a formalin-inactivated hepatitis A vaccine in healthy children. *N. Eng. J. Med., 327*, 453–457

Ye, J. Y. (1990) Outcome of pregnancy complicated by hepatitis A in the urban districts of Shanghai. *Chung-Hua-Fu-Chan-Ko-Tsa-Chih, 25*, 219–221

Yong, P. (1992) Epidemiology of hepatitis A. (*Proceedings of the satellite symposium of the IX Asian-Pacific Congress of Gastroenterology and the VI Asian-Pacific Congress of Digestive Endoscopy*). Bangkok, Thailand, p 8

Zuckerman, J. N., Cockcroft, A. and Griffiths, P. (1991) Hepatitis A immunization. *Br. Med. J., 303*, 247

Hepatitis B

Beasley, R. P., Hwang, L. Y., Lin, C. C. *et al.* (1982) Incidence of hepatitis B virus infections in preschool children in Taiwan. *J. Infect Dis., 142*, 198–204

Beasley, R. P., Hwang, L. Y., Lee, G. C. Y. *et al.* (1983) Prevention of perinatally transmitted hepatitis B virus infection with hepatitis B immune globulin and hepatitis B vaccine. *Lancet,* **2,** 1099–1102

Berris, B. and Feinman, S. V. (1991) Thyroid dysfunction and liver injury following alpha-interferon treatment of chronic viral hepatitis. *Dig. Dis. Sci.,* **36,** 1657–1660

Bhota, J. F., Ritchie, M. J. J., Dusheko, J. M., Mouton, H. W. K. and Kew, M. C. (1984) Hepatitis B virus carrier state in black children in Ovamboland: role of perinatal and horizontal infection. *Lancet,* **1,** 1210–1212

Bortolitto, F., Cadrobbi, P., Crivellaro, C. *et al.* (1990) Long-term outcome of chronic Type B hepatitis in patients who acquire hepatitis B virus infection in childhood. *Gastroenterology,* **99,** 805–810

Bianchi, L. (1982) The immunopathology of acute type B hepatitis. In: *Immunological Aspects of Liver Disease,* (eds H. C. Thomas, P. A. Miescher and H. J. Mueller-Eberhard). Springer Verlag, Berlin, p. 141

Bortolotti, F., Caizia, R., Cadrobbi, P., Giacchini, R. and Ciravegna, B. (1986) Liver cirrhosis associated with chronic hepatitis B virus infection in childhood. *J. Pedatr.* **108,** 224

Bortolotti, F., Calzia, R., Vegnente, A. *et al.* (1988) Chronic hepatitis in childhood: the spectrum of the disease. *Gut,* **29,** 659–64

Bortolotti, F., Calzia, R., Cadrobbi, P., Crivellaro, C., Alberti, A. and Marazzi, G. (1990) Long-term evolution of chronic hepatitis B in children with antibody to hepatitis Be antigen. *J. Pediatr,* **116,** 552–555

Brown, J. L., Carman, W. F. and Thomas, H. C. (1992) The clinical significance of molecular variation within the hepatitis B virus genome, *Hepatology,* **15,** 144–8

Cadrobbi, P., Bortolotti, M., Zaccheloo, Z. *et al.* (1985). Hepatitis B virus replication in acute glomerulo-nephritis with chronic, aggressive hepatitis. *Arch. Dis. Childh.* **65,** 83

Carman, W. F. and Thomas, H. C. (1992) Genetic variation in hepatitis B virus. *Gastroenterology,* **102,** 711–19

Carman, W. F., Zanetti, A. R., Karayiannis, P. *et al.* (1990) Vaccine-induced escape mutant of hepatitis B virus. *Lancet,* **2,** 325–329

Chang, M. H., Lee, C. Y., Chen Ding-Shinn, Hsu, H. C. and Lai, M. Y. (1987) Fulminant hepatitis in children in Taiwan: the important role of hepatitis B virus. *J. Pediatr.,* **111,** 34–39

Chang, M. H., Sung, J. L., Lee, C. Y. *et al.* (1989) Factors affecting clearance of hepatitis B e antigen in hepatitis B surface antigen carrier children. *J. Pediatr,* **115,** 385–90

Chow, C. B., Lau, T. T. Y., Leung, N. K. and Chang, W. K. (1989) Acute viral hepatitis: aetiology and evolution. *Arch. Dis Childh.,* **64,** 211–213

Chu, C. M., Karayiannis, P., Fowler, M. J., Monjardino, J., Liaw, Y. F. and Thomas, H. C . (1985) Natural history of chronic hepatitis B virus infection in Taiwan: studies of hepatitis B virus DNA in serum. *Hepatology,* **5,** 431–434

Draelos, Z. K., Hansen, R. C., Tuscon, M. A. J. and James, W. D. (1986) Gianotti Crosti Syndrome associated with infections other than hepatitis B. *J. Am. Med. Assc.,* **256,** 2386–2388

Dusheiko, G. and Hoofnagle, J. (1991) Hepatitis B. In: *Oxford Textbook of Clinical Hepatology* (Eds. McIntyre N, Benhamou JP, Bircher J, Rizzetto M, Rodes J). Oxford University Press, Oxford

Egea, E., Iglesias, A., Salazar, M. *et al.* (1991) The cellular basis for lack of antibody response to hepatitis B vaccine in humans, *J. Exp. Med.,* **173,** 531–538

Ewing, C. I. and Davidson, D. C. (1985). Fatal hepatitis B in infant born to a HB$_s$Ag carrier with HB$_e$Ab. *Arch. Dis. Childh.* **60,** 265

Fattovich, G., Cadrobbi, P., Crivellaro, C. *et al.* (1982) Virological changes in chronic hepatitis type B treated with laevamisole. *Digestion,* **25,** 131–135

Friede, A., Harris, J. R., Kobayashi, J. M., Shaw, F. E., Shoemaker-Nawas, P. C., Kane, M. A. (1988) Transmission of hepatitis B virus from adopted Asian children to their American families. *Am. J. Public Health,* **78,** 26–29

Ganem, D. andVarmus, H. E. (1987) The molecular biology of the hepatitis B viruses *Annu Rev Biochem,* **56,** 651–693

Giusti, G., Piccinino, F., Sagnelli, E., Ruggiero, G., Galanti, B. and Gallo, C. (1988) Immunosuppressive therapy of HBsAg positive chronic active hepatitis in childhood: a multicentre retrospective study on 139 patients. *J. Pediatr. Gastroenterol. and Nutr.,* **7,** 17–21

Grathwohl, J., Ndumbe, P., Leke, R., Uy, A., Gerlich, W. H. and Repp, R. (1992) Perinatale hepatitis-B-virus-ubertragung, Monatsschrift Kinderheilkunde **140,** 366–368

Gussetti, N., Lagaiolli, G. and D'Elia, R. (1988) Absence of maternal antibodies to hepatitis B core antigen and HBV vertical transmission: one cause of infection not withstanding passive-active prophylaxis. *Infection,* **16,** 167–170

Hadziyannis, S. (1991) Diagnostic flow chart in the hepatitis B carrier. In: *Oxford Textbook of Clinical Hepatology* (Eds. N. McIntyre, J. P. Benhamou, J. Bircher, M. Rizzetto, J. Rodes). Oxford University Press, Oxford

Hashida, T., Sawada, T., Esumi, N., Kinugasa, A., Kusunoki, T. and Kishida, T. (1985) Therapeutic effects of human leukocyte interferon on chronic active hepatitis B in children. *J. Pediatr. Gastroenterol. Nutr.,* **4**, 20–25

Hofmann, H., Tuma, W., Heinz, FX. and Kunz, C. (1990) Relevance of hepatitis B DNA detection in patient's serum. *Int. J. Med. Microbiol.,* **272**, 485–497

Hsu, H. C., Wu, M. Z., Chang, M. J., Su, I. J. and Chen, D. S. (1987) Childhood hepatocellular carcinoma develops exclusively in hepatitis B surface antigen carriers in three decades in Taiwan: a report of 51 cases strongly associated with rapid development of liver cirrhosis. *J. Hepatol,* **5**, 260–267

Hsu, H. C., Lin, Y. H., Chang, M. H., Su, I. J. and Chen, D. S. (1988) Pathology of chronic hepatitis B virus infection in children with special reference to the intrahepatic expression of hepatitis virus antigens. *Hepatology,* **8**, 378–382

Hsu, H. C., Chang, M. H., Lee, C. Y. and Chen, D. S. (1988) Fulminant hepatitis in infants in Taiwan: strong association with hepatitis Be antigen-negative but antibody-positive maternal hepatitis B surface antigen carriage. *J. Gastroenterol. Hepatol.,* **3**, 1–7

Hsu, H. Y., Chan, M. H., Chen, D. S. and Lee, C. Y. (1988) Hepatitis D virus infection in children with acute or chronic hepatitis B virus infection in Taiwan. *J. Pediatr.,* **112**, 888–892

Hsu, H. Y., Chang, M. H., Lee, C. Y., Chen, J. S., Hsu, H. C. and Chen, D. S. (1992) Spontaneous loss of HBsAg in children with chronic hepatitis B virus infection. *Hepatology,* **15**, 382–386

Immunization Practices Advisory Committee (1988) Prevention of perinatal transmission of hepatitis B virus: prenatal screening of all pregnant women for hepatitis B surface antigen. *MMWR,* **37**, 341–351

Jacyna, M. R. and Thomas, H. C. (1990) Antiviral therapy: hepatitis B. *Brit. Med. Bull.,* **46**, 368–382

Jonas, M. M., Ragin, L. and Silva, M. O. (1991) Membranous glomerulonephritis and chronic persistent hepatitis B in a child: treatment with recombinant iterferon alfa. *J. Pediatr.,* **119**, 818–820.

Keller, K. M., Poralla, T., Dienes, H. P., Wirth, S. and Baumann, W. (1990) Cellular cytotoxicity against autologous hepatocytes in children with different forms of chronic hepatitis B, *Eu.r J. Pediatr.,* **149**, 829–832

Kiire, C. F. (1990) Hepatitis B infection in sub-Saharan Africa. The African Regional Study Group. *Vaccine,* **8**, S107–112

Kojima, M., Shimizu, M., Tsuchimochi, T. *et al.* (1991) Posttransfusion fulminant hepatitis B associated with precore-defective HBV mutants. *Vox Sang,* **60**, 34–39

Kosaka, Y., Takase, K., Kojima, M. *et al.* (1991) Fulminant hepatitis B: Induction by hepatitis B virus mutants defective in the precore region and incapable of encoding e antigen. *Gastroenterology,* **100**, 1087–1094

La Banda, F., Ruiz-Moreno, M., Carreno, V. *et al.* (1988) Recombinant alpha 2-interferon treatment in children with chronic hepatitis B. *Lancet,* **1**, 25

La Manna, A., Polito, C., Del Gado, R., Olivieri, A. N. and Di Toro, R. (1985) Hepatitis B surface antigenaemia and glomerulopathies in children. *Acta. Paediatr. Scand.,* **74**, 122–125

Lai, C. L., Lok, A. S. F, Lin, H. J. *et al* (1987) Placebo controlled trial of recombinant -interferon in Chinese HBsAg carrier children. *Lancet,* **ii**, 877–880

Lai, C. L., Lin, H. J., Lau, J. Y. N. *et al.* (1991) Effect of recombinant α2 interferon with or without prednisolone in Chinese HBsAg carrier children. *Q. J. Med.,* **78**, 155–163

Lau, J. Y. N., Bain, V. G., Davies, S. E. *et al.* (1992) High-level expression of hepatitis B viral antigens in fibrosing cholestatic hepatitis. *Gastroenterology,* **102**, 956–962

Lee, S. D., Lo, K. J., Tsai, Y. T. *et al.* (1989) HBsAg carrier infants with serum anti-HBc negativity, *Hepatology,* **9**, 102–4.

Lee, S. D., Lo, K. J., Tsai, Y. T. *et al.* (1988) Role of caesarian section in the prevention of mother-infant transmission of hepatitis B. *Lancet,* **ii**, 833

Leuschner, I., Harms, D. and Schmidt, D. (1988) The association of hepatocellular carcinoma in childhood with hepatitis B virus infection. *Cancer,* **62**, 2363–2369

Lok, A. S. F. and Lai, C. L. (1988) A longitudinal follow-up of asymptomatic hepatitis B surface antigen positive Chinese children. *Hepatology,* **8**, 1130–1133

Lok, A. S. F., Liang, R. H. S., Chiu, E. K. W., Wong, K. L., Chan, T. K. and Todd, D. (1991) Reactivation of hepatitis B virus replication in patients receiving cytotoxic therapy, *Gastroenterology,* **100**, 182–188.

Lok, A. S. F., Wu, P-C., Lai, C-L. *et al.* (1992) A controlled trial of interferon with or without prednisone priming for chronic hepatitis B. *Gastroenterology,* **102**, 2091–2097

Maynard, J. E., Kane, M. A., Alter, M. J. and Hadler, S. C. (1988) Control of hepatitis B by immunization: global perspectives. In: *Viral Hepatitis and Liver Disease* (Ed. A. J. Zuckerman). Alan R Liss, New York, 967–969

Mondelli, M. and Eddleston, A. L. W. F. (1984) Mechanisms of liver cell injury in acute and chronic hepatitis B. *Sem. Liver Dis.,* **4**, 47–58

Mondelli, M. U., Bortolotti, F., Pontisso, P. *et al.* (1987) Definition of hepatitis B virus (HBV)-specific target antigens recognised by cytotoxic T cells in acute HBV infection. *Clin. Exp. Immunol.,* **68**, 242–250

Mondelli, M., Mieli-Vergani, G., Bortolotti, F. *et al.* (1985) Different mechanisms responsible for in vitro cell-mediated cytotoxicity to autologous hepatocytes in children with autoimmune and HBsAg positive chronic liver disease. *J. Pediatrics,* **106**, 899–906

Moriyama, K., Nakajima, E., Hohjoh, H., Asayama, R. and Okochi, K. (1991) immunoselected hepatitis B virus mutant (letter). *Lancet,* **337**, 8733

Naoumov, N. V., Schneider, R., Grotzinger, T. *et al.* (1992) Precore mutant hepatitis B virus infection and liver disease. *Gastroenterology.* **102**, 538–543

O'Grady, J. G., Smith, H. M., Davies, S. E. *et al.* (1992) Hepatitis B virus reinfection after orthotopic liver transplantation serological and clinical implications, *J. Hepatology,* **14**, 104–111.

Omata, M., Ehata, T., Yokosuka, O., Hosoda, K. and Ohto, M. (1991) Mutations in the precore region of hepatitis B virus DNA in patients with fulminant and severe hepatitis. *New Engl. J. Med.,* **324**, 1699–1704

Penna, A., Fowler, P., Bertoletti, A. *et al.* (1992) Hepatitis B Virus (HBV)-specific cytotoxic T-cell (CTL) response in humans: characterization of HLA class II-restricted CTLs that recognize endogenously synthesized HBV envelope antigens, *J. Virology,* **66**, 1193–1198.

Pignatelli, M., Waters, J., Lever, A., Iwarson, S., Gerety, R. and Thomas, H. C. (1987) Cytotoxic T-cell responses to the nucleocapsid proteins of HBV in chronic hepatitis. Evidence that antibody modulation may cause protracted infection. *J. Hepatol.,* **4**, 15–21

Pontisso, P., Morsica, G., Ruvoletto, MG. *et al.* (1991) Latent hepatitis B virus infection in childhood hepatocellular carcinoma. In: *HBV in HBsAg-Negative Hepatocellular Carcinoma.* Universita di Padova, Italy.

Rossetti, F., Cesaro, S., Pizzocchero, P., Cadrobbi, P., Guido, M. and Zanesco, L. (1992) Chronic hepatitis B surface antigen-negative hepatitis after treatment of malignancy. *J. Pediatr.,* **121**, 39–43

Ruiz-Moreno, M., Camps, T., Aguardo, J. G. *et al.* (1989) Serological and histological follow up of chronic hepatitis infection. *Arch. Dis. Childh.,* **64**, 1165–1169.

Ruiz-Moreno, M., Rua, M. J., Molina, J. *et al.,* (1991) Prospective randomized controlled trial of interferon-α in children with chronic hepatitis B. *Hepatology,* **13**, 1035–1039

Ruiz-Moreno, M., Rua, M. J., Moraleda, G., Guardia, L., Moreno, A. and Carreno, V. (1992) Treatment with interferon gamma versus interferon alfa and gamma in children with chronic hepatitis B. *Pediatrics,* **90**, 254–258

Schalm, S. W., Mazel, J. A., de Gast, G. C. *et al.* (1989) Prevention of hepatitis B infection in newborns through mass screening and delayed vaccination of all infants of mothers with hepatis B surface antigen. *Pediatrics,* **83**, 1041–1048

Schmacher, H. R. and Ball, E. P. (1974) Arthritis in acute and chronic hepatitis. *Am. J. Med.,* **57**, 655

Schoub, B. D., Johnson, S., McAnerney, J. M. *et al.* (1991) Intergration of hepatitis B vaccination into rural Africa primary health care programmes. *Br. Med. J.,* **302**, 313–316

Shafritz, D. A., Shouval, D., Sherman, H. I. *et al.* (1981). Integration of hepatitis B virus DNA into the genome of liver cells in chronic liver disease and hepatocellular carcinoma. *N. Engl. J. Med.* **305**, 1067

Shakhgil'dian, I. V., Farber, N. A., Kuzin, S. N. *et al.* (1990) Perinatal transmission with hepatitis B virus and the problem of its specific prevention. *Vestn-Akad-Med-Nauk-SSSR,* **7**, 29–32

Shiraki, K., Yohihara, N., Sakuri, M., Eto, T. and Kawana, T. (1980) Acute hepatitis B in infants born to carrier mothers with the antibody to hepatitis B e antigen. *J. Pediatr.,* **97**, 768–770

Sinatra, F. R., Shah, P., Weissman, J. Y., Thomas, D. W., Merritt, R. J. and Tong, M. J. (1982) Perinatal transmitted acute icteric hepatitis B in infants born to hepatitis B surface antigen-positive and anti-hepatitis B e-positive carrier mothers. *Pediatrics,* **70**, 557–559

Sokal, E. M., Ulla, L. and Otte, J. B. (1992) Hepatitis B vaccine response before and after transplantation in 55 extrahepatic biliary atresia children. *Dig. Dis. Sci.,* **37**, 1250–1252

Stevens, C. E., Neurath, R. E., Beasley, R. P. *et al.* (1979) HBeAg and antiHBe detection by radioimmunoassay: correlation with vertical transmission of hepatitis B virus in Taiwan. *J. Med. Virol.,* **3**, 237–241

Stevens, C. E., Taylor, P. E., Tong, M. J. *et al.* (1987) Yeast recombinant hepatitis B vaccine. Efficacy with hepatitis B immune globulin in prevention of perinatal hepatitis B virus transmission. *J. Am. Med. Ass.,* **257**, 2612–2616

Stroffolini, T., Franco, E., Romano, G. *et al.* (1989) Hepatitis B virus infection in children in Sardinia, Italy. *Eur. J. Epidemiol.,* **5**, 202–206

Tan, K. L., Oon, C. J., Goh, K. T., Wong, L. Y. M and Chan, S. H. (1990) Immunogenicity and safety of low doses of recombinant yeast derived hepatitis B vaccine. *Acta. Paediatr. Scand.,*79, 593–598

Terazawa, S., Kojima, M., Yamanaka, T. *et al.* (1991) Hepatitis B virus mutants with precore-region defects in two babies with fulminant hepatitis and their mothers positive for antibody to hepatitis B e antigen. *Pediatr. Res.,* **29**, 5–9

Tsai, S. L., Chen, P. J., Lai, M. Y. *et al.* (1992) Acute exacerbations of chronic type B hepatitis are accompanied by increased T-cell responses to hepatitis B core and e antigens, *J. Clin. Invest.,* **89**, 87

Tsen, Y. J., Chang, M. J., Hsu, H. Y., Lee, C. Y., Sung, J. L. and Chen, D. S. (1991) Seroprevalence of hepatitis B virus infection in children in Taipei, 1989: five years after a mass hepatitis B vaccination program. *J. Med. Virol.,* **34**, 96–99

Twu, J. S., Lee, C. H., Lin, M. P. and Schloemer, R. H. (1988) Hepatitis B virus suppresses expression of human β-interferon. *Proc. Natl. Acad. Sci.,* **85**, 252–256

Vajro, P., Orso, G., D'Antonio, A. *et al.* (1985) Inefficacy of immunosuppressive treatment in HBsAg-positive, α-negative moderate chronic active hepatitis in children. *J. Pediatr. Gastroenterol. Nutr.,* **4**, 26–31

Van Ditzhuijsen, T. J., de Witte van der Shoot, E., Van Loon, A. M., Rijntjes, P. J. and Yap, S. H. (1988) Hepatitis B virus infection in an institution for the mentally retarded. *Am. J. Epidemiol.,* **128**, 629–638

Van Thiel, D. H. and Dindzans, V. (1988) Are steroids contraindicated in HBsAg-positive individuals with liver disease? *J. Pediatr. Gastroenterol. Nutr.,* **7**, 3–6

Vanclaire, J., Cornu, C. H. and Sokol, E. M. (1991) Fulminant hepatitis B in an infant born to a hepatitis Be antibody positive, DNA negative carrier. *Arch. Dis. Childh.,***66**, 983–985

Vegnente, A., Guida, S., Lobo-Yeo, A. *et al.* (1990) T lymphocyte activation is associated with viral replication in chronic hepatitis B virus infection of childhood. *Clin. Exp. Immunol.,* **84**, 190–194

Vento, S., Hegarty, J. E., Alberti, A. *et al.* (1985) T lymphocyte sensitization to HBcAg in hepatitis B virus mediated unresponsiveness to HBsAg in hepatitis B virus related chronic liver disease. *Hepatology,* **5**, 192–197

Vyas, G. N. and Ulrich, P. P. (1991) Molecular characterization of genetic variants of hepatitis B virus. In: *Viral Hepatitis and Liver Disease* (Eds F. B. Hollinger, S. M. Lemon, H. S. Margolis). Williams and Wilkins, Baltimore, 135–148.

Wang, J-T., Wang, T-H., Sheu, J-C., Shih, L-N., Lin, J-T. and Chen, D-S. (1991) Detection of hepatitis B virus DNA by polymerase chain reaction in plasma of volunteer blood donors negative for hepatitis B surface antigen. *J. Infect. Dis.,* **163**, 397–99

Whittle, H., Inskip, H., Bradley, A. K. *et al.* (1990) The pattern of childhood hepatitis B infection in two Gambian villages. *J.Infect. Dis.,* **161**, 1112–1115

Williams, C., Weber, T. F., Cullen, J. and Kane, M. (1983). Hepatitis B transmission in school contacts of retarded HBsAg carrier students. *J. Pediatr.* **103**, 192

Wirth, S., Keller, K. M., Schaefer, E. and Zabel, B. (1992) Hepatitis B virus DNA in liver tissue of chronic HBsAg carriers in childhood and its relationship to other viral markers, *J. Pediatr. Gastroenterol. Nutr.,* **14**, 431–435

Wong, V. C. W, Ip, H. M. H., Reesink, H. W. *et al.* (1984) Prevention of the HBsAg carrier rate in newborn infants of mothers who are chronic carriers of HBsAg and HBeAg by administration of hepatitis-B vaccine and hepatitis-B immunoglobulin. Double-blind randomised placebo-controlled study. *Lancet,* **1**, 921–926

World Health Organization (1983) *Meeting on Prevention of Liver Cancer:* report of a WHO meeting, technical report series 691. World Health Organization, Geneva, 1–29

Wrzolkowa, T., Zurowska, A., Uszycka-Karcz, M. and Picken, M. M. (1991) Hepatitis B virus-associated glomerulonephritis: electron microscopic studies in 98 children, *Am. J. Kidney Dis.,* **18**, 306–12

Yamanaka, T., Takayanagi, N., Nakao, T. *et al.* (1991) Seroepidemiological study of hepatitis B virus (HBV) infection in the rural community in Kenya – changing pattern of transmission model of HBV in Kenya. *Kansenshogaku-Zasshi,* **65**, 26–34

Hepatitis C

Alberti, A. (1991) Diagnosis of hepatitis C; Facts and perspectives. *J. Hepatol,* **12**, 279–282

Alberti, A. and Realdi, G. (1991) Parenterally-acquired non-A, non-B (type C) hepatitis. In: *Oxford Textbook of Clinical Hepatology* (Eds. N. McIntyre, J. P. Benhamou, J. Bircher, M. Rizzetto, J. Rodes). Oxford University Press, Oxford

Al-Faleh, F. Z., Ayoola, E. A., Al-Jeffry, M. *et al.* (1991) Prevalence of antibody to hepatitis C virus among Saudi Arabian children: a community based study. *Hepatology,* **14**: 215–18

Alter, H. J. (1992) New Kit on the block: Evaluation of second generation assays for the detection of antibody to the heaptitis C virus. *Hepatology,* **15**, 229–233

Blanchette, V. S., Vortsman, E., Shore, A. *et al.* (1991) Hepatitis C infection in children with hemophilia A and B. *Blood,* **78**, 285–289

Bortolotti, F., Vajro, P., Cadrobbi, P. *et al.* (1992) Cryptogenic chronic liver disease and hepatitis C virus infection in children. *J. Hepatol,* **15**, 73–76

Chen, D-S., Kuo, G. C., Sung, J-L. *et al.* (1991) Hepatitis C virus infection in an area hyperendemic for hepatitis B and chronic liver disease: The Taiwan experience. *J. Infect. Dis.,* **162**, 817–822

Choo, Q. L., Kuo, G., Weiner, A. J., Overby, L. R., Bradley, D. W. and Houghton, M. (1989) Isolation of a cDNA clone derived from a blood-borne Non-A, Non-B viral hepatitis genome. *Science,* **244**, 359–362

Davis, G. L., Balart, L. A., Schiff, E. R. *et al.* (1989) Treatment of chronic hepatitis C with recombinant interferon alfa. A multicenter randomised, controlled trial. *N. Engl. J. Med.,* **321**, 1501–1506

de Virgilis, S., Clemente, M. G., Congia, M. *et al.* (1992) Recombinant interferon alpha treatment in thalassemia major children with chronic hepatitis C and liver iron overload. (*Proceedings of the second joint meeting of the British and Italian Societies of the Paediatric Gastroenterology and Nutrition*). Harwood Academic Publishers, Newmarket, UK, 65

Di Bisceglie, A. M., Martin P., Kassianides, C. *et al.* (1989) Recombinant interferon alfa therapy for chronic hepatitis C. A randomised, double-blind, placebo-controlled trial. *N. Engl. J. Med.,* **321**, 1506–1510

Ding-Shinn, C., Kuo, G. C., Juei-Low, S. *et al.* (1991) Hepatitis C virus infection in an area hyperendemic for hepatitis B and chronic liver disease: the Taiwan experience. *J. Infect. Dis.,* **162**, 817–822

Feinman, S. V., Berris, B. and Herst, R. (1991) Anti-HCV in posttransfusion hepatitis: deductions from a prospective study. *J. Hepatol.,* **12**, 377–381

Feray, C., Samuel, D., Thiers, V. *et al.* (1992) Reinfection of liver graft by hepatitis C virus after liver transplantation, *J. Clin. Invest.,* **89**, 1361–1365.

Garson, J. A., Clewley, J. P., Sommonds, P. *et al.* (1992) Hepatitis C viraemia in United Kingdom blood donors. *Vox Sang,* **62**, 218–223

Iorio, R., Guida, S., Fariello, I., de Rosa, E., Porzio, S. and Vegnente, A. (1992) Alpha lymphoblastoid interferon (α-Ly-IFN) therapy in 12 children with chronic non-A, non-B hepatitis (CNANBH) (7 anti HCV+) (*Proceedings of the second joint meeting of the British and Italian Societies of the Paediatric Gastroenterology and Nutrition*). Harwood Academic Publishers, Newmarket, UK, p65

Jonas, M. M., Zilleruelo, G. E., La Rue, S. I., Abitbol, C., Strauss, J. and Lu, Y. (1992) Hepatitis C infection in a pediatric dialysis population. *Pediatrics,* **89**, 707–709

Kiyosawa, K., Sodeyama, T., Tanaka, E. *et al.* (1991) Intrafamilial transmission of hepatitis C virus in Japan. *J. Med. Virol.,* **33**, 114–116

Lenzi, M., Ballardini, G., Fusconi, M. *et al.* (1990) Type 2 autoimmune hepatitis and hepatitis C virus infection. *Lancet,* **335**, 258–259

Locasciulli, A., Gornati, G., Tagger, A. *et al.* (1991) Hepatitis C virus infection and chronic liver disease in children with leukemia in long term remission. *Blood,* **78**, 1619–1622

Loreto, M. D., Ferrante, M., Panaro, A., Sorino, P., Collela, V. and Caringella, D. A. (1992) Hepatitis C virus antibodies in dialysis pediatric patients. *Nephron,* **61**, 365–366

Ma, Y., Peakman, M., Lenzi, M. *et al.* (1993) The case against sub-classification of type II autoimmune chronic active hepatitis. *Lancet,* **341**, p.60

Makris, M., Preston, F. E., Triger, D. R. *et al.* (1990) Hepatitis C antibody and chronic liver disease in haemophilia. *Lancet,* **335**, 1117–1119

Ngatchu, T., Stroffolini, T., Rapicetta, M., Chionne, P., Lantum, D. and Chiaramonte, M. (1992) Seroprevalence of anti-HCV in an urban child population: a pilot survey in a developing area, Cameroon. *J. Trop. Med. Hyg.,* **95**, 57–61

Novati, R., Thiers, V., Monforte, A. D. *et al.* (1992) Mother-to-child transmission of hepatitis C virus detected by polymerase chain reaction. *J. Infect. Dis.,* **165**, 720–723

Pereira, B. J. G., Milford, E. L., Kirkman, R. L. and Levey, A. S. (1991) Transmission of hepatitis C virus by organ transplantation. *New Engl J. Med.,* **325**, 454–460.

Plagemann, P. G. (1991) Hepatitis C virus. *Arch. Virol.,* **120**, 165–180

Ruiz-Moreno, M., Rua, M. J., Castillo, I. *et al.* (1992) Treatment of children with chronic hepatitis with recombinant interferon-alpha: a pilot study. *Hepatology,* **16**, 882–885.

Shah, G., Demetris, A. J., Gavaler, S. *et al.* (1991) Incidence prevalence and clinical course of hepatitis following liver transplantation. *Gastroenterology,* **103**, 323–329

Sherlock, S. and Dusheiko, G. (1991) Hepatitis C virus update. *Gut,* **32**, 965–967

Shun-Chien, H., Mei-Hwei, C., Ding-Shinn, C., Hey-Chi, H. and Chin-Yun, L. (1991) Non-A, non-B hepatitis in children. *J. Med. Virol.,* **35**, 1–6

Thaler, M. M., Park, C-K., Landers, D. V. *et al.* (1991) Vertical transmission of hepatitis C virus. *Lancet,* **338**, 17–18

Ulrich, P. P., Romeo, J. M., Lane, P. K., Kelly, I., Daniel, L. J. and Vyas, G. N. (1990) Detection, semiquantitation, and genetic variation in hepatitis C sequences amplified from plasma of blood donors with elevated alanine aminotransferase. *J. Clin. Invest.,* **86**, 1609–1614

Van Der Poel, C. L., Cuypers, H. T. M., Reesink, H. W. *et al.* (1991) Confirmation of hepatitis C virus infection by new four-antigen recombinant immunoblot assay. *Lancet,* **337**, 317–319

Weintrub, P. S., Veereman-Wauters, G., Cowan, M. J. and Thaler, M. M. (1991) Hepatitis C virus infection in infants whose mothers took street drugs intravenously. *J. Pediatr.,* **119**, 869–874

Wright, T. L., Donegan, E., Hsu, H. H. *et al.* (1992) Recurrent and acquired hepatitis C viral infection in liver transplant recipients, *Gastroenterology,* **103**, 317–322

Hepatitis D

Benhamou, J-P. (1991) Fulminant and subfulminant liver failure: definition and causes. In *Acute Liver Failure* (eds) R. Williams and R. D. Hughes, Mitre Press, London, 6–10

Bensabath, G., Hadler, S. C., Soares, M. C. *et al.* (1987) Hepatitis delta virus infection and Labrea hepatitis. Prevalence and role in fulminant hepatitis in the Amazon Basin. *J. Med. Assoc.,* **258**, 479–483

Buitrago, B., Hadler, S. C., Popper, H. *et al.* (1986) Epidemiologic aspects of Santa Marta hepatitis over a 40-year period. *Hepatology,* **6**, 1292–1296

Chen, G. H., Zhang, M. D. and Huang, W. (1990) Hepatitis delta virus superinfection in Guangzhou area. *China Med. J.,* **103**, 451–454

Farci, P., Barbera, C., Navone, C. *et al.* (1985) Infection with the delta agent in children. *Gut,* **26**, 4–7

Hadziyannis, S. J. (1991) Use of alpha-interferon in the treatment of chronic delta hepatitis, *J. Hepatol,* **13**, S21–26.

Hsu, H. Y., Chang, M. H., Chen, D. S. and Lee, C. Y. (1988) Hepatitis D virus infection in children with acute or chronic hepatitis B virus infection in Taiwan. *J. Pediatr.,* **112**, 888–892

Monjardino, J. P. and Saldanha, J. A. (1990) Delta hepatitis: the disease and the virus. *Br. Med. Bull.,* **46**, 399–407

Pacchioni, D., Negro, F., Chiaberge, E., Rizzetto, M., Bonino, F. and Bussolati, G. (1992) Detection of hepatitis delta virus RNA by a non-radioactive in situ hybridization procedure. *Hum. Pathol.,* **23**, 557–561.

Rizzetto, M. (1983) The delta agent. *Hepatology,* **3**, 729–737

Rizzetto, M. and Verme, G. (1991) Hepatitis D. (1991) In: *Oxford Textbook of Clinical Hepatology* (Eds. N. McIntyre, J. P. Benhamou, J. Bircher, M. Rizzetto, J. Rodes). Oxford University Press, Oxford, 592–599

Rizzetto, M., Canese, M. G., Arico, S. *et al.* (1977) Immunofluorescence detection of a new antigen/antibody system (delta/anti-delta) associated with hepatitis B virus in liver and serum of HBsAg carriers. *Gut,* **18**, 997–1003

Rizzetto, M., Ponzetto, A., Bonino, F. and Smedile, A. (1988) Hepatitis delta virus infection: clinical and epidemiological aspects. In (Ed. A. J. Zuckerman) *Viral Hepatitis and Liver Disease.* Alan R Liss, New York, 389–394

Rizzetto, M. and Durazzo, M. (1991) Hepatitis delta virus (HDV) infections; epidemiological and clinical heterogeneity. *J. Hepatol.,* **13**, S116–118.

Rosina, F., Saracco, G., Lattore, P. *et al.* (1988) Treatment of chronic delta hepatitis with alpha-2 recombinant interferon. In *Viral Hepatitis and Liver Disease* (ed. A. J. Zuckerman). Alan R Liss, New York, 857

Sagnelli, E., Stroffolini, T., Ascione, A. *et al.* (1992) The epidemiology of hepatitis delta infection in Italy. *J Hepatol.,* **15**, 211–215

Saracco, G., Macagno, S., Rosina, F., Caredda, F., Antinori, S. and Rizzetto, M. (1988) Serologic markers with fulminant hepatitis in persons positive for hepatitis B surface antigen: a worldwide epidemiologic and clinical survey. *Ann. Intern. Med.,* **108**, 380–383

Smedile, A., Dentico, P., Zanetti, A *.et al.* (1981) Infection with HBV associated delta agent in HBsAg carriers. *Gastroenterology,* **81**, 992–997

Taylor, J. M., Chao, M., Hieh, S. Y., Luo, G. and Ryo, W. S. (1991) Structure and replication of hepatitis delta virus. In *Viral Hepatitis and Liver Disease* (eds. F. B. Hollinger, S. M. Lemon, H. S. Margolis). Williams and Wilkins, Baltimore, 460–463.

Torres, J. R., Mondolfi, A. (1991) Protracted outbreak of severe delta hepatitis: experience in an isolated Amerindian population of the Upper Orinco basin. *Rev. Infect. Dis.,* **13**, 52–55

Hepatitis E

Bradley, D. W. (1990) Enterically-transmitted non-A, non-B hepatitis. *Br. Med. Bull.,* **46**, 442–461.

Bradley, D. W., Krawczynski, K., Cook, E. H. *et al.* (1988) Enterically transmitted non-A, non-B hepatitis: etiology of the disease and laboratory studies in non-human primates. In: (ed. A. J. Zuckerman) *Viral Hepatitis and Liver Disease.* Alan R Liss, New York, 138–147

De Cock, K. M., Bradley, D. W., Sandford, N. L., Govindarajan, S., Maynard, J. E. and Redeker, A. G. (1987) Epidemic non-A, non-B hepatitis in patients from Pakistan. *Ann. Intern. Med.,* **106**, 227–230

Goldsmith, R., Yarbough, P. O., Reyes, G. R. *et al.* (1992) Enzyme-linked immunosorbent assay for diagnosis of acute sporadic hepatitis E in Egyptian children. *Lancet,* **339**, 328–331

Hyams, K. C., Purdy, M. A., Kaur, M. *et al.* (1992) Acute sporadic hepatitis E in Sudanese children: analysis based on a new western blot assay. *J. Infect. Dis.,* **165**, 1001–1005.

Krawczynski, K. (1991) Hepatitis type E-enterically transmitted (epidemic) non-A, non-B hepatitis. In *Oxford Textbook of Clinical Hepatology* (Eds. N. McIntyre, J. P. Benhamou, J. Bircher, M. Rizzetto, J. Rodes). Oxford University Press, Oxford

Molinie, C., Saliou, P., Roue, R. *et al.* (1988) Acute epidemic non-A, non-B hepatitis: study of 38 cases in Chad. In *Viral Hepatitis and Liver Disease* (Ed. A. J. Zuckerman). Alan R Liss, New York, 154–157

Pillot, J., Lazizi, Y., Diallo, Y. and Leguenno, B. (1992) Frequent sporadic hepatitis E in West Africa as evidenced by characterization of a virus-associated antigen in stool. *J. Hepatol.,* **15**, 420–421.

Ramalingaswami, V. and Purcell, R. H. (1988) Waterborne non-A, non-B hepatitis. *Lancet, i*, 571–573

Reyes, G. R., Huang, C-C., Yarborough, P. O. and Tam, A. W. (1991) Hepatitis E virus. Comparison of 'New and Old World' isolates. *J. Hepatol.,* **13**, s155–161.

Robson, S. C., Adams, S., Brink, N., Woodruff, B. and Bradley, D. (1992) Hospital outbreak of hepatitis E. *Lancet,* **339**, 1424–1425

Tsega, E., Hansson, B.-G., Krawczynski, K. and Nordenfelt, E. (1992) Acute sporadic viral hepatitis in Ethiopia: causes, risk factors and effects on pregnancy. *Clinical Infectious Disease,* **14**: 961–65

Epstein-Barr virus

Anderson, J. P. (1991) Clinical aspects of Epstein-Barr virus infection. *Scand. J. Infect. Dis. Suppl.,* **80**, 90–104

Chen, R. L., Su, I. J., Lin, K. H. *et al.* (1991) Fulminant childhood hemophagocytic syndrome mimicking histiocytic medullary reticulosis. An atypical form of Epstein-Barr virus infection. *Am. J. Clin. Path.,* **96**, 171–176

Giller, R. H. and Grose, C. (1989) Epstein-Barr virus: the hematologic and oncologic consequences of virus-host interaction. *Crit. Rev. Oncol. Hematol.,* **9**, 149–195

Grierson, H. (1987) Epstein-Barr Virus infections in males with the X-linked lymphoproliferative syndrome. *Ann. Intern. Med.,* **106**, 538–545.

Ho, M., Jaffe, R., Miller, G. *et al.* (1988) The frequency of Epstein-Barr infection and associated lymphoproliferative syndrome after transplantation and its manifestation in children. *Transplantation,* **45**, 719–727

Okano, M., Matsumoto, S., Osato, T., Sakiyama, Y., Thiele, G. M. and Purtilo, D. T. (1991) Severe chronic active Epstein-Barr virus infection syndrome. *Clin. Microbiol. Rev.,* **4**, 129–135

Su, I. J., Lin, D. T., Hsieh, H. C. *et al.* (1990) Fatal primary Epstein-Barr virus infection masquerading as histiocytic medullary reticulosis in young children in Taiwan. *Hematol. Pathol.,* **4**, 189–195

Tanaka, K., Shimada, M., Sasahara, A., Yamamoto, H., Naruto, T. and Tomida, Y. (1986) Chronic hepatitis associated with Epstein-Barr virus infection in an infant. *J. Pediatr. Gastroenterol. Nutr.,* **5**, 467–471

Cytomegalovirus

Alford, C. A., Stagno, S., Pass, R. F. and Britt, W. J. (1990) Congenital and perinatal CMV infections. *Rev. Infect. Dis.,* **12**, S745–753

Berge, P., Stagno, S., Federer, W. *et al.* (1990) Impact of asymptomatic congenital cytomegalovirus infection on size at birth and gestational duration. *Pediatr. Infect. Dis. J.,* **9**, 170–175

Boppana, S. B., Pass, R. F., Britt, W., Stagno, S. and Alford, C. A. (1992) Symptomatic congenital cytomegalovirus infection: neonatal morbidity and mortality. *Pediatr. Infect. Dis. J.,* **11**, 93–99

Freise, C. E., Pons, V., Lake, J. *et al.* (1991) Comparison of three regimens for cytomegalovirus prophylaxis in 147 liver transplant recipients. *Transplant. Proc.,* **23**, 1498–1500

Gershon, A. A. (1990) Viral vaccines of the future. *Pediatr. Clin. N. Am.,* **37**, 689–707

Griffiths, P. D., Baboonian, C., Rutter, D. and Peckham, C. (1991) Congenital and maternal cytomegalovirus infections in a London population. *Br. J. Obstet. Gynaecol.,* **98**, 135–140

Kosai, K., Kage, M. and Kojiro, M. (1991) Clinicopathological study of liver involvement in cytomegalovirus infection in infant autopsy case. *J. Gastroenterol. Hepatol.,* **6**, 603–608

Levy, I., Shoshat, M., Levy, Y., Alpert, G. and Nitzhan, M. (1989) Recurrent ascites in an infant with perinatally acquired cytomegalovirus infection. *Eur. J. Pediatr.,* **148**, 531–532

Lurie, M., Elmalach, I., Schuger, L. and Weintraub, Z. (1987) Liver findings in infantile cytomegalovirus infection: similarity to extrahepatic biliary obstruction. *Histopathology ,* **11**, 1171–1180

Paya, C. V., Holley, K. E., Wiesner, R. H. *et al.* (1990) Early diagnosis of cytomegalovirus hepatitis in liver transplant recipients: role of immunostaining, DNA hybridization and culture of hepatic tissue. *Hepatology,* **12**, 119–126

Peckham, C. S. (1991) Cytomegalovirus infection: congenital and neonatal disease. *Scand. J. Infect. Dis. (Suppl.),* **80**, 82–87

Salt, A., Sutehall, G., Sargaison, M. *et al.* (1990) Viral and toxoplasma gondii infections in children after liver transplantation. *J. Clin. Pathol.,* **43**, 63–67

Shaefer, M. S., Stratta, R. J., Markin, R. S. *et al.* (1991) Ganciclovir therapy for cytomegalovirus disease in liver transplant recipients. *Transplant. Proc.,* **23**, 1515–1516

Stratta, R. J., Shaeffer, M. S., Cushing, K. A., Markin, R. S., Wood, R. P. and Langnas, A. N. (1991) Successful prophylaxis of cytomegalovirus disease after primary CMV exposure in liver transplant recipients. *Transplantation,* **51**, 90–97

Herpes simplex virus

Benador, N., Mannhardt, W., Schranz, D. *et al.* (1990) Three cases of neonatal herpes simplex virus infection presenting as fulminant hepatitis. *Eur. J. Pediatr.,* **149**, 555–559

Brooks, S. E., Taylor, E., Golden, M. H. and Golden B. E. (1991) Electron microscopy of herpes simplex hepatitis with hepatocyte pulmonary embolization in kwashiorkor. *Archives of Pathology and Laboratory Medicine,* **115**: 1247–49

Koskiniemi, M., Happonen, J. M., Jarvenpaa, A. I., Pettay, O. and Vaheri, A. (1989) Neonatal herpes simplex virus (HSV) infection: a report of 43 patients. *Pediatric Infectious Disease,* **8**: 30–35

Mannhardt, W. and Schumacher, R. (1991) Progressive calcifications of lung and liver in neonatal herpes simplex virus infection. *Pediatr. Radiol.,* **21**, 236–237

Phillips, M. J., Blendis, L. M., Poucell, S. *et al.* (1991) Syncytial giant-cell hepatitis: sporadic hepatitis with distinctive pathological features, a severe clinical course and paramyxoviral features. *New England Journal of Medicine,* **324**: 455–60

Human immunodeficiency virus (HIV)

Cappell, M. S. (1991) Hepatobiliary manifestations of the acquired immune deficiency syndrome. *Am. J. Gastroenterol.,* **86**, 1–15

Jonas, M. M., Roldan, E. O., Lyons, H. J. *et al.* (1989) Histopathologic features of the liver in acquired immunodeficiency syndrome. *J. Pediatr. Gastroenterol. Nutr.,* **9**, 73–76

Kahn, E., Greco, A., Daum, F. *et al.* (1991) Hepatic pathology in Pediatric Acquired Immunodeficiency Syndrome. *Human Pathol.,* **22**, 1111–1119

Lefkowitch, J. (1991) Pathologic aspects of the liver in human immunodeficiency virus (HIV) infection. In: *Oxford Textbook of Clinical Hepatology* (Eds. N. McIntyre, J. P. Benhamou, J. Bircher, M. Rizzetto, J.Rodes). Oxford University Press, Oxford

Ninane, J., Moulin, D., Latinne, D. *et al.* (1985) AIDS in two African children – one with fibrosarcoma of the liver. *Eur. J. Pediatr.,* **144**, 385–388

Witzleben, C. L., Marshall, G. S., Wenner, W., Piccoli, D. A. and Barbour, S. D. (1988) HIV as a cause of giant cell hepatitis. *Human Pathol.,* **19**, 603–05

Other viruses

Rizzetto M. (1991) Systemic virosis producing hepatitis occasionally, or as an opportunistic infection in the immunocompromised host. In: *Oxford Textbook of Clinical Hepatology* (Ed. N. McIntyre, J. P. Benhamou, J. Bircher, M. Rizzetto, J. Rodes). Oxford University Press, Oxford

Adenovirus

Abzug, M. J. and Levin, M. J. (1991) Neonatal adenovirus infection: four patients and review of the literature. *Pediatrics,* **87**, 890–896

Cames, B., Rahier, J., Burtomboy, G. *et al.* (1992) Acute adenovirus hepatitis in liver transplant recipients. *J. Pediatr.,* **120**, 33–37

Krilov, L. R., Rubin, L. G., Frogel, M. *et al.* (1990) Disseminated adenovirus infection with hepatic necrosis in patients with human immunodeficiency virus infection and other immunodeficiency states. *Rev. Infect. Dis.,* **12**, 303–307

Salt, A., Sutehall, G., Sargaison, M. *et al.* (1990) Viral and toxoplasma gondii infections in children after liver transplantation. *J. Clin. Pathol.,* **43**, 63–67

Coxsackie virus

Begovac, J., Puntaric, B., Borcic, D. *et al.* (1988) Mononucleosis-like syndrome associated with a multisystem Coxsackie virus type B3 infection in adolescent. *Eur. J. Pediatr.,* **147**, 426–427

Read, R. B., Ede, R. J., Morgan-Capner, P., Moscoso, G., Portmann, B. and Williams, R. (1985) Myocarditis and fulminant hepatic failure from Coxsackie virus B infection. *Postgrad. Med. J.,* **61**, 749–752

Measles virus

Shalev-Zimels, H., Weizman, Z., Lotan, C., Gavish, D., Ackerman, Z. and Morag, A. (1988) Extent of measles hepatitis in various ages. *Hepatology*, **8**, 1138–1139

Reovirus

Morecki, R., Glaser, J. (1989) Reovirus 3 and neonatal biliary disease: discussion of divergent results. *Hepatology*, **10**, 515–517

Rubella

Sugaya, N., Nirasawa, M., Mitamura, K. and Murata, A. (1988) Hepatitis in acquired rubella infection in children. *Am. J. Dis. Child.*, **142**, 817–818

Varicella zoster

McGregor, R. S., Zitelli, B. J., Urbach, A. H., Malatack, J. J. and Cartner, J. C. (1989) Varicella in pediatric orthotopic liver transplant recipients. *Pediatrics*, **83**, 256–261

Schiller, G. J., Nimer, S. D., Gajewski, J. L. and Golde, D. W. (1991) Abdominal presentation of varicella-zoster infection in recipients of allogenic bone marrow transplantation. *Bone Marrow Transplantation*, **7**, 489–491

Dengue virus

Alvarez, M. E. and Ramirez-Ronda, C. H. (1985) Dengue and hepatic failure. *Am. J. Med.*, **79**, 670–674

George, R., Liam, C. K., Chua, C. T. *et al.* (1988) Unusual clinical manifestations of dengue virus infection. *Southeast Asian Journal of Tropical Medicine and Public Health*, **19**: 585–90

Wang, L. Y., Chang, W. Y., Lu, S. N. *et al.* (1990) Sequential changes of serum transaminase and abdominal sonography in patients with suspected dengue fever. *Kao-Hsiung-I-Hsueh-Ko-Hsueh-Tsa-Chih*, **6**, 483–489

Yellow fever virus

de Cock, K. M., Monath, T. P., Nasidi, A. *et al.* (1988) Epidemic yellow fever in Eastern Nigeria, 1986. *Lancet*, **1**, 630–632

Enzootic 'exotic' viral hepatitides

Draelos, Z. K., Hansen, R. C., Tucson, M. A. J. and James, W. D. (1986) Gianotti-Crosti syndrome associated with infections other than hepatitis B. *JAMA*, **256**: 2386–88

Lucia, H. L., Coppenhaver, D. H., Harrison, R. L. and Baron, S. (1990) The effect of an arenavirus infection on liver morphology and function. *Am. J. Trop.Med. Hyg.*, **43**, 93–98

McCormick, J. B., Walker, D. H., King, I. J. *et al.* (1986) Lassa virus hepatitis: a study of fatal Lassa fever in humans. *Am. J. Trop. Med. Hyg.*, **35**, 401–407

Price, M. E., Fisher-Hoch, S. P., Craven, R. B. and McCormick, J. B. (1988) A prospective study of maternal and foetal outcome in acute Lassa fever infection during pregnancy. *Br. Med. J.*, **297**, 584–587

Snell, N. (1988) Ribavirin therapy for Lassa fever. *Practitioner*, **232**, 432

van-Eeden, P. J., Joubert, J. R., van de Wal, B. W., King, J. B., de Kock, A. and Groenewald, J. H. (1985) A nosocomial outbreak of Crimean Congo haemorrhagic fever at Tygerberg hospital. *South Afr. Med. J.*, **68**, 711–732

Woodruff, P. W., Morrill, J. C., Burans, J. P., Hyams, K. C. and Woody, J. N. (1988) A study of viral and rickettsial exposure and causes of fever in Juba, southern Sudan. *Trans. Roy. Soc. Trop. Med. Hyg.*, **82**, 761–766

Zuckerman, A. and Ellis, D. (1991) Exotic virus infections of the liver. In *Oxford Textbook of Clinical Hepatology* (eds. N. McIntyre, J.-P. Benhamou, J. Bricher, Rizzetto and J. Rodes). Oxford Medical Publications, Oxford. pp.638–646

Chapter 7

Bacterial, protozoal, fungal and helminthic infections of the liver

Hepatomegaly and impaired hepatic function with abnormal biochemical tests of liver function occur during the course of many non-viral microbial infections which usually have their main manifestation outside the hepatobiliary system. Jaundice is particularly common in the first month of life. Liver dysfunction arises both as a result of a direct invasion of the parenchyma and biliary system or from toxins elaborated by the infecting agent. Anaemia, hypoxia, inadequate food intake, dehydration and hepatotoxic agents contribute. Haemolysis may add to the jaundice. Factors involved in liver cell injury include endotoxin, thromboxane B2 and leukotrienes. Primary and secondary immuno-suppression including acute liver failure increase susceptibility.

The *pathological* features range from marked hyperplasia of the reticulo-endothelial system through various degrees of hepatocellular damage, the most minor of which may only be manifest on electron microscopy, to portal tract infiltration, features of bile duct obstruction or widespread hepatocellular necrosis with liver failure. Cholestasis is frequent. There may be fatty infiltration. If shock supervenes there is ischaemic necrosis. Perihepatitis occurs with *N. gonorrhoea* or *Chlamydia trachomatis*, usually occurring in association with pelvic inflammatory disease in adolescence. Granulomata may occur in tuberculosis, atypical mycobacterial infections including BCG and lepromatous leprosy and in fungal infections. Iron overload predisposes to *Yersinia*, which like *Listeria monocytogenes* and Q fever may also cause granulomata.

In malaria, leishmaniasis and toxoplasmosis there is pronounced hyperplasia of Kupffer cells. In parasitic infection with *Ascaris, Trichinella* and liver flukes (*Clonorchis sinensis* and *Fasciola hepatica*), there is direct invasion of the biliary system with tissue damage and obstruction.

Antimicrobial therapy will be dictated by the results of blood or liver biopsy culture but should be started empirically bearing in mind that Gram-negative, Gram-positive or anaerobic bacteria may be responsible. Rarely, supportive measures may be necessary if there is marked hepatocellular necrosis. Parasites in the biliary tree may require surgical removal.

Pyogenic abscess of the liver

Abscesses may form in the hepatic parenchyma or in ectatic bile ducts or cysts. Because there are usually no liver-specific clinical or laboratory features, the clinician may be slow to consider this site of infection and diagnosis is delayed.

Aetiology

Abscesses may occur as a complication of generalized septicaemia particularly in children with depressed immunity. These are often children with serious underlying disease, such as leukaemia, who are also receiving immunosuppressive drugs. In some instances, defective leucocyte function (chronic granulomatous disease), dysgammaglobulinaemia or sickle cell disease are predisposing factors. Intra-abdominal sepsis, such as peritonitis following perforated appendicitis, are now rarely complicated by hepatic abscess formation presumably because of improved surgical techniques and the effective use of antibiotics. Abscess formation still occurs following suppurative cholangitis usually associated with abnormalities of the biliary tree including surgically corrected biliary atresia or choledochal cyst, penetrating injuries of the liver and direct extension of infection from neighbouring organs. They may complicate hepatic malignancy. Cysts may become infected.

The infecting organisms include *Staphylococcus, Streptococcus* (aerobic and anaerobic), *E. coli, Klebsiella* and Enterobacteriaceae species, *Pseudomonas aeruginosa* and *Proteus*. In some parts of the world *Salmonella typhi* is frequently responsible. Mixed infections also occur. *Actinomyces, Nocardia* and *Candida albicans, Bacteroides clostridium* species, *Streptococcus millerei* and *Yersinia* are occasional causes.

Pathology

Abscesses may be large, single and well encapsulated with fibrous tissue. If multiple, they are usually close to the portal tracts. Where infection has occurred via the bile ducts the lesions are concentrated around the bile tracts. They cause disintegration of the surrounding hepatic structures. The majority of the abscesses arising from intra-abdominal causes or from septicaemia are in the right lobe of the liver. When there is a pyelonephritis the portal vein may contain pus and blood clots. There are frequently perihepatitis and ascites.

Clinical features

The initial clinical features are often very non-specific such as malaise, nausea, weight loss, fever, and vague upper abdominal discomfort or distension. Shoulder or pleuritic pain may occur. Onset may be insidious or with rigors. A previous history of intra-abdominal sepsis, trauma to the abdomen or surgery to the biliary tree should raise suspicion of the diagnosis. However, 25% have no clinical or laboratory features that indicate hepatic involvement. Unfortunately, many cases are still first diagnosed at autopsy. Complications include rupture into the peritoneum or biliary system, haemobilia, septicaemia empyema and curiously endophthalmitis.

Hepatomegaly with tenderness on deep palpation is the most useful clinical sign. A decreased range of respiratory movements may be noted.

Laboratory investigations

Standard tests of liver function are relatively unhelpful. In some instances the serum bilirubin is raised, the albumin depressed and the alkaline phosphatase raised. The white cell count may be raised with an increased proportion of polymorphonuclear neutrophil leucocytes but this is not invariable. Repeated blood culture may show the causative organism. On X-rays the diaphragm may be seen to be raised and a pleural effusion or gas-containing lesion in the liver demonstrated. Ultrasonic scanning is the most useful imaging investigation, demonstrating a fluid-filled lesion. Computed tomography (CT) scanning has slightly higher sensitivity and is helpful in localization but the appearance is not specific even with contrast enhancement.

Treatment

Treatment is by prolonged appropriate antibiotic therapy and drainage by aspiration under ultrasound control or rarely by an open surgical technique. Aspirated pus is cultured and an appropriate antibiotic regimen selected. Antibiotics are continued until the abscess cavity has disappeared on ultrasonography and the patient has been afebrile for 1–2 weeks. Small abscesses of less than 3–4 cm may resolve with prolonged antibiotic therapy with only diagnostic aspiration. Drainage must be repeated if the abscess cavity is not seen to progressively contract on ultrasonography repeated at 1–4-day intervals. An alternative is continuous drainage via a percutaneous catheter placed in the abscess cavity under ultrasound control. Even multiple abscesses can be controlled in this fashion but deeply placed abscesses may present difficulty. Surgical management is mandatory if there is associated peritonitis or bile duct obstruction. Surgical drainage may also be required for chronic abscesses which have developed a firm wall. Patients may require general supportive therapy with transfusions of blood, plasma, albumin and enteral or parenteral nutritional support.

Leptospirosis

Leptospirosis is an acute infectious disease of very varying severity caused by any one of over 130 serovars (formerly serotypes) of *Leptospira interrogans*, for example *L. icterohaemorrhagiae* (Weil's disease), *L. canicola* (canicola fever) and *L. autumnalis* (pre-tibial fever).

Epidemiology

Rats, cattle, household pets such as dogs and hamsters, and many wild animals, reptiles and birds are the sources of the disease. Many are persistent, healthy excreters. Excreta, particularly urine, are infected. Leptospiral spirochaetes can survive for a long period outside their animal vectors, so infection can occur without direct contact. Infection is transmitted to humans in food, drinking and bathing water or via abrasions. Children are frequently infected.

Pathology

Leptospirosis is characterized by an extensive vasculitis affecting small blood vessels of all organs. Increased permeability and tissue ischaemia results. The hepatic changes are those of a mild and diffuse hepatitis with Kupffer cell hyperplasia, portal tract infiltration and focal centrilobular necrosis with leucocyte infiltration. Acalculous cholecystitis and pancreatitis may also occur.

Clinical features

The incubation period ranges from 2 to 26 (average 10) days. Contrary to earlier reports, the course of the disease is not related to the leptospira serotype. Many infections are asymptomatic. Others cause biphasic illnesses which are self-limited and are not unlike many other viral or bacterial illnesses. Only 10% of recognized cases are icteric.

The overt disease is characterized by any or all of the following. There is an abrupt onset of a septicaemic phase with fever, muscular pains, headache and vomiting. A maculopapular petechial or purpuric rash may develop. Albuminuria with casts, red and white cells and uraemia may occur because of renal involvement. Pneumonitis and myocarditis may be evident. An aseptic meningitis may be found. From 4 to 30 days later these features may settle but in some cases damage to the myocardium, kidneys or liver becomes more severe during the period of marked immune response. Death may occur due to renal failure or arrhythmia. Jaundice starts on day 2 or 3 and lasts up to 4 weeks.

Laboratory findings

Laboratory tests reflect the degree of organ involvement with a high alkaline phosphatase the main abnormality in liver disease. In 50% creatinine phosphokinase is elevated due to muscle involvement. Leptospira can be recovered in the blood or cerebrospinal fluid in the first 10 days of the illness and in the urine from day 7–30. The diagnosis may be by leptospira antibody tests using a complement fixation technique or an enzyme-linked immunosorbent assay (ELISA). A rising antibody titre can usually be demonstrated although this can be suppressed by therapy.

Treatment

If given within 7 days of onset, penicillin, erythromycin, tetracycline or deoxycyline may be effective in limiting development of the disease. They are ineffective once jaundice develops. Supportive therapy will be required for congestive heart failure, renal failure or hepatic failure. If the vasculitis causes gangrene, amputation may be required.

Hepatic amoebiasis

The protozoal parasite *Entamoeba histolytica* causes liver damage when it is carried to the liver in the portal venous system from ulcerative lesions in the colon.

The amoebae multiply and block small intrahepatic portal vein branches causing focal necrosis and lysis of liver tissue. The necrotic areas vary in size from a few millimetres up to 10 cm in diameter. The large ones contain thick, red-brown liquid. The lesions are focal, not generalized. Surrounding liver tissue is normal. The lesions heal with some scar formation but cirrhosis does not develop.

Epidemiology

Although the amoebae have a worldwide distribution, the disease appears to occur principally in the tropics and subtropics. In part this is due to poor sanitary conditions. What determines whether the *E. histolytica* remains a luminal commensal or becomes an invasive pathogen is clear. Different strains may exist with different powers of invasion. Invasion may occur only in the presence of some other unrecognized factor.

Clinical features

Although *E. histolytica* infection of the liver occurs secondary to the trophozoite entering the mucosa of the large bowel, patients frequently give no history of significant gastrointestinal symptoms. High fever, rigors and profuse sweating are the main symptoms. Pain in the shoulder, neck and upper abdomen are occasional complaints.

Physical examination shows an ill-looking febrile child. Diminished respiratory movements, hepatomegaly with tenderness on palpation and percussion and anaemia are usual. Jaundice is rare. There may be no features suggesting liver involvement particularly in infancy. The clinical outcome is adversely affected by unnecessary surgery or rupture of the abscess into the chest, peritoneum or other intra-abdominal organs.

Laboratory investigations

Liver function tests are usually normal. The leucocyte count is raised with a predominance of polymorphonuclear neutrophil leucocytes. There may be mild anaemia. In less than 25% of cases cysts and vegetative forms of *E. histolytica* may be found in fresh stool specimens. Anti-amoebic antibodies are detected in over 95% of cases. Antibodies persist for many years after acute infection. The abscess may be delineated by ultrasound hepatic scintiscanning, CT scanning or angiography.

Treatment

Metronidazole (50 mg/kg/24 hours for 10 days) or tinidazole (60 mg/kg/day for 5 days) is the treatment of choice. Surgical drainage or aspiration under ultrasonographic control is indicated for lesions with secondary infection, and when rupture to other organs is imminent or has occurred or when the lesion continues to enlarge in spite of drug treatment. The disease can be prevented by good sewage disposal facilities, adequate filtration of the water supply and simple hygienic measures.

Helminthic diseases of the liver and biliary system

Hydatid disease

Hydatid disease is usually caused by the larval stage of infection by the dog tapeworm *Echinococcus granulosus*. Humans are infected by contact with the excreta of dogs. Sheep, pigs and camels, like man, are intermediate hosts. Rarely, the fox tapeworm, *E. multilocularis*, may be responsible.

The ova are ingested, burrow through the intestinal mucosa and are carried in the portal vein to the liver where they develop into adult cysts. A few ova will bypass the liver and be trapped in the lungs. A few will get into the general systemic circulation.

Pathology

Within the liver, the *Echinococcus* produces a slowly growing cyst surrounded by thickened compressed tissue which may eventually calcify. In some growth will stop and the cyst disappear. The surrounding layer of fibrous tissue is thin, however, and frequently daughter cysts are formed around the main cyst and eventually multiloculated cysts develop. These are usually found in the right lobe of the liver. The cyst may rupture into the peritoneum or into the biliary tree. E. multilocularis produces an invasive necrosis with multiple cysts surrounded by dense fibrous tissue.

Epidemiology

The disease is common in sheep-grazing countries. It is also frequently found in southern Europe, particularly in the Mediterranean Basin. The disease appears to be rare in the UK, but cases are reported from Wales and the Scottish islands.

Clinical features

An *Echinococcus* cyst is suspected when hepatomegaly is discovered and/or a cyst is found on ultrasound in a patient who may have had contact with infected dogs. There may be a distinct round and smooth swelling affecting part of the liver. The patient is not ill but may have a dull ache in the right upper quadrant. Urticaria or anaphylactic shock may occur if hydatid fluid is released into the peritoneum or into the circulation. The peripheral blood count may show an eosinophilia. Ultrasonic scanning shows this to be a fluid-filled cavity which may contain daughter cysts. A plain radiograph of the abdomen may show a calcified lesion. *E. multilocularis* produces features similar to liver cancer.

The diagnosis may be confirmed by serological tests in up to 80% of cases. A latex fixation test and an indirect haemagglutination test are more specific and more sensitive than the intradermal (Casoni) test which has been abandoned.

Treatment

Uncomplicated hepatic hydatid cysts carry a good prognosis. The risks of complications are always present. The risks of rupture and secondary infection are such that the cysts should be removed surgically. It is important that they be removed completely without contaminating the peritoneum. In patients who are too ill for surgery mebendazole (20–40 mg/kg/day) or albendazole(10–20 mg/kg/day) for 4 to 8 weeks may be effective. In *E. multilocularis* albendazole in larger doses or praziquantil may complement surgical treatment. Liver transplantation was successful in 70% in one series (Vuitton, 1990).

Schistosomiasis and liver flukes

The schistosomiasis and liver flukes are trematodes whose *life-cycle* includes fresh water snail intermediate hosts and a mammalian host including man. Parasite eggs passed in mammalian faeces gain entry to the snail emerging as thousands of free swimming cercariae. Those of schistosomes enter the mammalian host by penetrating skin. The cercariae of the liver fluke *Fasciola hepatica* (main mammalian hosts: sheep and cattle) are ingested attached to plants such as watercress. Those of *Clonorchis sinensis* and *Opisthorchis felineus* and *Opisthorchis viverrini* (main host cat) enter freshwater fish. Humans are infected if the fish is eaten undercooked.

Schistosomiasis (bilharziasis)

This disorder which affects at least 200 million people worldwide is caused by chronic infestation with one of three trematodes. *Schistosoma mansoni*, *S. japonicum* and *S. mekongi*. The cercariae penetrate unbroken skin or buccal mucosa and pass via the bloodstream and lungs to the liver where they develop within about 2 months into adult male and female worms. These migrate in the portal venous system against the blood flow to take up positions in intestinal venous plexuses. There they produce many eggs some of which are passed in the faeces, others are carried in the portal blood to the portal tracts where they cause pathological changes.

Epidemiology

These trematodes are widely distributed throughout the world. *S. mansoni* occurs in sub-Sahara Africa, the Arabian Gulf, the Caribbean and Brazil, *S. japonicum* in China, Philippines and Indonesia with *S. mekongi* occurring along the Mekong river. *S. mansoni* infects only humans, the others are zoonoses affecting many domestic and wild animals. Infestation occurs by contact with cercariae containing waters usually starting in childhood. Prevalence may reach 100% with the highest intensity of infection usually in the teens.

Pathology

Eggs produce granulomata with intense infiltration by round cells, eosinophils and some giant cells around portal tracts. The severity of disease is related to the intensity of the inflammatory response which is of a delayed hypersensitivity type as well as to the parasite load. Healing takes place with the production of fibrous tissue. In the liver the lesions are around and in the portal tracts. The portal tract becomes enlarged and fibrotic with little or no bile duct proliferation. There is little or no nodular regeneration, although there may be some disturbance of the hepatic architecture. As portal venous obstruction becomes more diffuse portal pressure rises, the spleen enlarges and portosystemic collaterals develop. When this occurs eggs may be carried to lungs and the central nervous system where they induce granuloma formation.

Clinical features

Schistosomiasis can occur in any age group. It is rare in the first 18 months of life, but in endemic areas most children become infected during childhood. The course is extremely variable.

The first stage is characterized by itching around the area of the entry of the organism into the skin. This stage is commonly missed. In the second stage, there may be features suggesting serum sickness; fever urticaria and eosinophilia are the most prominent features as well as vague symptoms such as malaise, lack of interest in school work, weight loss and poor appetite. The third stage may see a continuation of these symptoms but with, in addition, features due to involvement of the liver. The hepatic features are those of portal hypertension with splenomegaly, ascites and haematemesis. Hepatomegaly may be present in the early stages. Hepatocellular function is usually well maintained.

The diagnosis is suspected on the basis of history of exposure to possibly infected water. It is confirmed and its intensity assessed by the recovery of ova in the stool or rectal biopsy. Highly specific immunodiagnostic tests (ELISA) have been developed.

Treatment

The response to treatment depends a great deal on the degree of infestation of the individual, the duration of the illness and the severity of complications. Praziquantel (20 mg/kg twice for *S. mansoni* and three times for *S. japonicum* and *S. mekongi*) for one-day cures between 66 and 97% and diminishes morbidity in the remainder (Shekhar,

1991). Periodic re-treatment may be required but even in highly epidemic areas significant hepatobiliary schistosomiasis may not recur (King and Mahmoud,1989). Complications such as anaemia, ascites and portal hypertension may require specific management. Encephalopathy may develop after shunts in spite of the good hepatocellular function. Injection sclerotherapy may therefore be a better treatment option if there are bleeding oesophageal varices.

Prevention

Measures to prevent primary and re-infection should include avoiding skin contact with possibly infected fresh water, draining the habitat of the intermediate host, efficient sewage disposal and treatment of whole communities with praziquantel.

Liver flukes

These trematodes produce disease by infestation of the biliary system. *Fasciola hepatica* occurs worldwide in sheep- and cattle-rearing communities. *Opisthorchis felineus* has wide distribution outside the Americas. *Opisthorchis viverrini* and *Clonorchis sinensis* occurs in east Asia. Heavy infestations interfere with biliary flow. Cholangitis with fever, right upper quadrant pain, hepatomegaly and eosinophilia are the main features. There may be complicating suppurative cholangitis. Calculi and bile duct carcinoma may occur in association with *C. sinensis* infestation.

Diagnosis

Fever, evidence of biliary disease, eosinophilia and a history of ingestion of possibly contaminated watercress (*Fasciola*) or raw freshwater fish (*Clonorchis*) raise diagnostic suspicion. Diagnosis is established by recovery of the ova in the faeces or duodenal aspirate. Fascioliasis may be diagnosed by immunoelectrophoresis and indirect haemagglutination.

Treatment

For *fascioliasis*, bithionol (25 mg/kg for 10 days) is the treatment of choice. Opisthorchis and *Clonorchis* can be successfully treated with praziquantel 25 mg/kg three times daily for 2 days. Suppurative cholangitis may require antibiotic treatment. Surgery or endoprostheses inserted transhepatically or endoscopically may be required for biliary obstruction secondary to *Clonorchis* infestation.

Nematode (round worm) infestation

Ascaris lumbricoides

It has been estimated that between 0.6 and 1 billion people worldwide, living in areas of substandard hygiene, are infected by *Ascaris lumbricoides* which causes 20 000 deaths per annum. The adult worm lives in the small intestine but may enter the bile duct via the ampulla of Vater. There they persist for up to 1 month before they die and disintegrate. They cause bile duct obstruction, calculi formation with their sequelae and intrahepatic pyogenic abscesses. Ultrasound may be diagnostic demonstrating linear sometimes mobile echogenic structures in the bile ducts or gall bladder. Levamisole in a single dose of 5 mg/kg and mebendazole 100 mg in two doses at 12-hour intervals for intestinal parasitosis is often effective. Endoscopic removal of parasites may be required.

Visceral larva migrans

Visceral larva migrans is caused in humans primarily by *toxocara canis* the dog asteroid. Eggs eliminated by the dog develop into infective embryos which on ingestion by humans hatch into larvae which enter the portal circulation and are arrested in various organs including the liver. They produce necrosis with an intense inflammatory infiltrate composed predominantly of eosinophils. Fever, hepatomegaly, urticarial rashes, respiratory symptoms and a history of pica in a patient with eosinophilia and contact with dog excreta should suggest the diagnosis. The diagnosis can be confirmed by positive serological tests. Treatment with thiabendazole in a dose of 25 mg/kg twice daily for 5 days kills the larvae. Corticosteroids may be required for hypersensitivity reactions.

Malaria

Malaria is an infection by one or more species of *Plasmodium* (*P. falciparum, vivax, ovale* and *malariae*). Sporozoites injected by the *Anopheles* mosquito invade and multiply in hepatocytes without impairing function. Infected red cells in the erythrocytic stage are phagocytosed by Kupffer cells, endothelial cells and macrophages. In *P. falciparum* erythrocytes are sequestered in the sinusoids by interaction of malarial antigens on their surface with adherence molecules on the endothelial cells, reducing blood flow by 50%. Hepatic sequelae include tender hepatosplenomegaly with, in severe infections, jaundice, hypoglycaemia and lactic acidosis. In chronic infections *tropical splenomegaly syndrome* develops with severe sinusoidal lymphocytosis, variable chronic inflammation in portal tracts, splenomegaly, hypersplenism and elevation of serum IgM. Treatment is supportive and antimalarials dictated by the species of malaria and its geographical area of origin.

Hepatic granuloma

Granulomata are found in the liver in association with a wide range of acute and chronic infections, infestations and toxins. They occur in many other generalized diseases including malignant disease and in the immunosuppressed patient. Finding granulomata in the liver biopsy is thus an indication of a systemic disease.

Pathology

A granuloma is a circumscribed organized proliferative focal inflammatory lesion with a mature macrophage (which may be large and multinucleated) at its centre surrounded by lymphocytes and fibroblasts. Sometimes other inflammatory cells are present. The

Table 7.1 Causes of hepatic granulomas

Infectious diseases:	*Malignant disease*:	*Miscellaneous*:
Bacterial	Hodgkin's disease	Sarcoidosis
Tuberculosis	Non-Hodgkin's lymphoma	Chronic granulomatous disease
BCG vaccination	? other intra-abdominal neoplasms	Hypogammaglobulinaemia
Atypical mycobacterial infection		Erythema nodosum
Brucellosis		Vasculitis
Leprosy		Drug reactions
Francisella		
Yersinia prorrioni treponema		
Fungal		
Candidiasis		
Histoplasmosis		
Coccidiomycosis		
Aspergillosis		
Actinomycosis		
Nocardiosis		
Cryptococcosis		
Parasitic		
Schistosoma		
Ascaris		
Toxocara		
Protozoa		
Toxoplasmosis		
Leishmaniasis		
Viral		
Cytomegalovirus		
Epstein–Barr virus		
Rickettsial		
Q fever		
AIDS		
Spirochaetal		
Syphilis		

macrophage frequently contains inclusion bodies and may undergo generative necrotic or caseating change. Healing is by sclerosis and fibrosis. The many possible causes are given in Table 7.1.

Clinical and laboratory features

These are the features of the underlying disease. Hepatomegaly, sometimes tender, may be noted. Liver function tests are usually normal but there may be elevated serum alkaline phosphatase and gamma-glutamyl transpeptidase particularly if granulomata are frequent. Jaundice is unusual. Ultrasound or CT scans may show multiple focal lesions. Liver biopsy with culture for microbes may be invaluable in identifying the cause and in planning treatment.

Differential diagnosis

Infective causes to be considered in children are cytomegalovirus infection, infectious mononucleosis, tuberculosis, BCG immunization, brucellosis, leprosy, *Toxocara, Schistosoma* and *Ascaris* infestation. Candidiasis, particularly in patients with primary or

Table 7.2 Investigations to be considered in hepatic granuloma

Full blood count
IgM antibodies for infectious causes
Culture blood, secretions, urine, stools or tissue
Stool microscopy for parasites and ova
Tuberculin skin test
Chest X-ray
Serum immunoglobulins
Nitroblue tetrazolium test
Serum angiotensin converting enzyme activity (for sarcoidosis)
Bone marrow aspiration
Lymph node biopsy
Barium enema
Colonoscopy

secondary immune defects, histoplasmosis, coccidiomycosis and blastomycosis may also be responsible. *Listeria* in neonates may be the cause. Granulomata occur also in chronic granulomatous disease and in hypergammaglobulinaemia. They are seen also with erythema nodosa, Crohn's disease and with reticulo-endothelial malignancy, particularly Hodgkin's disease. Rarely they are seen in association with reactions to drugs such as sulphonamides. The investigations which should be considered in the diagnosis of hepatic granuloma are shown in Table 7.2.

Sarcoidosis

Sarcoidosis, a generalized granulomatous disease of unknown cause, affecting particularly the lung, eyes, lymph nodes, skin and central nervous system, involves the liver in over 60% of cases. Granulomata are most frequent in the portal zones. They usually have a central area of eosinophilic necrosis, conspicuous giant cell transformation, inclusion bodies and a very thin ring of lymphocytes, but there are no pathognomonic features. Healing is by sclerosis. With massive involvement liver function tests may be deranged and, exceptionally, jaundice or portal hypertension may occur.

Bibliography and references

van Allan, R. J., Katz, M. D., Johnson, M. B., Laine, L. A., Lin, Y. and Ralls, P. W. (1992) Uncomplicated amebic liver abscess: prospective evaluation of percutaneous therapeutic aspiration. *Radiology*, **183**: 827–30
Vuitton, D. (1990) Alveolar echinococcosis of the liver: a parasitic disease in search of a treatment. *Hepatology*, **12**: 617–18

Bacterial

Khosla, S. N. (1990) Typhoid hepatitis. *Postgrad. Med. J.,* **66**, 923–5
Kibbler, C. (1991) Bacterial infection and the liver. In *Oxford Textbook of Clinical Hepatology* (Ed. N. McIntyre, J. P. Benhamou, J. Bircher, M. Rizzetto, J. Rodes). Oxford University Press, Oxford
Mongenstern, R. and Hayes, P. C. (1991) The liver in typhoid fever: always affected, not just a complication. *Am. J. Gastroenterol.,* **86**, 1235–1239
Paton, A. (1984) Sepsis in cholestasis. *Br. Med. J.,* **289**, 857
Saebo, A. and Lassen, J. (1992) Acute and chronic liver disease associated with *Yersinia enterocolitica* infection: a Norwegian 10-year follow-up study of 458 hospitalized patients. J. Int. Med., **231**, 531–535

Fungal

Rolando, N., Harvery, F., Brahm, J., Philpott-Howard, J., Alexander, G., Casewell, M. and Fagan, E. (1991) Fungal infection: a common, unrecognised complication of acute liver failure. *J. Hepatol.*, **12**, 1–9

Pyogenic abscesses

Barnes, P. F., de Cock, K. M., Reynolds, T. N. and Ralls, P. W. (1987) A comparison of amebic and pyogenic abscess of the liver. *Medicine*, **66**, 472–483.
Bergamini, T. M., Larson, G. M., Malangoni, M. A. and Richardson, J. D. (1987) Liver abscess: review of a 12-year experience, *Am. Surg.*, **53**, 596–9
Donovan, A. J., Yellin, A. E. and Ralls, P. W. (1991) Hepatic abscess, *World J. Surg.*, **15**, 162–169
Khalil, A., Chadha, V., Mandapati, R. *et al.* (1991) Hemobilia in a child with liver abscess. *J .Paed . Gastroenterol. Nutr.*, **12**, 136–138
Maltz, G. and Knauer, C. M. (1991) Amebic liver abscess: a 15-year experience. *Am. J. Gastroenterol.*, **86**, 704–710
Pineiro-Carrero, V. M. and Andres, J. M. (1989) Morbidity and mortality in children with pyogenic liver abscess. *Am. J. Dis Child*, **143**, 1424–1427
Saing, H., Tam, P. K. H., Choi, T. K., Wong, J. (1988) Childhood recurrent pyogenic cholangitis. *J. Pediatr. Surg.*, **23**, 424–9
Stain, S. C., Yellin, A. E., Donovan, A. J. and Brien, H. W. (1991) Pyogenic liver abscess: modern treatment. *Arch Surg.*, **126**, 991–996
Taguchi, T., Ikeda, K., Yakabe, S. and Kimura, S. (1988) Percutaneous drainage for post-traumatic hepatic abscess in children under ultrasound imaging. *Pediatr Radiol*, **18**, 85–87
Vachon, L., Diament, M. J. and Stanley, P. (1986). Percutaneous drainage of hepatic abscesses in children. *J. Pediatr. Surg.*, **21**, 366–8
Vock, P., Kehrer, B. and Tschaeppeler, H. (1986) Blunt liver trauma in children: the role of computed tomography in diagnosis and treatment. *J. Pediatr. Surg.* **21**, 413–418

Leptospirosis

Da C. Gayotto, L., Da Silva, L. C. (1991) Leptospirosis. In *Oxford Textbook of Clinical Hepatology* (Ed. N. McIntyre, J. P. Benhamou, J. Bircher, M. Rizzetto, J. Rodes). Oxford University Press, Oxford
Ferguson, I. R. (1991) Leptospirosis update. *Br. Med. J,* **302**, 128–129.
Lindenbaum, I., Eylan, E. and Shenberg, E. (1984). Leptospirosis in Israel: a report of 14 cases caused by icterohaemorrhagiae sera group (1968–1982). *Isr. J. Med. Sci.,* **20**, 132

Hepatic amoebiases

Ahmad, M., Khan, A. H. and Mubarik, A. (1991) Fatal amoebic liver abscess: an autopsy study. *J. Gastroenterol. Hepatol.*, **6**, 67–70.
Jessee, W. F., Ryan, J. M, Fitzgerald, J. F. and Grosfeld, J. L. (1985) Amebic liver abscess in childhood. *Clin. Pediatr.*, **14**, 134–145.
Knight, R. (1984) Hepatic amoebiasis. *Semin. Liver Dis.,* **4**, 277
van Allan, R. J., Katz, M. D., Johnson, M. B., Laine, L. A., Liu, Y. and Ralls, P. W. (1992) Uncomplicated amebic liver abscess: prospective evaluation of percutaneous therapeutic aspiration. *Radiology,* **183**, 827-30

Hydatid disease

Davis, A., Dixon, H. and Pawlowski, Z. S. (1989) Multicentre clinical trials of benzimidazole-carbonates in human cystic echinococcus (phase 2). *Bull WHO,* **67**, 503–508.
Erdener, A., Ozok, G. and Demircan, M. (1992) Surgical treatment of hepatic hydatid disease in children. *Eur. J. Pediatr. Surg.*, **2**, 87–89
Filice, C., Pirola, F., Brunetti, E., Dughetti, S., Strosselli, M. and Foglieni, C. S. (1990) A new therapeutic approach for hydatid liver cysts. *Gastroenterology,* **98** 1366-1368
Gonzalez, E. M., Selas, P. R., Martinez, B., Garcia, I. G., Carazo, F. P. and Pascual, M. H. (1991) Results of surgical treatment of hepatic hydatidosis: current therapeutic modifications. *World J. Surg.,* **15**, 254–263.
Miguet, J. P., Bresson-Hadni, S., Vuitton, D. (1991) Echinococcosis of the liver. In *Oxford Textbook of Clinical Hepatology* (Ed. N. McIntyre, J. P. Benhamou, J. Bircher, M. Rizzetto, J. Rodes). Oxford University Press, Oxford

Morris, D. L., Smith, P. G. (1987) Albendazole in hydatid disease – hepatocellular toxicity. *Trans. Roy. Soc. Trop. Med. Hyg.,* **87**, 343–344
Murty, T. V. M., Sood, K. C., Fawzi, S. R. (1989) Biliary obstruction due to ruptured hydatid cyst. J. Paediatr. Surg., **24**, 401–403
Ovnat, A., Peiser, J., Oravinoah, E. *et al.* (1984). Acute cholangitis caused by ruptured hydatid cyst. *Surgery,* **95**, 497

Liver flukes

Bacq, Y., Besnier, J-M., Duong, T-H., Pavie, G., Metman, E-H. and Choutet, P. (1991) Successful treatment of acute fasciolasias with Biothionol. *Hepatology,* **14**, 1066–1069.
Carmona, R. S., Crass, R. A., Limb, R. C. and Trunkley, D. D. (1984) Oriental cholangitis. *Am. J. Surg.,* **148**, 117
Jones, A. E., Kay, J. M., Milligan, H. P. *et al.* (1977) Massive infecton with *Fasciola hepatica* in man. *Am. J. Med,* **63**, 836
Navab, R., Diner, W.C., Westbrooke, K. C. *el al.* (1984) endoscopic biliary lavage in a case of *clonorchis sinensis, Gastrointest. Endosc.,* **30**, 292
Uflacker, R., Wholey, M. H., Amaran. N. H. *et al.,* (1982) Parasitic and mycotic causes of biliary obstruction. *Gastrointest. Radiol.* **7**, 173
Warren, K. S. (1991) Blood flukes (schistosomes) and liver flukes. In *Oxford Textbook of Clinical Hepatology* (Ed. N. McIntyre, J. P. Benhamou, J. Bircher, M. Rizzetto, J. Rodes). Oxford University Press, Oxford

Schistosomiasis

Andrade, Z. A., Peixoto, E., Guerret, S. and Grimaud, J.-A. (1992) Hepatic connective tissue changes in hepatosplenic schistosomiasis. *Hum. Pathol.,* **23**, 566–573.
King, C. H. and Mahmoud, A. A. F. (1989) Drugs five years later, prazaquintel. *Ann. Inter. Med.,* **110**, 290–296.
Mitchell, G. F., Premier, R. R., Garcia, E. G. *et al.* (1983) Hybridoma antibody-based competitive ELISA in *Schistosoma japonicum* infection. *Am. J. Trop. Med. Hyg.,* **32**, 114
Nash, T. E. (1982) Schistosome infection in humans; perspectives and recent findings. *Am. Inter. Med.* **97**, 740
Shekhar, K. C. (1991) Schistomiasis: drug therapy and treatment considerations. Drugs, **42**, 379–405

Hepatic granuloma

James. D. G. and Jones-Williams. W. (1985). *Sarcoidosis and other Granulomatous Disorders.* W. B. Saunders, Philadelphia
James, D. G. and Scheuer, P. (1991) Hepatic granulomas. In: *Oxford Textbook of Clinical Hepatology* (Ed. N. McIntyre, J. P. Benhamou, J. Bircher, M. Rizzetto, J. Rodes). Oxford University Press, Oxford
Keteste, H., Latour. F. and Levitt, R. E. (1984). Portal hypertension complicting sarcoid liver disease: Case report and review of the literature. *Am. J. Gastroenterol.,* **79**, 389
Mills. P. R. and Russell. R. I. (1983) Diagnosis of hepatic granulomas: a review. *J. R.. Soc. Med.,* **76**, 393
Zoutman, D. E., Ralph, D. E. and Frei, J. V. (1991) Granulomatous hepatitis and fever of unknown origin: an 11-year experience of 23 cases with three years' follow-up. *J.Clin. Gastroenterol.,* **13**, 69–75

Nematodes

Da C. Gayotto, L. and Da Silva, L. C. (1991) Ascariasis, visceral larva migrans, capillariasis, strongyloidiasis, and pentastomiasis. In: *Oxford Textbook of Clinical Hepatology* (Ed. N. McIntyre, J. P. Benhamou, J. Bircher, M. Rizzetto, J. Rodes). Oxford University Press, Oxford
Khuroo, M. S., Zargar, S. A., Mahajan, R., Bhat, R. L. and Javid, G. (1987) Sonographic appearances in biliary ascariasis. *Gastroenterol.,* **93**, 267–272
Taylor, M. R. H., Keane, C. T., O'Connor, P. *et al.* (1988) The expanded spectrum of toxacaral disease. *Lancet,* **1**, 692–695

Chapter 8

Fulminant and severe acute liver failure

Definition

Acute liver failure is a rare, clinically heterogeneous and complex multi-system disorder in which severe impairment of liver function occurs in association with hepatocellular necrosis in a patient with no recognized underlying chronic liver disease. When associated with encephalopathy the term fulminant is applied. In the absence of encephalopathy the severity of the liver impairment is best assessed by the severity of coagulopathy. Factors II, V, VII, IX and X at values less than 50% of normal or an international normalized ratio of more than 4 (prothrombin time >50 seconds) after intravenous vitamin K implies life-threatening disease. The mortality ranges from 30 to 90% depending on the cause and age at onset. If the child survives, liver function and structure are likely to return to a near normal state and the long-term prognosis is good. A critical life-threatening complication is cerebral oedema with increased intracranial pressure which may lead to medullary coning. Modern management requires early appreciation of the severity of the illness, skilled intensive care and, in those children in whom death is probable, emergency liver transplantation before irreversible brain damage has occurred.

Categories of acute, life-threatening liver failure

'Severe' liver failure   In these patients the prothrombin ratio is greater than 4 but there is no apparent encephalopathy. This occurs particularly commonly in infants. The prognosis is that of fulminant liver failure

Fulminant liver failure   By convention acute liver disease with hepatic encephalopathy starting within 8 weeks of the first sign of liver disease is termed fulminant liver failure (Trey and Davidson, 1970). A number of confusing definitions which relate to the time between the first features of liver disease and the onset of encephalopathy have been adopted in an effort to identify subgroups with differing prognosis. The term fulminant liver failure is restricted to those patients with onset of encephalopathy within 2 weeks by French authors who define those with onset between 2 weeks and 3 months as *'subfulminant'* liver failure (Berneau *et al.*, 1986). Others have termed those in whom the encephalopathy starts between 8 and 24 weeks *'late-onset'* liver failure (Gimson *et al.*, 1986)

Acute on chronic   It is important to recognize that hepatic encephalopathy may be a presenting feature in patients with previously asymptomatic undiagnosed chronic liver disease such as Wilson's disease or autoimmune chronic liver disease. There are important differences in the prognosis and management of such patients (see Chapters 11, 12 and 17).

Pathology

Liver biopsy during life, or immediately following death, shows widespread hepato-cellular necrosis or absence of hepatocytes, except for a cuff of cells surviving in periportal zones. The area on the slide occupied by hepatocytes, normally accounting for approximately 85% of the section is frequently reduced to between 15 and 35% of the section. Little or no regeneration may be evident. Numerous bile ducts are seen because of the collapse of the reticulin framework allowing marked crowding of portal tracts. Bile ducts may also be prominent because of regeneration. There may be a marked acute inflammatory cell infiltrate, both in the portal tracts and in the hepatic parenchyma. There may be prominent pigment-laden macrophages.

Brain oedema may be detected at post mortem in up to 40% of fatal cases. In some there may be an increase in Alzheimer Type II astrocytes but otherwise there are no neuropathological abnormalities unless ischaemia has occurred.

Causes

The causes are given in Tables 8.1–8.4. In most paediatric series hepatitis A, B (which may include superinfection with D hepatitis), sporadic non-A, non-B (which may include HBsAg negative cases which have not been tested for anti-HBc and fatal cases due to

Table 8.1. Causes of fulminant liver failure

Infective:

Viral hepatitis:
A, B, B+ delta, C, E (enteric non-A, non-B)
Epstein-Barr virus
Cytomegalovirus
Adenovirus
Echo virus
Varicella
Measles
Yellow fever
Lassa
Ebola
Marburg
Dengue
Haemorrhagic fevers
(Bunyaviridae family of viruses)
Toga viruses
(HIV viruses)
Septicaemia
Leptospirosis
Malaria

Table 8.2 Causes of fulminant liver failure

Toxic or drug-related:
   Amanita phalloides
   Carbon tetrachloride
   Paracetamol
   Halothane
   Valproate
   Carbamazepine
   Phenytoin
   Isoniazid
   Amiodarone
   Cytotoxics
   Monoamine oxidase inhibitors

Irradiation

Table 8.3 Causes of fulminant liver failure

Inherited/Metabolic:

Galactosaemia
Fructosaemia
Tyrosinaemia
Familial erythrophagocytic reticulosis
Alpha-1 antitrypsin deficiency
Neonatal haemochromatosis
Niemann–Pick II (C)
Wilson's Disease

Table 8.4 Causes of fulminant liver failure

Ischaemic:

Budd–Chiari syndrome
Acute circulatory failure
Septicaemia with shock
Heat stroke

Infiltrative:

Leukaemia
Haemophagocytic lymphohistiocytosis
Haemangioendiothelioma
Lymphangioendiothelioma

Autoimmune:

Smooth muscle antibody or Liver kidney microsomes +ve hepatitis
Giant cell hepatitis with haemolytic anaemia in early childhood

hepatitis in whom serological testing has been performed before antibodies can be detected with current techniques) and drug-related liver damage account for up to 90% of cases. Of the more than 200 drugs and toxins implicated only those more commonly encountered are given.

Pathogenesis

Although the cause of the liver damage has a major role in determining outcome when acute liver failure occurs, what determines the severity of liver damage with many of these causes is largely unknown. With toxins such as paracetamol the degree of liver injury is related to the dose of the toxin. In 'idiosyncratic' drug-induced injury continued drug administration after the onset of jaundice often causes a fatal outcome. What determines the severity of liver damage in infection is largely obscure (see below). Both the age of the patient and the competence of the immune system influence prognosis. In severe hepatitis B infection with encephalopathy there is a vigorous immune response with rapid clearance of the virus. HBsAg is not detected in the serum in up to 50%. Diagnosis requires demonstration of high titre IgM anti-HBc antibodies. Infants born to HBsAg positive mothers who are either anti-HBe positive or neither anti-HBe nor HBe positive are at particular risk of severe hepatitis B including acute liver failure. In some instances this has been attributed to a mutant HBV. Super- or co-infection with hepatitis D (delta) may cause a similarly severe hepatitis but in children this has as yet only been recognized commonly in Venezuela. There is insufficient evidence on serologically proven hepatitis C or E in children to comment on the relative frequency of acute liver failure. The newborn and immunocompromised patients are particularly at risk from herpes simplex viruses 1 and 2, cytomegalovirus, Epstein–Barr virus, varicella, and adenovirises and echoviruses. Note that in herpes infection there may not be cutaneous or mucosal evidence of infection. Endotoxaemia is often present but its contribution to further tissue necrosis is uncertain.

What limits the liver's ability to recover or regenerate is enigmatic. If part of the liver is resected either in the experimental animal or in humans, because of trauma or tumour, rapid regeneration occurs. In fulminant hepatic failure in many cases no signs of regeneration are found.

Early recognition of acute liver failure.

Features of liver disease may have been present for hours or weeks. The course may be one of progressive or increasingly severe jaundice, anorexia and vomiting, followed by clouding of consciousness. In other patients after a typical initial onset of hepatitis, there is a period of improvement followed by the recurrence of fever, anorexia, abdominal pain and vomiting. In such patients rapid decrease in liver size in the absence of clinical improvement is a very serious sign. Rarely encephalopathy may develop before jaundice is apparent. The respiratory rate usually increases early in the encephalopathy, with typically deep and forceful respiration which may lead to a respiratory alkalosis.

In an icteric patient with suspected or confirmed viral hepatitis the clinician should be alerted to the possibility of acute liver failure by a number of clinical features such as persisting anorexia, progressively deepening jaundice, spontaneous bleeding or bleeding from injections sites, hypoglycaemia, the development of ascites and, particularly, *a reduction in liver size to less than normal.* A prothrombin time which remains prolonged by more than 5 seconds after parenteral vitamin K should forewarn its onset. In the patient with encephalopathy without prior features of liver disease icterus, a bleeding tendency, hepatomegaly or a reduction of liver size should indicate a hepatic cause of encephalopathy. The finding of abnormal biochemical tests of liver function with progressively disturbed clotting and/or hypoglycaemia and/or raised blood ammonia confirms it. Note that the ammonia may be normal.

Chronic liver disease, with underlying cirrhosis, due to Wilson's disease or autoimmune chronic active hepatitis may present in a similar fashion and with no features to suggest chronicity (see Chapters 11 and 17). Although both of these conditions may improve with specific therapy, the liver structure will not return to normal but remain scarred or cirrhotic.

Established encephalopathy

Any change from normal behaviour for age, however slight, such as disinterest in play or television must be regarded as a sign of encephalopathy. In some instances encephalopathy may proceed or start simultaneously with other features of liver disease.

The initial neurological features may be lethargy, verbal confusion or combative,

Table 8.5 Grades of acute hepatic encephalopathy

1 Minor disturbances of consciousness or motor function
2 Drowsy but responsive to commands
3 Stuporous but responsive to pain
4 Unresponsive to pain

irritability, irrational hyperactivity. Infants may regress to more immature behaviour. Restlessness, disorientation, repeated yawning and sucking movements progress to apathy, stupor and coma. Eventually, the respiratory and vasomotor centres fail.

The neuromuscular state varies with the degree of encephalopathy (Table 8.5). In minor degrees, incoordination and tremor may be evident. Asterixis or flapping tremor, that is, rapid flexion and extension movements of the wrist and metacarpal phalangeal joints on sustained extension of the wrists with the forearm fixed, is often present only transiently. Tendon reflexes may be increased and as the coma deepens the Babinski response becomes positive. Clonus can be demonstrated. Eventually, decerebrate rigidity or decorticate posture may occur. With progressive brain stem involvement 'doll's-eye' movements are lost, the pupils become fixed and unresponsive. Hypotonia and areflexia occur terminally.

Clinical features of mild encephalopathy are lethargy with minor disturbances of cerebration or motor function. In the next stage (Grade 2) the child is drowsy but responds to verbal commands. In both of these stages the child may become restless with hallucinations, irrational hyperactivity or combative behaviour. Repeated vomiting and hyperventilation may occur. Stupor in which the child is responsive only to painful stimuli is the next grade (3). In grade 4 there is no response to painful stimuli, no extensor posturing and rigidity, and finally irreversible brain stem depression with failure of respiratory and vasomotor centres occurs.

Convulsions can occur in any grade. Patients commonly have a period of days in which less severe encephalopathy is recognized before irreversible cerebral oedema occurs, but in a small proportion it develops in a few hours. CT brain scan, and toxicological studies may be required to exclude other causes of encephalopathy.

Table 8.6 Aggravating factors in hepatic encephalopathy

Gastrointestinal haemorrhage	Uraemia
Hypovolaemia	Infection
Potassium depletion	High protein intake
Hypoglycaemia	Constipation
Sedatives and anaesthetics	

The mechanisms of hepatic encephalopathy

The absence of structural changes within the brain (other than oedema), the rapid onset of coma and its reversibility suggest a metabolic origin. In spite of intensive study of the complex biochemical features of this syndrome, as yet there is no adequate explanation for such features, nor have the biochemical data provided a rational basis for the comprehensive management of this disorder and its complications.

Hepatic encephalopathy is usually attributed to the abnormal retention of nitrogenous metabolites or toxins secondary to impaired hepatic function. There is considerable evidence that substances involved in causing the syndrome arise from the gut. In addition, intrahepatic shunting of portal blood directly into the systemic circulation, without contact with hepatocytes, may be important. Intestinal bacteria, ingested protein and the presence of blood in the alimentary tract play a major part in the production of encephalopathy by increasing ammonia absorption and mercaptan production. Serum ammonia levels determined in venous blood are elevated to a degree which reflects the cerebral state but is not directly correlated with it. However, some patients who are in deep coma have normal serum ammonia. Current experimental evidence indicates that although ammonia is possibly a major factor in the pathogenesis of coma it is not responsible for all the neuropsychiatric symptoms and signs.

In addition to alimentary factors causing the coma the continuing hepatic necrosis with incomplete hepatic metabolism and the effects of the initiating illness on other organs, makes the metabolic consequences of this syndrome very different from those of subtotal hepatectomy. Other metabolic factors which have been implicated in the pathogenesis include short-chain fatty acids as butyrate valerate and octanoate, which are increased in the blood and cerebrospinal fluid in hepatic encephalopathy, possibly because of ineffective hepatic metabolism. The levels attained are not in themselves sufficient to cause coma, but they may do so by acting synergistically with ammonia.

Considerable interest has recently been directed to abnormalities in serum amino acid concentrations in fulminant hepatic failure and to the possible role of changes in the concentration within the brain of neurotransmitters. The straight chain amino acids phenylalanine, tyrosine, methionine and tryptophan are increased, while the branched chain amino acids valine, leucine and isoleucine are decreased.

Neurotransmitters are chemicals which mediate the post-synaptic action of neurons. The 'false' neurotransmitters are chemicals structurally related to neurotransmitters but interfering with synaptic function. Neurotransmitters are metabolized from amino acids. Thus, the abnormalities in amino acids may lead to secondary changes in neuro-transmitters. Data relating to the concentration of these true or false neurotransmitters in blood or cerebrospinal fluid must be interpreted with caution. There may be wide variation in the concentration of these substances in various parts of the brain. The site of critical concentration of these metabolites is not known, but it is considered that an important site of action may be the reticular formation. The inhibitory neurotransmitter gamma-amino butyric acid may also increase.

A very important metabolic abnormality which may complicate the encephalopathy is profound hypoglycaemia. In addition, changes in the serum concentration of hydrogen ion, sodium, potassium, phosphate, magnesium and calcium may contribute. In the initial stages there is commonly a respiratory alkalosis due to hyperventilation, leading to a decrease in cerebral perfusion and oxygen consumption. A metabolic alkalosis may arise secondary to hypokalaemia which is often present early in the course. Alkalosis increases the cerebral uptake of ammonia.

Tissue necrosis both within the liver and in sites of secondary infection and tissue hypoxia may give rise to a metabolic acidosis. Hyponatraemia may develop spontaneously or be aggravated by salt-losing diuretics. Osmotic diuretics such as hypertonic glucose, given for nutritional reasons or to reduce intracranial pressure, may cause hypernatraemia, particularly if the urinary sodium excretion is low.

Cerebral blood flow may be decreased in part due to hypocapnia. Encephalopathy has been attributed to both reduced cerebral blood flow and reduced glucose utilization, but the data relating to this do not indicate whether these changes are primary or secondary.

Management

The essentials in management are:

(1) accurate diagnosis of the cause of the liver injury and of the cause of the encephalopathy;
(2) skilled intensive care to minimize aggravating factors and complications until liver function recovers or transplantation can be performed; and
(3) liver transplantation in patients in whom the chances of recovery are worse than outcome of emergency liver transplantation.

Components of intensive care include full circulatory support, with monitoring of pressure in the systemic circulation, central veins, pulmonary artery and within the skull. Note that central venous pressure may be misleading and for optimum fluid balance control measuring pressure continually in the pulmonary artery with a Swan-Ganz catheter is desirable in selecting those requiring inotropes, haemodialysis or liver transplantation. The maintenance of tissue perfusion and oxygenation is essential. Particularly important is adequate cerebral perfusion. Haemodialysis or ultrafiltration is required in patients with renal failure.

Particular therapeutic measures are applicable for specific causes and at different stages in the development of the disorder. The care of the patient with fulminant hepatic failure requires intensive observation, support and care by nursing and medical staff familiar with the range of metabolic abnormalities and complications which have to be anticipated and prevented or minimized. Earliest possible contact should be made with senior staff of a liver failure unit so that an appropriate regimen of management and indications for and the timing and mode of transfer be agreed.

Initial assessment

A careful history of family illnesses, consanguinity, contact with patients with liver, parenteral infusions or exposure to drugs or toxins as well as mode of onset of the illness is essential. Thorough complete clinical examination is required to look for diagnostic clues such as herpetic vesicles or Kayser Fleischer rings (by slit-lamp examination) as well as to document features of liver disease, the patient's general condition and to grade semiquantitatively the severity of the encephalopathy (see Table 8.6). A battery of aetiological investigations requires consideration (Table 8.7). In early infancy the infections indicated in Table 8.1 require particular attention as well as inherited metabolic disorders other than Wilson's disease.

Serial determination of pulse, blood pressure, central venous pressure, body weight, serum and urinary concentration of electrolytes, urea, creatinine and osmolarity, blood pH and concentrations of glucose, phosphate, calcium and magnesium is essential every few hours. Standard tests of liver function, serum amylase, peripheral blood count, prothrombin time and chest X-ray should be performed daily.

An electrocardiogram should be performed to assess the intracellular potassium status with continuous recording to detect arrhythmias. Electroencephalogram monitoring adds to information available on the state of the central nervous system.

General measures

Irrespective of the cause of liver damage the following regimen is recommended. If the child is resting quietly in grade I or II coma he/she should be nursed in a quite room with

Table 8.7 Investigations in infants and children with acute liver failure

---

Biochemical tests of liver function
Blood sugar
Serum sodium, potassium, calcium, phosphate and magnesium
Serum ammonia
Uric acid
Cholesterol
Triglyceride
Amylase

Full blood count
Reticulocyte count
Prothrombin time
Blood group
Red blood cell antibodies
(Coomb's test)

Chest X-ray
ECG
Echocardiography
Ultrasound of abdomen particularly liver, portal and hepatic vein, inferior vena cava and biliary system
Technetium-99m colloid liver scan
EEG

Blood gases

Urine: chemical analysis, including toxicology, osmolality, urea and electrolyte content

Bacterial cultures: urine, blood, ascitic fluid if present, stool, throat swab, sputum and skin lesions

Viral studies: hepatitis BsAg, IgM antibodies to hepatitis A, hepatitis B core (D Ag and Ab if positive), C,
   and E, CMV, EB, HIV, measles, varicella, adenovirus, herpes 1, 2 and 6 and echoviruses
Viral culture of urine for CMV and of vesicles if present

Serological studies for toxoplasmosis, leptospirosis and listeriosis

Alpha-1-antitrypsin phenotype
Urinary succinylacetone

Immunoglobulins
Tissue autoantibodies
Complement C3 and C4
Antibodies to liver specific lipoprotein
Antibodies to liver asialoglycoprotein receptor
T-cell subsets and activation markers
Lymphokines

NB: Save 5 ml of serum and aliquot of initial urine for possible subsequent toxicological, serological or
   chemical investigation

Infants only:
Galactose-1-phosphate uridyl transferase

Children over 3 years of age:
Serum copper
        caeruloplasmin
24 hour urinary copper (baseline)
        with penicillamine 0.5 g twice daily

Consider
Bone marrow to exclude infiltrative/neoplastic and storage disorders
CT brain scan for other cause of coma
CSF examination for evidence of haemophagocytic lymphoreticulosis

If liver transplantation is a possibility
HLA typing
Screening of throat, nose, axillae, perineum, wounds or other skin lesions for multiple resistant *Staph aureus*
Immunization record

---

as little stimulation or painful intervention as possible to minimize acute increases in intracranial pressure. A nurse should be present at all times recording vital signs, blood pressure and neurological status at frequent intervals. Blood sugar should be checked before meals and 2 hourly while asleep. *Sedatives aggravate encephalopathy and may precipitate respiratory failure. They must not be given unless the patient is to be mechanically ventilated.* Hypoglycaemia must be prevented and excessive breakdown of endogenous protein minimized by intravenous glucose or oral glucose polymers. Unless the patient is dehydrated fluid intake should initially be limited to 60% of normal maintenance in the hope that this may limit the risk of cerebral oedema while maintaining normal tissue perfusion, blood pressure and a central venous pressure of 6–10 cm H_2O. Fluid will normally be given as 10–20% glucose infusion with added potassium at a minimum rate of 3 mmol/kg/24 hours if there is no renal failure. It may be necessary to add magnesium, phosphate or bicarbonate. The volume of all urine passed should be carefully measured and its blood, protein, electrolyte and sugar content recorded. Diuretics should be avoided since they aggravate fluid and electrolyte problems. Protein feeds are stopped initially to minimize the contribution of nitrogenous metabolites to encephalopathy. When the encephalopathy stabilizes and the prothrombin time improves protein intake is gradually resumed. Lactulose is given to produce three to four loose stools per day but it is probably counterproductive to give it when the patient is incontinent, irritable or uncooperative.

Cimetidine 30 mg/kg/24 hours in divided doses at 6-hourly intervals and vitamin K 1 mg/day both given intravenously may prevent bleeding from gastric erosion. Ranitidine may cause less inhibition of liver regeneration than cimetidine but its dose in children is less well established (0.35 mg/kg over 2 hours and repeated every 6–8 hours, but increases if the gastric pH < 5). If fresh frozen plasma or other clotting factors are given it does make assessment of the progression of liver disease difficult in the next 4 to 6 hours. These should only be given if there is bleeding, if a decision has been made to proceed to transplantation or if the patient is at particular risk, for example, during transport. Careful consideration should be given to the use of acyclovir if herpes has not been excluded and to the use of antibiotics. Any confirmed infection must be treated with appropriate antimicrobials (see below). A prophylactic selective parenteral and enteral antimicrobial regimen (cefuroxime intravenously; amphotericin B, tobramycin and polymyxin E for the sterilization of the gut and mupirocin to the nose) significantly reduces infective episodes but the reduction in mortality is not significant (Rolando, 1991a). If antibiotics are used topical oral anti-candidal treatment is essential.

In *paracetamol poisoning* monitoring the prothrombin time (PT) at 12-hourly intervals is the best marker of severity of liver damage. If the PT is normal at 48 hours recovery is the rule. The mortality is greater than 80% if the pH is < 7.3 or if the PT is greater than 50 seconds and the creatinine > 300 μmol/litre.

Such fatalities may be prevented by gastric lavage within 4 hours of ingestion or with intravenous N-acetyl cysteine begun within 15 hours of ingestion. N-acetyl cysteine is metabolized to glutathione which is conjugated with toxic paracetamol metabolites. The earlier it is given the better. It may be worth giving it later than 15 hours if the PT is still normal. Such treatment is required if a plasma concentration is above a line joining 200 μg/ml (1.32 mmol/litre) at 4 hours and 60 μg/ml (0.39 mmol/litre) at 12 hours after ingestion, plotted on a semi-log graph of concentration *versus* time. The dose is 150 mg/kg given over 15 minutes, followed by 50 mg/kg over 4 hours and 100 mg/kg over the next 16 hours given in appropriate volumes of 5% dextrose. Urticaria, bronchospasm, anaphylaxis, rashes, nausea and vomiting are the main side-effects.

Indications for transfer to a specialized unit

In all but the mildest cases it is advisable to transfer the patient to an intensive care facility with the experience to anticipate and minimize the multisystem complications and to proceed to liver transplantation before irreversible brain damage occurs. It must be stressed that in viral hepatitis the level of coma in the first hours of encephalopathy is no guide to the eventual outcome.

If encephalopathy progresses to grade II or the patient becomes agitated in the absence of hypoglycaemia transfer is essential. It may be necessary to institute some components of intensive care locally while optimum arrangements for transfer are made. Mechanical ventilation is necessary if there is hypoxia, if the patient is agitated in grade I-II coma or if in coma grades III and IV. Ventilation is maintained at minimal pressures and oxygen concentrations to give a normal PaO_2 with rates adjusted to give a $PaCO_2$ of 26–34 mmHg. The conventional teaching is that if the blood pressure is normal the patient should be nursed with the upper trunk and head elevated if possible at 45°, with no neck flexion, to minimize intracerebral pressure. If the blood pressure is low the patient should be nursed flat and if the central venous pressure is low colloid or fresh frozen plasma or whole blood given (depending on the serum protein, clotting factor and haemoglobin concentrations). Recent observations suggest that elevation of the head has minimal effects on intracranial pressure but may significantly diminish cerebral perfusion. Cerebral oedema may be exacerbated by tactile stimuli, noise, hypoxia, hypercapnia, hypotension, and hypoglycaemia.

If the blood pressure is low, with a normal central venous pressure, dopamine may help but full intensive care with intracranial pressure monitoring is mandatory to optimize cerebral perfusion. It is usually prudent to establish ventilation and sedation and secure measures to prevent hypoglycaemia and minimize the risks of cerebral oedema prior to transfer. Full consultation with the receiving specialist unit is essential.

Patient monitoring

Acute hepatic failure is a syndrome of considerable variability. Different therapeutic measures are applicable in different patients and different stages in the development of the disorder. The care of the patient with fulminant hepatic failure requires intensive nursing support and observation by medical staff familiar with the range of metabolic abnormalities and complications which have to be anticipated or prevented. As part of supportive therapy, intensive monitoring of the cardiovascular, respiratory and central nervous systems, and of fluid and electrolyte balance is essential. As well as clinical assessment, this requires continuous monitoring of pulse, blood pressure, central venous and intracranial pressure, with repeated determination of body weight, serum and urinary concentration of electrolytes, urea, creatinine and osmolarity. The blood pH and concentrations of glucose, phosphate, calcium, magnesium and PT must be measured at 4 to 8 hourly intervals until the patient's condition stabilizes. Standard tests of liver function, serum amylase, peripheral blood count and chest X-ray should be performed daily.

An ECG should be performed to assess the intracellular potassium status with continuous recording to detect arrhythmia. EEG monitoring may show progressive slowing with increased amplitude of electrical activity in the early stages. With deterioration there are paroxysmal bursts of triphasic waves on a background of ever decreasing amplitude, until a flat EEG occurs.

Indications for urgent consideration of orthotopic liver transplantation

Irrespective of the severity of encephalopathy if the PT is prolonged by more than 90 seconds after intravenous vitamin K the mortality is virtually 100%, and urgent liver transplantation is necessary. In a recent analysis of 54 children admitted to our unit between 1982 and 1991 with acute liver failure of diverse causes, the mortality was 90% in those with an prothrombin ratio (international normalized ratio, INR) >4, while 15 of 17 aged less than 2 years died.

Based on experience largely in adults, mortality is more than 80% if the prothrombin exceeds 50 seconds time. In HBV, non-A, non-B, drug-induced or late onset acute liver failure. With a factor V concentration of less than 15% of normal the mortality is 85% in type A hepatitis and paracetamol ingestion and more than 90% in other causes of liver failure. The development of cerebral oedema or renal failure gives a mortality of 50% and 70% respectively in patients with grade 3 or 4 encephalopathy irrespective of the severity of the coagulopathy. In patients who develop encephalopathy grade 3 or 4 within 7 days of onset a survival rate of 34% was recorded compared with 7% with later onset.

Outcome with liver transplantation The success rate with liver transplantation in children is steadily improving, with 1 year survival rates of between 75 and 90% being reported in those transplanted for end-stage chronic liver disease. One year survival rates of 55–70% have been reported in five series of adults transplanted for acute liver failure. Survival rates of 60% and 64% have been reported in two small paediatric series. The technique of reduction hepatectomy which allows a child to be grafted with part of a liver from an larger donor should increase the chances of children being transplanted before intractable cerebral oedema occurs. In a few adults heterotopic liver transplantation with the transplanted liver segment draining to the infrarenal inferior vena cava has been used successfully.

Major complications

A full list of complications to be anticipated are given in Table 8.8. Major ones are discussed in detail below.

Table 8.8 Complications

Hypoglycaemia
Cerebral oedema
Renal failure
Acid-base disturbances
Fluid and electrolyte disturbances
Bleeding diathesis
Hypoxia
Circulatory problems
Secondary bacterial and fungal infection
Pancreatitis
Bone marrow depression

Cerebral oedema   Cerebral oedema is a frequent complication, documented at post mortem in between 30 and 40% of fatal cases. Increased intracranial pressure is to be suspected in any patient in whom tendon reflexes are abnormally brisk and is certainly present when spasticity, rigidity or if clinical features of brain stem involvement can be demonstrated. Rapid rises in systolic blood pressure, pulse or respiratory rate or changes in pupillary reflexes are also indicative. Although the intracranial pressure is raised, papilloedema rarely occurs. The CT brain scan is often unhelpful in diagnosing cerebral oedema.

Optimum monitoring requires continuous measurement of arterial pressure and of intracranial pressure with an extradural monitor. The cerebral perfusion pressure (mean arterial pressure minus intracranial pressure) should be maintained at more than 50 mmHg, with the cerebral pressure ideally less than 20 mmHg (normal less than 10). If the perfusion falls check that the $PaCO_2$ is in the region of 3.3–3.4 kPa (26–34 mmHg), sedation and paralysis are adequate, that the serum osmolality is 300–310 mOsm/litre and that the CVP is 6–10 cmH$_2$O. In the meantime hyperventilate temporarily and give intravenous mannitol 0.5 g/kg as a 20% solution over a 15-minute period. This is usually effective and may be repeated if the osmolarity is not greater than 320 mOsm/litre and a diuresis occurs. If there is renal failure haem-ultrafiltration will be necessary removing 200 ml of water for each 100 ml of mannitol solution. In mannitol-resistant poor cerebral perfusion intravenous thiopentone may be tried in a bolus dose of 2–4 mg/kg over 15 minutes followed by a slow intravenous infusion of between 1–2 mg/kg/hour, while planning for transplantation. Arterial hypotension is a major risk with thiopentone.

Circulatory problems   Circulatory disturbances are common. A high cardiac output is required because of decreased peripheral resistance. Sinus tachycardia occurs in 75% of cases. The blood pressure must be maintained to achieve maximum hepatic perfusion. Patients are extremely sensitive to volume depletion. If there is hypovolaemia salt-poor albumin, fresh frozen plasma or whole blood, depending on the serum albumin concentration, prothrombin time and haemoglobin concentration, should be carefully infused. A Swan-Ganz catheter may provide early evidence of failing cardiac output due to myocardial dysfunction. Inotropic drugs and correction of any cardiac arrhythmia may be helpful. The use of epoprostenol and or *N*-acetyl cysteine to improve cardiac output (>4.5 l/min/M^2), microcirculatory flow, and oxygen delivery of >800/min/M^2 and oxygen consumption >150 ml/min/M^2 in shock associated with acute liver failure seems to improve survival while measures to increase arterial pressure alone such as epinephrine may be detrimental.

Bradycardia is a late development. In the late stages, unexplained hypotension is very common. It may arise from central vasomotor depression. Sudden, unexpected cardiac arrest occurs in up to 25% of cases.

Bleeding diathesis   A bleeding diathesis is almost always present. Its severity varies from patient to patient. The incidence of clinical haemorrhage varies in reported series from between 40 and 70% and is a contributory factor to death in between 10 and 60%. The most common coagulation defect is a decrease in Factors II, V, VII, IX and X; all except V are measured by the prothrombin time. An increase in Factor VIII is occasionally seen and is unexplained. Severe hypofibrinogenaemia is rare and the mechanism of the decrease is uncertain. Although evidence of disseminated intravascular coagulation has been found, heparin therapy is not helpful. Severe gastrointestinal haemorrhage is frequently a major contributory factor to death. It may occur when the generalized bleeding diathesis is improving. Severe thrombocytopenia may contribute to this. Many patients bleed from localized erosions in the oesophagus, stomach or duodenum. Prophylactic H_2 antagonists help but platelet concentrates and fresh frozen plasma are required if there is overt bleeding.

Renal failure   Renal failure with severe oliguria, inappropriately low sodium excretion, or anuria, often develops, particularly in the later stages. Both acute tubular necrosis and functional renal failure may occur. The mechanism leading to functional renal failure is not known. It is essential to correct hypovolaemia and to maintain renal perfusion. Dopamine in a dose of 2 µg/kg/min may be helpful. Frusemide by infusion (1 mg/ml) in a dose of 1–3 mg/kg may stimulate urine production but if repeated carries the risk of electrolyte depletion, particularly potassium. Mannitol used likewise in a dose of 0.75 g/kg carries the risk of hypervolaemia if it fails to produce a diuresis. Haemodialysis is required if the creatinine exceeds 400 µmol/l, if the pH is <7.3 or if the K^+ exceeds 6 mmol/litre. Ultrafiltration may be required if there is fluid overload.

Hypoxia   Hypoxia occurs frequently. As well as central depression of respiratory drive it may be due to pulmonary infection, aspiration, pulmonary collapse or pulmonary oedema occurring secondary to abnormal capillary permeability or fluid retention. Intrapulmonary shunts may contribute to the hypoxia. A respiratory acidosis may occur. Physiotherapy, turning the patient or bronchoscopy may be required but additional sedation is needed during these procedures to minimize rises in intracranial pressure.

Acid-base and electrolyte disturbances   These occur in nearly all cases. Hyperventilation is a constant feature during the early stages of coma, causing a respiratory alkalosis. Metabolic alkalosis also occurs due to potassium deficiency, administration of alkalis or continuous gastric aspiration. Lactic acidosis may occur in association with hypoglycaemia. Hypokalaemia and hypophosphotaemia require careful correction because of the risk of renal failure. Hyponatraemia usually reflects dilution and is best treated by fluid restriction. Additional sodium may aggravate cerebral oedema.

Susceptibility to infection   Bacterial and fungal infections occur commonly and contribute to the morbidity and mortality. Associated endotoxaemia exacerbates the liver injury and may cause renal impairment. Increased metabolic demands and tissue breakdown may lead to increased accumulation of amino acids and short-chain fatty acids which aggravate the encephalopathy. Factors contributing to infection include defective opsonization, low complement levels, impaired polymorphonuclear neutrophil leucocyte function and the need for invasive monitoring. In the unconscious state, inadequate ventilation favours respiratory tract infection. Awareness of this danger with asepsis as far as practicable, is essential. Prophylactic parenteral and enteric broad-spectrum antimicrobials reduce the frequency of infective episodes.

Infection in the respiratory or urinary system, septicaemia or peritonitis may be present *with few overt signs*. The main effects are a deterioration in liver function and in the level of consciousness. There may be no fever. A high index of suspicion and frequent bacteriological investigations are necessary for early diagnosis. Gram-negative organisms or *Staphylococcus Aureus* are often responsible. If the patient deteriorates and no other parameters have changed it is essential to use a combination of broad-spectrum antibiotics while awaiting the results of bacteriological investigations. If this occurs after 3–6 days of broad-spectrum antibiotics a fungal infection is likely, particularly if the total white cell count is greater than $20 \times 10^9/l$ or if there are signs of otherwise unexplained renal impairment.

Bone marrow depression   It may affect all components or only platelets, white blood series or the red blood cell series. It occurs rarely but is usually irreversible. Bone marrow transplantation may be required. Granulocyte colony stimulating factor and granulocyte macrophage colony stimulating factor should be considered although their effects on platelet and red cell production are controversial.

Bibliography and references

Arora, A., Sharma, M. P., Buch, P. and Mathur, M. (1990) Paroxysmal nocturnal hemoglobinuria with hepatic vein thrombosis presenting as hepatic encephalopathy. *Indian J. Gastroenterol.,* **9**, 91–92

Asano, Y., Yoshikawa, T., Suga, S., Yazaki, T., Kondo, K. and Yamanishi, K. (1990) Fatal fulminant hepatitis in an infant with human herpesvirus-6 infection [letter]. *Lancet,* **335**, 862–863

Baglin, T. P., Harper, P. and Marcus, R. E. (1990) Veno-occlusive disease of the liver complicating ABMT successfully treated with recombinant tissue plasminogen activator (rt-PA). *Bone Marrow Transplant,* **5**, 439–441

Basile, A. S., Hughes, R. D., Harrison, P. M. *et al.* (1991) Elevated brain concentrations of 1,4-benzodiazepines in fulminant hepatic failure. *N. Eng. J. Med.* **325**, 473–478

Berman, D. H., Leventhal, R. I., Gavaler, J. S., Cadoff, E. M. and Van Thiel, D. H. (1991) Clinical differentiation of fulminant Wilsonian hepatitis from other causes of hepatic failure. *Gastroenterology,* **100**, 1129–1134

Berneau, J., Rueff, B. and Benhamou, J. P. (1986) Fulminant and subfulminant liver failure, definition and causes. *Sem. Liver dis.,* **6**, 97–106

Berneau, J. and Benhamou, J.-P. (1991) Fulminant and subfulminant liver failure. In: *Oxford Textbook of Clinical Hepatology* (eds N. McIntyre, J.-P. Benhamou, J. Bricher, M. Rizzetto and J. Rodes). Oxford Medical Publications, Oxford. 924–942

Bismuth, H., Samuel, D., Gugenheim, J. *et al.* (1987) Emergency liver transplantation for fulminant hepatitis. *Ann. Int. Med.* **107**, 337–341

Blei, A. T. (1991) Cerebral oedema and intracranial hypertension in acute liver failure: distinct aspects of the same problem. *Hepatology,* **13**, 376–379

Bosman, D. K., Deutz, N. E. P., deGraaf, A. A. *et al.* (1990) Changes in Brain metabolism during hyperammonnia and acute liver failure, results of a comparative $_1$H-NMR spectroscopy and biochemical study. *Hepatology,* **123**, 281–290

Brusillo, S. W. and Traystman, R. (1986) Hepatic Encephalopathy. *New Engl. J. Med.* **314**, 768

Butterworth, R. F. and Pomier-Layrargues, G. (1990) Benzodiazepine receptors and hepatic encephalopathy. *Hepatology,* **11**, 499–501

Chu, C. M. and Liaw, Y. F. (1990) The incidence of fulminant hepatic failure in acute viral hepatitis in Taiwan: increased risk in patients with pre-existing HBsAg carrier state. *Infection,* **18**, 200–203

Davenport, A., Will, E. J. and Davison, A. M. (1990) Effect of posture on intracranial pressure and cerebral perfusion pressure in patients with fulminant hepatic and renal failure after acetaminophen self-poisoning. *Crit. Care Med.,* **18**, 286–289

Davenport, A., Will, E. J. and Losowsky, M. S. (1989) Rebound surges of intracranial pressure as a consequence of forced ultrafiltration used to control intracranial pressure in patients with severe hepatorenal failure. *Am. J. Kidney Dis.,* **14**, 516–519

DeVictor, D., Desplanques, L., Debray, E. *et al.* (1992) Emergency liver transplantation for fulminant liver failure in infants and children. *Hepatology,* **16**, 1156–1162

Dioguardi, F. S., Brigatti, M., Dell'Oca, M., Ferrario, E. and Abbiati, R. (1990) Effects of chronic oral branched-chain amino acid supplementation in a subpopulation of cirrhotics. *Clin. Physiol. Biochem.,* **8**, 101–107

Dirix, L. Y., Polson, R. J., Richardson, A. and Williams, R. (1989) Primary sepsis presenting as fulminant hepatic failure. *Q. J. Med.,* **73**, 1037–1043

Ede, R.J. and Williams, R. (1986) Hepatic encephalopathy and cerebral oedema. *Sem. Liver Dis.,* **6**, 107–118

Egbring, R. and Seitz, R. (1990) Improved prognosis of fulminant hepatic failure (FHF) after plasma derivative replacement therapy. Enhanced proteolysis of hemostatic proteins confirmed by proteinase-inhibitor complexes determination. *Z Gastroenterol,* **28**, 104–109

Emond, J. C., Aran, P. P., Whitington, P. F., Broelsch, C. E. and Baker, A. L. (1989) Liver transplantation in the management of fulminant hepatic failure. *Gastroenterology,* **96**, 1583–1588

Fagan, E. A. and Williams, R. (1990) Fulminant viral hepatitis. *Br. Med. Bull.,* **46**, 462–480

Ferenci, P., Grimm, G., Meryn, S. and Gangl, A. (1989) Successful long-term treatment of portal-systemic encephalopathy by the benzodiazepine antagonist flumazenil. *Gastroenterology,* **96**, 240–243

Forbes, A., Alexander, G. J., O'Grady, J. G. *et al.* (1989) Thiopental infusion in the treatment of intracranial hypertension complicating fulminant hepatic failure. *Hepatology,* **10**, 306–310

Gammal, S. H. and Jones, E. A. (1989) Hepatic encephalopathy. *Med. Clin. North Am.,* **73**, 793–813

Gimson, A. E. S., O'Grady, J., Ede, R. J., Portmann, B. and Williams, R. (1986) Late onset hepatic failure: clinical, serological and histological features. *Hepatology,* **6**, 288–294

Gregorious, J. B., Moses, L. W. and Norenberg, M. D. (1985) Morphologic effects of ammonia on primary astrocyte cultures: electromicroscopic studies. *J. Neuropathol. Exp. Neurol.* **34**, 397–403, 404–411

Grisolia, S., Felipo, V. and Minana, M. D. (1991) *Cirrhosis, Hepatic Encephalopathy and Ammonium toxicity.* Plenum Press, New York

Grungreiff, K., Presser, H.J., Franke, D., Lossner, B., Abicht, K. and Kleine, F. D. (1989) Correlations between zinc, amino acids and ammonia in liver cirrhosis. *Z Gastroenterol,* **27**, 731–735

Hadzic, N., Portmann, B., Davies, E. T., Mowat, A. P. and Mieli-Vergani, G. (1990) Carbamazepine-induced acute liver failure. *Arch. Dis. Child,* **65**, 315–317

Harrison, P. M., Keays, R., Bray, G. P., Alexander, G. J. and Williams, R. (1990) Improved outcome of paracetamol-induced fulminant hepatic failure by late administration of acetylcysteine. *Lancet,* **335**, 1572–1573

Jones, E. A. (1991) Benzodiazepine receptor ligands and hepatic encephalopathy: further unfolding of the GABA story. *Hepatology,* **14**, 1286–1290

Jones, E. A. and Gammel, S. H. (1980) Hepatic Encephalopathy, In: *The Liver: Biology and Pathobiology,* 2nd Edn. (eds I. M. Arias, W. B. Jacoby, H. Popper, D. Schachter and D. A. Shefritz). Raven Press, New York, 985–1005

Joo, F. and Klatzo, I. (1989) Role of cerebral endothelium in brain oedema. *Neurol Res.,* **11**, 67–75

Kato, M., Hughes, R. D., Keays, R. T. and Williams, R. (1992) Electron microscopic study of brain capillaries in cerebral edema from fulminant hepatic failure. *Hepatology,* **15**, 1060–1066

Kinmond, S., Carter, R., Skeoch, C. H. and Morton, N. S. (1990) Nephroblastoma presenting with acute hepatic encephalopathy. *Arch. Dis. Child,* **65 (5)**, 542–543

Kirkland, J. L. (1990) Propylthiouracil-induced hepatic failure and encephalopathy in a child. *DICP,* **24**, 470–471

Krishnamoorthy, M. S., Sundaravalli, N., Soundar, S. and Karthikeyan, S. (1989) Biogenic amine status in acute fulminant hepatocellular failure in children. *Ind. J. Physiol. Pharmacol.* **33**, 15–20

Lenn, N. J., Ellis, W. G., Washburn, E. R. and Ruebner, B. (1990) Fatal hepatocerebral syndrome in siblings discordant for exposure to valproate. *Epilepsia,* **31**, 578–583

Michalopoulos, G. K. and Zarnegar, R. (1992) Hepatocyte growth factor. *Hepatology,* **15**, 149–155

Mockli, G., Crowley, M., Stern, R., Warnock, M. L. (1989) Massive Hepatic necrosis in a child after administration of phenobarbital. *Am. J. Gastro.,* **84**, 820–822

Mondragon, R., Mieli-Vergani, G., Heaton, N. D., Mowat, A. P., Vougas, V., Williams, R. and Tan, K. C. (1992) Results of liver transplantation for fulminant hepatic failure in children. *Transplant Int.,* **5**, S206–S208

Moritz, M. J., Jarrell, B. E., Armenti, V. *et al.* (1990) Heterotopic liver transplantation for fulminant hepatic failure–a bridge to recovery. *Transplantation,* **50**, 524–526

Mowat, A. P. (1993) Hepatic encephalopathy: acute and chronic. In: *Coma* (ed J. Eyre) *Bailliere's Clinical Paediatrics,* Harcourt Brace Jovanovich, London

Mullen, K. D. (1991) Benzodiazepine compounds and hepatic encepahlopathy. *N. Engl. J. Med.,* **325**, 509–511

Munoz, S. J., Robinson, M., Northtup, B. *et al.* (1991) Elevated intracranial pressure and computed tomography of the brain in fulminant hepatic failure. *Hepatology,* **13**, 209–212

O'Grady, J. G., Gimson, A. E. S., O'Brien, C. J. *et al.* (1988) Controlled trials of charcoal haemoperfusion and prognostic factors in fulminant hepatic failure. *Gastroenterology,* **94**, 1186–1192

O'Grady, J. and Williams, R. (1989) Acute liver failure. *Bailliere's Clin. Gastroenterol.,* **3**, 75–98

O'Grady, J. G., Alexander, G. J. M., Hallyer, K. M. and Williams R. (1989) Early prognostic indicators of prognosos in fulminant hepatic failure. *Gastroenterology,* **97**, 439–445

Parker, D., White, J. P., Paton, D., Routledge, P. A. (1990) Safety of late acetylcysteine treatment in paracetamol poisoning. *Hum. Exp. Toxicol.,* **9**, 25–27

Pinson, C. W., Daya, M. R., Benner, K. G. *et al.* (1990) Liver transplantation for severe Amanita phalloides mushroom poisoning. *Am. J. Surg.,* **159**, 493–499

Rolando, N., Gimson, A. E. S. and Wade, G. J. M. *et al.* (1991a) Prospective study of SPEAR (Selective parenteral and enteral antimicrobial regimen) in patients with acute liver failure. *J. Hepatol.,* **13**, S65

Rolando, N., Harvey, F., Brahm, J. *et al.* (1991b) Fungal infection: a common, unrecognised complication of acute liver failure. *J. Hepatol.,* **12**, 1–9

Rolando, N., Harvey, F., Brahm, J. *et al.* (1990) Prospective study of bacterial infection in acute liver failure, an analysis of fifty patients. *Hepatology,* **11**, 49–53

Russell, G. J., Fitzgerald, J. F., Clark, J. H. (1987) Fulminant hepatic failure. *J. Pediatr,* **111**, 313–319

Sari, A., Yamashita, S., Ohosita, S. *et al.* (1990) Cerebrovascular reactivity to CO2 in patients with hepatic or septic encephalopathy. *Resuscitation,* **19**, 125–134

Shin, K., Nagai, Y., Hirano, C. *et al.* (1989) Survival rate in children with fulminant hepatitis improved by a combination of twice daily plasmapheresis and intensive conservative therapy. *J. Pediatr. Gastroenterol. Nutr.,* **9**, 163–166

Sinclair, S. B. and Levy, G. A. (1991) Treatment of fulminant viral hepatic failure with prostaglandin E: a preliminary report. *Dig. Dis. Sci.,* **36**, 791–800

Trey, C. and Davidson, C. S. (1970) The management of fulminant hepatic failure. In *Progress in Liver Diseases* (eds. B. Popper and F. Schaffner). Grune and Stratton, New York. p. 282

van Saene, H. K. F., Stoutenbeek, C. P., Faber-Nijholt, R., van Saene, J. J. M. (1992) Selective decontamination of the digestive tract contributes to the control of disseminated intravascular coagulation in severe liver impairment. *J. Pediatr. Gastroenterol. Nutr.,* **14**, 436–442

Vickers, Ch., Neuberger, J., Buckels, J., McMaster, P. and Elias, E. (1988) Transplantation of the liver in adults and children with fulminant hepatic failure. *J. Hepatol.,* **7**, 143–150

Wendon, J. A., Harrison, P. M., Keays, R., Gimson, A. E., Alexander, G. J. M. and Williams, R. (1992) Effects of vasopressor agents and epoprostenol on systemic haemodynamics and oxygen transport in fulminant hepatic failure. *Hepatology,* **15**, 1067–1071

Yohannan, M. D., Arif, M. and Ramia, S. (1990) Aetiology of icteric hepatitis and fulminant hepatic failure in children and the possible predisposition to hepatic failure by sickle cell disease. *Acta. Paediatr. Scand.,* **79**, 201–205

Yokota, K. (1990) Cerebrovascular reactivity to CO_2 in patients with hepatic or septic encephalopathy. *Resuscitation,* **19**, 125–134

Chapter 9

Reye's syndrome

Introduction

Reye's syndrome, an acute, life-threatening encephalopathy associated with acute liver dysfunction but with minimal or no clinical signs of liver involvement, is a clinically useful aggregate of symptoms, signs and laboratory findings. Suspicion of the syndrome should prompt immediate measures to control cerebral oedema and to minimize metabolic abnormalities which aggravate the primary pathology. Classic (cryptogenic) cases are most effectively treated if recognized in the early stages. An increasing range of inborn errors of metabolism which are now recognized as presenting with these features must be identified rapidly since these require more specific treatment. Although there has been a dramatic decline in recognized or reported cases in the USA and Britain in the last 10 years, reasons for this are not clear and the frequency could again increase. At present it seems that a child presenting with the features of Reye's syndrome is as likely to have a inborn error of metabolism as to have classic Reye's syndrome. Up to 20–60% of recognized cases die. As many as 50% of survivors have permanent brain damage. The mortality rate is particularly high in infancy.

Definition

Reye's syndrome is an acute sporadic encephalopathy without encephalitis occurring in association with acute liver dysfunction. Although standard laboratory tests for liver disease and of coagulation are abnormal only rarely are there clinical signs of liver involvement.

Classic Reye's syndrome

In the cryptogenic form the pathogenesis is unique. The principal abnormality is a severe self-limiting disturbance of hepatic mitochondrial structure with decreased mitochondrial enzymatic activity lasting up to 6 days. The structure and function of other subcellular organelles within hepatocytes are minimally affected. There is no hepatocellular necrosis but there is marked panlobular microvesicular fat deposition. Similar mitochondrial changes may occur in muscle and neural tissue but are less well documented. Mitochondrial enzymatic activity is well preserved in these tissues.

The second abnormality is an acute intense catabolic state which aggravates the mitochondrial dysfunction and its sequelae. Typically the disorder occurs within a few

Table 9.1 Genetic Disorders or familial disorders which have presented with Reye's syndrome.

Defects in mitochondrial fatty acid oxidation (Acyl-CoA dehydrogenase deficiency: six forms)
Organic acidurias
Urea cycle defects
Disorders of branch-chain amino acid metabolism
Systemic carnitine deficiency
Fructosaemia
Fructose-1,6-diphosphatase deficiency
Alpha-1 antitrypsin deficiency
Glycerol kinase deficiency
Familial haemophagocytic lymphohistiocytosis
Cystic fibrosis

days of onset of what seems to be an unremarkable viral infection of the respiratory or gastrointestinal tract or an exanthematous illness such as chicken pox.

Death or permanent brain damage are caused by cerebral oedema without encephalitis or meningitis. The relationship between the liver lesion and the central nervous system manifestations is obscure. If cerebral oedema is controlled there is completed recovery.

Reye-like illnesses

An ever increasing number of inherited metabolic disorders have been recognized as presenting with similar clinical and laboratory features (Table 9.1). The differential diagnosis also includes many acquired infectious or toxic conditions in which both liver and brain function are affected. Some will have grossly similar histological features. These conditions have been labelled cumbersomely, 'Reye's syndrome-like illnesses'.

Epidemiology

Reye's syndrome occurs predominantly in children aged 6 months to 15 years but has been reported at ages ranging from 4 days to 29 years. The first reported case was probably in 1929. Until Reye and others highlighted the disorder in 1962–63 it was rarely recognized. The number of cases thereafter increased reaching a peak in voluntary reporting systems in the USA in 1980 (555 cases) and in the UK in 1983 (91 cases). The incidence in different communities ranged from 0.2 to 4.0 per 100 000 children under the age of 18 years, with a death to case ratio of 0.2 to 0.6. The numbers reported have fallen progressively to 20 in the USA in 1989 and to 13 in the UK in 1990. With no practical sensitive specific diagnostic feature or test for the classic syndrome these figures must be regarded as estimates of incidence. To what extent the fall is due to a decreased frequency of the condition, possibly related to a decreased use of aspirin in childhood, waning interest in reporting or to more frequent early recognition of metabolic disorders mimicking the syndrome is unclear. The sex incidence is equal. The geographical distribution is worldwide. Case prevalence may be increased in rural and suburban areas. The frequency of recognition of cases in any one area increases from time to time, sometimes in relation to epidemics of viral infection, particularly influenza. In Britain the epidemiology of Reye's syndrome differs from that in the USA in that the median age of cases is 14 months as opposed to 11 years and there is no clear association with influenza.

Genetic factors have been implicated because Reye's syndrome has been reported in twins, siblings and in the offspring of first cousin marriages. Such cases are probably due to distinct genetic abnormalities such as defects in the fatty acid oxidation which have become well documented only in the last decade. These present typically in an episodic fashion similar to Reye's syndrome and are similarly aggravated by starvation.

Classic Reye's syndrome

Pathology

Hepatic changes

In the first 24 hours after the onset of vomiting or neurological abnormalities hepatic abnormalities seen on light microscopy are limited to glycogen depletion and cytoplasmic swelling, most evident at the periphery of the hepatic lobule. In severe cases the glycogen depletion may be panlobular and is likely to be associated with a high incidence of hypoglycaemia and a high death rate.

If frozen sections are stained with Sudan red, tiny lipid droplets are found throughout the hepatic parenchyma. These cannot be detected by stains performed on paraffin-fixed tissues. Over the course of 1 to 4 days the fat droplets coalesce and become evident as microvacuolization in the periphery of the hepatocytes. Mitotic activity may be evident in the periphery of the lobule within 10 hours of onset, but is more evident 3 days later. Hepatic necrosis is absent or inconspicuous. In severe cases mild portal tract inflammation is evident. Lipid may clear in 2 to 5 days in mild cases, but persists up to 9 days in severe ones. By 1 month the liver is histologically normal.

Electron microscopy of liver tissues obtained within 24 hours of the onset of encephalopathy shows loss of glycogen, proliferation of the smooth endoplasmic reticulum and an increase in peroxisomes. The mitochondria are swollen, deformed and pleomorphic but at this stage still have an intact matrix. Ultrastructural alterations appear first in individual cells. Contiguous cells may be near normal. In comatose patients virtually all liver cells are affected. The mitochondrial matrix is less dense and disorganized. The outer membranes of the mitochondria are often disrupted. Some hepatocytes lose electron density except in residual bodies and peroxisomes. In fulminant cases such clear cells dominate the liver histology. Although in general the degree of pathological change mirrors the severity of the clinical illness, marked and diffuse changes have been reported with grade 1 encephalopathy. After 4 to 5 days of the illness the mitochondrial injury resolves, glycogen is restored, small fat droplets coalesce to large globules. The ultrastructural diagnosis of Reye's syndrome is then impossible.

Histochemical techniques or biochemical assays in the first 2–6 days of the illness show a severe reduction in activity of all mitochondrial enzymes (e.g. cytochrome oxidase or succinate dehydrogenase). Within 4 to 8 days of onset enzymatic activity is restored. Activity of cytoplasmic enzymes is normal.

Cerebral lesions

In fatal cases the brain is swollen with flattened gyri and narrow sulci. There may be herniation of the brain stem through the foramen magnum and secondary compression. There is no significant inflammatory reaction in the brain or meninges. The cerebrospinal fluid is normal. Microscopic changes secondary to cerebral oedema and hypoxia are prominent.

Ultrastructural studies of the few brain biopsies performed at the time of craniotomy, a manoeuvre sometimes necessary for alleviating severe cerebral oedema, have shown unusual diffuse pleomorphic mitochondrial swelling in neurons, somewhat similar to that seen in hepatocytes. The foot processes of astrocytes are swollen, devoid of granules and vaculated. Small blebs or vesicles may be found in the myelin sheath.

Skeletal muscle

Glycogen deposition and fat deposition are apparent. The mitochondria show matrix expansion and a degree of pleomorphism.

Fatty changes are also seen in the epithelial cells of the loop of Henle and of the proximal convoluted tubule of the kidney, in the heart, the pancreas and the lymph nodes.

Clinical features

Typically Reye's syndrome occurs in a child with a previously unremarkable medical history a few days after the onset or during the recovery phase of what seems to be an unexceptional or ordinary viral infection. This may take the form of a respiratory or gastrointestinal tract infection or an exanthematous illness such as chicken pox.

The clinical features are usually dominated by pernicious vomiting and disturbed consciousness – the main signs of encephalopathy. In some instances perfuse and persistent vomiting is the first feature. It may be associated or rapidly followed by neurological changes. Rarely there may be no vomiting. Tachypnoea may be noted. The severity and rate of progress of the encephalopathy vary greatly. The initial neurological abnormality may be a quiet, withdrawn state with disinterest in play and normal activities. There may be confused, argumentative, combative irrational behaviour, sometimes with visual hallucinations and agitated delirium. There are no focal neurological signs and no meningeal irritation. Ophthalmological features of increased intracranial pressure are rarely evident. Thirty percent of cases develop convulsions. In progressive cases deepening coma is associated with decerebrate posturing, opisthotonos, dilated or unequal and slowly responsive or unresponsive pupils. There is deep, rapid respiration and variations in pulse rate and finally a flaccid apnoeic state with fixed dilated pupils. This may occur over a course extending from 4 to 60 hours. The neurological status may stabilize or improve spontaneously or with therapy, at any stage short of brain death 6 hours to 5 days after the onset of the encephalopathy.

In contrast to the overt encephalopathy and vomiting the acute disturbance of liver function has little or no clinical features. It is suspected by the finding of disturbed coagulation (prolonged prothrombin time) and abnormal biochemical tests of liver function, particularly raised serum transaminases, ammonia and hypoglycaemia. Rarely the liver is clinically enlarged. Jaundice is very exceptional. If the patient does not die of cerebral oedema laboratory evidence of liver involvement resolves within 4 to 6 days.

Infants

Infants with Reye's syndrome have a somewhat different presentation. Initial features are respiratory, namely tachypnoea, respiratory distress, hyperinflation and apnoea. There may be temperature instability. Seizures are more common. Vomiting is often absent and is rarely pernicious. Hypoglycaemia and hepatomegaly are more commonly identified than in older children. A history of preceding viral infection is less common.

Laboratory features

Biochemical evidence of liver dysfunction is always found. Serum transaminase values are elevated from levels of between twice normal to over 100 times normal. Hyperammonaemia is present in almost all cases of more than minimal severity but it may be transient.

The prothrombin time is usually prolonged but sometimes only by a few seconds. Elevated serum bilirubin levels are most unusual. Hypoglycaemia is a feature of severe cases particularly in children under 2 years of age.

Table 9.2 Diagnosis of Reye's syndrome

Mild antecedent illness
Profuse vomiting
Objective central nervous system dysfunction
Biochemical evidence of hepatic dysfunction
Absence of other possible causes
Characteristic liver biopsy findings (see text)

Table 9.3 Disorders causing coma and abnormal liver function tests

Septicaemia with shock
Salmonellosis
Shigellosis
Meningitis
Fulminant hepatitis, particularly in early infancy
Severe generalised viral illnesses, e.g. Varicella or adenoviruses
Severe acute illnesses
   hypoxic brain and liver damage
Severe dehydration
Encephalopathies causing convulsions
   requiring intramuscular infections
'Near-miss' sudden infant death syndrome
Haemorrhagic shock encephalopathy syndrome

Table 9.4 Drugs or toxins which will mimic Reye's syndrome

Aflatoxin
Emulsifiers
Endotoxin
Hornet stings
Hypoglycins
Insecticides
Isopropyl alcohol
Margosa oil
Pentenoic acid
Pteridines
Salicylates
Outdated teracyclines
Valproate
Warfarin

The cerebrospinal fluid is normal apart from a low sugar concentration in some cases. Because of the high risk of brain swelling lumbar puncture is contraindicated in the typical case. If it is considered necessary to exclude meningitis lumbar puncture should be delayed until the patient is ventilated and it has been shown that the intracranial ventricles are not compressed on CT scanning.

These clinical features and laboratory findings are sufficiently distinctive to allow a presumptive diagnosis of Reye's syndrome until liver biopsy can be performed (Table 9.2). However, there are other encephalopathies which may mimic Reye's syndrome without having the distinctive hepatic pathology (Tables 9.3 and 9.4).

Secondary metabolic events

A major factor in the pathogenesis of the many metabolic aberrations is the transient depression of all mitochondrial function. These include enzymes essential for urea synthesis, gluconeogenesis, organic acid oxidation and oxidative phosphorylation, and in drug detoxification.

Massive tissue breakdown occurs in Reye's syndrome. Enormous losses of protein and nitrogen occur. Serum amino acids increase including substrates of the urea cycle. Among these is carbamyl phosphate. This diffuses from mitochondria into the cytoplasm where it is changed to orotic acid, a substance which, in some species at least, decreases lipoprotein synthesis and may thereby contribute to fatty acid retention within the liver.

Another important factor is increased lipolysis from adipose tissue stores, associated with very high serum concentration of glucocorticoids, growth hormones and glucagon. Lipolysis causes high concentrations of fatty acids in serum and a raised serum glycerol level. The presentation of these to a liver incapable of fully metabolizing them may result in an accumulation of triglycerides in the parenchymal cells. There is frequently a defect in beta-oxidation of fatty acids with accumulation of fatty acids and acyl-CoA esters in plasma and liver. Omega oxidation may occur with the production of dicarboxylic acids. Very long chain dicarboxylic acids may aggravate the primary mitochondrial injury by acting as uncouplers of oxidative phosphorylation. Thus, mitochondrial energy production will be decreased as are all mitochondrial processes which are energy dependent.

The abnormal products of the amino acid or fatty acid metabolism may undergo reversible conjugation with glycine and carnitine. Relative carnitine deficiency may develop with insufficient carnitine being available to transfer fatty acids into mitochondria. Thus energy production in mitochondria is further decreased.

Aetiology of classic Reye's syndrome

Reye's syndrome is a very rare sequela of common viral infections. The cause is unknown. Epidemiological observations in humans and experimental studies in small laboratory rodents suggest that Reye's syndrome is a stereotyped reversible reaction in mitochondria arising from an interaction of viral and toxic environmental factors occurring most commonly during the growing period.

Limitations of epidemiological studies

The low incidence has resulted in all epidemiological attempts to identify contributory factors being *retrospective* case-control studies. Biases are difficult to avoid in such circumstances, even with meticulous planning, and well-trained investigators. A major difficulty is the lack of a specific practical diagnostic laboratory test, positive at all stages of the illness and in all grades of severity. As a result epidemiologists have had to use relatively non-specific measures for case definition, namely, encephalopathy of unknown cause with no sign of infection or inflammation in the central nervous system in the presence of raised serum transaminases, blood ammonia and more rarely microvesicular fatty infiltration in liver biopsy (Table 9.2). There should be no other reasonable explanation for the condition.

The vast majority of cases in epidemiological studies have not had a liver biopsy. Very few have had the necessary highly technical diagnostic investigations to identify recently recognized inborn errors of metabolism. No study includes grade 1 cases such as those recognized during prospective studies in an area with a very high public and professional awareness of Reye's syndrome. Eighty-five children with a preceding viral upper respiratory tract infection or chicken pox and vomiting, who had on investigation a threefold rise in serum aspartate aminotransferase but none of the neurological features of Reye's syndrome had typical liver mitochondrial changes of Reye's syndrome on percutaneous liver biopsy. Of the 83 patients treated with only glucose and electrolyte infusion, five progressed to a deeper grade of coma. These five had significant elevation of blood ammonia or prolongation of the prothrombin time at presentation. Finally, epidemiologists must rely on voluntary reporting of cases.

Viral factors in the aetiology

At least 19 different viruses have been implicated in the prodromal illness. These virus include examples of the major groups of DNA- and RNA-containing viruses with the sole exception of measles. Viral vaccines have also been implicated. The frequency of recognized cases of Reye's syndrome in any one area increases from time to time sometimes in relation to epidemics of viral infection particularly influenza A and influenza B. From these observations an estimated attack rate of 3 and 0.3 per 10 000 cases of influenza have been calculated. Varicella with its distinct clinical feature is also commonly implicated that the attack rate is lower at 0.3 instances per 100 000 cases. Viruses are rarely recovered from the affected tissues.

The sera of patients with Reye's syndrome have both complement and fibronectin depletion. Interferon production by the lymphocytes is decreased. Whether these immune changes are primary or secondary is unclear.

Exogenous chemical or toxic factors

Case reports and epidemiological studies have implicated with varying degrees of frequency a wide range of exogenous factors. These include aspirin, aflatoxin, latex paints, pesticides, pesticide emulsifiers, insect repellents, paracetamol (acetaminophen), pteridines, isopropyl alcohol, margosa oil, products of akee fruits including hypoglycin-A and 4-pentanoic acid. The evidence associating any of these with Reye's syndrome is at present contentious.

Aspirin   The most intensively investigated is salicylate usually in the form of aspirin. Four case-control studies from North America showed that patients with Reye's syndrome had taken aspirin significantly more frequently prior to, or early in, the illness than had controls with prodromal illnesses that were similar. These studies were severely criticized because of bias in case and control selection and in data collection.

To resolve these difficulties and to determine any implication of medication in Reye's syndrome three further studies were commissioned in the USA but stopped prematurely because of the increasing rarity of Reye's syndrome and the consequent expense and difficulty in enroling additional patients in a reasonable period of time. Nevertheless all found a strong statistical association with the ingestion of salicylates, mainly aspirin, in the antecedent illness of Reye's syndrome. In Britain a case-comparison study suggested that an association between Reye's syndrome and aspirin ingestion may exist. In contrast, an epidemiological study in Japan failed to confirm the association. Cases of fully confirmed Reye's syndrome do occur in which there is no evidence of aspirin ingestion. Further data cited as evidence in support of an association between salicylates and Reye's syndrome include the occurrence of the syndrome among children on long-term salicylate therapy for connective tissue disorders.

The second piece of evidence relating aspirin to Reye's syndrome was the finding of apparent histopathological similarities between liver changes in Reye's syndrome and those associated with salicylate poisoning. This was not confirmed in a subsequent study. The third piece of evidence, elevated serum salicylate levels in Reye's syndrome, was based on non-specific techniques and was not confirmed with appropriate methodology.

Could aspirin administration aggravate the effects of mitochondrial injury? In both Reye's syndrome and disorders such as organic aciduria and defects in fatty acid oxidation, secondary deficiency of carnitine can occur with accumulation of metabolites which form toxic CoA compounds. There may be an additional load on glycine conjugation, a process which requires ATP and acetyl CoA. Aspirin is metabolized by conjugation with glycine. It has a higher affinity for the conjugating enzyme than many of the endogenous products that accumulate in genetic disorders, such as valeric acidaemia, and can accumulate in Reye's syndrome particularity if there is relative deficiency of carnitine. Thus it can be speculated that aspirin given to a child with relative carnitine deficiency (carnitine production is increased in Reye's syndrome) could change what had been a potential grade 1 Reye's syndrome into a more severe grade which would be more easily recognizable clinically.

Despite concerns about the epidemiological evidence, government agencies in many countries took measures, in the mid 1980s, to limit the use of aspirin in children age 12 or less, except when specifically indicated for chronic rheumatic disorders. Given the reported age range of Reye's syndrome an age limit of 18 years might have been more appropriate.

Experimental studies are limited by the absence of an animal model which accurately mimics the idiopathic disorder in humans (Mowat, 1992). They do provide many examples of the adverse effects on mitochondrial functions of exogenous factors such as aspirin, paracetamol, insecticides, solvents and emulsifiers in the presence of viral infections in the growing animal. These effects are aggravated by dietary factors and, particularly, by starvation. In some studies only particular genetic strains are affected. Just how these chemicals interact with viruses to cause functional or structural changes in mitochondria is unclear.

Thus both epidemiological and experimental studies are compatible with the hypothesis that 'cryptogenic' Reye's syndrome arises from an unusual response to viral infection, possibly determined by host genetic factors but modified by a range of exogenous agents of which aspirin could be one. It must remain an open question whether aspirin acts alone or in the presence of some additional cause of mitochondrial injury such as an emulsifiers or insecticide. It is hard to challenge the conclusion of Dr Susan Hall and her coworkers in 1988, 'If aspirin has an aetiological role there must be an exceptional unpredictable combination of circumstances that act as trigger.'

Cause of the encephalopathy

The cause of the encephalopathy is undetermined. There is no evidence of primary central nervous system infection. It is unclear whether the neural mitochondrial lesions occur as part of the primary disease mechanism or are secondary to metabolic changes elsewhere. Nor is it certain whether the cerebral effects are all due to mitochondrial dysfunction in the brain. Inhibition of fatty acid oxidation in the endothelial cells of the cerebral vessels may underlie the development of cerebral oedema and defective oxidative phosphorylation within the cells may interfere in the transport of glucose from the blood to the brain. Hypoglycaemia may be an important contributory factor together with hyperammonaemia and increased fatty acids acting singly or in combination.

Diagnosis

It is essential to assume that an inborn error of metabolism is responsible for Reye's syndrome particularly in any child of less than 4 years. Plasma (lithium heparin 5 ml and fluoride 1 ml), whole blood (5 ml in EDTA in plastic tube for DNA studies) and urine *collected at the time of presentation and* stored at −20°C, may be invaluable in providing evidence for the diagnosis, particularly of organic acidurias and disorders of ketogenesis. Plasma amino acids, 3-hydroxybutyrate, free fatty acids, lactate and urinary ketones and organic acids analysed by gas chromatography/mass spectrometry in addition to the

Table 9.5 Investigations required at initial assessment (see Diagnosis) and to monitor progress

Serum
   sodium
   potassium
   chloride
   bicarbonate
   magnesium
   calcium
   phosphate
Blood sugar
Serum osmolality
Blood ammonia
Creatine phosphokinase
Standard biochemical tests of liver function
Nonesterified fatty acid concentration
Prothrombin time
Haemoglobin, total white count, platelet count
Blood gas and hydrogen ion concentration

investigations in Table 9.5 allow the rapid identification of these disorders and urea cycle defects. Skin fibroblasts cultured for enzymatic studies may be essential. Any biopsy tissues should be stored at −70°C. It is important to consider the wide range of disorders which can cause coma with abnormal biochemical test of liver function (see Tables 9.3, 9.4).

Management

Therapy in Reye's syndrome is aimed at preventing, minimizing and correcting identified metabolic abnormalities and at controlling increased intracranial pressure. Details of therapy must be modified depending on clinical assessment, including the grade of encephalopathy (Table 9.6) and laboratory findings (Table 9.5). It is essential that treatment be instituted before irreversible brain damage occurs. Cases identified early and treated in units with full intensive care facilities including the monitoring and control of intracranial pressure have the best prognosis. Factors associated with a poor prognosis are given in Table 9.7.

Table 9.6 Clinical assessment of severity of encephalopathy in Reye's syndrome

	Mild (1)	Moderate (2)	Severe (3)	Very severe (4)	Brain death (5)
Mental state	Quiet, normal response to verbal commands	Lethargic, slow mental processes such as difficulty in counting	Agitated delirium, out of contact with environment, but responds to pain	Coma, decerebrate rigidity, pain produces exacerbation of decerebrate posture	Coma, spinal reflexes preserved
Muscular activity	Wishes to lie down but no other abnormality	Clumsy	Poorly controlled, gross movements, intermittent clonus	Opisthotonos, extensor spasms of arms and legs	Flaccid paralysis
Respiration	Normal	Normal or increased rate	Normal or increased rate	Increased rate and depth	None
Pupillary responses	Normal	Normal	Dilated, but rapidly responsive	Dilated but slowly responsive	Dilated and unresponsive
Fundi	Normal	Normal	Venous engorgement	Marked venous engorgement, discs blurred, papilloedema	Variable

Table 9.7 Factors indicating poor prognosis

Age less than 1 year
Rapid progression of symptoms to grade 4 encephalopathy
Ammonia more than six times normal
Creatinine phosphokinase greater than 10 times normal
SGOT/SGPT (AST/ALT) ratio less than 1
EEG: marked slowing
Non-esterified fatty acids greater than 71 mEq/litre
Marked increases in long chain dicarboxylic acids

SGOT = aspartate aminotransferase   AST = serum aspartate transaminase
SGPT = alanine aminotransferase   ALT = alanine transaminase

Treatment at suspicion of diagnosis

Glucose Infusion An intravenous glucose infusion should be started immediately. It minimizes protein breakdown and lipolysis and thereby the accumulation of ammonia and fatty acids as well as correcting hypoglycaemia. The exact concentration of glucose is a matter of debate, some groups use a 10% solution while others use 20–30% aiming at blood sugar levels of between 11 mmol/litre and 22 mmol/litre (200–400 mg/100 ml) rather than 8–11 mmol/litre (150–200 mg/ml). It is argued that the higher concentrations will have an additive effect in decreasing proteolysis and promoting the uptake of amino acids by muscle and directly diminished cerebral oedema. After correcting dehydration the infusion rate should be restricted to provide 60% of normal fluid maintenance requirements; additional bicarbonate may be required.

Encephalopathy If the blood pressure is normal the patient should be nursed with head and upper trunk elevated at an angle of 40 degrees. Unnecessary handling or stimulation must be avoided since this increases intracranial pressure. If the coma is more than grade 1 the patient should be given intravenous mannitol at a dose of 1–2 g/kg of body weight over a 20-minute period and ventilation established with endotracheal intubation to maintain the PaO_2 at between 130 and 170 mmHg (12–23 kPa) and the PCO_2 should be between 25 and 30 mmHg (3.5–4.0 kPa). The patient should be transferred to an intensive care unit in which continuous intracranial pressure monitoring is possible. The objective is to maintain the intracranial pressure at less than 20 mmHg and a cerebral perfusion pressure in the range of 50–90 mmHg.

Intravenous diazepam and phenytoin may be required to control convulsions. Continuous clinical and biochemical monitoring is essential (Tables 9.5 and 9.6). Intravenous lignocaine 1.0 mg/kg over 5 minutes may be required before endotracheal suction. A rise in intracranial pressure with the serum osmolarity of less than 300 mOsmol/kg should be treated with mannitol 0.5 g/kg, repeated if necessary after 40 minutes. If the osmolarity is greater than 300 mOsmol/kg intravenous thiopentone should be given but this may produce a fall in arterial blood pressure requiring the giving of inotropes such as dopamine in a dose of 5–20 μg/kg per minute. If the intracranial pressure remains elevated in spite of these measures consideration should be given to cerebral decompression by bifrontal craniotomy and hypothermia, reducing the body temperature to 30–31°C, thereby reducing the cerebral metabolic rate and oxygen requirement. Recovery with good neurological function has been reported in a few patients treated in this manner.

Recovery stage When the intracranial pressure has been normal and stable for 24 hours, sedation and hyperventilation are gradually ceased and after a further 12-hour period of observations spontaneous respiration should be re-established. If anticonvulsants have been used these are continued for at least 6 months.

Physiotherapy may be required for the motor disability that frequently complicates this disorder or its treatment. Follow-up is essential to determine the need for continuing anticonvulsant therapy and for special educational provision to compensate for neurological deficits. It is essential that the complete case record is scrutinized to ascertain that all currently known metabolic disorders which mimic Reye's syndrome have been excluded. If there is no evidence of such conditions the family should be advised that the recurrence of the syndrome is unlikely but at the onset of any features suggesting a possible recurrence intravenous glucose infusions should be initiated immediately.

References and bibliography

Andreou, A., Bonora, G., Luciani, L. and Peretti, L. (1988) Reyes syndrome and aspirin. *Lancet,* **ii**, 684

Anonymous (1991) Reyes syndrome surveillance – United States, 1989. *J. Am. Med. Assoc.,* **265**, 960

Anonymous (1982) Reye's syndrome – epidemiological considerations. *Lancet,* **i**, 941–943

Blisard, K. S. and Davis, L. E. (1990) The sequence of changes in liver and brain in the Influenza B mouse model of Reyes Syndrome. *J. Neuropath. Exp. Neurol.,* **49**, 498–508

Brown, A. K., Fikrig, S. and Findberg, L. (1983) Aspirin and Reye's syndrome. *J. Pediatr.,* **102**, 157–178

Centres for Disease Control (1980) Reye's syndrome – Ohio, Michigan. *MMWR,* **29**, 537–539

Corkey, B. E., Hale, D. E., Glennon, M. C., Kelley, R. I., Coates, P. M. and Kilpatrick L. (1988) Relationship between unusual hepatic acyl coenzyme A profiles and the pathogenesis of Reye Syndrome. *J. Clin. Invest.,* **82**, 782–788

Crocker, J. F. S., Lee, S. H. S., Love, J. A. *et al.* (1991) Surfactant-potentiated increases in intracranial pressure in a mouse model of Reye's syndrome. *Exp. Neurol,* **111**, 95–97

Crocker, J. F. (1982) Reye's syndrome. *Sem. Liver Dis.,* **2**, 240–52

Davis, L. E., Blisard, K. S. and Kornfeld (1990) The Influenza B mouse model of Reyes Syndrome: clinical, virologic and morphologic studies of the encephalopathy. *J. Neurol. Sci.,* **97**, 221–231

Ede, R. J. and Williams, R. (1988) Reye's syndrome in adults. *Br. Med. J.,* **296**, 518–519

Elpeleg, O. N., Christensen, E., Hurvitz, H. and Branski, D. (1990) Recurrent, familial Reye-like syndrome with a new complex amino and organic aciduria. *Eur. J. Pediatr.,* **149**, 709–712

Forsyth, B. W., Horwitz, R. I., Acamora, D. *et al.*(1989) New Epidemiologic evidence confirming that bias does not explain the aspirin/Reye's syndrome association. *J. Am. Med. Assoc.,* **261**, 2517–2524

Glasgow, J. F. T. (1984) Clinical features and prognosis of Reye's syndrome. *Arch. Dis. Child.,* **59**, 230–235

Green, A. and Hall, S. M. (1992) Investigation of metabolic disorders resembling Reye's syndrome. *Arch. Dis. Child.,* **67**, 1313–1317.

Hall, S. M., Plaster, P. A., Glasgow, J. F. T. and Hancock, P. (1988) Preadmission antipyretics in Reye's syndrome. *Arch. Dis. Child.,* **63**, 857–866

Hall, S. M. (1986) Reye's syndrome and aspirin. A review. *J. R. Soc. Med.,* **79**, 596–598

Halpin, T. J., Holtzhauer, F. J., Campbell, R. J. *et al.* (1982) Reye's syndrome and medication use. *J. Am. Med. Assoc.,* **248**, 687–691

Heubi, J. E., Daugherty, C. C., Partin, J. S., Partin, J. C. and Schubert, W. K. (1984) Grade 1 Reye's syndrome - outcome and predictors of progression to deeper coma grades. *N. Engl. J. Med.,* **311**, 1539–1542

Hurwitz, E. S., Barrett, M. J., Bergman, D. *et al.* (1987) Public health service study on Reye's syndrome and medication. *J. Am. Med. Assoc.,* **257**, 1905–1911

Hurwitz, E. S., Barrett, M. J., Bergman, D. *et al.* (1985) Public health service study on Reye's syndrome and medications. Report of the pilot phase. *N. Engl. J. Med.,* **313**, 849–857

Hurwitz, E. S. (1989) Reye's Syndrome. *Epidemiol. Rev.,* **11**, 249–253

Huttenlocher, P. R, Trauner, D. A. (1978) Reye's syndrome in infancy. *Pediatrics,* **62**, 84

Johnson, G. M., Sucrelitis, T. D. and Carroll, N. B. (1963) A study of 16 fatal cases of encephalitis-like disease in North Carolina children. *NC Med. J.,* **24**, 464–473

Kang, A. S., Crocker, J. F. S. and Johnson, G. M. (1986) Reye's syndrome and salicylates. *N. Eng. J. Med.,* **314**, 920–921

Kilpatrick-Smith, L., Hale, D. E. and Douglas, S. D. (1989) Progress in Reye syndrome: epidemiology, biochemical mechanism and animal models. *Dig. Dis.,* **7**, 135–46

Kilpatrick-Smith, L., Hale, D. E. and Douglas, S. D. (1989) Progress in Reye Syndrome: Epidemiology, biochemical mechanisms and animal models. *Dig. Dis.,* **7**, 135–146

Krieger, I. and Tanaka, K. (1976) Therapeutic effects of glycine in isovalericacidemia. *Pediatr. Res.,* **10**, 25–28

Martens, M. E., Lee, C. P. (1984) Reyes syndrome. Salicylates and mitochondrial functions. *Biochem. Pharmacol.,* **33**, 2869–2876

Mowat, A. P. (1988) Endogenous factors in Reye' syndrome. In *Reye's syndrome – Royal Society of Medicine Symposium,* No 8 (ed. C. Wood). Royal Society of Medicine, London

Mowat, A. P. (1986) Reye's syndrome and aspirin. In *Aspirin and other Salicylates* (Eds. J. R. Vane and R. M. Botting). Chapman and Hall Medical, London, 531–547.

Mowat, A. P. (1992) Reye's Syndrome and Aspirin. In *Aspirin and other salicylates* (eds. J. R. Vane and R. M. Botting). Chapman and Hall Medical, London. pp. 531–547

Partin, J. S. (1988) The ultrastructural changes in the liver, muscle and brain in Reye's syndrome. In *Reye's syndrome – Royal Society of Medicine Round Table Symposium,* no 8 (ed. C. Wood). Royal Society of Medicine, London

Partin, J. S., Partin, J. C., Schubert, W. K. and Hammond, J. G. (1982) Serum salicylate concentrations in Reye's disease. A study of 130 biopsy-proven cases. *Lancet,* **i**, 191–194

Partin, J. S., Daugherty, C., McAdams, A. J., Partin, J. C. and Schubert, W. K. (1984) A comparison of liver ultrastructure and salicylate intoxication in Reye's syndrome. *Hepatology,* **4**, 697–690

Porter, J. D. H., Robinson, P. H., Glasgow, J. F. T., Banks, J. H. and Hall, S. M. (1990) Trends in the incidence of Reye's syndrome and the use of aspirin. *Arch. Dis. Child.,* **65**, 826–829

Rennebohm, R. M., Heubi, J. E., Daugherty, C. C. and Daniels, S. R. (1985) Reye's syndrome and children receiving salicylate therapy for connective tissue disease. *J. Pediatr.,* **107**, 877–880

Reye, R. D. K., Morgan, G. and Baral, J. (1963) Encephalopathy and fatty degeneration of the viscera: a disease entity in childhood. *Lancet,* **ii**, 749–752

Roe, C. R., Billington, D. S., Maltby, D. A. and Kinnebrew, P. (1986) Recognition of medium chain acyl CoA dehydrogenase deficiency in asymptomatic siblings of children dying of sudden infant death or Reye-like syndromes. *J. Pediatr.,* **108**, 13–18

Rozee, K. R., Lee, S. H., Crocker, J. F., Digout, S. and Arciue, E. (1982) Is a compromised interferon response an etiological factor in Reye's syndrome? *Can. Med. Assoc. J.,* **126**, 798–802

Starko, K. M., Ray, C. G., Dominguez, L. B., Stromberg, W. L. and Woodall, D. F. (1980) Reye's syndrome and salicylate use. *Pediatrics,* **66**, 859–864

Sullivan-Bolya, J. S. and Corey, L. (1981) Epidemiology of Reye's syndrome. *Epidemiol. Rev.,* **3**, 1–31

Tonsgard, J. H. (1989) Effect of Reye's syndrome serum on the ultrastructure of isolated liver mitochondria. *Lab. Invest.,* **60**,568–573

Waldman, R. J., Hall, W. N., McGee, H. and Van Amburg, G. (1982) Aspirin as a risk factor in Reye's syndrome. *J. Am. Med. Assoc.,* **247**, 3089–3094

Williams, F. M., Ferner, R. E., Graham, M., Blain, P. G., Alberti, K. G. M. M. and Rawlins, M. D. (1990) The metabolic effects of aspirin in fasting and fed subjects: relevance to the aetiology of Reye's syndrome. *Eur. J. Clin. Pharmacol.,* **38**, 519–521

Wood, C. (ed) (1988) *Reye's syndrome – Royal Society of Medicine Round Table Symposium,* No 8. Royal Society of Medicine, London

Yamashita, N. F., Eiichiro, O., Kimura, A. and Yoshida, I. (1985) Reye's syndrome in Asian countries. In *Reye's syndrome 4* (ed. J. D. Pollak). National Reye's Syndrome Foundation, Ohio, 47–60

Chapter 10

Chronic hepatitis

Chronic hepatitis is an important concept, since it implies a continuing inflammatory process which can become irreversible. If the inflammation leads to the progressive accumulation of intrahepatic fibrous tissue this may cause impairment of liver cell function, distortion of the hepatic architecture and ultimately cirrhosis and all its sequelae (Chapter 13). Chronic hepatitis thus has major diagnostic, prognostic and therapeutic implications. Thorough investigation is mandatory to discover the cause of liver damage, assess its severity and plan treatment.

Definition

Chronic hepatitis has been defined as a continuing inflammatory lesion of the liver with the potential to either progress to more severe disease (including cirrhosis), to continue unchanged or to subside, spontaneously or with treatment. This definition thus covers any inflammatory disease of the liver not due to acute self-limiting infection (viral, rickettsial, bacterial, spirochaetal, mycotic, protozoal or helminthic) or to past drug exposure. Such causes of acute liver damage (e.g. hepatitis A viral infection) may occur in patients with chronic forms. The possibility of chronic liver disease should be considered again if clinical and biochemical abnormalities persist beyond the expected period of recovery from the acute liver disease.

In chronic hepatitis, the inflammatory reaction is demonstrated by persistently abnormal laboratory tests for liver disease, e.g. raised serum aspartate aminotransaminase, and by a range of histological abnormalities which cannot be assessed accurately from clinical and laboratory features. Percutaneous liver biopsy is therefore essential in the initial assessment of patients with suspected chronic hepatitis. Unfortunately irreversible chronic liver damage can occur before any symptoms of liver disease develop and in the absence of clinical or laboratory features of chronic liver disease. Conversely although the transaminases may have been abnormal for years the histological features may show no changes of chronicity.

The apparent duration of disease at presentation is therefore of little or no importance. The only exception at present is hepatitis B viral infection. In HBc IgM+ hepatitis B infection, it seems reasonable to not to regard this as chronic for at least 6 months, since this will avoid unnecessarily early liver biopsy. As we learn more about chronic hepatitis C infection it too may have a similar caveat. In other forms of chronic hepatitis, the 6-month definition is unhelpful since irreversible inflammatory liver disease may found when symptoms have been present for as little as 1 week.

Pathology

Chronic hepatitis is arbitrarily divided into the three major pathological categories: chronic persistent hepatitis, chronic aggressive hepatitis and the rarer chronic lobular hepatitis. In all three forms there is hepatocellular damage, lymphocyte infiltration, and a degree of regeneration and repair. In some circumstances the severity can change from one category to another both spontaneously and with specific therapies. It is therefore essential to qualify the pathological categorization by aetiological (e.g. hepatitis C) or associated factors (e.g. autoimmune phenomena) (Table 10.1).

Table 10.1 Forms of chronic hepatitis in childhood

Chronic active hepatitis auto-immune, viral, idiopathic
Chronic persistent hepatitis viral, idiopathic
Wilson's disease
Liver disease associated with alpha-1 antitrypsin deficiency
Other genetic disorders
Sclerosing cholangitis
Budd–Chiari syndrome
Drug therapy: isoniazid, methyldopa, antimitotic agents, oxyphenisatin
Sequelae of hepatitis in infancy: metabolic, familial progressive and idiopathic
Bile duct lesions: choledochal cyst (*see* cirrhosis)
Parasitic infections – schistosomiasis
Ulcerative colitis or regional ileitis

A semiquantitative assessment of inflammation, necrosis and fibrosis in both portal tracts and lobules and of the degree of alteration of architecture is particularly helpful (Scheuer, 1991).

Chronic persistent hepatitis

Chronic persistent hepatitis is characterized by an inflammatory infiltrate mainly of mononuclear cells, which may include a few plasma cells and macrophages virtually confined to slightly widened portal tracts. There is minimal erosion of the limiting plate where hepatic parenchyma meets the portal tract. There may be minimal portal tract fibrosis with small fibrous septa extending out from the tracts but the liver architecture is preserved. There may be small infrequent foci of liver cell necrosis with inflammatory cells in the parenchyma and prominent Kupffer cells (Figure 10.1).

The aetiology includes non-specific reactive hepatitis due to systemic illness or gastrointestinal disease: in these the liver cells are likely to show variation in cell size with increased Kupffer cell proliferation and some intralobular inflammation, malignancy, leukaemia and lymphosarcoma. Viral hepatitis type B, C, non-A, non-B, non-C hepatitis and residual severe viral hepatitis type A may be responsible. Bowel disorders include Crohn's disease. ulcerative colitis, *schistosoma mansoni*, salmonellosis and bacterial gastroenteritis. In leukaemia and lymphoma focal dense cellular infiltrate occurs also in the sinusoids. Biliary tract disease may show very similar inflammatory infiltrate but there are usually some polymorphonuclear leucocytes present and more marked bile duct proliferation.

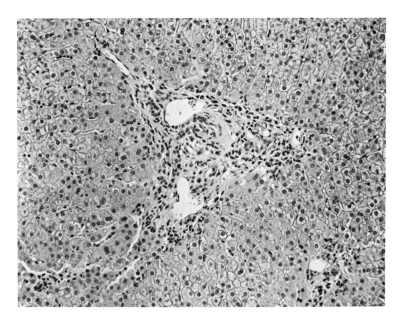

Figure 10.1 Chronic persistent hepatitis. There is a mononuclear inflammatory cell infiltrate in the slightly swollen portal tract. The limiting plate at the junction of the portal tract and the hepatic parenchyma is virtually intact. The cells with elongated nuclei in the portal tract are fibroblasts which are present in a slight excess. A few inflammatory cells are seen in the hepatic parenchyma – in the lower left corner. No other abnormalities are seen in the hepatic parenchyma (percutaneous liver biopsy: haematoxylin and eosin × 125, reduced to two-thirds in reproduction)

Chronic aggressive hepatitis

Chronic aggressive hepatitis (CAH) is characterized by the presence of a perilobular hepatitis with an inflammatory cell infiltrate of lymphocytes and plasma cells extending from the portal tracts into the adjacent hepatic parenchyma and causing hepatocellular necrosis and marked fibroblastic activity. Hepatocytes undergoing necrosis are surrounded by lymphocytes and fibroblasts in a process termed piecemeal necrosis. The liver cells are swollen and may assume pseudoductular arrangements. This process is associated with marked proliferation of fibroblasts and collagen deposition (Figure 10.2). These changes disturb the lobular architecture but true cirrhosis is, by definition absent. The presence of so-called 'bridging' lesions, in which proliferating fibroblasts and inflammatory cell aggregates are found in fibrous septa linking the portal tracts to each other and to the hepatic vein is a pathological feature which indicates severe CAH. There may be parenchymal cellular infiltrate similar to acute hepatitis. Regeneration may take the form of twinning of liver cell plates or giant cell transformation of hepatocytes which contain four or more nuclei. The histological findings in the liver may vary from lobule to lobule and from time to time. It is often difficult to discern whether or not cirrhosis is present. In the late stages cirrhosis, with or without the features of chronic aggressive hepatitis, is an invariable finding (Table 10.2). If, however, the disease is controlled by drugs or undergoes complete spontaneous resolution, only residual scarring may be found. These histological changes which are commonly associated with autoimmune chronic active

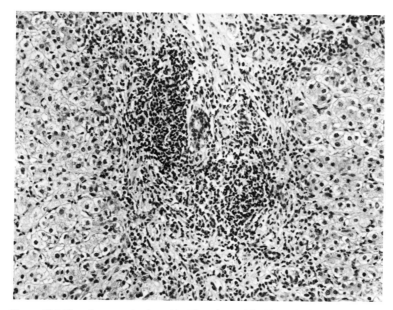

Figure 10.2 Chronic aggressive hepatitis. There is considerable widening of the portal tracts with an intense mononuclear cell infiltrate. The junction between the portal tract and hepatic parenchyma is irregular and inflammatory cells extend from the portal tract out into the parenchyma. In the upper part of the portal tract there is increased fibrosis. The hepatocytes show some vacuolation and there is patchy inflammatory cell infiltrate throughout the parenchyma (percutaneous liver biopsy: haematoxylin and eosin × 125, reduced to two-thirds in reproduction)

Table 10.2 Pathological features in liver biopsy

Chronic persistent hepatitis	Chronic actve hepatitis
Chronic inflammatory cell infiltrate in widened portal tracts sharply demarcated from hepatic parenchyma	Chronic inflammatory cell infiltrate in portal tracts with marked perilobular hepatitis and 'piecemeal' hepatocellular necrosis
Minimal erosion of limiting plate	Marked fibroblastic proliferation
Normal hepatic parenchyma	Distortion of architecture
± Slight fibrosis of portal tracts	Inflammatory cell infiltrate in parenchyma
Fine fibrous septa in parenchyma	± Signs of actute hepatitis
Areas of liver cell necrosis with inflammatory cell infiltrate	Liver cell 'rosettes' at the periphery of lobules
Kupffer cell prominence	Inflamed intralobular fibrous septa

hepatitis may also be found in sclerosing cholangitis, Wilson's disease and in chronic liver damage due to drugs such as methyldopa. They are said to occur in alpha-1 antitrypsin deficiency (PIZZ).

Chronic lobular hepatitis

Chronic lobular hepatitis is a poorly documented entity in which the hepatic architecture is preserved but there are scattered throughout the hepatic parenchyma histological changes similar to those seen in acute viral hepatitis; namely, focal liver cell degeneration and necrosis maximal around the central veins with infiltration by inflammatory cells and Kupffer cell proliferation. There may be focal groups of hepatocytes, two to three cells thick, indicating hepatocellular regeneration. Occasionally, such features may be present months or years after the onset of an acute hepatitis or may be found in the presence of relapsing hepatitis. Occasionally, these histological features are also found in association with the perilobular changes characteristic of chronic aggressive hepatitis. Hepatitis B virus infection or non-A, non-B hepatitis is the most common association with these pathological features.

Clinical aspects

Some patients with an apparent acute hepatitis have the features of chronic liver disease detailed below including alimentary bleeding from portal hypertension. In others it is the laboratory investigation results which first suggest a chronic liver disorder. Yet others will have no clinical or laboratory features suggesting chronicity and chronic hepatitis is suspected when no cause of acute liver damage can be found or when the serum transaminase values fail to return to normal as rapidly as expected in acute disorders. On occasions the condition is discovered in patients with no current or past clinical evidence of liver disease when biochemical tests of liver function, particularly the aspartate amino transferase or gamma-glutamyl transferase, performed as part of a routine medical examination, or in the investigation of some unrelated complaint, are found to be persistently abnormal. Physical examination may show no abnormality or there may be slight hepatomegaly without any features suggestive of chronic liver disease.

Clinical features suggesting chronicity

Chronic hepatitis should be suspected in the patient with hepatitis in the following circumstances:

(1) History of conjugated hyperbilirubinaemia in infancy.
(2) Family history of chronic liver disease, inherited or auto-immune disorders
(3) A relapse of apparent acute hepatitis.
(4) Persistence of clinical features of acute hepatitis for more than three months.
(5) Previous history of Hepatitis B, C or non-A,non-B hepatitis.

Features of chronic liver disease at presentation, include:

small liver
enlarged left lobe of liver
hard or nodular liver

firm splenomegaly
ascites
oedema
cutaneous portosystemic shunts
bleeding from portal hypertension
growth failure
muscle wasting
cutaneous features of chronic liver disease (facial telangiectasia, spider angiomata, clubbing or palmar erythema).
extrahepatic manifestations of autoimmune chronic active hepatitis
presence of Kayser-Fleischer rings
papular acrodermatitis

Investigative features suggesting chronicity

Chronic hepatitis should be suspected if the serum albumin is less than 35 g/litre, the prothrombin time prolonged by more than 3 seconds and not corrected by parenteral vitamin K administration and if the serum gammaglobulin is raised. Ultrasonic demonstration of a nodular liver with impaired portal vein flow velocity, flat venous wave form in the hepatic vein and increased arterial pulsatility are indicative. A technetium–99m colloid liver scan showing relatively poor hepatic uptake, enhanced splenic uptake and particularly uptake by the bone marrow, is also suggestive of severe liver disease which may be chronic.

Percutaneous liver biopsy is essential in all cases to define the severity of morphological change and to provide material for histological and biochemical analysis to confirm the diagnosis. In some cases the prothrombin time may be so prolonged that liver biopsy is contraindicated. If a treatable cause such as autoimmune disease or Wilson's disease is found biopsy can be delayed until the coagulation abnormalities correct with specific therapy for these disorders.

Differential diagnosis

A detailed past and family history with particular emphasis on liver disease, inherited or autoimmune disorders is essential. Are there features suggesting chronic inflammatory bowel disease? A careful history should be taken with special attention given to exposure to drugs or possible hepatotoxins and/or opportunities of contracting chronic infections affecting the liver. This may include a variety of parasitic infections such as *Schistosoma mansoni* and liver flukes as well as the more familiar viral hepatitis types B, C and D. Careful clinical examination should include a search for features of constrictive pericarditis. Remember that a raised serum transaminase may be due to myopathy rather than liver disease.

Investigations   Serological tests will detect the chronic infections mentioned above. In all patients it is essential to exclude other treatable disorders (Table 10.3).

These include Wilson's disease diagnosed by examination for Kayser-Fleischer ring and studies of copper metabolism. These should include 24-hour urinary copper excretion with and without penicillamine challenge as well as caeruloplasmin and serum copper. To exclude autoimmune disorders the concentration of serum immunoglobulins IgG, IgA, IgM, complement components C3 and C4 together with auto-antibodies to antinuclear factor, smooth muscle antigens and liver kidney microsomes (Chapters 11 and 12) should

Table 10.3 Investigations in suspected chronic hepatitis

Standard biochemical tests of liver function
Prothrombin time
Ultrasound of liver, its vessels and biliary system
Technetium-99m colloid liver scan
Alpha-1 antitrypsin phenotype
Serum caeruloplasmin
24-hour urinary copper excretion with penicillamine
Serum immunoglobulins
Tissue autoantibodies
Serological tests for HBV, HCV
Alpha-fetoprotein
Chest X-ray
ECG
Echocardiogram

be determined. Remember that endoscopic cholangiography is required to distinguish autoimmune primary sclerosing cholangitis from chronic active hepatitis in childhood. An ultrasound scan should be performed to exclude choledochal cyst or other surgical disorders of the biliary system. Dilated or obliterated hepatic veins on ultrasound indicate the necessity to perform cardiac catheterization and cannulation of the hepatic veins with pressure measurement and angiography to delineate the various causes of Budd–Chiari syndrome. Among inherited causes of chronic liver disease presenting without diagnostically helpful clinical features are alpha-1 antitrypsin PIZZ, determined by protease inhibitor phenotyping, tyrosinaemia, Niemann-Pick type 2 and, rarely, cystic fibrosis.

Bibliography

Arias, I. M., Jacoby, W. B., Popper, H., Schachter, D. and Shafritz, D. A. (eds.) (1988) *The Liver – Biology and Pathobiology,* 2nd edn. Raven Press, New York

Bianchi, L. (1986) Necro-inflammatory liver diseases. *Semin. Liver Dis.,* **6**, 185–198

Colucci, G., Colombo, M., Del Ninno, E. and Paronetto, F. (1983) In situ characterization by monoclonal antibodies of the mononuclear cell infiltrate in chronic active hepatitis. *Gastroenterology,* **85**, 1138–1145

De Grotte, J., Desmet, V. J., Gedigk, P. *et al.* (1968) A classification of chronic hepatitis. *Lancet,* **ii**, 626–628

International Group (1977). Acute and chronic hepatitis revisited. *Lancet,* **ii**, 914

Kelsall, A. R., Stewart, A. and Witts, L. J. (1947) Subacute and chronic hepatitis. *Lancet,* **ii**, 195–198

Knodell, R. G., Ishak, K. G., Black, *et al.* (1981) Formulation and application of a numerical scoring system for assessing histological activity in asymptomatic chronic active hepatitis. *Hepatology,* **1**, 431–435.

Martin, G. R. and Kleinmann, H. K. (1985) The extracellular matrix in development and disease. *Sem. Liver Dis.,* **5**, 147–159

Mowat, A. P. (1989) Chronic hepatitis and cirrhosis. In *Paediatric Gastroenterology and Nutrition in Early Childhood.* 2nd edn. (ed. E. Lebenthal) Raven Press, New York 1017–1043

Popper, H. and Schaffner, F. (1971) The vocabulary of chronic hepatitis. *New Engl. J. Med.,* **284**, 1154–1156

Scheuer, P. J. (1987) Cirrhosis. In *Pathology of the Liver*, 2nd edn (eds. R. N. M. MacSween, P. P. Anthony and P. J. Scheuer) Churchill-Livingstone, Edinburgh, 274–302

Scheuer, P. J. (1991) Classification of chronic viral hepatitis: a need for reassessment. *J. Hepatology,* **13**, 372–374

Senaldi, G., Portmann, B., Mowat, A. P., Mieli-Vergani, G. and Vergani, D. (1992) Immunohistochemical features of the portal tract mononuclear cell infiltrate in chronic aggressive hepatitis. *Arch. Dis. Childh.,* **67**, 1447–1453

Sherlock, S. (1989) Classifying chronic hepatitis. *Lancet,* **ii**, 1168–1170

Wilkinson, S. P., Portmann, B., Cochrane, A. M. G. *et al.* (1978). Clinical course in chronic lobular hepatitis. *Q.. J. Med.,* **47**, 421

Chapter 11

Autoimmune chronic active hepatitis

Definition

Autoimmune chronic active hepatitis (AiCAH) is characterized by chronic aggressive hepatitis with or without cirrhosis, high concentrations of serum immunoglobulins and the presence of non-organ specific autoantibodies. Other causes of chronic liver disease must be excluded. These include chronic hepatitis B virus infection, sclerosing cholangitis, particularly the primary autoimmune form, Wilson's disease, alpha-1 antitrypsin deficiency and exposure to hepatotoxic drugs. AiCAH can usually be controlled by immunosuppressive therapy. Treatment should be started at presentation, not after observing the patient for months to be convinced that the disease is indeed chronic. Rarely, emergency liver transplantation is necessary. The recently suggested designation *autoimmune hepatitis* (Johnson *et al*, 1993) is particularly appropriate since in the majority the disease presents acutely.

Epidemiology

The age at diagnosis has ranged from 6 months to 75 years. In the paediatric age group it rarely occurs before the age of 6 years but increases in frequency thereafter with a maximum age incidence between 10 and 30 years. Over 70% of cases are females. There may be a family history of autoimmune disorders.

Aetiology and pathogenesis

The aetiology of AiCAH is unknown. A genetically determined defect in immunoregulation, similar to that occurring in other immune-mediated disorders, is thought to play a part in pathogenesis. Evidence for such a defect initially took the form of high serum concentrations of immunoglobulin G (IgG) and of high titres of non-organ specific autoantibodies in both patients and their close relatives. More recently, a number of authors have reported persistently high titres of antibodies against liver membrane antigens (LMA), hepatocyte membrane antigen (HMA) and liver-specific lipoprotein (LSP). LMA and HMA are detected using immunofluorescence techniques which show immunoglobulin G deposits on the surface of liver cells obtained from liver biopsies of patients with AiCAH. LSP is a complex heterogeneous macrolipoprotein containing many antigens. Some are liver specific, e.g. the chemically well-characterised asialoglycoprotein receptor (ASGPR). Antibodies to LMA, HMA and LSP are present in AiCAH and in other acute and chronic liver disorders. Antibodies to ASGPR found in acute hepatitis type A and B and chronic liver disorders are not specific for AiCAH. Not all patients with anti-LSP have antibody to ASGPR. A close relationship has been demonstrated between the serum concentration of anti-LSP, measured by radioimmunoassay, and the extent of periportal inflammation and necrosis in liver biopsy. These liver specific autoantibodies are thought to be target antigens involved in mediating liver damage.

Mechanisms of liver damage (Figure 11.1)

These observations are consistent with the hypothesis that liver damage in AiCAH is likely to stem from the interaction of helper/inducer T lymphocytes (CD4-positive) with a self antigen (e.g. ASGPR) which has been mistakenly recognized as foreign. The antigen, in association with human leucocyte antigens (HLA) class II, may be presented to the helper/inducer T cells by the hepatocyte itself and/or by antigen presenting cells (APC). The T helper cell becomes activated and initiates a cascade of immune reactions by producing cytokines, activating cytotoxic T cells and inducing autoantibody production by B lymphocytes. This hypothesis is supported by the observations that hepatocytes from patients with active AiCAH express class II HLA antigens, not normally expressed on liver cells; that circulating levels of the cytokines interleukin 1 and 6, tumour necrosis factor and interferon-gamma are increased in AiCAH patients with active disease; that CD4-positive and activated lymphocytes are present in areas of piecemeal necrosis; that these patients have a high proportion of circulating activated helper T lymphocytes expressing the activation marker interleukin 2 receptor (IL-2R).

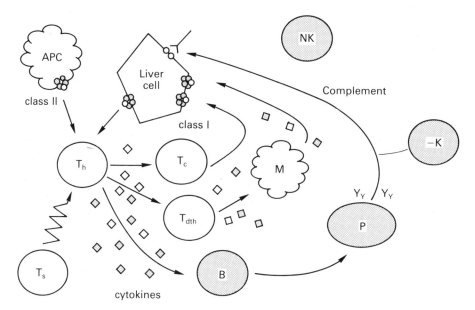

Figure 11.1 Liver cell autoimmune attack. A normal component of the liver cell membrane is presented to T helper (Th) lymphocytes either directly or by an antigen presenting cell (APC), in the context of class II HLA antigens. If T suppressor (Ts) lymphocytes do not oppose, then a variety of effector mechanisms are triggered. Liver cell destruction could derive from the action of: T cytotoxic (Tc) lymphocytes which react with the self antigen(s) in the context of class I HLA antigens; cytokines produced by T helper (Th), T delayed type hypersensitivity (Tdth) lymphocytes and recruited macrophages; autoantibody production by B lymphocytes with activation of complement and/or engagement of killer (K) lymphocytes. (*Reproduced by kind permission of G. Mieli-Vergani and D. Vergani*, 1993)

Once the autoimmune reaction is initiated, hepatocytes can be destroyed by various mechanisms. These include direct T cell cytotoxicity, cytokine action or autoantibody-driven complement or killer (K) cell mediated lysis. Liver-specific autoantibodies may initiate the recruitment of cytotoxic lymphocytes. Using an *in vitro* technique in which lymphocytes and hepatocytes from the same patients are incubated together, Mieli-Vergani and co-workers (1979) have shown that lymphocytes from children with AiCAH are cytotoxic to the hepatocytes. Cytotoxicity is blocked by LSP and aggregated IgG. Experiments using subpopulations of T and non-T lymphocytes indicate that the cytotoxicity is caused by non-T lymphocytes. These observations suggest that lymphocyte cytotoxicity in AiCAH is an antibody-dependent phenomenon in which K lymphocytes bind through their Fc receptor to an antibody reacting with an antigen on the hepatocyte surface and thus cause cell damage. Studies have failed to demonstrate complement activation in AiCAH.

Using monoclonal antibodies and various *in vitro* assays it has been possible to show reduced T suppressor numbers and reduced T suppressor function in circulating lymphocytes in both adults and children with this disorder. In one of these studies it was possible to correct, *in vitro*, the defect in suppressor T cell function by incubation of the lymphocytes with concentrations of prednisolone akin to those found in the plasma of patients on maintenance treatment. It is suggested that impairment of T suppressor function allows persistence of autoimmune reaction by failing to suppress antibody production from B cells and perhaps T cell cytotoxicity (see Figure 11.1).

The female sex predilection is unexplained. Recent research has highlighted some possible genetic factors that may contribute to this disorder. The HLA antigen B8 DR3 occurs in over 80% of young females with AiCAH. HLA B8 DR3 increases susceptibility to a wide range of autoimmune disorders.

In a recently reported family with multiple occurrence of AiCAH, female sex and possession of DR3 were more important than B8 in conferring susceptibility to the disease, suggesting that a defective antigen recognition by T cells in the context of class II HLA molecules plays a central role in generating autoimmunity, in association with gender determined factors (genes and hormones).

Recently, it has been shown that susceptibility to AiCAH is conferred independently by two genes within the major histocompatibility complex linked to the DR3 and DR4 genes (Doherty *et al.*, 1991). When compared with the DR4-positive patients, those with A1/B8/DR3 were shown to present at an earlier age, to relapse more frequently and to be more frequently referred for liver transplantation. Haplotypes conferring susceptibility to the juvenile or mature form of AiCAH have been further characterized. The DR3 haplotype predisposing to the juvenile form is DRB1*0301–DRB3*0101–DQA1*0501–DQB1*0201 with the individual alleles DRB3*0101 and DQA1*0501 exerting the greatest predisposing effect.

An additional genetic factor which might contribute to the development of AiCAH is the immunoglobulin GM allotype, *Gm ax* determined by the immunoglobulin locus on chromosome 14. The presence of both HLA B8 DR3 and *Gm ax* confers a 40-fold increased risk of disease. How this occurs is not clear.

Genetic deficiency of the complement component C4 (associated with a silent gene C4AQ0) has also been demonstrated in children with AiCAH. C4 deficiency has been reported in association with other autoimmune disorders. Since C4 is coded for by genes closely linked to the HLA genes it is possible that the association with low C4 derives from linkage disequilibrium between the C4 genes and the true disease susceptibility gene (or genes). Alternatively genetically-determined C4 deficiency might be a predisposing factor to autoimmunity.

All the above data suggest that AiCAH conforms to a multifactorial model in which a disease develops when a threshold is exceeded by environmental factors interacting with multiple genetic factors. What environmental factors are necessary to initiate the disease are unknown. Measles which has been implicated in adults does not appear to be a factor in children. Hepatitis A may have been a factor in two cases (Vento *et al.*, 1991). An unexplained association, in some adults, is anti-LKM-1 and Hepatitis C and LKM-2 and Hepatitis D.

Clinical features

Chronic hepatitis may present with features of an *acute* hepatitis; namely anorexia, malaise, nausea and vomiting, proceeding to jaundice with dark urine and pale stools. A large, hard liver, splenomegaly, ascites or cutaneous manifestations of liver disease such as spider angiomata and palmar erythema should suggest the diagnosis even if the duration of symptoms is short and the onset apparently acute. Some rapidly develop acute hepatic encephalopathy. In patients presenting without features of chronic liver disease it is only when causes of acute disease have been excluded or hepatitis has persisted for more than 8 weeks that the possibility of chronic liver disease must be considered. Less frequently the presentation is insidious with non-specific symptoms such as lethargy and anorexia and the diagnosis is suggested by clinical examination findings of a large firm liver. Some patients present with *complications of cirrhosis* such as ascites, haematemesis or hepatic coma. Rarely, investigations are initiated by the incidental finding of abnormal biochemical tests of liver function. At presentation hepatomegaly is found in over 90% of cases with splenomegaly in 60%. Approximately 25% have the systemic disorders listed in Table 11.1.

Some children at presentation are acutely ill with anorexia, loss of subcutaneous fat and muscle, malaise and fever as well as features of hepatocellular failure. Rarely the picture may be that of acute liver failure (Porta *et al.*, 1990). Epistaxis, bleeding gums and bruising with minimal trauma are frequent complaints. Other children are surprisingly active, well nourished and of normal stature. The diagnosis has been made as a result of finding abnormal tests of liver function in a child with no abnormal features (Peeters *et al.*, 1993). The condition is aggravated by interferon therapy. Spider naevi are found in nearly every patient. Amenorrhoea is usual. Ascites, oedema and hepatic encephalopathy are late features. Some patients develop hepatocellular carcinoma.

Table 11.1 Systemic disorders associated with autoimmune chronic active hepatitis

Site	Manifestation
Skin	Spider angiomata, malar flush, acne, inflammatory papules, striae gravidarum, urticaria, lupus erythematosis, vitiligo, alopecia
Locomotor system	Arthralgia, arthritis
Renal system	Albuminuria, haematuria, glomerulonephritis, renal tubular acidosis
Gastrointestinal system	Ulcerative colitis
Pulmonary system	Pleurisy, pleural effusion, multiple pulmonary arteriovenous anastomosis, fibrosing alveolitis
Endocrine system	Cushinoid features, gynaecomastia in males, amenorrhoea, thyroiditis
Cardiovascular system	Polyarthritis nodosa
Reticulo-endothelial system	Coombs' positive haemolytic anaemia, cryoglobulinaemia
Ocular system	Iridocyclitis

Laboratory investigations

Increased serum transaminase values and hypergammaglobulinaemia are the characteristic abnormalities. At presentation serum transaminases are raised to values of between two and 30 times normal. In contrast, the serum alkaline phosphatase and gamma-glutamyl transpeptidase are only modestly elevated 0.2–0.3 and 1–2 times normal respectively. Hyperbilirubinaemia is present except in those with an insidious onset. The serum albumin concentration is usually low. The prothrombin time is usually prolonged by at least 4 seconds at an early stage, with more marked prolongation occurring if liver damage is more advanced.

A characteristic almost constant abnormality is hypergammaglobulinaemia with levels greater than 20 g/litre. The serum IgG is usually elevated above 16 g/litre. In 15–20% of cases the serum IgM is also elevated. In up to 10% serum IgA levels are low. Complement component C4 concentrations may be low. C3 may also be low if liver damage is severe.

Non-organ specific IgG autoantibodies to internal components of cells are present in nearly every case at presentation but we have seen one case in which they appeared only after immunosuppression was started.

Three patterns of autoantibody response are seen, antibodies:

1. To smooth muscle alone or with antinuclear factor.
2. To liver/kidney microsomes (LKM-1, also called endoplasmic reticulum antibody since it reacts with cytochrome P-450IID6 and related antigens of the mono-oxygenase complex).
3. To a soluble liver antigen.

In addition gastric parietal cell antibodies, thyroid autoantibodies, rheumatoid factor or a Coomb's positive haemolytic anaemia is detected. There is no evidence of HBV infection. Given that some adult patients with hepatitis C have antibodies to the P-450-IID6 component of LKM-1, it seems prudent to exclude HCV infection by the most sensitive technique available (Vergani and Mieli-Vergani, 1993).

Endoscopic cholangiography and sigmoidoscopy are necessary to exclude sclerosing cholangitis and colitis.

Liver biopsy

Ideally this should be performed at presentation. If the prothrombin time is too prolonged it may be postponed for 4–10 weeks while liver function improves with treatment. The histological features will remain those of chronic aggressive hepatitis (Figure 11.2). Part of the liver biopsy should be analysed for copper content. Orcein staining usually shows no copper-associated protein while this is likely to be positive in primary sclerosing cholangitis. Other causes are considered in Chapter 10.

Drug treatment

Three prospective randomized controlled clinical trials in adults have shown that immunosuppressive treatment reduces morbidity and prolongs survival. No similar studies have been reported in children but observations in more than 200 suggest a similar response to treatment. Prednisolone in a dose of 2 mg/kg/day up to a maximum of 60 mg/day is given initially. The aim of treatment is to induce clinical and

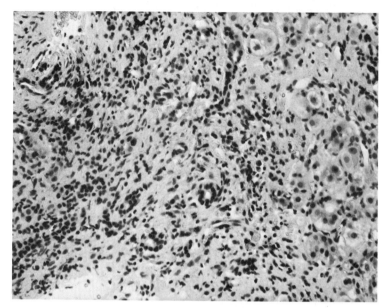

Figure 11.2 Chronic aggressive hepatitis. A section of portal tract and the adjacent hepatic parenchyma is shown. There is typical piecemeal necrosis of the hepatic parenchyma on the right. The interface between the portal tract and hepatic parenchyma is almost completely lost. Hepatocytes are swollen and have assumed abnormal configurations, such as rosettes. They are surrounded by lymphocytes and some groups of hepatocytes are isolated from other parts of the hepatic lobule. Within the portal tract the elongated nuclei of fibroblasts can be seen. These represent an integral part of the hepatic reaction in chronic aggressive hepatitis (percutaneous liver biopsy: haematoxylin and eosin × 320, reduced to two-thirds in reproduction)

biochemical remission while avoiding side-effects from steroids. Excessive weight gain, sometimes with ascites occurs in the first weeks of treatment. Some patients have behaviour problems. Full doses are maintained for the first 4 weeks of treatment by which time clinical features will have improved and the elevation of transaminase will be less marked. Over the course of 2–3 months the dose of steroids is gradually reduced to that which will give no side effects while maintaining a normal transaminase value. If reduction of the steroid dose is associated with a rise in transaminase or a recurrence of symptoms, azathioprine is added for steroid-sparing effect. A dose of 0.5–2.0 mg/kg/day is used. The lower dose is advisable initially, particularly in patients with low total white blood cell count or thrombocytopenia. Weekly full blood counts and platelet counts are essential following the addition of this medication. A dose of 1.5–2 mg/kg/day is usually tolerated.

Standard biochemical tests of liver function, serum immunoglobulins, tissue autoantibodies and prothrombin time are checked at 4-weekly intervals until stable but thereafter testing at 3-monthly intervals suffices, if asymptomatic. Serum immunoglobulin concentrations fall to normal in most cases but more frequently non-organ specific autoantibodies remain detectable in serum. If therapy is fully effective antibodies to liver components disappear and biochemical test for liver damage become normal. When these

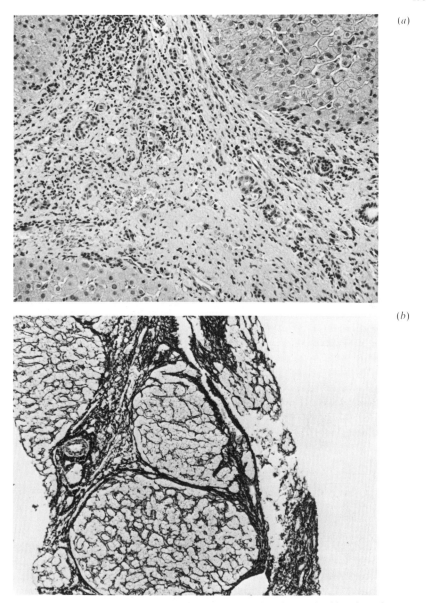

(*a*)

(*b*)

Figure 11.3 (*a*) Chronic aggressive hepatitis suppressed by drug therapy. A widened portal tract with intense fibrosis and patchy mononuclear cell infiltrate is shown. The junction between hepatic parenchyma and portal tract is now clear-cut (percutaneous liver biopsy: haematoxylin and eosin × 125, reduced to two-thirds in reproduction). (*b*) A reticulin stained biopsy (× 80, reduced to two-thirds in reproduction) shows distortion of the hepatic parenchyma by fibrous septa. Widened portal tract is shown with islets of hepatocytes without hepatic veins surrounded by fibrous tissue, cirrhosis having supervened. These biopsies are from a girl aged 12 years who had had two episodes of jaundice between the age of eight and ten years when investigations showed she had the full syndrome of chronic active hepatitis. Symptoms and liver function tests returned to normal within one year of commencing treatment and had been normal for one year prior to the above biopsies. Unfortunately, cirrhosis is now present

have been normal for 1 year a repeat liver biopsy should be performed to confirm that there is no evidence of aggressive hepatitis (Figure 11.3). If this persists. therapy must be maintained. If the disease is histologically inactive, immunosuppressive therapy may be gradually withdrawn but with monthly checks of standard biochemical tests of liver function serum immunoglobulins and tissue autoantibodies. The frequency with which relapse occurs is difficult to assess. It is almost universal in adults: only two of 17 children reported by Maggiore *et al.* (1984) were able to cease treatment as were seven of 28 in our series (Vegnente *et al.*, 1984) but 19 of 26 children reported by Arasu *et al.* in 1979 were able to stop treatment. It should be noted that one adult died of fulminant hepatic failure following drug withdrawal.

In rare instances the autoimmune process cannot be controlled by these measures. A trial of cyclosporin A in doses less than those which prevent rejection following liver transplant may be effective.

Liver transplantation

In patients with autoantibodies to LKM antigens and a prothrombin time prolonged by more than 20 seconds at presentation, liver transplantation should be considered if there is no evidence of improvement within 4 weeks of corticosteroids. If encephalopathy is present liver transplantation may be required earlier. Rarely it is necessary at a later stage (see below).

Prognosis

Our knowledge of the natural history of AiCAH in children is incomplete. In adults without treatment the disease usually runs a progressive downhill course, punctuated by periods of exacerbation of hepatic dysfunction, leading ultimately to cirrhosis and death in 50% of cases within 5 years of onset. In a review of paediatric series up to 1975, approximately one-third were dead at the time of reporting (Silverberg, 1979). In three more recent series (Arasu *et al.*, 1979: Maggiore *et al.*, 1984: Vegnente *et al.*, 1984) only four of 71 children died but over 50% in the latter two reports had proved or suspected cirrhosis. Vegnente *et al.* demonstrated an increased incidence of cirrhosis at diagnosis and follow-up the longer the duration of symptoms before treatment was started. At the time of reporting no patient had developed ascites, encephalopathy, bleeding oesophageal varices or died while on treatment or during follow-up. Two have subsequently required liver transplantation because of complications of end stage of liver disease. In at least two instances patients stopped immunosuppressive therapy without informing their parents or medical advisers. Concern about drug side-affects particularly cosmetic complications of steroids may have been a factor. Children with LKM autoantibodies tend to have more severe, even fulminant, liver disease at presentation and to respond less satisfactorily to immunosuppression than other subgroups.

In adults, a similarly high incidence of cirrhosis occurs but with a 93% 5-year survival in patients in remission or with disease controlled by immunosuppressants. These observations reinforce the contention that any child with a hepatitis not due to acute type A or B viral infection, as demonstrated by the presence of IgM antibodies to hepatitis A virus or the hepatitis B virus core, be immediately assessed for causes of possible chronic liver disease, including AiCAH, with a view to instituting immunosuppressive therapy irrespective of the apparent duration of symptoms.

References and bibliography

Acha-Orbea, H., Mitchell, D. J., Timmermann, L. *et al.* (1988) Limited heterogeneity of T cell receptors from lymphocytes mediating autoimmune encephalomyelitis allows specific immune intervention. *Cell,* **54,** 263–273

Arasu, T. S., Wyllie, R., Hatch, T. F. and Fitzgerald, I. F. (1979). Management of chronic aggressive hepatitis in children and adolescents *J. Pediatr.,* **95,** 514

Bearn, A. G., Kunkel, H. G. and Salter, R. J. (1956). The problem of chronic liver disease in young women. *Am. J. Med.,* **21,** 3

Berzofsky, J. A. (1988) Structural basis of antigen recognition by T lymphocytes: Implications for vaccines. *J. Clin. Invest.,* **82,** 1811–71

Bianchi, L. (1986) Necro-inflammatory liver diseases.*Sem. Liver Dis.,* **6,** 185–198

Chandra, R. K. and Silverberg, M. (1979). Chronic liver disease in children. In *Liver and Biliary System in Infants and Children,* (ed. R. K. Chandra), Churchill Livingstone, Edinburgh, p. 174

Chaves, V., Paunier, L., Berclaz, R., Deleze, G., Abuaf, N. and Belli, D. C. (1991) Anti-liver-kidney microsomal antibody-positive autoimmune hepatitis associated with alopecia. *J. Pediatr. Gastroenterol. Nutr.,* **12,** 288–290

Codoner-Franch, P., Paradis, K., Guen, M., Bernard, O., Costesec, A. A. and Alvarez, F. (1989) A new antigen recognised by antiliver-kidney microsome antibody (LKMA). *Clin. Exp. Immunol.,* **75,** 354–358.

Colucci, G., Colombo, M., Del Ninno, E. and Paronetto, F. (1983) In Situ characterization by monoclonal antibodies of the mononuclear cell infiltrate in chronic active hepatitis. *Gastroenterology,* **85,** 1138–1145

Doherty, D. J., Donaldson, P. T., Farrant, J. M. *et al.* (1991) Strong association between HLA-DQA, DQB and DRB3 alleles and autoimmune chronic active hepatitis demonstrated by PCR oligonucleotide analysis [Abstract]. *J. Hepatol.,* **13,** S25

Donaldson, P. T., Hussain, M. J., Mieli-Vergani, G., Mowat, A. P. and Vergani, D. (1989) Anti-lymphocytic antibodies in autoimmune chronic hepatitis starting in childhood. *Clin. Exp. Immunol.,* **75,** 41–46

Donaldson, P. T., Doherty, D. G., Hayllar, K. M., McFarlane, I. G., Johnson, P. J. and Williams, R. (1990) Susceptibility to autoimmune chronic active hepatitis: human leukocyte antigens DR4 and A1-B8-DR3 are independent risk factors. *Hepatology,* **13,** 701–706

Hegarty, J. E., Nouri, A. K T., Portmann, B. *et al.* (1983). Relapse following treatment withdrawal in patients with autoimmune chronic active hepatitis. *Hepatology,* **3,** 685

Hodges, S., Lobo-Yeo, A., Donaldson, P., Tanner, M. S. and Vergani, D. (1991) Autoimmune chronic active hepatitis in a family. *Gut,* **32,** 299–302

Homberg, J. C., Abuaf, N., Bernard, O. *et al.* (1987) Chronic active hepatitis associated with anti liver/kidney microsome antibody type 1, a second type of 'autoimmune' hepatitis. *Hepatology,* **7,** 1333–1339

International Group (1977) Acute and chronic hepatitis revisited. *Lancet,* **ii,** 914

Jensen, D. M., Mcfarlane, I. G., Portmann, B. S. *et al.* (1978) Detection of antibodies directed against a liver specific membrane lipoprotein in patients with acute and chronic active hepatitis. *New Engl. J. Med.,* **299,** 1

Johnson, G. D., Holborow, E. J., Glynn, L. E. (1965) Antibody to smooth muscle in patients with liver disease. *Lancet,* **ii,** 878–879

Johnson, P. J. and McFarlane (1993). Meeting report: International Autoimmune Hepatitis Group. *Hepatology,* **18,** 998–1005

Kelsall, A. R., Stewart, A. and Witts, L. J. (1947) Subacute and chronic hepatitis. *Lancet,* **ii,** 195–198

Kirk, A. P., Jain, S., Pocock, S. *et al.* (1980) Late results of The Royal Free Hospital controlled trial of prednisolone therapy in Hepatitis B surface antigen negative chronic active hepatitis. *Gut,* **21,** 78

Li, W., Peakman, M., Lobo-Yeo, A. *et al.* (1990) T-cell-directed hepatocyte damage in autoimmune chronic active hepatitis. *Lancet,* **336,** 1527–1530

Lobo-Yeo, A., Alviggi, L., Mieli-Vergani, G., Portmann, B., Mowat, A. P. and Vergani, D. (1987) Preferential activation of helper/inducer T lymphocytes in children with autoimmune chronic active hepatitis. *Clin. Exp. Immunol.,* **67,** 95–104

Lobo-Yeo, A., McSorley, C., McFarlane, B., Mieli-Vergani, G., Mowat, A. P. and Vergani, D. (1989) Detection of anti-liver cell membrane antibody using a human hepatocellular carcinoma cell line. *Hepatology,* **9,** 201–214

Lobo-Yeo, A., Mieli-Vergani, G., Mowat, A. P. and Vergani, D. (1990) Soluble interleukin 2 receptors in autoimmune chronic active hepatitis. *Gut,* **31,** 690–693

Lobo-Yeo, A., Senaldi, G., Portmann, B., Mowat, A. P., Mieli-Vergani, G. and Vergani, D. (1990) Class I and class II major histocompatibility complex antigen expression on hepatocytes. A study in children with liver disease. *Hepatology,* **12,** 224–232

McFarlane, I. G., McFarlane, B. M., Major, G. N., Tolley, P. and Williams, R. (1984) Identification of the hepatic asialoglycoprotein receptor (hepatic lectin) as a component of liver specific membrane lipoprotein (LSP). *Clin. Exp. Immunol.,* **55,** 347–354

McFarlane, I. G., Smith, H. M., Johnson, P. J., Bray, G. P., Vergani, D. and Williams, R. (1990) Hepatitis C virus antibodies in chronic active hepatitis: pathogenetic factor of false-positive result? *Lancet,* **335,** 754–757

Maggiore, G., Bernard, O., Homberg, J. C. *et al.* (1986.) Liver disease associated with anti-liver-kidney microsome antibody in children. *J. Pediatr.,* **108,** 399–404

Maggiore, G., Bernard, O., Hadchouel, M. *et al.* (1984). Treatment of chronic activie hepatitis in childhood. *J. Pediatr.*, **104**, 839

Manns, M., Gerken, G., Kyriatsoulis, A., Staritz, M. and Meyer zum Buschenfelde, K. H. (1987) Characterization of a new subgroup of autoimmune chronic active hepatitis by autoantibodies against a soluble liver antigen. *Lancet*, **i**, 292–294

Mieli-Vergani, G., Vergani, D., Jenkins, P. J. *et al.* (1979). Lymphocyte cytotoxicity to autologous hepatocytes in HB/sAg negative chronic active hepatitis. *Clin. Exp. Immunol.*, **83**, 16

Mieli-Vergani, G. and Mowat, A. P. (1986). The immunology of autoimmune chronic active hepatitis. In *Paediatric Gastroenterology, Aspects of Immunology and Infections* (eds. D. Branski, G. Dinari, P. Rosen, J. A. Walker-Smith). Karger, Basel. 286

Mieli-Vergani, G., Sutherland, S. and Mowat, A. P. (1989) Measles and autoimmune chronic active hepatitis. *Lancet*, **2**, 688

Mieli-Vergani, G., Lobo-Yeo, A., Mcfarlane, B. M., Mcfarlane, I. G., Mowat, A. P. and Vergani, D. (1989) Different immune mechanisms leading to autoimmunity in primary sclerosing cholangitis and autoimmune chronic active hepatitis of childhood. *Hepatology*, **9**, 198–203

Mowat, A. P. (1989) Chronic hepatitis and cirrhosis. In *Paediatric Gastroenterology and Nutrition in Early Childhood*. 2nd edn, (ed. E. Lebenthal) Raven Press, New York. 1017–1043

Nouri, A. K. T., Lobo-Yeo, A., Vergani, D. *et al.* (1985). T-suppressor cell function and number in children with liver disease. *Clin. Exp. Immunol.*, **61**, 283

Nouri, A. K. T. Donaldson, P. T., Hegarty, J. E. *et al.* (1985). HLA A1 B8 DR3 and suppressor cell function in first-degree relatives of patients with autoimmune chronic active hepatitis. *J. Hepatol.*, **1**, 235

Peakman, M., Bevis, L., Mieli-Vergani, G., Mowat, A. P. and Vergani, D. (1989) Double stranded DNA binding in autoimmune chronic active hepatitis and primary sclerosing cholangitis starting in childhood. *Autoimmunity*, **3**, 271–280

Peeters, S., Blecker, U., De Valck, J., Goossens, A., Hautekeete, M., Devis, G. and Vandenplas, Y. (1993) Asymptomatic autoimmune chronis active hepatitis in a male adolescent. *J. Pediatr. Gastroenterol. Nutr.* (In press)

Poralla, T., Treichel, U., Lohr, H. and Fleischer, B. (1991) The asialoglycoprotein receptor as target structure in autoimmune liver diseases. *Sem. Liver Dis.*, **11**, 215–222

Porta, G., Carlos de Costa Gayotto, L. and Alvarez, F. (1990) Anti-liver-kidney microsome antibody-positive autoimmune hepatitis presenting as fulminant liver failure. *J. Pediatr. Gastroenterol. Nutr.*, **11**, 138–140

Rizzetto, M., Swana, G. and Doniach, D. (1973) Microsomal antibodies in active chronic hepatitis and other disorders. *Clin. Exp. Immunol.* **15**, 331–344

Ruiz-Moreno, M., Rua, M. J., Carreno, V., Quiroga, J. A., Manns, M., Meyer zum Buschenfelde, K. H. (1991) Autoimmune chronic hepatitis type 2 manifested during interferon therapy in children. *J. Hepatology*, **12**, 265–266

Senaldi, G., Mieli-Vergani, G., Mowat, A. P. and Vergani, D. (1989) C4 function in children with autoimmune chronic active hepatitis. *Hepatology*, (letter) **9**, 345

Senaldi, G. (1990) Mononuclear cell infiltrate characterisation and hepatocyte expression analysis of class I and II major histocompatibility complex molecules in liver biopsies from children with hepatic disorders. PhD thesis, University of London, pp. 132–152

Senaldi, G., Portmann, B., Mowat, A. P., Mieli-Vergani, G. and Vergani, D. (1992) Immunohistochemical features of the portal tract mononuclear cell infiltrate in chronic aggressive hepatitis. *Arch. Dis. Childh.*, **67**, 1447–1453.

Sheron, N. and Eddleston, A. (1991) Autoimmune chronic active hepatitis. In: *Oxford Textbook of Clinical Hepatology* (ed. N. McIntyre, J. P. Benhamou, J. Bircher, M. Rizzetto, J. Rodes). Oxford University Press, Oxford, 758–767

Vegnente, A., Larcher, V.E., Mowat, A. P. *et al.* (1984). Duration of chronic active hepatitis and development of cirrhosis. *Arch. Dis. Childh.*, **59**, 330

Vento, S., Garofano, T., Di Perri, G., Dolci, L., Concia, E. and Bassetti, G. (1991). Identification of hepatitis A virus as a trigger for autoimmune chronic hepatitis type 1 in susceptible individuals. *Lancet*, **337**, 1183–1187.

Vergani, D. and Mieli-Vergani, G. (1993) Type II autoimmune hepatitis. What is the role of the hepatitis C virus? *Gastroenterology*, **104**, 1870–73

Vergani, D., Mieli-Vergani, G., Mondelli, M., Portmann, B. and Eddleston, A. L. W. F. (1987) Immunoglobulin on the surface of isolated hepatocytes is associated with antibody-dependent cell-mediated cytotoxicity and liver damage. *Liver*, **7**, 307–315

Vergani, D., Wells, L., Larcher, V. F. *et al.* (1985) Genetically determined low C4: a predisposing factor to autoimmune chronic active hepatitis. *Lancet*, **2**, 294–298

Wen, L., Peakman, M., Mowat, A. P., Mieli-Vergani, G. and Vergani, D. (1991) T cell clones from liver biopsies of children with autoimmune chronic active hepatitis (aCAH) and primary sclerosing cholangitis (aPSC) are cytotoxic to human liver target cells [Abstract]. *J. Hepatol.*, **13**, S80

Wen, L., Peakman, M., Lobo-Yeo, A. *et al.* (1990) T-cell-directed hepatocyte damage in autoimmune chronic active hepatitis. *Lancet*, **336**, 1527–1530

Wright, E. C., Seeff, L. B., Berk, P. D. *et al.* (1977). Treatment of chronic active hepatitis: An analysis of three control trials. *Gastroenterology*, **73**, 1422

Chapter 12

Sclerosing cholangitis

Sclerosing cholangitis was first described in 1924 by Delbet. Until the advent of endoscopic retrograde cholangiopancreatography (ERCP) and percutaneous transhepatic cholangiography (PTHC) recognition was rare, being made at laparotomy in patients with persistent jaundice. With the advent of cholangiography the disease is now recognized in anicteric patients and its apparent prevalence in both adults and children is increasing. It may be a more common cause of chronic liver disease in children than the few cases reported to date would suggest.

Definition

Sclerosing cholangitis (SC) is characterized by a chronic inflammation which produces multifocal fibrotic narrowing and dilatation of the intrahepatic and extrahepatic bile ducts (La Russo et al., 1991). The diagnosis is made on the basis of the cholangiographic appearances. The characteristic features are irregularities in the outline of the intrahepatic and extrahepatic bile ducts with areas of annular strictures, intervening areas of normal calibre or dilatation (beading) and sometimes short band-like strictures and small diverticulae. Sections of the intrahepatic bile ducts may retain the same calibre over excessive lengths (El Shabrawi et al., 1987). In some patients the disease appears to involve only the intrahepatic ducts, in others only the extrahepatic ducts. The extrahepatic bile duct may be dilated. The gall bladder is frequently very large. The appearances of the ducts in SC must be distinguished from the 'attenuated' intrahepatic ducts seen in cirrhosis.

Primary sclerosing cholangitis must be distinguished from *secondary sclerosing cholangitis* which may occur in association with a lesions in the biliary system or with generalized disease processes (Sisto et al., 1987; Sharpe and Freese, 1987). (Table 12.1). A recently recognized form occurs as a sequela of cryptogenic neonatal hepatitis (Amedee-Manesme et al., 1987).

Pathology

Percutaneous liver biopsies show features of a chronic or an acute cholangitis. Polymorphs infiltrate the bile duct epithelium and may be found in the bile duct lumen. Portal tract swelling with oedema, increased fibrosis and periductular inflammation is characteristic. The inflammatory cell infiltrate is composed of lymphocytes, polymorphs, plasma cells, histiocytes and occasionally eosinophils. The fibrosis is concentrated around the ducts. In approximately 50% of biopsies it takes the form of 'onion skin' type fibrosis

Table 12.1 Categories of sclerosing cholangitis

Classic cholangiographic features
    Affecting: Intra- and extrahepatic ducts
                Intrahepatic only
                Extrahepatic only

Compatible liver histology
    + or − cirrhosis

Primary:
    (A) commencing with cholestasis in infancy.
    (B) autoimmune
        associated with high serum immunoglobulins and non-organ specific autoantibodies. (C4
        concentration normal unless liver disease is decompensated. Circulating T lymphocytes displaying
        IL 2R. <5%)
            1. with or without chronic inflammatory bowel disease
    (C) with normal serum immunoglobulins and no autoantibodies
            1. with or without chronic inflammatory bowel disease
    (D) With systemic diseases
        Langerhans cell histiocytosis (histiocytosis X)
        Immune deficiency states
        HIV infection
        Neutropenic states
        Cystic fibrosis
        Graft versus host disease
        Chronic pancreatitis
        Riedel's thyroiditis
        Submandibular gland fibrosis
        Weber-Christian disease
        Sickle cell anaemia
        Reticular cell sarcoma

Secondary to other biliary lesions:
    Biliary surgery or trauma
    Choledochal cyst
    Congenital hepatic fibrosis
    Caroli's syndrome
    Liver rejection

encircling bile duct branches in one or more portal tracts. Bile ducts are obliterated and may disappear completely. Orcein-positive copper-associated protein is present in periportal hepatocytes. There may be conspicuous piecemeal necrosis leading to an inaccurate diagnosis of chronic aggressive hepatitis if the bile duct lesion is overlooked. Portal phlebitis or phlebosclerosis has been found in over 20% of liver biopsy specimens from adults (Ludwig *et al.*, 1986). The biliary damage leads to cirrhosis and death from complications of cirrhosis (Figure 12.1). About 20% of patients with primary sclerosing cholangitis have cirrhosis at the time of diagnosis.

A similar fibrosing cholangitis is found in interlobular, septal and segmental bile ducts. In addition these show segments of cholangiectasis with the diameter of the bile channel exceeding that of the accompanying artery by between two and 10 times. These dilated ducts have lacunae in their epithelial lining and little evidence of ongoing inflammation. There is excessive mucus production from epithelial cells and from glands in the walls of larger ducts. In contrast other bile ducts are replaced by solid fibrous cords. These obliterative ducts are responsible for the 'pruned tree' effect seen in cholangiograms. Biopsies of gall bladder or extrahepatic bile ducts show chronic

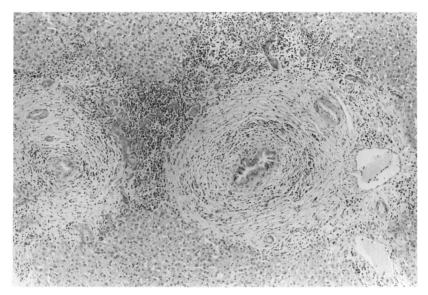

Figure 12.1 Two intralobular bile ducts in the liver biopsy of a 14-year-old boy with primary sclerosing cholangitis and colitis. The bile ducts are encircled by fibrous tissue with a mild, inflammatory cell infiltrate. At the periphery of the portal tracts there is a focal dense inflammatory cell infiltrate causing piecemeal necrosis of areas of surrounding hepatic parenchyma. (Haematoxylin and eosin, magnification × 100, reduced to two-thirds in reproduction)

inflammatory cell infiltrates and fibrosis. Cholangiocarcinoma is a recognized complication in adults.

Primary sclerosing cholangitis

Epidemiology, aetiology and pathogenesis

The aetiology of primary sclerosing cholangitis (PSC) is unknown and little is understood of its pathogenesis. PSC has been associated with a number of diseased states. The most common in both children (50%) and adults (70%) is chronic inflammatory bowel disease. The prevalence of PSC in adults with ulcerative colitis ranges from 1% to 5%. Colitis usually predates the PSC, the colitis is frequently mild although the degree of involvement is extensive. There is no relation between the severity or relapses of colitis and the cholangitis. The prevalence of PSC in children with ulcerative colitis is unknown but in up to 5% advanced liver disease is present which could be due to PSC.

The association with Crohn's disease is extremely rare. In adults, PSC has been associated with retroperitoneal and mediastinal fibrosis. Seventy percent of adult patients are male, with a median age at diagnosis of 40 years. In childhood symptoms may start at any age but most frequently in the second year with and equal male/female frequency.

An early aetiological hypothesis was chronic low-grade biliary infection. Bile, however, is usually sterile. An unusual response to bile infection, e.g. by Reo, CMV or hepatitis C is not excluded. Later hypotheses have sought to incriminate toxic factors such as bile acids or disordered immune mechanisms. The familial occurrence of PSC supports the hypothesis that genetic factors may play a role in aetiology. The increased frequency of HLA-B8 antigen and the A1 B8 DR3 DQW2 DRW52a haplotype in patients with PSC compared with patients with ulcerative colitis or healthy controls suggests that the susceptibility gene for PSC may be associated with the B loci of the major histocompatibility complex (Prochazka *et al.*, 1990, Donaldson *et al.*, 1991). Low IgA concentrations in bile have been suggested as a possible contributory factor.

There is some evidence that suggests that immune mechanisms may be implicated in the pathogenesis of PSC although not necessarily primarily (Chapman, 1991). In adults, raised serum IgM occurs in up to 50% of patients but elevations of serum IgA and IgG are relatively uncommon. Positive antinuclear antibodies have been reported in 8% to 32% of adults. Circulating immune complexes were found in 16 of 20 adults with PSC (Bodenheimer *et al.*, 1983).

In recent paediatric series, very high IgG levels and positive smooth muscle and/or antinuclear antibodies were found in nearly all patients (El Shabrawi, 1987; Classen *et al.*, 1987, Mieli-Vergani *et al.*, 1989). None have been reported with LKM antibodies. The other immunological findings were similar to those in autoimmune chronic active hepatitis in childhood except as detailed in Table 12.2.

Table 12.2 Laboratory features distinguishing autoimmune chronic active hepatitis (AiCAH) from autoimmune primary sclerosing cholangitis (AiPSC)

	AiCAH	*AiPSC*
IL 2R +ve T lymphocytes	>6%	<5%
T suppressor cell numbers	low	normal
T suppressor cell function	low	normal
Complement C4	low	normal
Orcein positive granules in liver biopsy	absent	present

In our own unit we have studied a series of regulatory and effector immune mechanisms in eight children with PSC, comparing them with 14 children with autoimmune chronic active hepatitis (Mieli-Vergani *et al.*, 1989) (Table 12.2). Two important differences were found. T suppressor cell numbers and T suppressor function were normal in patients with PSC but significantly decreased in patients with AiCAH. The percentage of T lymphocytes expressing interleukin 2 receptors was greatly increased in AiCAH but normal in PSC. The frequency of auto-antibodies to a liver membrane protein preparation (LSP) and to asialoglycoprotein receptor were similar as was the degree of lymphocyte cytotoxicity to autologous hepatocytes. Autoaggression in PSC seems to result from direct activation of B lymphocytes by an unknown stimulus which is able to override T cell control. Whether the persistently increased numbers of IL-2R positive T lymphocytes present in AiCAH derives from the presence of a continuous activating stimulus or from a genetic factor causing impairment of regulating mechanisms is a matter for speculation. Eight of 10 with PSC had in serum an anti-neutrophil antibody as had three of eight with AiCAH (Lo *et al.*, 1993). These observation suggest many pathophysiological similarities in what may transpire to be a spectrum of autoimmune hepatobiliary disease rather than two distinct conditions.

Clinical features

In recent paediatric series the majority of patients have presented with non-specific symptoms such as abdominal pain or fever. Less than 50% have had jaundice. A minority had pruritus, arthralgia or complications of liver disease at presentation. In the majority liver disease was suspected by the finding of hepatomegaly or hepatosplenomegaly on clinical examination. In others it was the presence of abnormal liver function tests in a patient with inflammatory bowel disease that provoked further investigation and ultimately diagnosis. The age of onset of symptoms has ranged from 1 to 16 years with an equal incidence in males and females. In the majority of patients with inflammatory bowel disease gastrointestinal symptoms have preceded the identification of liver involvement but in a minority the liver disease has preceded inflammatory bowel disease.

Investigative findings

In the above paediatric series liver function tests show a raised serum bilirubin value in a minority of patients. Aspartate aminotransferase is usually raised to values of between 1.5 and 48 times the upper limit of normal. Gamma-glutamyl transpeptidase activity is increased to values of between 1.5 and 85 times the upper limit of normal. Some patients had normal aspartate aminotransferase or normal gamma-glutamyl transpeptidase. Alkaline phosphatase is raised in the majority of cases to values of between two and 16 times the upper limit of normal. The serum albumin is normal early in the disease. Peripheral blood eosinophilia was noted in five of 13 patients in one series. Immunological findings are discussed above.

Cholangiographic features

In the majority of reported cases both intra- and extrahepatic ducts had been involved at the time of reporting. In a few only the intrahepatic ducts had been abnormal while in others only extrahepatic ducts. In seven of 21 studies the gall bladder was reported to be abnormally large. Sigmoidoscopy and/or colonoscopy with mucosal biopsies is essential to exclude inflammatory bowel disease, usually ulcerative colitis (see Table 12.3), which

Table 12.3 Hepatobiliary complications of ulcerative colitis or Chrohn's disease

Pericholangitis
Fatty liver
Primary sclerosing cholangitis
Chronic active hepatitis
Biliary cirrhosis
Amyloidosis (Crohn's disease only)
Hepatic abscess
Hepatic granulomata
Cholelithiasis
Carcinoma of the biliary tree
Benign duct neoplasia
Portal vein thrombosis
Hepatic venous occlusion

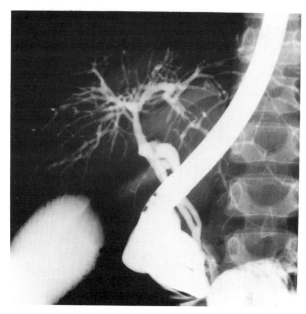

Figure 12.2 Endoscopic retrograde cholangiopancreatogram of a
7-year-old with primary sclerosing cholangitis without associated
bowel disease. The gall bladder is large, the extrahepatic bile ducts
are normal, there is a narrowing via the junction of the right and left
hepatic duct with dilatation of the main left duct and numerous areas
of strictures and dilatations of the right and left duct system. Both
the strictured and dilated ducts show typically parallel borders with
no tapering.

was present in seven of 10 recent cases in our service. The clinical, investigative and liver
biopsy findings are indistinguishable from AiCAH without endoscopic retrograde
cholangiography (Figure 12.2).

Prognosis

Because of the infrequency with which the disease is recognized the natural history of
PSC is poorly defined. There have been no prospective long-term follow-up studies even
in adults. Patients diagnosed prior to the availability of cholangiography (pre-1976) form
a different data base to those diagnosed since then. Nevertheless from six recent adult
series, it seems that the majority of patients with PSC when followed prospectively for 4
to 6 years from the time of diagnosis show progression of their liver disease accompanied
by morbidity and mortality. The medial survival was in the range of 8–14 years.

Complications include malabsorption, osteoporosis, stones in the gall bladder or bile
ducts, cholangitis and those of cirrhosis. Cholangiocarcinoma develops in up to 23%. In
a study of 180 patients with PSC followed for a mean period of 6 years, 70% of
asymptomatic patients developed symptoms during the period of follow-up and 25%
developed hepatic decompensation or died (Weisner *et al.*, 1988). In the symptomatic
patients approximately 50% died or required liver transplantation. The mean time from
diagnosis of PSC to liver transplantation was 5.8 years (range 1 to 16 years) (Marsh *et al.*,
1988).

There is a paucity of long-term follow-up studies in children. In eight patients followed for 1 month to 6 years, there was no evidence of progression of the disease (Classen et al., 1987). Two of three patients in a further study had end-stage liver disease within a few months and 2 years of onset (Sisto et al., 1987).

Treatment

There is no specific effective medical treatment for PSC. Choleretics, immuno-suppressives and antifibrotics singly or in combination have been shown to produce improvements in some of the laboratory features and to decrease inflammatory changes in liver biopsy tissues. Their effect on hepatic fibrosis and the long-term prognosis have yet to be established. In a recently reported randomized double blind controlled trial of ursodeoxycholic acid in 18 adults, a dose of 10 mg/kg/day produced an insignificant improvement in liver biochemical tests but no histological improvement (O'Brien et al., 1991). In 12 adults prednisolone in a dose of 10 mg/day and colchicine, 0.6 mg twice daily were associated with improvement in liver function test at 6 and 12 months but not at 24 months (Lindor et al., 1991). Low dose methotrexate in another uncontrolled study caused improvement in biochemical tests for liver disease and liver histology with in one patient the ERCP reverting to normal. Penicillamine had no effect on the progression of symptoms, hepatic laboratory values or histological change in sequential liver biopsies in a controlled study (La Russo et al., 1988). No prospective or randomized studies have been done in children or adults with disordered immune function in whom corticosteroids or other immunosuppressants, theoretically, may have value. In an uncontrolled study in our own unit 18 children were followed-up for 9 months to 10 years (median 2.5 years), 17 receiving immunosuppressants. All showed symptomatic improvement. In 14 the mean aspartate aminotransferase level fell, becoming normal, however, in only six. In eight the IgG values returned to normal with the auto-antibodies becoming negative. In five of nine follow-up biopsies periductular inflammation decreased while on seven lobular hepatitis decreased. In a study of six children treated with 'above conventional' doses of steroids, 6-mercaptopurine or colectomy liver function tests became normal and liver biopsies showed no inflammation but residual fibrosis in five patients. It was observed that the inflammatory activity in rectal biopsies correlated with abnormalities in the liver function tests. There was no reduction of hepatic fibrosis. Sharpe and Freese (1987) reported broadly similar results.

These observations have led to the suggestion that immunosuppressive treatment of PSC coupled with effective control of ulcerative colitis before the liver pathology is advanced may be successful in arresting the progression of the disorder whereas treatment given in the presence of advanced disease may be ineffective.

Other measures

Attacks of bacterial cholangitis require appropriate antibiotic treatment. Dietary supplements with fat soluble vitamins, calcium and phosphate are required if there is significant cholestasis. Cholestyramine, phototherapy or rifampicin may be helpful in relieving itching. There is no evidence that surgical dilatation of biliary strictures and long-term drainage through T tubes prolong survival and they should be avoided since they may make surgery for orthotopic liver transplantation more difficult. Biliary tract surgery is frequently complicated by biliary or hepatic sepsis. If a biliary drainage procedure is required an endoscopically placed stent tube is to be preferred since it makes liver transplantation less hazardous.

Liver transplantation

End-stage liver disease due to PSC is, in adults, the most frequent indication of orthotopic liver transplantation in North America. The 1 year survival rate in patients without prior surgery is between 70–80%. The issue of recurrence of PSC after liver transplantation remains unsettled. Radiologically demonstrated biliary tract findings identical to PSC have been seen in liver transplantation recipients irrespective of the initial disorder.

Sclerosing cholangitis with immune deficiencies and rare disorders

Cholangiographic features of sclerosing cholangitis have been seen in children with a range of immunodeficiency syndromes. The majority of these patients have had chronic diarrhoea with clinical and biochemical features similar to PSC associated with inflammatory bowel disease. In some instances the liver histology has been normal, others have had features of cholangitis. Over periods of observation of 2 to 5 years the disease

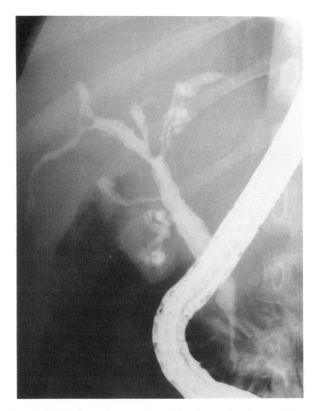

Figure 12.3 Endoscopic retrograde cholangiogram in a 9-year-old boy with X-linked agammaglobulinaemia. There is mild dilatation of the common duct with narrowing of the terminal 1.5 cm. There is marked irregularity of the walls of the extrahepatic and intrahepatic ducts, stenosis at the junction of the intrahepatic ducts and multiple filling defects compatible with debris within the ducts

appears to be stable or slowly progressive. Sclerosing cholangitis associated with Langerhans cell histiocytosis (histiocytosis X) progresses more rapidly to a biliary cirrhosis which may require liver transplantation by 6 years of age (Rand and Whitington, 1992) (Figure 12.3).

Sclerosing cholangitis with neonatal onset

Fourteen children, including two siblings, have been described with typical cholangiographic features of sclerosing cholangitis all having presented with jaundice in the neonatal period, the stools being acholic in all six in which this was recorded. The serum bilirubin value falls to near normal by 1 year of age but rises as cirrhosis develops. All patients had persistently abnormal biochemical tests for liver disease. Cirrhosis was documented in six patients aged between 3 months and 9 years. By that age some of the children had developed increasing serum bilirubin concentrations. None of these patients had symptoms of chronic inflammatory bowel disease but few have had colonoscopy or large bowel biopsies. Immunological investigations were normal in the one case in which they were reported (Mulberg *et al.*, 1992; Baker *et al.*, 1993).

References and bibliography

Amedee-Manesme, O., Bernard, O., Brunelle, F. *et al.* (1987) Sclerosing cholangitis with neonatal onset. *J. Pediatr.*, **111**, 225–229

Baker, A., Portmann, B., Westaby, D., Wilkinson, S., Karani, J. and Mowat, A. P. (1993) Neonatal sclerosisng cholangitis in 2 siblings: a category of progressive intrahepatic cholestasis. *J. Paediatr. Gastroenterol. Nutr.*, (in press)

Barton, J. R. and Ferguson, A. (1990) Clinical features, morbidity and mortality of Scottish children with inflammatory bowel disease. *Q. J. Med*, **75**, 423–439.

Bodenheimer, J. C., La Russo, N. F., Thayer, W. R., Charland, C., Stapel, P. and Ludwig, J. (1983) Elevated circulating immune complexes in primary sclerosing cholangitis. *Hepatology*, **3**, 150–154

Chapman, R. W. (1991) Role of immune factors in the pathogenesis of primary sclerosing cholangitis. *Sem. Liver Dis.*, **11**, 1–4

Chong, S. K. F. and Walker-Smith, J. A. (1984). Ulcerative colitis in childhood. *J. Roy. Soc. Med.*, **77**, 21

Classen, M., Goetze, H., Richter, H. J. and Bender, F (1987) Primary sclerosing cholangitis in children. *J. Pediatr. Gastroenterol. Nutr.*, **6**, 197–202

Dayer, E., Roux-Lombard, P., Huber, O. and Dayer, J-M. (1991) Chronic sclerosing cholangitis and recurrent pulmonary infections in two brothers associated with cellular immunodeficiency and increased cytokine production. *Pediatr. Allergy Immunol.*, **2**, 87–92

Delbet, P. (1924) Retrecissement du choledoque: cholecystoduodenostomie. *Bull. Mem. Soc. Nat. Chir.*, **50**, 1144

Donaldson, P. T., Farrant, J. M., Wilkinson, M. L., Hayllar, K., Portmann, B. C. and Williams, R. (1991) Dual association of HLA DR2 and DR3 with primary sclerosing cholangitis. *Hepatology*, **13**, 129–133

Duerr, R. H., Targan, S. R., Landers, C. J. *et al.* (1991) Neutrophil cytoplasmic antibodies: a link between primary sclerosing cholangitis and ulcerative colitis. *Gastroenterology*, **100**, 1385–1391

El Shabrawi, M., Wilkinson, M. L., Portmann, B. *et al.* (1987) Primary sclerosing cholangitis. *Gastroenterology*, **92**, 1226–1235.

Farrant, J. M., Hayllar, K. M., Wilkinson, M. L. *et al.* (1991) Natural history and prognostic variabes in primary sclerosing cholangitis. *Gastroenterology*, **100**, 1710–1717

Helzberg, J. H., Petersen, J. M. and Boyer, J. L. (1987) Improved survival with primary sclerosing cholangitis. *Gastroenterology*, **92**, 1869–1875

Kaplan, M. M. (1991) Medical approaches to primary sclerosing cholangitis. *Sem. Liver Dis.*, **11**, 56–63

Knox, T. A. and Kaplan, M. M. V. (1991) Treatment of primary sclerosing cholangitis with oral methotrexate. *Am. J. Gastroenterol.*, **86**, 546–552

La Russo, N. F., Wiesner, R. H. and Ludwig, J. (1991) Sclerosing cholangitis. In: *Oxford Textbook of Clinical Hepatology* (Eds. N. McIntyre, J. P. Benhamou, J. Bircher, M. Rizzetto, J. Rodes). Oxford University Press, Oxford, p 767–776

La Russo, N. F., Wiesner, R. H., Ludwig, J. *et al.* (1988) Prospective trial of penicillamine in primary sclerosing cholangitis. *Gastroenterology*, **95**, 1036–1042

Lebovics, E., Palmer, M., Woo, J. and Schaffner, F. (1987) Outcome of primary sclerosing cholangitis: analysis of long term observation of 38 patients. *Arch. Intern. Med.,* **147,** 729–731

Lindor, K. D., Wiesner, R. H., Colwell, L. J., Steiner, B., Beaver, S. and La Russo, N. F. (1991) The combination of prednisone and colchicine in patients with primary sclerosing cholangitis. *Am. J. Gastroenterol.,* **85,** 57–61

Lo, S. K., Chapman, R. W. G., Chessman, P. *et al.* (1993) Anti-neutrophil antibody – A test for autoimmune primary sclerosing cholangitis in childhood. (in press)

Ludwig, J., MacCarty, R. L., La Russo, N. F. *et al.* (1986) Intrahepatic cholangiectases and large duct obliteration in primary sclerosing cholangitis. *Hepatology,* **6,** 560–568

MacCarty, R. L., La Russo, N. E. and Wiesner, R. H. (1983). Cholangiographic and pancreographic features of primary sclerosing cholangitis. *Radiology,* **149,** 39

Maggiore, G., De Giacomo, C. and Ugazio, A. G. (1988) Sclerosing cholangitis in childhood. *Gastroenterology,* **94,** 551

Margin, S., Nouri-Aria, K. T., Donaldson, P. T. *et al.* (1989) The relationship between HLA-DR3 and T-cell regulation of immunoglobulin production in primary sclerosing cholangitis. *Clin. Immunol. Immunopathol.,* **50,** 205–212

Marsh, J. W., Iwatsuki, S., Makowka, L. *et al.* (1988) Orthotopic liver transplantation for primary sclerosing cholangitis. *Ann. Surg.,* **207,** 21–25

Mieli-Vergani, G., Lobo-Yeo, A., Mcfarlane, B. M., Mcfarlane, I. G., Mowat, A. P. and Vergani, D. (1989) Different immune mechanisms leading to autoimmunity in primary sclerosing cholangitis and autoimmune chronic active hepatitis of childhood. *Hepatology,* **9,** 198–203

Mulberg, A. E., Arora, S., Grand, R. J. and Vinton, N. (1992) Expanding the spectrum of neonatal cholestatic liver disease. *Hepatology,* **16,** 192a

Nemeth, A., Ejderhamn, J., Glaumann, H. and Strandvik, B. (1990) Liver damage in juvenile inflammatory bowel disease. *Liver,* **10,** 239–248

Neveu, I., Labrune, P., Huguet, P., Musset, D., Chaussain, J. L., Odievre, M. (1990) Cholangite seclerosante revelatrice d'une histiocytose X. *Arch. Fr. Pediatr.,* **47,** 197–199

O'Brien, C. B., Senior, J. R., Arora-Mirchandani, R., Batta, A. K. and Salen, G. (1991) Ursodeoxycholic acid for the treatment of primary sclerosing cholangitis: a 30-month pilot study. *Hepatology,* **14,** 838–847

Olsson, R., Danielsson, A., Jarnerot, G. *et al.* (1991) Prevalence of primary sclerosing cholangitis in patients with ulcerative colitis. *Gastroenterology,* 1319–1323

Pirovino, M., Jeanneret, C., Lang, R. H., Luisier, J., Bianchi, L. and Spichtin, H. (1988) Liver cirrhosis in histiocytosis X. *Liver,* 293–298

Porayko, M. K., Wiesmer, R. H., La Russo, N. F. *et al.* (1990) Patients with asymptomatic primary sclerosing cholangitis frequently have progressive disease. *Gastroenterology,* **98,** 1594–1602

Prochazka, E. J., Terasaki, P. I., Park, M. S., Goldstein, L. I. and Busuttil, R. W. (1990) Association of primary sclerosing cholangitis with HLA-DRw52a. *New Engl. J. Med.,* **322,** 1842–1844

Rand, E. B. and Whitington, P.F. (1992) Successful orthotopic liver transplantation in two patients with liver failure due to sclerosing cholangitis with Langerhans Cell Histiocytosis. *J. Paediatr. Gastroenterol. Nutr.,* **15,** 202–207

Rosen, C. B., Nagorney, D. M., Wiesner, R. H., Coffey, R. J. and La Russo, N. F. (1991) Cholangiocarcinoma complicating primary sclerosing cholangitis. *Ann. Surg.,* **213,** 21–25

Sharp, H. L. and Freese, D. K. (1987) What is Primary Sclerosing Cholangitis? *J. Paediatr. Gastroenterol. Nutr.,* **6,** 161–163

Sherlock, S. (1991) Pathogenesis of sclerosing cholangitis: the role of nonimmune factors. *Sem. Liver Dis.,* **11,** 5–8

Sisto, A., Feldman, P., Garell, *et al.* (1987) Primary sclerosing cholangitis in children: a study of 5 cases and review of the literature. *Pediatrics,* **80,** 918–923

Spivatk, W., Grand, R. J. and Eraklis, A. (1982). A case of primary sclerosing cholangitis in childhood. *Gastronenterology,* **82,** 129

Stephen, T. C., Younoszai, M. K., Tyson, R. W., Groff, D. B. (1992) Fibrosing pancreatitis associated with pericholangitis and cholangitis in a child. *J. Paediatr. Gastroenterology Nutr,* **15,** 208–212

Toghil, P. J., Benton, P. and Smith, P. G. (1974). Chronic liver disease associated with childhood ulcerative colitis. *Postgrad. Med. J.,* **59,** 72

Werlin, S. L., Glicklich, M., Jona, J. and Starshak, R. J. (1980). Sclerosing cholangitis in childhood. *J. Pediatr.,* **96,** 544

Wiesner, R. H., Grambsch, P., La Russo, N. F. and Dixon, E. R. (1988) Is primary sclerosing cholangitis a progressive disease or not? *Hepatology,* **8,** 971–972

Chapter 13

Cirrhosis and its complications

Cirrhosis is the irreversible end stage of many forms of liver injury. The main pathophysiological effects are impaired hepatic function and portal hypertension. Cirrhosis may be complicated by the development of hepatocellular carcinoma.

Definition

Cirrhosis is defined pathologically as a diffuse process affecting the whole liver in which normal architecture is replaced by structurally abnormal nodules surrounded by prominent fibrous tissue. Accumulation of fibrous connective tissue within the portal tracts and in septa extending between portal tracts interferes with hepatic blood flow and contributes to the development of portal hypertension. This is aggravated by the development of anastomotic channels within large fibrous septa which shunt blood from the hepatic artery to portal vein branches. In addition, sinusoidal blood flow is impeded by perisinusoidal fibrosis. In large fibrous septa linking portal tracts and central veins, anastomotic channels developing between hepatic artery branches and hepatic vein tributaries carry blood which completely bypasses the sinusoids. Such circulatory disturbances compromise many aspects of liver function and may lead to liver cell death, thereby perpetuating accumulation of connective tissue; thus a vicious circle is established.

In regenerative nodules normal acinar structure is lost. Hepatocytes are in plates two, three or four cells thick, with irregularly placed or inconspicuous hepatic vein tributaries. The hepatocytes, even in a single nodule, often show considerable pleomorphism, some cells appearing normal, others having both cellular and nuclear enlargement. These changes may be due to a combination of the primary aetiology, vascular effects and changes in extracellular matrix components which interact with specific receptors on hepatocytes to influence their metabolism. The normal zonal distribution of enzymatic activity is changed. Although the diagnosis of cirrhosis implies an irreversible or even progressive pathological change it may still be compatible with normal growth and activity for many years.

Nodules without fibrosis, as in regenerative nodular hyperplasia, or fibrosis without nodule formation as in hepatoportal sclerosis are not cirrhosis.

Classification

Classification is based on morphology, the stage of development, aetiology, severity of hepatocellular necrosis and the clinical effects.

Pathological classification

Micronodular cirrhosis is characterized by nodules of approximately equal size, usually less than 3 mm but up to 1 cm in diameter, surrounded by fine bands of fibrous tissue of equal width. Very few hepatic veins and portal tracts are seen. In micro-micronodular cirrhosis fibrous tissue is increased in all parts of the acinus and isolates subacinar areas of parenchyma. Macronodular cirrhosis is characterized by nodules of various size up to 5 cm in diameter, many being multilobular. Broad, fibrous septa surround these nodules. The liver may be shrunken and deformed. In incomplete septal cirrhosis fine fibrous bands with little inflammation are clearly demarcated from large regeneration nodules. Some blind-ending fine fibrous bands occur.

In defining aetiology and planning management two other pathological forms are more helpful.

Biliary cirrhosis   In chronic bile duct obstruction increasing fibrosis develops within the portal tracts initially, then extends out into the parenchyma and finally links adjacent portal tracts. The hepatic parenchyma is relatively unchanged initially, and central (hepatic) veins persist in their normal position.

Hepatic venous outflow block   In this form of cirrhosis, caused by cardiac lesions and by the causes of Budd-Chiari syndrome, fibrosis extends from central veins to portal tracts. In both forms true regeneration nodules eventually, develop and gradually the distinguishing features may be obliterated.

All forms may be subdivided into *active* or *inactive cirrhosis* depending on the presence of biochemical or histological evidence of hepatocellular necrosis and inflammation. In *compensated* cirrhosis there are no clinical or laboratory features of hepatocellular failure, but these are present in the *decompensated* stage.

Changes on liver biopsy

In percutaneous needle liver biopsy specimens it is frequently difficult to demonstrate all the features described above, particularly if the specimen is taken from a large macronodule or if a fragmented specimen is obtained. In the absence of such changes the following suggest cirrhosis: (1) the liver feels hard; (2) the specimen is of unequal width or fragments in the needle or during processing, in spite of careful handling; (3) on histological examination there may be hyperplasia of hepatocytes with enlarged nuclei or cytoplasm; (4) the liver cell plates may be two to four cells thick; (5) areas of parenchyma without discernible hepatic veins or portal tracts may be seen bordered by an incomplete thin layer of connective tissue, best seen with a reticulin stain; (6) there may be fragments of fibrous tissue with an excessive number of bile ducts, attached to part of the biopsy; (7) a relative excess of hepatic vein branches suggests a macronodule.

Pathogenesis

The liver, like other tissues, responds to injury with a complex series of events involving inflammation, the release of cytokines, increased turnover of components of the extracellular matrix (ECM) and regeneration. Following severe hepatic injury due to infection, toxins such as paracetamol, or following hepatic resection the liver is capable of phenomenal regrowth with preservation of normal hepatic architecture. Why an apparently similar insult in one patient will be followed by return to functional and structural integrity, while in others it is followed by cirrhosis, is uncertain. The genotype of the patient, the nature of the noxious agent, its duration, intensity and frequency of exposure and the nature of the immune response appear to be critical. Together these initiate increased metabolism and accumulation of connective tissue components and ineffective hepatocellular regeneration.

Changes in extracellular matrix component metabolism

Transformation of Ito cells to myofibroblasts is an important development with major pathophysiological consequences. These sinusoidal cells, which in normal liver are devoted primarily to the storage and metabolism of retinoids, become activated during tissue injury. Paracrine mechanisms and autocrine loops transform them into myofibroblasts. Their metabolism increases causing them to develop fine tentacle-like projections, with contractile properties, which encircle the sinusoids. They become the main cell producing excessive amounts of collagens and other connective tissue components at sites of damage (Figure 13,1).

In cirrhosis there are increased amounts of all five genetically distinct types of *collagen* found in normal liver. Types I, III and VI are increased particularly in portal tracts and in fibrous septa while types IV and V increase especially along the sinusoids. The biosynthesis of collagens requires a number of specific, complex post-translational modifications. These include the hydroxylation of proline and lysine residues in nascent

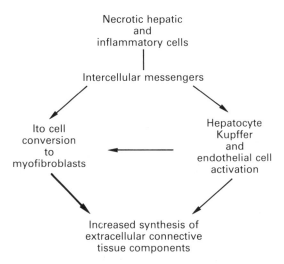

Figure 13.1 Fibrogenesis within the liver. Hepatocyte injury produced by infection, toxins or metabolic abnormalities causes reactions in the Kupffer cell and in migratory macrophages, T lymphocytes and neutrophils. These produce poorly characterized intercellular messengers such as fibroblast chemotactic factor, macrophage and lymphocyte fibroblast activating and growth factors which act on hepatocytes and endothelial cells causing them to produce connective tissue proteins. Perhaps of more importance is the action of these messengers on the fat-storing (Ito) cells in the space of Disse which are thought to proliferate as myofibroblasts and to be the main cell involved in increased fiobrogenesis

polypeptide protocollagen chains, glycosylation of hydroxylysine and formation of procollagen as a triple helix. These contain, in the case of the major fibre-forming collagens, peptide extensions which are removed extracellularly by specific peptidases. The collagen fibrils then become aligned and cross-linked by lysyl oxidase into high-tensile strength collagen fibres.

Collagen degradation is an equally complex process involving both intra- and extracellular steps. Intracellular degradation occurs in lysosomes, endoplasmic reticulin and the Golgi apparatus. Extracellular degradation involves several enzymes, particularly the neutral metalloproteinases. In cirrhosis, increases are seen in five of the six structural *glycoproteins* found in liver. Fibronectin, which attracts fibroblasts to the site of injury and assists in fibroblast adhesion, vitronectin, nidogen (entactin) and tenascin are diffusely increased. Laminin increases significantly around the sinusoids where a continuous basement membrane is formed (sinusoidal capillarization). In contrast, undulin (which is normally associated with mature collagen fibres) appears to be diminished and disrupted in irreversible fibrosis. All proteoglycans increase, but in disproportionate amounts resulting in a pattern which is markedly altered from normal. Factors from activated Kupffer cells stimulate the synthesis of hyaluronan by transformed lipocytes resulting in up to 10-fold increases in hepatic hyaluronan concentration.

Hepatocyte regeneration

From the infrequency of mitosis in human liver biopsies it has been estimated that the hepatocyte population is replaced no more than twice in adult life. Knowledge of factors controlling the regeneration of human hepatocytes is derived mainly from animal studies. There are three essential requirements for normal hepatocyte regeneration: an adequate supply of nutrients, energy and oxygen; extracellular matrix components present in appropriate concentration and the correct balance of circulating and locally active growth controlling factors.

Hepatotropic agents

A variety of factors with stimulatory, inhibitory or multifunctional effects on hepatocyte growth and differentiation have been identified and partially characterized. *In vitro* nanogram quantities of the following stimulate hepatocyte proliferation: epidermal growth factor (EGF), glucagon, insulin, insulin-like growth factors alpha and beta (IGF-α1, IGF-β) and somatostatin C. The first three of these are non-covalently bound to specific, saturable, high affinity receptors on the sinusoidal membrane. Binding activates complex biochemical mechanisms that promote cell growth and differentiation. A major effect is to activate membrane ion fluxes that promote active energy-dependent amino acid transport into the cell, stimulating messenger RNA and protein synthesis. There is increased cyclic AMP production which facilitates DNA replication. Kupffer cells produce hepatocyte-stimulating factors like interleukin 1 (IL-1) which induce production of alpha$_2$-macroglobulin and decrease albumin synthesis. Platelets store a hepatocyte growth factor and a heat-labile inhibitory factor.

Hepatocytes are also affected by multifunctional macromolecules such as interleukin 1, tumour necrosis factor and transforming growth factor beta (TGF-β). TGF-β opposes the effect of platelet-derived growth factor, EGF and IL-1 and down-regulates DNA synthesis and cell growth and, depending on the balance of other growth factors, can stimulate or inhibit cell proliferation and differentiation. Developmental factors also influence response to growth factors. For example, in cultured fetal hepatocytes glucagon and insulin stimulate synergistically alpha-fetoprotein production but have no affect on albumin synthesis. In the adult rat hepatocytes the converse is found. Although it is true that in general growth-stimulating factors suppress specialized hepatocyte function, this is not a universal finding.

Thus changes can be demonstrated in a whole array of adverse interacting factors affecting extracellular matrix components and hepatocyte regeneration. What the critical or rate limiting factors are is unclear. A situation is created so that, whatever the primary cause of liver damage, excessive connective tissue formation leads to hypoxic or nutritive damage to liver cells, causing more hepatocellular necrosis, inflammation and even more fibrosis and vascular changes.

Clinical features of cirrhosis

Compensated disease

The clinical features of cirrhosis are those of chronic hepatocellular failure and portal hypertension. In compensated cirrhosis there may be no symptoms. The principal features will a hard or nodular liver, with in some patients a small right lobe or splenomegaly. Commonly the liver is small and even impalpable. Hepatic dullness is reduced to a small area in the right anterolateral chest wall, above the costal margin. The liver is likely to be enlarged in biliary cirrhosis. There may be marked abdominal distension particularly if there is ascites. Inguinal and umbilical hernia may develop. Portal blood may be deviated via the paraumbilical veins to the umbilicus, and prominent collateral veins radiating from the umbilicus towards the systemic circulation may develop. Malnutrition with little subcutaneous fat and poor muscle bulk and growth failure may be present. There may be features of the underlying cause, e.g. haemolytic anaemia in Wilson's disease. Where jaundice has followed biliary disease pruritus, jaundice, xanthelasma, malabsorption and deficiency of fat-soluble vitamins (particularly vitamin D and X) may be prominent features.

Cutaneous features   Spider angiomata are frequently observed in the vascular territory of the superior vena cava. They contain a central arteriole from which radiates numerous fine vessels superficially resembling spiders' legs. They range in size from a pinhead up to 0.5 cm in diameter. Pressure on the centre of the lesion with a pin causes blanching of the whole lesion. They disappear if the blood pressure falls due to shock or haemorrhage.

Spiders occur also in normal persons, particularly children, and unless more than five are present these should not be taken as indicative of liver disease. The appearance of new spiders or the increasing size of older ones is suggestive of progressive liver damage. White spots which, when examined with a lens, show in the centre the beginnings of a spider, are also typical of cirrhosis. These are most prominent on the buttocks and arms. Palmar erythema, an exaggeration of the ordinary speckled mottling of the palm may be found on the hands or feet. There may be fine telangiectasia on the face and upper back. Clubbing of the fingers may be found, particularly in patients with biliary cirrhosis. White nails are a prominent feature of cirrhosis in adults but this is less frequently seen in children.

Circulatory changes

The main vascular abnormality associated with cirrhosis is portal hypertension. This is associated with the development of collateral vessels which bypass the liver and by a reduction in effective hepatic blood flow. Cirrhosis may also be associated with changes in systemic, visceral and pulmonary circulation. Underlying the first two, at least, is arteriolar vasodilatation causing a decrease in peripheral resistance. The blood volume is also elevated. A hyperkinetic circulatory state with increased cardiac output develops. The mechanisms causing these changes are not fully understood but changes in nitric oxide metabolism have recently been implicated (Moncada *et al.*, 1991). They are major factors in causing the complications discussed below.

Features indicating decompensation

The major signs of diminished hepatocellular function and decompensation are the development of ascites, peripheral oedema, hepatic encephalopathy or alimentary bleeding from portal hypertension. The appearance of jaundice in a patient with other than biliary cirrhosis is also indicative of very advanced disease. Spontaneous bruising and epitaxis, caused by both deficiency of platelets due to hypersplenism and by impaired hepatic production of clotting factors, are also a grave sign. In advanced disease, patients may develop septicaemia and/or peritonitis caused by both Gram-positive and Gram-negative bacteria. Fever may be inconspicuous and there may be little leucocytosis. It may be a terminal event. Cyanosis due to intrapulmonary shunting may occur in the absence of other features of decompensation.

Investigative findings

Laboratory investigations

Routine laboratory tests of liver function may be entirely normal. The albumins may be low and gamma-globulins increased due to a polyclonal increase in immunoglobulins. Serum complement component C3 may decrease, particularly late in the disease. Serum alkaline phosphatase and gamma-glutamyl transpeptidase are often elevated, particularly in biliary cirrhosis. In this form the total serum cholesterol may be elevated. In decompensated cirrhosis the cholesterol concentration falls. The prothrombin time is frequently prolonged. The serum transaminases may be increased, indicating active disease, but often to a value of only 50% above the upper limit of normal. In many instances transaminases will be normal.

Particularly in patients with marked splenomegaly the peripheral blood count will often show a modest decrease in the haemoglobin concentration with levels of 2–3 g below normal. Red cells are frequently normochromic and normocytic. The total white blood count is frequently decreased to a level of less than 5×10^9/litre and the platelet count, too, is frequently low, often with levels of less than 100×10^9/litre. In advanced disease the red blood cells show marked acanthocytosis (Burr cells).

A respiratory alkalosis may develop in cirrhosis. In addition, potassium depletion caused by hyperaldosteronism may also cause a metabolic alkalosis.

Imaging, endoscopic and radiological investigations

Ultrasonic scanning confirms the degree of hepatosplenomegaly. The liver may be nodular with increased echogenicity but similar findings may be caused by increased hepatic fat. Doppler studies may show flattening of the wave form in the hepatic vein, reduced blood flow velocity or even reversed blood flow in the portal vein and reduced diastolic flow in the hepatic artery (Figure 13.2).

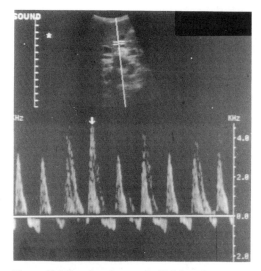

Figure 13.2 Doppler ultrasound of left hepatic artery showing reversed diastolic flow due to high vascular resistance in a cirrhotic liver

It also can show enlargement of the portal or splenic veins if there is significant portal hypertension. If there are associated gall-stones, dense echoes may be seen in the gallbladder.

Liver scintiscans following the intravenous injection of isotopes such as technetium-99m confirm liver and spleen size. The liver has a mottled isotope uptake with a reduced peak count rate which may be less than the uptake by the spleen. In advanced disease there is prominent uptake by bone marrow. This technique provides little additional information to that provided by skilled ultrasonography and is largely abandoned.

Endoscopy or a barium meal may show varices in the oesophagus, stomach or duodenum. If the varices are small they may only be visible using a double contrast technique. Laparoscopy, allowing the visualization of the upper and lower surfaces of the liver, has been found to be useful in confirming cirrhosis in adults. It is particularly valuable when there is a focal abnormality on ultrasound, in that the biopsy needle can be directed visually to the suspicious lesion. The investigation does cause considerable discomfort and can only be done in children under a general anaesthetic. It rarely needs to be performed.

Diagnosis

The diagnosis of cirrhosis is a two-step process: (a) confirming the presence of cirrhosis, and (b) determining its cause (Tables 13.1 – 13.3). The provisional diagnosis of cirrhosis may frequently be made on the basis of a history of liver damage and the physical findings, without recourse to any laboratory investigations. Typical biochemical and ultrasonic changes and the presence of varices provide valuable supporting evidence. Confirmation will ultimately rest with interpretation of the liver biopsy findings. This will also establish the type of cirrhosis, its severity and the degree of activity. It may help in determining the cause of the cirrhosis. There may be features of biliary disease or hepatic

Table 13.1 Causes of biliary cirrhosis

Extrahepatic biliary atresia
Intrahepatic biliary hypoplasia
Choledochal cyst
Cystic fibrosis
Progressive intrahepatic cholestasis
Bile duct stenosis or obstruction
Choledocholithiasis
Pancreatic fibrosis
Pancreatic tumours
Sclerosing cholangitis
Familial intrahepatic cholestasis
Ascending pyogenic cholangitis
Cholangitis due to *Fasciola, Clonorchis sinensis, Ascaris*, cytomegalovirus infection
Langerhans cell histiocytosis (histiocytosis X)

Table 13.2 Post-necrotic cirrhosis

Post-hepatic	Hepatitis in infancy
	Autoimmune chronic liver disease
	Viral hepatitis (viral hepatitis B ± Delta hepatitis, hepatitis C, non-A, non-B)
	Hepatitis due to drugs e.g. actinomycin D, methotrexate
	Toxins e.g. aflatoxin
	Radiation
Venous congestion	Constrictive pericarditis
	Ebstein's anomaly
	Budd–Chiari syndrome
	Congestive cardiac failure
	Venacaval webs
Veno-occlusive disease	
Indian childhood cirrhosis	
Ulcerative colitis	

Table 13.3 Genetic disorders associated with cirrhosis

Wilson's disease	Gaucher's disease
Galactosaemia	Wolman's disease
Fructosaemia	Defects in fatty acid oxidation
Glycogen storage disease Type IV	Abetalipoproteinaemia
Glycogen storage disease Type III	Sickle cell disease
Hurler's syndrome	Thalassaemia
Cystic fibrosis	Hepatic porphyria
Alpha-1 antitrypsin deficiency	Haemochromatosis, idiopathic and neonatal
Tyrosinosis	Haemochromatosis secondary to chronic haemolytic disease
Orthinine transcarbamylase deficiency	Zellweger's syndrome
Cystinosis	Byler's disease
Niemann–Pick disease Type C	Coprostanic acidaemia
Cholesterol ester storage disease	Shwachmann's syndrome
	Hereditary hypofibrinogemia

Table 13.4 Investigation of patients with suspected cirrhosis

All cases

Serum proteins including electrophoresis	Full blood count
Serum immunoglobulins	Serum urea or creatinin
Bilirubin	Electrolytes and bicarbonate
Aspartate aminotransaminase	Ultrasound scan of liver and kidney
Alkaline phosphatase	Blood gases
Cholesterol	Alpha-fetoprotein
Prothrombin time	Barium meal or endoscopy

Selected patients
Peripheral blood tests
Alpha-1 antitrypsin phenotype
Caeruloplasmin
Fasting blood sugar, pyruvate and lactate
Red cell glycogen content
Red blood cell galactose-1-phosphate uridyl transferase
Haemoglobin electrophoresis
Serum iron and total iron binding capacity
Serum amino acids
Serum cholesterol and lipoproteins
Serum bile acids
Hepatitis B surface antigen, antibody to hepatitis BsAg, antibody to hepatitis B core
Antibody to hepatitis C virus
Antibody to hepatitis A virus, AB virus, CMV toxoplasmosis
Serum immunoglobulins
Serum complement

Urine tests
24-hour copper excretion with penicillamine challenge
Porphyrins
Amino acids
Non-glucose reducing substances
Mucopolysaccharides
Fatty acid degradation products
Radiological investigations
Intravenous pyelogram
Endoscopic retrograde cholangiography
Percutaneous cholangiography
Inferior venacavagram
Hepatic venogram
CT scan of liver and biliary system

Miscellaneous
Sweat electrolytes
Technetium 99m methyl bromo IDA biliary excretion scan
Fibroblast culture for enzyme studies
Liver biopsy

venous outflow block or features specific for particular inherited or infective conditions.

Problems in interpretation arise more commonly from small samples rather than because of heterogeneous liver involvement. Both congenital hepatic fibrosis and areas of severe parenchymal collapse with prominent bile ducts in fibrous tissue can be interpreted as biliary cirrhosis. Before performing a biopsy, however, an attempt must be made to try to determine which of the many causes of liver damage may have been responsible, so that the liver tissue may be subjected to appropriate histological and biochemical analysis to determine the cause. This is particularly important in those genetic disorders such as fructosaemia, in which liver biopsy is the only means by which a definite diagnosis may be established (Tables 13.4).

Diagnostic difficulties

Many disorders causing portal hypertension or liver dysfunction need to be considered. The following seem to cause most diagnostic difficulties. In congenital hepatic fibrosis the liver is usually enlarged and hard, but liver function tests are normal, although occasionally the alkaline phosphatase may be raised. Ultrasonography or pyelography showing the typical renal anomaly provides a clue to the diagnosis.

Hepatoportal sclerosis and regenerative nodular hyperplasia can also cause difficulties. Difficulty may occur with constrictive pericarditis if abdominal manifestations greatly exceed the cardiac features, particularly if the raised jugular venous pressure is overlooked or absent. Infiltrative disorders such as reticulosis may also cause difficulties. The peripheral blood count may not be diagnostic and may be complicated by portal hypertension. In portal hypertension due to portal vein obstruction the liver is small, liver function tests are normal, but typically there is a prolongation of the prothrombin time by 4 or 5 seconds. There may be portal fibrosis on liver biopsy. Ultrasonographic demonstration of a normal sized portal vein and of good blood flow by Doppler techniques excludes this diagnosis.

Aetiological diagnosis

In many instances the cause of the liver damage will be evident on the basis of the history and examination findings. This is particularly so with biliary type cirrhosis, but there are exceptions. In some patients with ulcerative colitis liver damage may be severe although gastrointestinal symptoms are mild. Rarely, cirrhosis may be a presenting feature in cystic fibrosis. Patients with both choledochal cyst and tumours of the biliary tree may present with few of the classic features and have advanced liver disease when first coming to medical attention.

In considering the genetic disorders, principal consideration must be given to those conditions in which treatment if started early is effective, for example, Wilson's disease, galactosaemia, fructosaemia, glycogen storage disease and tyrosinaemia. Although therapy will not reverse cirrhosis it may have a significant ameliorating effect at least for a time. In other genetic disorders, for example, thalassaemia, precise assessment may have therapeutic implications, such as the administration of desferrioxamine. Unfortunately for many genetic disorders such as alpha-1 antitrypsin deficiency, precise diagnosis is important only in that it allows appropriate genetic advice to be given and as a guide to prognosis.

In post-necrotic cirrhosis reversal of the features is of course impossible. Where it is due to autoimmune chronic liver disease considerable symptomatic improvement may occur if the disease process is controlled by immunosuppressants. Similarly, if liver damage is caused by drugs (see Chapter 10), symptomatic improvement may follow their withdrawal.

Management

Having made a histological diagnosis of cirrhosis and confirmed the aetiology, the aim of management is to minimize further liver damage by treating the cause of liver disease, if

Table 13.5 Complications of cirrhosis

Portal hypertension
Ascites
Hepatic encephalopathy
Hyperdynamic circulation
Endocrine changes
Impaired hepatic metabolism of drugs and hormones
Bleeding diathesis
Increased susceptibility to infection
Spontaneous bacterial peritonitis
Hypoxaemia
Impaired fat absorption
Malnutrition
Growth failure
Hepatoma
Renal failure
Gall stone formation
Impaired fat absorption
Malignant hepatoma
Renal failure

this is possible, and to prevent or control the complications (Table 13.5). If complications are difficult to control, there is growth failure or a poor quality of life, liver transplantation should be performed.

Nutritional management

The aim should be to provide sufficient calories, protein, essential fatty acids, minerals, trace elements and vitamins for growth and normal activities. This may be difficult if the patient is restricted in fluid or salt intake. In addition, a degree of fat malabsorption is almost invariable. Anorexia is frequently a problem. Overnight nasogastric feeding may be invaluable in supplying a calorie requirement which seems to be as much as 50% above normal in children awaiting transplantation after failed surgery for biliary atresia. Rarely in these circumstances intravenous feeding is required.

Vitamin supplements containing both water-soluble and fat-soluble vitamins should be taken daily. Deficiency of fat-soluble vitamins A, D, K and E will develop unless oral vitamin supplements are given in a dose of at least twice normal. If steatorrhoea is marked it will be necessary to give vitamin K 5 mg intramuscularly weekly. A vitamin D dose of 10 000 units intramuscularly at monthly intervals may be sufficient to prevent the development of rickets, but this must be controlled by regular clinical assessment, radiographs of the wrist and by measuring the serum phosphate, calcium and alkaline phosphatase. Vitamin E deficiency should be monitored by regular determination of the vitamin E/total lipid ratio. If it is low increased oral vitamin E supplements may suffice, but patients with severe cholestasis will require parenteral vitamin supplements

The calorie intake may be increased with glucose polymers (e.g. Maxijul, Caloreen). In an effort to decrease steatorrhoea and to improve nutrition medium-chain triglycerides should be given since these can be absorbed without bile salts. These may aggravate hepatic encephalopathy the dietary management of which is discussed below. Pancreatic supplements may reduce steatorrhoea. If the serum cholesterol is high or xanthelasma develops, a low cholesterol diet is advisable. Cholestyramine in a dose of 4–8 g given three times daily with meals helps to prevent and control this complication. It is important, however, to ascertain that essential fatty acid intake is adequate. Cholestyramine is also helpful in controlling pruritus in biliary cirrhosis. It has also been claimed that it may improve liver function in patients with post-necrotic cirrhosis. It does, however, aggravate steatorrhoea and may cause deficiency of trace elements. Other drugs which may cause nutritional difficulties are penicillamine which may lead to zinc, copper and pyridoxine deficiency and diuretics which increase the urinary excretion of metals. There is no evidence that the avoidance of or adherence to any particular type of food has any influence on the progression of established cirrhosis.

Portal hypertension

Portal hypertension causes splenomegaly, alimentary bleeding and contributes to ascites. Splenomegaly and hypersplenism rarely require intervention. Major problems are bleeding from oesophageal varices (see p. 387) and ascites, considered in detail below.

Ascites and oedema

Ascites may develop insidiously or be precipitated by acute events such as alimentary bleeding, intra-abdominal surgery, anaesthesia or the development of hepatoma. It may be associated with peripheral oedema, pleural effusions and basal atelectasis. Hernias may develop. Other complications are listed in Table 13.5.

Pathophysiology of ascites formation

Mechanisms leading to the formation of ascites and oedema in chronic liver disease are complex and imperfectly understood. Nevertheless, a knowledge of established pathophysiological changes is essential to optimize treatment. A necessary requirement is portal hypertension. Arteriolar vasodilatation, particularly splanchnic, causing arteriolar hypotension, is thought to be the second major underlying factor. Together they lead to two distinct but interrelated processes: (a) a redistribution of fluid within the body, and (b) an increase in the sodium and water content of the body. Hypoalbuminaemia may also contribute.

Fluid redistribution

The exchange of fluid between capillaries and tissue spaces including the peritoneal cavity is dependent on the hydrostatic and osmotic pressures inside and outside the blood vessels. Two factors in liver disease favour the development of ascites: (a) hypertension in the hepatic sinusoids, and (b) hypertension in the portal venous system. Both may be aggravated by increased splanchnic blood flow associated with arteriolar hypotension.

Where hepatic vein obstruction occurs, for example, in the Budd-Chiari syndrome, there is a marked increase in sinusoidal pressure. Ascites is severe and often intractable. In advanced cirrhosis the sinusoidal pressure is increased to a variable but lesser extent. Excessive fluid with a high protein content exudes into the perisinusoidal spaces to be taken up by the hepatic lymphatics. In cirrhosis dilated lymphatic channels which drain to the portahepatis carry much lymph to the thoracic duct. When the carrying capacity of the lymphatic system is saturated, extravascular fluid with a very high protein content weeps from the liver surface. This small spillover of hepatic lymph is believed to be an important factor in causing ascites. Ascitic fluid rarely has a protein content as high as that found in the thoracic duct, presumably because of dilution by fluid from the serosal surface of the gut. This also arises only when the production of tissue fluid in the intestine exceeds the capacity of the lymphatics to transport it. If hypertension is limited to the extrahepatic portal system, ascites is likely to be minimal unless the albumin concentration drops.

Increased sodium and water retention

Renal excretion of sodium and water is less than that ingested. The factors leading to increased fluid and salt retention are complex. Splanchnic arteriolar vasodilatation produces underfilling of the vascular compartment. This invokes baroreceptor-mediated stimulation of three endogenous vasoconstrictive systems. In patients with ascites increased plasma renin and aldosterone are found with highest levels in those with marked sodium retention. Plasma noradrenaline is also increased reflecting increased sympathetic activity. Both promote increased sodium reabsorption by renal tubules. Antidiuretic hormone increases water reabsorption in the distal tubule by its action on V-2 (vasopressin-2) receptors. Its concentration is increased in cirrhotics with ascites, contributing to the maintenance of arterial pressure. These changes which are an upregulation of mechanisms functioning in compensated cirrhosis cause increased blood volume, hyperdynamic circulation and a high cardiac index. When ascites develops activation is greater. Renal blood flow and glomerular filtration are maintained at normal or only slightly reduced rates by vasodilatory prostaglandins E_2 and I_2 until functional renal failure develops. Increased production and increased plasma levels of atrial natriuretic hormone have been reported in cirrhosis. Plasma activity of a poorly characterized natriuretic hormone also appears to be increased. These are evidently ineffective in the face of the above changes.

There seems to be considerable evidence of redistribution of blood flow within the renal substance. Blood flow to the outer cortex where most of the functioning glomeruli are to be found is reduced. There is increased blood flow to the juxtamedullary nephrons which have increased capacity for sodium reabsorption. The mechanisms leading to this redistribution of blood flow within the kidney are not fully understood.

Hypoalbuminaemia   Hypoalbuminaemia, due to reduced albumin synthesis in the liver, lowers the intercapillary colloid osmotic force allowing the transfer of fluid into the tissue spaces causing oedema in dependent parts and contributing to ascites. This effect in itself is probably of minor importance compared with the effect of the high hydrostatic pressure in the hepatic sinusoids and the portal venous system.

Treatment

Mild ascites causing no discomfort or difficulties with mobility or breathing requires no treatment unless the patient has had an episode of spontaneous peritonitis. As in all branches of medicine, it is essential to remember the vow: *primum non nocere* (first do no harm), particularly since treatment will not influence the underlying disease process. If treatment is necessary, avoiding excessive salt and fluid intake and judicious use of spironolactone are effective in most circumstances. If these fail liver transplantation must be considered. Careful monitoring of weight, blood pressure, urinary output and concentration of serum and urinary electrolytes and creatinine is essential. It is important to try to reduce weight slowly at a rate less than 1% per day unless paracentesis is performed.

Sodium restriction   In adults, sodium and water restriction are the keystone of treatment. In children a very low sodium diet is rarely tolerable, particularly if the child is already anorexic. It is rarely possible to reduce intake to less than 1 mmol/kg per day. Similarly water restriction to less than normal intake is unnecessary unless there is hyponatraemia or spironolactone resistance. The volume of water may be restricted to 70–80% of normal in these circumstances.

Diuretics   Currently available diuretics have revolutionized management. The diuretic of choice is the aldosterone antagonist spironolactone, having the advantage of causing potassium retention which is very desirable in cirrhotic patients, who are usually potassium depleted. Hyperkalaemia may occur if renal failure develops. Its disadvantage is that it has no effect for 2 to 4 days after starting treatment. Different patients have different degrees of hyperaldosteronism, so a flexible dosage regimen is required. Doses required in cirrhotic patients are considerably greater than in other disorders causing fluid retention.

The following are appropriate initial doses:

Age 1–3 years	12.5 mg four times a day
Age 4–7 years	25 mg four times a day
Age 8–11 years	27.5 mg four times a day
Age 12 years and older	50 mg four times a day

If there is no weight loss after 4 days the dose should be doubled. If diuresis still does not occur and sodium excretion in the urine is still low, the dose may be increased by a further 50% and in most instances diuresis will occur. The most serious side-effect of spironolactone therapy is hyponatraemia. This may be complicated by hepatic encephalopathy or renal failure. Occasionally a metabolic acidosis may develop. These complications and hyperkalaemia are indication for stopping spironolactone.

If spironolactone alone does not control ascites, a kaliuretic diuretic in small doses may be added to the regimen. These diuretics act on the proximal tubules. Thiazide derivatives, frusemide and ethacrynic acid are most commonly used. Their toxicity is largely due to the excessive urinary losses of potassium and chloride which they cause. This is closely related to the diuretic potency. Frusemide and ethacrynic acid have a greater effect on pH and also appear to increase ammonia production, and for that reason their use is more frequently complicated by hepatic encephalopathy.

Chlorothiazide in a dose of 25% of the recommended dose when used alone, should be given initially. This will often produce a very satisfactory diuresis. Some patients will be refractory to this dosage regimen and it must be increased slowly. It is important to assess the intracellular potassium state by means of an ECG. Muscle cramps sometimes relieved by magnesium or quinine may be major problems.

Refractory ascites

Albumin infusions   Salt-free albumin 0.5 g/kg infused over a 4–6 hour period with simultaneous frusemide, may sufficiently modify the intravascular volume to allow good urinary output and subsequent control of ascites by dietary and diuretic measures.

Paracentesis   A series of controlled trials in large numbers of adult patients, without renal failure and with prothrombin activity greater than 40% of normal, have demonstrated the relative safety of paracentesis in the management of ascites. It must be done with strict aseptic techniques as for a surgical procedure. Over a 20–90-minute period ascites is drained completely with a doctor in constant attendance. At the end of the procedure plasma expanders in the form of albumin 6–8 g/l of ascites or 125 ml of 5% Haemaccel/litre are given over a 4–6 hour period. The procedures were as effective and as free from complications as diuretic therapy.

Two further techniques frequently used in adults may be considered for very refractory ascites although their use has not been reported in children.

Paracentesis with reinfusions   In adults, an automated ultrafiltration apparatus has been used to concentrate ascitic fluid to give a protein concentration two or three times as much as in ascitic fluid. This is then reinfused intravenously. Urinary output increases and the patient becomes more responsive to diuretic drugs. Careful monitoring of the central venous pressure is necessary to detect overload which carries a risk of congestive heart failure and bleeding from oesophageal varices. Transient pyrexia, pulmonary oedema and intraperitoneal haemorrhage have also been reported.

Peritoneal-venous shunts (Le Veen Shunt)   A long perforated plastic tube within the peritoneal cavity drains to a special pressure sensitive valve lying extraperitoneally. The valve is connected to a further tube which is passed subcutaneously into the internal jugular vein. Its end lies in the superior vena cava. For a few patients the technique undoubtedly controls ascites for a long period. There are many complications however, and in patients with Child grade III cirrhosis the mortality of this procedure is prohibitive. For patients with less severe cirrhosis, traditional measures should suffice.

Renal failure

Oliguric renal failure without structural abnormalities in the kidney (functional renal failure) is frequently a terminal event in advanced cirrhosis. It presents in two forms. There may be a rapid increase in creatinine to very high levels over the course of a few days usually associated with a deterioration of liver function. Oliguria, dilutional hyponatraemia and a low urinary sodium concentration (less than 10 mmol/litre) and hyperkalaemia. The urine to plasma osmolality ratio is between 1.1 and 1.15. There is no proteinuria. It may be impossible to distinguish this from acute tubular necrosis. In other patients there is a slow development of azotaemia with a marked reduction of glomerular filtration rate. Note that a small further rise in creatinine indicates a large deterioration in renal function.

The cause of functional renal failure is not understood. There is substantial reduction in glomerular infiltration rate and of effective renal plasma flow. There may be increased urinary concentrations of the arachidonic acid vasoconstrictive metabolite thromboxane, while the vasodilatory metabolite prostaglandin E_2, concentration in the urine is decreased. Renal kallikrein synthesis may be impaired. Endotoxaemia may have a role. Functional renal failure is reversed by liver transplantation. Kidneys from patients with functional renal failure function well when transplanted to patients with chronic renal failure.

Functional renal failure may be aggravated by the development of ascites, over enthusiastic diuretic treatment, paracentesis or by gastrointestinal haemorrhage. There is no effective treatment except liver transplantation. The condition must be distinguished from other causes of renal failure in the cirrhotic patient such as plasma volume depletion with hypotension, electrolyte depletion secondary to diuretic therapy and potentially nephrotoxic antibiotics such as neomycin or aminoglycosides and non-steroidal anti-inflammatory drugs such as indomethacin. Septicaemia should be excluded. It may be distinguished from acute tubular necrosis by serial measurements of the urinary sodium and osmolality in both urine and plasma. In acute tubular necrosis the ratio is less than 1.1. Mannitol, frusemide, hypertonic saline and renal dialysis do not improve survival in renal failure complicating end-stage cirrhosis and may hasten death. Renal failure may occasionally be due to a progressive glomerulonephritis with haematuria, and proteinuria associated with glomerular IgA and complement deposition. Such deposits are not unusual in cirrhotic patients without renal impairment presumably representing gut-derived IgA and dietary antigens which have escaped capture by the hepatic and pulmonary reticuloendothelial systems.

Hepatic encephalopathy

Chronic hepatic encephalopathy is a complex neuropsychiatric syndrome, the features of which are aggravated by an increased protein intake and alleviated by a reduced protein intake. It occurs classically in cirrhosis with portosystemic shunting but it may occur following shunting for extrahepatic portal hypertension. Chronic hepatic encephalopathy is less commonly recognized in children than in adults. The advent of portoenterostomy for biliary atresia and liver transplantation for end-stage liver disease in infancy and childhood has stimulated studies of neurodevelopmental problems associated with liver disorders which previously caused death in early childhood. Studies of children requiring liver transplantation identified low IQ in nine of 21 in whom the liver disease had started in the first year of life compared with two of 15 with liver disease of later onset. Following liver transplant these children had difficulty with abstract thinking, logical analysis and flexibility of thought and memory (Stewart *et al.*, 1991). Although malnutrition from early infancy may have been a factor these problems could represent a form of hepatic encephalopathy.

Clinical features

Chronic hepatic encephalopathy causes intellectual impairment, personality change and clouding of consciousness which may progress to stupor and coma. The speech may be slurred and sleep pattern may be disturbed. Writing deteriorates and there is apraxia. The most characteristic neurological abnormality is the so-called 'flapping tremor'. This is elicited by asking the patient to attempt maximum dorsiflexion of the wrist with the arms extended. A rapid flexion–extension movement at the metacarpal phalangeal and wrist joint occurs every 1 or 2 seconds, sometimes accompanied by lateral movement of the digits. It is caused by a brief loss of neuromuscular conductivity to the extensors of the wrist. Tendon reflexes are increased early but later become reduced. There may be various neurological signs indicating organic cerebral disease. A particularly typical feature is the marked variability of severity in response to changes in the protein load. The behavioural changes commonly seen in children with end-stage liver disease, such as tiredness, irritability, listless and general disinterest in normal activities may be as much due to encephalopathy as to systemic weakness.

Pathogenesis

The brain in chronic hepatic encephalopathy may show no histological abnormality. There may be an increase in the number of protoplasmic astrocytes and, in the cerebral cortex, cerebellum and basal ganglia, rarely, neural degeneration and demyelination. It is therefore thought that the neural dysfunction is largely secondary to metabolic changes. The exact nature of these metabolic changes is not completely understood. Clinical observations and studies in experimental models emphasize the importance of nitrogenous products – particularly ammonia – derived from gut and its contents. Cerebral intoxication occurs when such substances are not metabolized by the liver. These speculative toxins are thought to be produced by bacterial action in the bowel since symptoms can often be relieved by oral, broad spectrum, non-absorbed antibiotics such as neomycin. As well as ammonia, methionine and some of its derivatives such as methylmercaptan have been implicated. Changes in intracellular metabolism due to the hypokalaemic alkalosis, so often present in cirrhosis, may also contribute. Other possible contributing factors are considered in Chapter 7.

Aggravating factors

Gastrointestinal haemorrhage aggravates in two ways; it puts more protein into the bowel which increases ammonia production while the hypovolaemia may compromise both hepatic and renal function. In infection, increased tissue metabolism leads to an increased endogenous nitrogen load and hence increases ammonia production while endotoxaemia aggravates liver dysfunction. It may also lead to dehydration. The development of hepatocellular carcinoma may be associated with encephalopathy. In portosystemic shunts it appears that the risk of encephalopathy increases with the severity of hepatocellular damage and diminution in portal blood flow.

Laboratory assessment of chronic hepatic encephalopathy

No single laboratory test is specific for encephalopathy. No biochemical test such as blood ammonia levels or the ratio of concentrations of branch chain amino acids to aromatic amino acids correlates with the grade of encephalopathy (Davies *et al.*, 1990). A good correlation has been reported between the cerebrospinal fluid concentration of glutamine and alpha-ketoglutarate. Although changes in EEGs, visual evoked responses and components of the auditory evoked responses provide objective evidence of brain dysfunction the changes are non-specific, and do not always correlate with the severity of the encephalopathy. In adults slow waves at 5–6 cycles/s are a prominent feature. Unfortunately they may occur in normal children (Yen and Liaw, 1990). Serial studies may be of value. In adults abnormal brain stem auditory evoked potentials are the most sensitive parameters for the detection of HE (Mehndiratta *et al.*, 1990). Although these EEG responses may be abnormal in latent encephalopathy psychometric testing will also be abnormal. Only if the abnormality varies with the protein intake can one conclude that changes are definitely due to hepatic encephalopathy.

Treatment

The basis of treatment is to improve liver function by treatment specific to the cause of liver damage and to remove or correct identifiable precipitating factors. If liver damage is irreversible or there is no specific treatment early consideration of liver transplantation is mandatory. It is important to prevent the accumulation of ammonia and other gut-derived nitrogenous products. There are two main methods of reducing ammonia production by the gut: (a) protein restriction; and (b) reducing bacterial flora in the gut. Protein restriction is of value possibly by reducing the total body urea pool. It may also be beneficial in that it reduces the production of urea and other potential toxic nitrogenous metabolites within the gut (Mullen and Weber, 1991). Lactulose, a non-absorbable synthetic disaccharide (4-*O*-β-D-galactopyranosyl-D-fructose) produces an osmotic fermentative diarrhoea with lactic and acetic acid production which causes a drop in pH in the colon and hence a reduction in ammonia reabsorption (Mortensen *et al.*, 1990).

Table 13.6 Precipitating causes of hepatic encephalopathy

Gastrointestinal haemorrhage
Potassium depletion
Systemic infection
High protein diet
Medium chain triglycerides
Hypoglycaemia
Diuretics
Acid-base disturbances
Hyponatraemia
Constipation
Sedatives
Renal failure
Development of hepatocellular carcinoma
Pancreatitis

Broad spectrum antibiotics act by reducing the amount of bacterial urease available by partial sterilization of the bowel. Neomycin is the antibiotic most commonly used with vancomycin for resistant cases (Tarao *et al.*, 1990). Both are potentially toxic and best avoided. Dietary supplements with medium-chain triglycerides may aggravate hepatic encephalopathy by increasing short-chain fatty acid concentration (Table 13.6). Double blind randomized studies of branched-chain amino acids for chronic hepatic encephalopathy in adults with cirrhosis give conflicting results (Dioguardi *et al.*, 1990; Marchesini *et al.*, 1990; Vilstrup *et al.*, 1990). There are no reported studies in children. Zinc repletion is advised (Mullen and Weber, 1991). Hypokalaemia, particularly if associated with alkalosis, must be corrected. It causes increased ammonia concentration by its effect on the kidney. Not only is ammonia formation by the kidney increased, but ammonia excretion is also decreased. All sedatives are potentially dangerous and best avoided. In unexplained coma, latent infections such as urinary tract infection, septicaemia or peritonitis must be excluded.

Acute hepatic encephalopathy with cerebral oedema is an increasingly identified complication of acute hepatic necrosis in patients with biliary atresia (Gartner et al., 1987).

Pulmonary complications

Although a range of restrictive and obstructive pulmonary abnormalities are well described in adults with cirrhosis the only abnormalities shown in children are low lung volumes (Greenough *et al.*, 1988). Some children with alpha-1 antitrypsin deficiency have high functional residual capacity (Hird *et al.*, 1991). Variceal sclerotherapy may have a deleterious effect on lung function.

Hepatopulmonary syndrome

Hypoxaemia with reduced arterial oxygen saturation is a relatively common complication of cirrhosis and other forms of chronic liver disease. It may be so severe as to cause cyanosis. Hypoxia (oxygen saturations 76–95%) was present in 20 (four with cyanosis) of 48 children with cirrhosis (McGuire *et al.*, 1993). The frequency was unrelated to the type of liver disorder, severity of liver damage, presence of cutaneous vascular lesions or portal hypertension. Intrapulmonary shunting was detected by ventilation/perfusion scans using technetium-99m macroaggregated albumin shunt studies (Figure 13.3) in 14 of 20 with hypoxia and in eight without, seven in each group had forced expiratory volume in 1 second (FEV_1) < 80% predicted, while eight hypoxic and four non-hypoxic had forced ventilatory capacity (FVC) <80% predicted. Our results demonstrate a high frequency (36%) of unsuspected hypoxia in children with cirrhosis and refute previous suggestions that hypoxia is caused only by intrapulmonary shunts. True arteriovenous shunts can rarely be demonstrated anatomically but precapillary arterioles and lung capillaries are dilated. There may be ventilation/perfusion mismatch and a reduction in diffusion capacity. The hypoxia may be reduced by breathing 100% oxygen.

A further cause of hypoxia may be portopulmonary venous anastomoses connecting paraoesophageal portosystemic collaterals with the pulmonary venous system. The degree of intrapulmonary change does not correlate with the severity of the liver damage. The mechanisms are unknown. Raised serum ferritin levels and vasoactive intestinal peptides bypassing the liver have been suggested as possible causes. The degree of cyanosis may be proportionally greater than the hypoxaemia due to the presence of systemic arteriovenous shunts and peripheral vasodilatation.

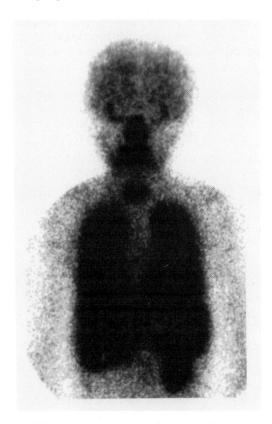

Figure 13.3 Following the intravenous injection of 50 mbq of technetium-99m macro-aggregated albumin, 46% of the dose bypassed the lungs and was trapped in the brain, thyroid and kidneys. The patient was cyanosed due to massive intrapulmonary shunting associated with cirrhosis secondary to chronic Budd-Chiari syndrome

Clinical features   Such patients present with breathlessness on effort but it may be noted at rest. Typically dyspnoea and hypoxia are most marked when upright and relieved by lying down (orthodeoxia), the converse of most cardiorespiratory causes of dyspnoea. It may aggravate hepatic encephalopathy. Postoperative hypoxaemia may markedly limit the patient's tolerance of anaesthesia, operative procedures and particularly liver transplantation. Although liver transplantation reverses many of the systemic and pulmonary vascular changes associated with cirrhosis, it does not reverse in the first year all pulmonary abnormalities.

Pulmonary hypertension   This is an uncommon complication of cirrhosis and occurs even more rarely in extrahepatic portal vein obstruction, in the absence of intrinsic liver disease. The basis for the association has not been defined. Pulmonary thromboemboli originating in the portal venous system or its collateral channels may reach the lungs via spontaneous or surgically created portosystemic anastomosis. There may also be a failure of metabolic degradation of toxic vasoactive substances, such as powerful vasoactive peptides, normally secreted by endothelial cells, i.e. endothelin and prostaglandin F2, arising in the splanchnic circulation. These may cause plexogenic pulmonary hypertension. The disorder may be overlooked clinically until cyanosis develops. Systematic screening for hypoxia, signs of right ventricular hypertrophy or accentuation of perihilar arteries on chest radiographs may allow its detection at a time which would allow liver and lung transplantation.

Pneumonia and effusions   Right-sided pleural effusions with or without ascites may develop if there are diaphragmatic defects. The above complications and the patient's decreased resistance to infection causes an increased incidence of lower respiratory tract infection.

Anaemia

A refractory, normocytic anaemia commonly develops in cirrhosis. There may be many contributory factors. There may be iron deficiency secondary to blood loss from oesophageal varices, poor iron absorption and low transferrin levels. Thrombocytopenia and deficiency of other clotting factors may aggravate blood loss. Other factors causing low haemoglobin concentrations include shortened red cell survival due to splenomegaly or haemolysis. Rarely, the haemolysis may be associated with a positive Coomb's test. In biliary cirrhosis, vitamin E deficiency may be a factor. Erythropoietic activity in the bone marrow may be decreased. This is commonly attributed to hypersplenism but the mechanism is not understood. Finally, the blood volume may be increased giving a low haemoglobin concentration although the total red blood cell mass is not decreased.

Treatment

Most of the above factors cannot be modified by therapy. If the serum iron is low and the total iron binding capacity elevated, oral iron will be helpful, but often the total iron binding capacity is within normal range and iron therapy is not beneficial. Vitamin E may help in biliary cirrhosis. Steroids should be considered in haemolytic anaemia if the anaemia is contributing to symptoms. Portocaval anastomosis without splenectomy rarely increases the haemoglobin concentration but if the spleen is removed and the bleeding stops the haemoglobin is likely to rise. It is rarely necessary to remove the spleen in a patient with cirrhosis because of hypersplenism.

Bacterial infections

The incidence of urinary and respiratory tract infections and bacteraemia is increased in cirrhosis. As well as impaired function of Kupffer cells, due to shunting or intrinsic changes, a generalized reduction in efficiency of bactericidal and opsonic mechanisms, complement deficiency, alterations in intestinal flora and in mucosal barriers may all contribute to pathogenesis. Iatrogenic factors, particularly surgical, also predispose. Pneumococcal and haemophilis influenza vaccination should be performed.

Spontaneous bacterial peritonitis

This potentially lethal complication occurs in patients in whom cirrhosis is complicated by ascites. Characteristically the patient develops increasing abdominal distension, fever, abdominal pain with vomiting or diarrhoea and often features of hepatic encephalopathy. Bowel sounds are absent or reduced and there is rebound tenderness. Occasionally spontaneous bacterial peritonitis may be asymptomatic, bowel sounds may be present and no rebound tenderness found or the pain may be localized. The diagnosis is established by a diagnostic ascitic tap which reveals cloudy, ascitic fluid with a white cell count of more than 500×10^6/litre. Cells are predominantly polymorphonuclear neutrophil leucocytes. The protein concentration is frequently low, less than 20 g/litre. The causative organism can be recovered from the ascitic fluid and often from blood cultures. In adult series, enteric bacteria account for approximately 60% of cases but in children *Streptococcus pneumoniae* predominated (Larcher *et al.*, 1985).

The disorder carries a high mortality. Early diagnosis and the institution of an antibiotic regimen effective against pneumococci, as well as Gram-negative organisms, may reduce the mortality. A third generation cephalosporin should be used initially, pending the results of bacteriological studies. When infection is controlled liver transplantation should be considered. Intestinal decontaminating regimens or norfloxacin in controlled studies have reduced the incidence of infections due to enteric organisms after gastrointestinal bleeding. Prophylactic flucloxacillin and co-trimoxazole may also be used.

Other complications include delayed sexual maturation and a higher prevalence of hyperglycaemia, peptic ulceration, gallstones and hepatocellular carcinoma.

Bibliography and references

Arroyo, V., Gines, P., Jimenez, W. and Rodes, J. (1991) Ascites, renal failure, and electrolyte disorders in cirrhosis. Pathogenesis, diagnosis and treatment. In: *Oxford Textbook of Clinical Hepatology* (eds. N. McIntyre, J. P. Benhamou, J. Bircher, M. Rizzetto, J. Rodes). Oxford University Press, Oxford, pp.427–470

Assadi, F. K., Gordon. T., Kacskes, S. E. and John. E. (1985). Treatment of refractory ascites by ultrafiltration reinfusion of ascitic fluid peritoneally. *J. Pediatr.*, **106**, 443

Barnes, P. F., Arevalo, C., Chan, L. S., Wong, S. F. and Reynolds, T. B. (1988) A prospective evaluation of bacteraemic patients with chronic liver disease. *Hepatology*, **8**, 612–616

Charlton, C. P. J., Buchanan, E., Holden, C. E. *et al.* (1992) Intensive enteral feeding in advanced cirrhosis: reversal of malnutrition without precipitation of hepatic encephalopathy. *Arch. Dis. Childh.*, **67**, 603–607

Cohen, M. D., Rubin, L. J., Taylor, W. E. and Cuthbert, J. A. (1983) Primary pulmonary hypertension: An unusual case associated with extrahepatic portal hypertension. *Hepatology*, **3**, 588

Davies, M. G., Rowan, M. J., MacMathuna, P., Keeling, P. W., Weir, D. G. and Feely, J. (1990) The auditory P300 event-related potential: an objective marker of the encephalopathy of chronic liver disease. *Hepatology*, **12** (4 Pt 1), 688–694

Dioguardi, F. S., Brigatti, M., Dell'Oca, M., Ferrario, E. and Abbiati, R. A. D. (1990) Effects of chronic oral branched-chain amino acid supplementation in a subpopulation of cirrhotics. *Clin. Physiol. Biochem.*, **8**, 101–107

Editorial (1992) Nitric oxide: the elusive mediator of the hyperdynamic circulation of cirrhosis. *Hepatology*, **16**, 1089–1092

Gartner, J. C., Jaffe, R., Malatack, J. J., Zitelli, B. J. and Urbach, A. H. (1987) Hepatic infarction and acute liver failure in children with extrahepatic biliary atresia and cirrhosis. *Journal of Pediatric Surgery,* **22,** 360–362

Greenough, A., Pool, J. B., Ball, C., Mieli-Vergani, G. and Mowat, A. P. (1988) Functional residual capacity related to hepatitic disease. *Arch. Dis. Child.* **63,** 850–852

Hird, M. F., Greenough, A., Mieli-Vergani, G. and Mowat, A. P. (1991) Hyperinflation in Children with liver disease due to Alpha-1 antitrypsin deficiency. *Pediatr. Pulmonol.,* **11,** 212–216

Hourani, J. M., Bellamy, P. E., Tashkin, D. P., Batra, P. and Simmons, M. S. (1991) Pulmonary dysfunction in advanced liver disease: frequent occurence of an abnormal diffusing capacity. *Am. J. Med.,* **90,** 693–700

Jervis, G. A. (1979) Encephalopathy in infantile hepatic cirrhosis. *Acta. Neuropathologica.,* **48,** 73–75

Keren, G., Boichis, H. Swas, T. S. and Frand, M. (1983). Pulmonary arterio-venous fistulae in hepatic cirrhosis. *Arch. Dis. Childh.,* **58,** 302

Larcher, V. F., Manolaki, N., Vegnente, A., Vergani, D. and Mowat, A. P. (1985) Spontaneous bacterial peritonitis in children with chronic liver disease: clinical features and aetiological factors. *J. Pediatr.,* **106,** 907

Maguire, S., Monahan, M. J., Sayed, J. M., Price, J. and Mowat, A. P. (1993) Mechanisms of hypoxia; a frequent complication in children with cirrhosis. (submitted for publication)

Marchesini, G. M., Dioguardi, F. S., Bianchi, G. P. *et al.* (1990) Long-term oral branched-chain amino acid treatment in chronic hepatic encephalopathy. A randomized double-blind casein-controlled trial. The Italian Multicenter Study Group. *J. Hepatol.,* **11,** 92–101

Matsubara, O., Nakamura, T., Uehara, T. and Kasuga, T. (1984). Histometrical investigations of the pulmonary artery in severe hepatic disease. *J. Pathol.,* **143,** 31

Moncada, S., Palmer, R. M. J. and Higgs, E. A. (1991) Nitric oxide: Physiology, pathophysiology and pharmacology. *Pharmacol. Rev.,* **43,** 109–142

Moore, K., Ward, P. S., Taylor, G. W. and Williams, R. (1991) Systemic and renal production of thromboxane A2 and prostacyclin in decompensated liver disease and hepatorenal syndrome. *Gastroenterology,* **100,** 1069–1077

Mortensen, P. B., Holtug, K., Bonnen, H. and Clausen, M. R. (1990) The degradation of amino acids, proteins, and blood to short-chain fatty acids in colon is prevented by lactulose. *Gastroenterology,* **98,** 353–360

Moscoso, G., Mieli-Vergani, G., Mowat, A. P. and Portmann, B. (1991) Sudden death caused by unsuspected pulmonary hypertension, 10 years after surgery for extrahepatic biliary atresia. *J. Ped. Gastroenterol. Nutr.,* **12,** 388–393

Mowat, A. P. (1993) Hepatic encephalopathy: Acute and Chronic. In *Coma* (ed. J. A. Eyre) *Bailliere's Clinical Paediatrics.* Bailliere Tindall, London, Ch. 5

Mowat, A. P. (1989) Chronic hepatitis and cirrhosis. In *Paediatric Gastroenterology and Nutrition in Early Childhood,* 2nd ed. (ed. E. Lebenthal) Raven Press, New York, 1017–1043

Mullen, K. D., Szauter, K. M. and Kaminsky-Russ, K. (1990) 'Endogenous' benzodiazepine activity in body fluids of patients with hepatic encephalopathy. *Lancet,* **336,** 81–83

Mullen, K. D. and Weber, F. L. (1991) Role of nutrition in hepatic encephalopathy. *Sem. Liver Dis.,* **11,** 292–304

Oellerich, M., Brudelski, M., Lautz, H-U., Schulz, M., Schmidt, F-W. and Herrmann, H. (1990) Lidocaine metabolite formation as a measure of liver function in patients with cirrhosis. *Ther. Drug Monitor.,* **12,** 219–226

Papadakis, M. A., Fraser, C. L. and Arieff, A. I. (1990) Hyponatraemia in patients with cirrhosis. *Q. J. Med.,* **76,** 675–688

Riggio, O., Balducci, G., Ariosto, F. *et al.* (1989) Lactitol in prevention of recurrent episodes of hepatic encephalopathy in cirrhotic patients with portal-systemic shunt. *Dig.Dis Sci.,* **34,** 823–829

Scheuer, P. J. (1987) Cirrhosis. In: *Pathology of the Liver,* 2nd edn. (eds. R. N. M. MacSween, P. P. Anthony and P. J. Scheuer). Churchill-Livingstone, Edinburgh, 274–302

Schrier, R. W. (1992) A unifying hypothesis of body fluid volume regulation. *J. Roy. Coll. Phys.,* **26,** 295–306

Stewart, S. M., Hiltebeitel, C., Nici, J., Waller, D. A., Uauy, R. and Andrews, W. S. (1991) Neuropsychological outcome of pediatric liver transplantation. *Pediatrics,* **87,** 367–376

Tarao, K., Ikeda, T., Hayashi, K., Sakurai, A., Okada, T., Ito, T., Karube, H., Nomoto, T., Mizuno, T. and Shindo, K. (1990) Successful use of vancomycin hydrochloride in the treatment of lactulose resistant chronic hepatic encephalopathy. *Gut,* **31,** 702–706

Vilstrup, H., Gluud, C., Hardt, F. *et al.* (1990) Branched chain enriched amino acid versus glucose treatment of hepatic encephalopathy. A double-blind study of 65 patients with cirrhosis. *J. Hepatol.,* **10,** 291–296

Vjaro, P., Hadchouel, P., Hadchouel, M., Bernard, O. and Alagille, D. (1990). Incidence of cirrhosis in children with chronic hepatitis. *J. Pediatr.,* **117,** 392–396

Wyke, R. J. (1989) Bacterial infections complicating liver disease. *Baillieres.Clin. Gastroenterol.,* **3,** 187–210

Yen, C. L. and Liaw, Y. F. (1990) Somatosensory evoked potentials and number connection test in the detection of subclinical hepatic encephalopathy. *Hepatogastroenterology,* **37,** 332–334

Chapter 14

Liver disorders caused by drugs or environmental toxins

Definition

Liver damage may be attributed to a drug or toxin when the agent produces liver damage in a *predictable dose-related fashion*, in all recipients, with its onset occurring within a fixed period after exposure. Where damage is due to a drug metabolite rather than the parent drug the rate of onset and the dose required to cause injury are influenced by metabolic rates.

In *non-predictable drug injury* a harmful effect on liver function is seen in only a very small proportion of individuals taking the drug. This may start 1 to 5 weeks after starting the drug or be delayed for many months. Other causes of liver disease should have been excluded. In acute disorders the liver damage may regress when the agent is withdrawn. Confirmation of the association comes when the dysfunction recurs when the drug is reintroduced. This is rarely clinically defensible. There is usually no specific test for such drug-induced idiosyncratic hepatic injury. The presence of antibodies reacting with drug-induced liver antigens may provide supportive evidence for an association (see Halothane hepatitis on p. 235). An *in vitro* toxic reaction in patients' lymphocytes when exposed to anticonvulsant metabolites appears to be a marker for anticonvulsant hypersensitivity including hepatitis (Shear and Spielberg, 1988).

In practice the clinician must be aware that over 600 drugs been incriminated in causing a wide range of hepatic disorders and that any sporadic unexplained liver damage could be due to drugs (Table 14.1).

Although drug-induced liver damage is more commonly recognized in adults than in children, it is worth recalling that the average child at home will take some form of drug as often as one day in 10. Having identified a possible drug cause the only safe course is to stop the drug and not use it again. If acute liver failure occurs the mortality is high and early referral for possible liver transplantation is essential.

Liver and drug or toxin metabolism

The great susceptibility of the liver to drug- or toxin-induced injury has a number of possible causes. The liver's strategic position astride the portal blood exposes it to absorbed pharmaceuticals, food additives and other xenobiotics. It has a marked ability to concentrate some of these and plays an important role in their metabolism and excretion.

Table 14.1 Drugs which may cause liver damage

Antibiotics
  Tetracycline
  Erythromycin estolate
  Nitrofurantoin
  Ampicillin
  Cloxacillin
  Oxacillin
  Carbenicillin
  Chloramphenicol
  Fusidic acid
  Lincomycin
  Oleandomycin
  Spiramycin
  Sulphonamides
  Trimethoprim-sulphamethoxazole
  Metronidazole
  Sulphasalazine
  Clindamycin
  Novobiocin
  Troleadomycin
  Amoxycillin/clavulanic aid (Augmentin)

Antituberculous drugs
  PAS
  Isoniazid
  Rifampicin
  Pyrazinamide
  Ethionamide
  Ethambutol
  Ethioacetazone

Other antimicrobials
  Ketoconazole
  Amphotericin
  Mebendazole
  Quinine
  Didanosine
  Griseofulvin
  Mepairine
  Idoxyuridene
  Amodiaquine
  Fansidar
  Hycanthone
  Dapsone

Antineoplastic and immunosuppressant agents
  Methotrexate
  6-mercaptopurine
  Azathioprine
  Mitomycin
  Vincristine
  Cyclosporin
  Dacarbazine
  Actinomycin
  Chlorambucil
  Busulphan

Anaesthetics
  Halothane
  Methoxyflurane
  Enflurane
  Chloroform
  Isofluane

Anticonvulsants and antidepressants
  Sodium valproate
  Phenobarbitone
  Diphenylhydantoin
  Trimethadione
  Chlordiazepoxide
  Tricyclic antidepressants (e.g. amitriptyline)
  Monoamine oxidase inhibitors (e.g. iproniazid)
  Phenothiazine
  Haloperidol
  Clotiazedam
  Progabide

Analgesic and anti-inflammatory agents
  Phenylbutazone
  Indomethacin
  Paracetamol (acetaminophen)
  Aspirin
  Benorylate
  Dextropropoxyphene
  Ibuprofen
  Naproxen
  Pirprofen
  Benoxaprofen

Anti-thyroid drugs
  Methimazole
  Carbimazole
  Thiouracil
  Propylthiouracil

Cardiovascular agents
  Methyldopa
  Propranolol
  Oxprenolol
  Hydrallazine
  Captopril
  Perhexiline
  Enalapril
  Benzothadiazine diuretics
  Amidodarone lisinopril
  Verapamil

Oral hypoglycaemic agents
  Chlorpropamide
  Tolbutamide

Hormones
  Methyltestosterone
  Anabolic steroids
  Oestrogens
  Oral contraceptives

Other agents
  Alcohol
  Oxyphenisatin
  Intravenous nutrients
  Vitamin A
  Cimetidine
  Ranitidine
  Penicillamine
  Tienilic acide (LKM-2)
  Gold
  Iron
  Dantrolene
  Total parenteral nutrition
  Benzodiazepine
  Phenelzine

Hepatic metabolism of drugs and toxins is mediated by a large, increasingly well characterized, variety of metabolic pathways. The major initial step in drug metabolism (phase 1) utilizes two classes of enzymes, oxidoreductases and hydrolyases, which often generate from the parent compound very reactive products since they introduce carboxyl, epoxide or hydroxyl groups (Table 14.2). These chemical groups serve as acceptors of glucuronic acid, sulphates, glutathione, acetate and amino acids in reactions catalysed by a series of transferases (phase 2). A single drug is often metabolized by more than one of these types of reactions. Many compounds can be metabolized by phase 2 reactions without undergoing a phase 1 reaction. Both phase 1 and phase 2 reactions usually increase polarity and water solubility of products. Phase 2 reactions generally produce less biologically active products. These metabolic changes occur in the endoplasmic reticulum, mitochondria and cell cytoplasm. The end product of metabolism is usually a water-soluble product which will be excreted in the bile if the molecular weight is greater than 400 and in urine if smaller.

The metabolic changes within the liver may convert a drug from a toxic to a non-toxic state or vice versa. This ability can be modified by more than 200 compounds, e.g. drugs such as barbiturates or polycyclic hydrocarbons such as insecticides or cigarette smoke, which non-specifically increase the activity of drug metabolizing enzymes in the liver (Table 14.3). Enzyme induction can increase or decrease the toxicity of drugs and environmental toxins.

The *mechanisms involved in hepatotoxicity* include the generation of free radicals which cause peroxidative degeneration of membrane-phospholipid and the generation of strong electrophilic centres which cause enzyme inactivation, decrease cellular protein

Table 14.2 Principal enzymatic pathways involved in metabolism of drugs and toxins

Phase 1	Phase 2

Oxidases
    Cytochrome P-450 system
    Mixed function amine oxidases
    Amine oxidases
    Alcohol dehydrogenase
    Aldehyde oxidases
	Transferases
	which conjugate with:
	
	    Glucuronides
	    Sulphates
	    Glutathiones
	    Acetyl Co-A
	    S-adenosyl methionine
	    Amino acids

Reductases
    Aldo-keto-reductase
    Azo-reductase	

Hydrolases
    Esterases
    Epoxide
    Hydrolase	

Enzymes involved are located in the endoplasmic reticulum, mitochondria, cell cytoplasm and cell membranes. Phase 1 reactions are catalysed by oxidoreductases and hydrolyses. Phase 2 reactions by transferases. A single drug may be metabolized by many reactions. Some cases of 'idiosyncratic' drug toxicity may be explained by differences in the relative rate of several alternative phase 1 pathways, producing metabolites of differing hepatotoxic potential, or the relative inefficiency of phase 2 reactions in 'detoxification' of these.

Table 14.3 Poisons affecting the liver

Biological	Chemical	Physical
Aflatoxin	Carbon tetrachloride	Hyperthermia
Senecio alkaloids	Tetrachlorethane	Burns
Hypoglycins (Ackee fruit)	Chlordecone	Irradiation
Amanita mushrooms	Chlorophenoxy herbicides	
Crotolaria	? Emulsifiers	
Lupinus	Benzyl alcohol	
Heletropium	Dichlorethane	
Mistletoe	Benzene derivatives	
Clove oil	Trinitrotoluene	
	Phosphorus	
	Iron	
	Copper	
	Cadmium	
	Beryllium	
	Vinyl chloride	
	Paraquat	
	Methylene diamine	
	Toluene solvents ('glue sniffing')	

concentration and induce cell necrosis. This is particularly likely to occur if there is depletion of glutathione or its precursor cysteine or n-acetylcysteine as occurs in protein depletion, fasting and in the presence of many substrates. These biochemical processes may induce antigenic changes in liver cell membranes which initiate immunological mechanisms of liver damage.

Drug metabolism can be influenced by *genetic* factors as illustrated by the rapid and slow acetylators of isoniazid but this is only one example of many drugs whose metabolism is influenced by genetic polymorphism.

Hepatic drug metabolism is also influenced by the state of *nutrition*, by the presence of liver disease and portosystemic shunting both through a direct effect on hepatic drug metabolism and the production of drug-binding proteins. *Age* also has a major effect. The human neonate (as opposed to many intensively studied laboratory animals) from the first day of life is well equipped with drug metabolizing enzymes with the exception of those involving glucuronide formation and possibly those oxidizing polycyclic aromatic hydrocarbons. Direct studies however are sparse. Drug metabolism, as evidenced by the half-life in serum, changes with age in a divergent and often unexpected fashion. Paracetamol, for example, has a half-life on the first day of life which is nearly that of the adult while that of phenobarbitone is around 200 hours, falling to 100 hours at 5–15 days of age and to 50 hours between 1 and 3 months. Theophylline, on the other hand, has a half-life of 100 hours at birth, falling to 3–4 hours at 1–4 years of age and extending to 5–6 hours in the adult. It must be stressed that these pharmacokinetic observations may be influenced by plasma protein binding, lipid content of membranes and by renal function as well as hepatic drug metabolizing activity.

While it cannot be excluded that differences in drug metabolizing enzymes in childhood account for the less frequent recognition of drug-related liver disease in children compared with adults, it also seems possible that a lower incidence of self-prescription of drugs and of drug dependence, as well as less alcohol intake may be equally important. Drugs and environmental factors must be considered in all types of unexplained liver disease.

Patterns of liver cell injury

Both the pattern of liver injury (Table 14.4) and its severity vary considerably. There may be alteration of only one metabolic function without structural change. It may range from asymptomatic elevation of transaminases to fulminant hepatic necrosis; from minor changes in the sinusoids to obstruction of major vessels; from mildly increased fibrosis to cirrhosis and malignant change.

Cholestasis without cellular change

17-Alpha-alkyl-substituted steroids such as methyltestosterone, anabolic steroids such as norethandrone, and oestrogens cause cholestasis without any hepatocellular necrosis or cellular change in the portal tract. The disorder appears to be rare and may only occur in those with a genetic predisposition. The mode of action is not known but it is thought to be because these agents cause a decrease in bile salt-dependent bile flow. There is complete recovery when the drug is withdrawn.

Hepatocellular damage due to direct cytotoxic injury

A wide range of hepatic cellular injury has been associated with drugs. The exact pathogenesis is frequently unknown. While certain patterns of injury can be recognized pathologically and clinically, there is often considerable overlap. The concomitant administration of drugs which induce microsomal enzymes involved in drug metabolism

Table 14.4 Histological patterns of drug- or poison-induced liver injury

Clincopathological features	Example of drug or poison
Cholestasis without cellular change	Anabolic steroids
Fatty liver:	
Macrovesicular	Corticosteroids, ethanol
Microvesicular	Valproate
Hepatocellular necrosis:	
Direct	Tetracycline
Metabolite related	Paracetamol
Metabolite + immunological mechanism	Isoniazid
Cholestatic hepatitis	Phenothiazines
Chronic active hepatitis	Mehtyldopa, nitrofurantoin
Granulomatous hepatitis	Phenylbutazone
Venous thrombosis	Senecio, irradiation, carbamazine
Peliosis	Anabolic steroids
Increased fibrosis	Methotrexate
Adenoma	Oral contraceptives, androgens
Focal nodular hyperplasia	Oral contraceptives
Carcinoma	Androgens
Angiosarcoma	Vinyl chloride
Gall stones	Oral contraceptives, clofibrate

may increase the frequency and severity of such liver injury, for example, when rifampicin is given with isoniazid.

Hepatocellular necrosis may occur as the result of a drug or its metabolites interfering directly with a vital function within the cell or by damaging intracellular membrane. Necrosis occurs without much inflammatory cell infiltration as, for example, in paracetamol overdosage and with carbon tetrachloride. The earliest change seen is an inhibition of protein synthesis associated with a fragmentation of the endoplasmic reticulum and mitochondrial injury leading to a loss of energy production.

Fat accumulates and as the effects of injury become more widespread within the cell, lysosomal membranes disintegrate releasing hydrolytic enzymes. General cell lysis follows. With some drugs such injury is proportional with dose and duration of administration occurring within days of starting the drug and can be reproduced in humans and experimental animals. With drugs or poisons causing direct injury it may be possible to demonstrate the drug in tissue or body fluids.

In other instances, the pathological process is more complex, with *immunological mechanisms* playing a part in cell damage. The drug or one of its metabolites may change cell membranes so that they become immunoreactive. It is postulated, for example, that isoniazid and methyldopa, both of which cause temporary elevation of transaminases with mild hepatocellular necrosis in up to 10% of individuals, cause liver injury only in those subjects who mount an inappropriate immunological response. With such drugs, significant liver disease rarely starts until the drug has been taken for 3 weeks and may not occur for as late as 12 months. The pathological changes within the liver can range from classic centrilobular necrosis, as occurs with paracetamol, to a subacute or chronic aggressive hepatitis, or even a periportal necrosis in association with antinuclear autoantibodies, for example, caused by propylthiouracil (Maggiore *et al.*, 1989). Autoimmune mechanisms have been implicated in halothane hepatitis.

Hepatocellular damage may also occur with features of *generalized hypersensitivity*. Fever, arthralgia, rash and eosinophilia with, sometimes, generalized lymph gland enlargement precede the onset of liver disease. The hepatic reaction may be predominantly of hepatocellular necrosis with cellular infiltrate. Occasionally granulomata will occur. The mechanism of this liver injury is imperfectly understood.

Some drugs appear to produce a predominantly *cholestatic* picture with an inflammatory infiltrate in widened portal tracts. There may be a high proportion of eosinophils in the infiltrate. There is only slight oedema and slight bile duct proliferation. Cholestasis is mainly centrilobular and is usually not accompanied by much liver cell necrosis or inflammatory cell infiltrate. The liver cells, however, may be swollen and show variation in nuclear size. Portal tract reaction tends to fade after a few weeks but in some instances appearances are those of chronic aggressive hepatitis. In other patients granulomata may appear in the portal tracts.

In adults further pathological changes have been reported. Androgens and oral contraceptives have been implicated in causing adenomas and hepatocellular *carcinoma*. Increased hepatic *fibrosis* and cirrhosis has followed the use of methotrexate for psoriasis and leukaemia. Hepatic fibrosis and angiosarcoma have occurred following ingestion of arsenic, inhalation of vinyl chloride and Thorotrast injection.

Clinical features

The essential clinical feature is a history of exposure to a drug or toxin. If the agent is hepatotoxic in a dose-related fashion, e.g. paracetamol or carbon tetrachloride, the diagnosis is rarely in doubt. Where the patient is taking a drug with known hepatotoxic effects, e.g. isoniazid for periods of 3–52 weeks, hepatotoxicity occurs so commonly that suspicion should be high. Where exposure has occurred at intervals of months or years, e.g. halothane anaesthesia, the association may not be so clear. The liver disorder may mimic almost any form of hepatic disease in childhood.

Causality may be based on five criteria:

(1) Specificity of the clinical and pathological features.
(2) A temporal relationship between the intake and onset and between the discontinuation and disappearance of hepatic injury.
(3) The simultaneous appearance of rash, fever, arthralgia, eosinophilia or non-organ specific autoantibodies when liver injury has an immune basis.
(4) The demonstration of antibodies or other immune phenomena in the presence of tissue damaged by the drug in question.
(5) Exclusion of other possible causes for the liver dysfunction.

There may be toxic effects on other organs such as the kidney, gastrointestinal tract, bone marrow or the brain which overshadow the hepatic features. Thus any drug under suspicion must be withdrawn and other causes of hepatic injury carefully excluded.

It is impossible to consider all hepatotoxic drug effects in such a text. Principal clinical features of commonly observed liver dysfunction caused by hepatotoxic drugs in children are considered below. The examples chosen also exemplify the difficulties in relating liver disease to drugs and illustrate some of the pathobiological mechanisms considered above. In all of these disorders the *prothrombin time* is the best guide to the severity of liver damage. If it is prolonged by more than 6 seconds after parenteral vitamin K or if there is any evidence of hepatic encephalopathy the mortality is likely to considerable and immediate contact with a centre able to perform liver transplantation is recommended. If the international normalized ratio (INR) is greater than 4 liver transplantation is advised.

Liver injury due to halothane and related anaesthetic agents

Halothane is generally a very safe anaesthetic but significant liver necrosis may occur very rarely following exposure. The majority of cases occur in patients who have had more than one exposure to halothane. The age of reported cases ranges from 11 months to 75 years. The severity of liver injury varies from asymptomatic hepatocellular necrosis detected by a rise in serum transaminase values to fulminant hepatic failure. A specific *in vitro test* for IgG antibodies to halothane-altered liver cell membranes is positive in 70% of cases. A similar form of liver damage has been reported to occur even more rarely following anaesthesia with the related, more recently introduced agents, methoxyflurane, enflurane and isoflurane.

Mechanisms of liver injury

Minor hepatic dysfunction may occur in 20% of halothane recipients. Major hepatocellular necrosis is so rare that its frequency can only be estimated from large retrospective studies being put at between 1 in 6000 to 1 in 100 000 administrations. The mode of such severe hepatocellular injury is uncertain. Current research suggests that halothane or one of its metabolites produced during oxidative metabolism may cause antigenic changes in liver cell membranes. Genetic factors, some HLA associated, may determine the nature of the immune response. It includes the production of IgG antibodies against halothane-altered liver cell membranes and antibodies against normal liver membrane components. These antibodies may bind to hepatocytes and induce lymphocyte-mediated cytotoxicity analogous to liver damage in chronic hepatitis B virus infection.

Pathology

The pathological features are those of acute viral hepatitis, indistinguishable morphologically from hepatitis A virus infection, through submassive confluent zonal necrosis to total necrosis. Fatty change may suggest a drug cause. Granulomatous hepatitis and chronic hepatitis are rare manifestations.

Clinical features

The patient typically has a number of surgical procedures requiring general anaesthesia. The interval between these exposures may be as long as 13 years. Symptoms start after a latent period of 2 or 4 days and rarely 1, 2 or even 4 weeks. Fever, lasting for a few days in the absence of sepsis, arthralgia, rash, malaise and non-specific gastrointestinal symptoms, followed rapidly by jaundice if liver damage is severe, is the typical story. If the significance of these features, particularly the fever or jaundice, is not appreciated and halothane is again given, symptoms recur but after a shorter latent period and severe hepatocellular necrosis is likely. If hepatic encephalopathy occurs the mortality is 75%.

Laboratory investigations

Laboratory investigation findings include aspartate aminotransferase values ranging from 300 to more than 4000 IU/litre. The prothrombin time is prolonged in severe cases. Eosinophilia and liver-kidney-microsomal autoantibodies may be found. The specific IgG antibody test against halothane-altered liver membrane antigens is positive in 70% of cases.

Treatment

There is no specific treatment. Corticosteroids have not been assessed in a systematic fashion. If the prothrombin time is prolonged by more than 50 seconds (INR >4) liver transplantation is recommended.

Patients requiring repeated anaesthesia should be given halothane on only one occasion. A history of unexplained jaundice, abnormal 'liver function tests' or unexplained fever after halothane anaesthesia are absolute contraindications to its future use in that child.

Hepatitis due to antituberculous drugs

Tuberculosis is probably the commonest condition in which paediatric patients develop signs of liver damage which can be confidently attributed to drugs. Streptomycin is the only commonly used antituberculous drug which has not been associated with hepatic injury. The range of injury extends from slight asymptomatic rises in the serum transaminases to fulminant hepatic necrosis. In most instances, the patient has been receiving more than one drug in order to minimize the risks of possible bacterial resistance to the antibiotics.

Isoniazid becomes hepatotoxic when it is acetylated. Hepatotoxicity is more likely to occur when the rate of acetylation is increased as may occur for genetic reasons, or be caused by drugs which induce the acetylating enzymes. Among these are rifampicin and phenobarbitone. Approximately 10% of individuals receiving isoniazid develop asymptomatic elevation of these serum transaminases and mild hepatitis. These abnormalities settle in the vast majority over the course of 2–3 weeks, but in a few patients the liver function tests remain abnormal. If this occurs, or the transaminase elevation is greater than six times normal, or if jaundice develops, the drug must be stopped, since isoniazid-induced hepatitis is likely to be present. It may progress to a chronic hepatitis or massive hepatic necrosis. There is no specific therapy. The mortality is as high as 10%.

Para-aminosalicylic acid (PAS) causes fever, rash and lymphadenopathy in approximately 5% of individuals; 2% of these are likely to have a raised transaminase. If the drug is not withdrawn at this stage a fulminant hepatitis may appear with a mortality of 20%.

Rifampicin causes a predictable impairment of bilirubin uptake by the liver, is an enzyme inducer, and may cause hepatitis. It causes an asymptomatic rise in transaminases in 20% of individuals, of whom 8% become jaundiced. The hepatitis is usually mild and resolves when the drug is withdrawn. When two drugs are given together the incidence of asymptomatic elevation of transaminases and hepatitis increases. For example, in patients treated with isoniazid and rifampicin, 35% develop raised transaminases. Some of these will be self-limited but a small percentage do go on to significant hepatitis. Ethambutol and isoniazid together cause elevated aspartate transaminases in some 12% of individuals. Pyrazinamide and ethionamide cause hepatitis in between 5 and 10% of recipients. It should be noted that isoniazid, pyrazinamide and ethionamide are chemically related and if one causes hepatic toxicity, the others should not be used.

Management

Should liver damage occur in a patient with tuberculosis on antituberculous treatment, the tuberculosis may be considered so severe that therapy must be continued. Streptomycin and either ethambutol, cycloserine or capromycin which have little propensity for liver damage, should be given.

If the tuberculosis seems well controlled, all drugs may be stopped and the patient watched until the transaminase returns to normal. Isoniazid, ethambutol and streptomycin should be started carefully. A single test dose of one drug should be given and liver function tests repeated every second day for 1 week. If no abnormalities are observed a full dose is given for a further week while monitoring of liver function tests is continued. This procedure is then repeated with each of the drugs under suspicion. When the offending agent has been identified it is best excluded from therapy but if it has to be used, desensitization with very small doses which are gradually increased if tolerated, may be successful.

Paracetamol

Paracetamol is a safe, well tolerated, mild analgesic and antipyretic which is increasingly recommended for children with febrile illnesses. Fatalities due to acute drug overdosage are well known in adolescents and adults but have now been reported in children, while self-limiting fulminant hepatic failure has been reported in infants of 6 and 7 weeks of age who had toxic drug levels after allegedly normal doses. Such fatalities may be prevented if treatment with intravenous *N*-acetyl cysteine is commenced within 8 hours of ingestion and may be minimized by later therapy. Fortunately most children with accidental overdoses present within a few hours of ingestion.

Such *treatment* is required if a plasma concentration is above a line joining 200 µg/ml (1.32 mmol/litre) at 4 hours and 30 µg/ml (0.16 mmol/litre) at 12 hours after ingestion, plotted on a semilog graph of concentration versus time. The dose is 150 mg/kg given over 15 minutes, followed by 50 mg/kg over four hours and 100 mg/kg over the next 16 hours given in appropriate volumes of 5% dextrose. Serum transaminases become abnormal 12 to 36 hours after ingestion and reach a maximum concentration at 3 or 4 days. If the prothrombin time is normal at 48 hours the liver injury is likely to be self-limiting and the patient can be discharged. If it is slightly prolonged treatment for acute liver failure is necessary. Liver transplantation is recommended if prolonged to 50 seconds and the patient's pH is <7.3, as the mortality is as high as 90% in such patients. Renal failure developing at 24–72 hours may require treatment with dialysis. Rarely liver damage can occur with the administration of therapeutic doses over a period of days particularly in ill patients taking enzyme-inducing drugs.

Anticonvulsants

Sodium valproate hepatotoxicity

Sodium valproate is widely used in the control of all forms of epilepsy. Approximately 10% of patients receiving the drug develop elevation of serum transaminases without other abnormalities in biochemical tests of liver function during the first 6 months of treatment. The rise is usually asymptomatic and reverses spontaneously or on reducing the drug dosage. Raised blood ammonia values without other abnormalities in liver function tests have been reported in approximately 1% of cases. In some instances there has been associated lethargy, vomiting and stupor. When the drug is withdrawn these symptoms remit.

Since 1978 a number of reports have indicated a possible association between sodium valproate therapy and fatal hepatitis. The majority of such fatalities have been in children under the age of 10 years. Fatality usually occurs within 6 months of initiating therapy. In these cases only rarely have other causes of liver failure been excluded. The majority were taking other anticonvulsants which may have influenced valproate metabolism.

Liver histology in the fatal cases is characterized by central lobular necrosis with approximately 50% of cases showing microvesicular steatosis. In four instances cirrhosis has been present. Three fatal cases with a Reye-like syndrome have also been recorded.

Valproate is a branched, medium-chain fatty acid. Its metabolite 2-propyl-4-pentanoic acid, an analogue of the active agent in Jamaican vomiting sickness, may cause inhibition of mitochondrial function and thus hepatic steatosis and necrosis while propionic acid may interfere with carbamyl phosphate synthetase to cause hyperammonaemia. Up to 30% of the fatal cases have had structural neurological abnormalities. Some may have had liver disease associated with familial progressive neuronal degeneration (see Chapter 11). At present it is impossible to predict which children will develop liver failure. It seems prudent not to use valproate in patients with abnormal liver function tests prior to therapy or in patients with inborn errors of mitochondrial function and to measure aspartate aminotransferase and blood ammonia levels regularly in the first 6 months of treatment, although there is as yet no evidence that such screening predicts the development of liver failure.

Phenobarbitone, phenytoin and carbamazepine

Many patients receiving therapeutic doses of any of these drugs, alone or as combined anticonvulsants, develop asymptomatic rises in transaminases, e.g. 6% of children taking carbamazepine, possibly due to a inherited defect in detoxification of arene oxides. A much smaller percentage, presumed to be derived from those with raised transaminases, develop a hypersensitivity syndrome. This is characterized by fever usually starting 3 weeks after therapy was begun and followed 1 or 2 days later by a skin rash which may take a variety of forms, and lymphadenopathy. Within 1 week the child may develop evidence of target organ disease, which can include liver involvement. There may be eosinophilia, raised serum immunoglobulins, particularly IgE and decreased complement levels, but these are not invariable. The liver injury may range from persistent elevations of transaminases to fulminant hepatic necrosis. Deterioration may continue for weeks after the drug has been stopped. Corticosteroids should be given since in some patients improvement follows, with relapse when it is withdrawn. Transplantation may be required.

Amanita mushroom poisoning

Amanita phalloides in Europe and *Amanita verna* in the USA exert their hepatotoxicity through the action of alpha-amanitin. Three medium-size mushrooms contain a dose of this heat-stable toxin which is lethal in an adult. Children are more susceptible. Following ingestion of such a dose there are no symptoms for 6 to 12 hours. Severe vomiting, diarrhoea and abdominal pain then develops, lasting 1 to 4 days. Features of liver involvement develop towards the end of this period. Therapy is supportive. Liver transplantation may be required, the indications being as in other forms of acute liver failure.

Radiation hepatitis

The liver is relatively resistant to damage by irradiation. If given with chemotherapeutic (cytotoxic) drugs damage may occur with doses as low as 12 Gy (1200 rad) and is very likely to occur with doses of 20 Gy (2000 rad). Drugs implicated in aggravating liver damage include Adriamycin (doxorubicin), actinomycin D, cytosine arabinoside, azathioprine, busulphan, 6-mercaptopurine, 6-thioguanine, mitomycin C, urethane, indicine-n-oxide and cyclophosphamide. Bone marrow transplant recipients may develop liver damage with total body irradiation of as little as 10 Gy (1000 rad) if there is pre-existing biochemical evidence of liver damage or underlying malignancy other than acute leukaemia.

Pathology

With irradiation alone the primary injury appears to be the walls of the hepatic venules. There is a loosely arranged fibroblastic reaction which spreads to the endothelium causing venous obstruction. Liver biopsy therefore shows extreme hepatic congestion with dilated sinusoids and haemorrhages into the walls of hepatic veins. With chemoirradiation damage there may be primary damage to hepatocytes around central venules and to hepatic venules. There is loss of hepatocytes with reticulum collapse particularly around the central area. The liver is frequently reduced in size. When healing occurs there is marked fibrosis which may be complicated by portal hypertension and the development of cirrhosis.

Clinical features

Clinical features of liver injury may occur between 7 days and 5 months following irradiation. With bone marrow grafting the onset is within 8–20 days of conditioning therapy. In acute cases there may be fever, anorexia, vomiting, followed by the rapid onset of jaundice and ascites which may proceed to fulminant hepatic failure. Serum aminotransferase values are raised with low serum albumin and the prothrombin time may be prolonged. Technetium colloid liver scan shows decreased liver size and hepatic uptake may be reduced generally or focally, mimicking metastasis. Delayed hepatic clearance of myelosuppressive drugs may cause pancytopenia and increase other toxic effects.

The disease may proceed to total hepatocellular necrosis but more commonly, particularly if hepatotoxic drugs are withdrawn, liver function improves over the course of 3–4 weeks returning to normal after 3–4 months. There may, however, be persistent reduction in the size of the right lobe of the liver with compensatory hypertrophy of the left. Features of portal hypertension may develop.

Liver disease following bone marrow transplantation

Bone marrow transplantation is being used to treat a wide variety of disorders including some forms of acute leukaemia, aplastic anaemia and metabolic abnormalities. Some recipients have liver pathology as part of the primary disorder. Many are exposed to a very wide range of potentially hepatotoxic drugs and viruses in the treatment of the underlying disease, during conditioning therapy and after grafting. Opportunistic infection and parenteral nutrition may contribute to liver damage. During the first 2 months after grafting, the majority of patients have mild elevation of biochemical tests of liver function which gradually resolve.

Two distinct complications with considerable morbidity and mortality may occur. *Veno-occlusive disease* (see p. 378) occurs particularly in the first 20 days after grafting. *Graft versus host disease* (GVHD) resulting from the response of donor immunocompetent cells to histocompatibility antigens of the recipient causes death in 50%. The acute form, which may start as early as 7 days but usually between 20 and 60 days, and chronic form (after 100 days) are equally serious. Liver involvement is usually associated with skin manifestations of GVHD, i.e. an erythematous, desquamating rash and intestinal GVHD manifest by diarrhoea which can be severe.

Biochemical tests of liver function become more abnormal, mild jaundice develops with hepatomegaly which may proceed to ascites and liver failure. The most striking pathological abnormality is extensive damage to septal and interlobular bile ducts which is seen 2 weeks after onset in almost 90% of cases. Less than 25% of the bile ducts will appear normal. Approximately one-third of cases show mild portal tract infiltration with lymphocytes, mild parenchymal necrosis and cholestasis. One-third of cases show lymphocytes adherent to the endothelial cells of the portal or hepatic vein branches. More than 50% of those surviving the acute form develop chronic form but others develop *de novo*. As the disease becomes chronic portal and bridging fibrosis develops proceeding to cirrhosis which may be micronodular. Diagnosis is based on the histological appearance in liver and skin biopsies and exclusion of drug and infective causes of liver damage.

Treatment is generally unsatisfactory but increased immunosuppressants or thalidomide may abrogate early changes. Death is frequently from infections rather than liver failure.

Bibliography and references

General

Mowat, A. P. (1984) Age related effects on drug metabolism. In *Liver Annual* Volume 4, (eds. I. M. Arias, M. Frenkel, and I. H. P. Wilson), Elsevier, Amsterdam, p. 322

Ormerod, L. P. (1990) Chemotherapy and management of tuberculosis in the United Kingdom. *Thorax,* **45**, 403–408

Pessayre, D. and Larrey, D. (1991) Drug-induced liver injury. In *Oxford Textbook of Clinical Hepatology* (eds. N. McIntyre, J. P. Benhamou, J. Bircher, M. Rizzetto, J. Rodes). Oxford University Press, Oxford, 873–903

Stricker, B. H. C. H. (1986). Hepatic injury by drugs and environmental agents. In *Liver Annual*, Volume 5, (eds. I. M. Arias, M. Frenkel and I. H. P. Wilson), p.419. Elsevier, Amsterdam

Stricker, B. H. C. A. and Spoelstra, P. (1985). *Drug-Induced Hepatic Injury*, 1st Ed. Elsevier, Amsterdam

Tucker, R. A. (1982). Drugs in liver disease: A tabular compilation of drugs and the histological changes that can occur in the liver. *Drug. Intell. Clin. Pharm.*, **16**, 569

Wilson, I. H. P. (1984). Drugs and the liver. In *Liver Annual* Volume 4, (eds. I. M. Arias, M. Frenkel, and I. H. P. Wilson), Elsevier, Amsterdam, p. 413

Halothane and related agents

Benjamin, S. B., Goodman, Z. D., Ishak, K. G., Zimmerman, H. I. and Irey, M. S. (1985). The morphological spectrum of halothane-induced hepatic injury: analysis of 77 cases. *Hepatology*, **5**, 11163

Brown, B. R. (1985). Halothane hepatitis revisited. *New Engl. J. Med.*, **21**, 1347

Degrot, H. and Noll, P. (1983). Halothane hepatotoxicity: relation between metabolic activation hypoxia, lipid peroxidation and liver cell damage. *Hepatology*, **3**, 601

Hassal, E., Israel, D. M., Gunaskaren, T. and Steward, D. (1990) Halothane Hepatitis in children. *J. Pediatr. Gastroenterol. Nutr.,* **11**, 553–557

Kenna, J. G., Neuberger, I. and Williams, R. (1984). Detection by ELISA of antibody specific halothane induced liver damage. *J. Immunol. Methods*, **75**, 3

Kenna, J. G., Neuberger, J., Mieli-Vergani, G., Mowat, A. P. and Williams, R. (1987). Halothane hepatitis in children.*Br. Med. J.*, **294**, 1209–1211

Mieli-Vergani, G., Vergani, D., Tredgar, I. M., Edelston, A. L. W., Davis, M. and Williams, R. (1980). Lymphocyte cytotoxicity to halothane-altered hepatocytes in patients with severe hepatic necrosis following halothane anaesthesia. *J. Clin. Lab. Immunol.*, **4**, 49

Neuberger, J. and Williams, R. (1984). Halothane anaesthesia in liver damage. *Br. Med. J.*, **4**, 1136

Neuberger, J., Mieli-Vergani, G., Mowat, A. P. and Williams, R. (1987) Halothane Hepatitis in Children. *Br. Med. J.*, **294**, 1209–1211

Otsuka, S., Yamamoto, M., Kasuya, S. *et al.* (1985). HLA antigens in patients with unexplained hepatitis following halothane anaesthesia. *Acta Anaesthesiol. Scand.*, **29**, 497

Vergani, D., Mieli-Vergani, G., Alberti, A., Neuberger, J., Edelston, A. L. W., Davis, M. and Williams. R. (1980). Antibodies to the surface of halothane-altered rabbit hepatocytes in patients with severe halothane-associated hepatitis. *New Engl. J. Med.*, **303**, 66

Wark, H. J. (1983). Postoperative jaundice in children. The influence of halothane anaesthesia. *Anaesthesia*, **38**, 237

Warner, W., Beech, T. P., Garvin, J.P. and Warner, E. J. (1984). Halothane in children – the first quarter century. *Anesth. Analg.*, **63**, 838

Paracetamol

Dixon, R. M., Angus, P. W., Rajagopalan, B. and Radda, G. K. (1992) ^{31}P magnetic resonance spectroscopy detects a functional abnormality in liver metabolism after acetaminophen poisoning. *Hepatology,* **16**, 943–948

Greene, J. W., Craft, S. and Ghishen, F. (1983). Acetaminophen poisoning in infancy. *Am. J. Dis. Child.*, **137**, 386

O'Grady, J. G., Alexander, G. J. M., Hallyer, K. M. and Williams, R. (1989) Early Prognostic indicators of prognosis in fulminant hepatic failure. *Gastroenterology*, **97**, 439–445

Parker, D., White, J. P., Paton, D. and Routledge, P. A. (1990) Safety of late acetylcysteine treatment in paracetamol poisoning. *Hum. Exp. Toxicol.*, **9**, 25–27

Prescott, L. F., Illingworth, R. M., Critchley, J. E. J. H. *et al.* (1979). Intravenous N-acetyl cysteine: The treatment of choice for paracetamol poisoning. *Br. Med. J.*, **2**, 1097

Irradiation and cytotoxic drugs

Bhanot, P., Cushing, B., Philippart, A., Das, L. and Farooki, Z. (1979). Hepatic irradiation and adriamycin. *J. Paediatr.*, **95**, 561

Fajardo, L. F. and Colby, T. V. (1980). Pathogenesis of venocclusive liver disease after irradiation. *Arch. Pathol. Lab. Med.*, **104**, 584

Johnson, F. L. and Balis, M. M. (1982). Hepatopathy following irradiation in chemotherapy for Wilm's tumour. *Am. J. Pediatr. Haematol. Oncol.*, **4**, 217

Post bone marrow transplantation

Baglin, T. P., Harper, P. and Marcus, R. E. (1990) Veno-occlusive disease of the liver complicating allogeneic bone marrow transplantation successfully treated with recombinant tissue plasminogen activator. *Bone Marrow Transplant*, **5**, 439–441

Farthing, M. J. G., Clark, M. L., Sloane, J. P., Powles, R. L. and McElwain, J.T. (1982). Liver disease after bone marrow transplantation. *Gut*, **23**, 465

Girardin, S. M. M. F., Vernanat, J. P., Dhumeaus, D. (1991) The liver in graft-versus-host disease In: *Oxford Textbook of Clinical Hepatology* (eds. N. McIntyre, J. P. Benhamou, J. Bircher, M. Rizzetto, J. Rodes). Oxford University Press, Oxford, 776–779

Gluckman, E., Jolivet, I., Scrobohaci, M. L. *et al.* (1990) Use of prostaglandin E1 for prevention of liver veno-occlusive disease in leukaemic patients treated by allogeneic bone marrow transplantation. *Brit. J. Haematol.*, **74**, 277–281

Hershko, C., Gale, R. P. (1980) GvHD scoring system for predicting survival and specific mortality in bone marrow transplant recipients. In: *Biology of bone marrow transplantation.* (eds. R. P. Gale, C. F. Fox). Academic Press, New York, 59–66

Jones, R. J., Lee, K. S. K., Beschorner, W. E. *et al.* (1987) Veno-occlusive disease of the liver following bone marrow transplantation. *Transplantation*, **44**, 778–783

McDonald, G. B., Sharma, P., Matthews, D. E., Shulman, H. M. and Thomas, E. D. (1984). Veno-occlusive disease of the liver after bone marrow transplantation: diagnosis, incidence and predisposing factors. *Hepatology*, **4**, 116

Shulman, H. M. and Hinterberg, W. (1992) Hepatic veno-occlusive disease – liver toxicity syndrome after bone marrow transplantation. *Bone Marrow Transplantation*, **10**, 197–214

Snover, D. C., Weisdorf, S. A., Ramsay, M. K., Mcglave, P. and Kersey, J. H. (1984). Hepatic graft versus host disease: A study in the predictive value of liver biopsy in diagnosis. *Hepatology*, **4**, 123

Anticonvulsants

Greene, S. H. (1984). Sodium valproate and routine liver function tests. *Arch. Dis. Childh.*, **59**, 813

Hadzic, N., Portmann, B., Davies, E. T., Mowat, A. P. and Mieli-Vergani, G. (1990) Carbamazepine-induced acute liver failure. *Arch. Dis. Child.*, **65**, 315–317

Harding, B. N., Egger, J., Portmann, B. and Erdohazi, N. (1986). Progressive neuronal degeneration of childhood with liver disease. *Brain*, **109**, 181

Lenn, N. J., Ellis, W. G., Washburn, E. R. and Ruebner, B. (1990) Fatal hepatocerebral syndrome in siblings discordant for exposure to valproate. *Epilepsia*, **31**, 578–583

Mockli, G., Crowley, M., Stern, R., Warnock, M. L. (1989) Massive hepatic necrosis in a child after administration of phenobarbital. *Amer. J. Gastro.*, **84**, 820–822

Powell-Jackson, P. R., Tredger, J. M. and Williams, R. (1984) Hepatotoxicity to sodium valproate: a review. *Gut*, **25**, 673

Shear, N. H. and Spielberg, S. P. (1988) Anticonvulsant hypersensitivity syndrome. *J. Clin. Invest.*, **82**, 1826–1832

Mushroom poisoning

Pinson, C. W., Daya, M. R, Benner, K. G. *et al.* (1990) Liver transplantation for severe Amanita phalloides mushroom poisoning. *Am. J. Surg.*, **159**, 493–499

Others

Jonas, M. M. and Edison, M. S. (1988) Propylthiouracil hepatotoxicity: two pediatric cases and review of the literature. *J. Pediatr. Gastroenterol. Nutr.*,**7**, 776–779

Kirkland, J. L. (1990) Propylthiouracil-induced hepatic failure and encephalopathy in a child. *DICP.*, **24**, 470–471

Maggiore, G., Larizza, D., Lorini, R., de Giacomo, C., Scotta, M. S. and Severi, F. (1989) Letters to the Editor: Propylthiouracil hepatotoxicity mimicking autoimmune chronic active hepatitis in a girl. *J. Pediatr. Gastroenterol. Nutr.*, **8**, 547–548

Roulet, M., Laurini, R., Rivier, L., Calame, A. (1988) Hepatic veno-occlusive disease in newborn infant of a woman drinking herbal tea. *Clin. Lab. Observ.*, **112**, 433–436

Shaefer, M. S., Edmunds, A. L., Markin, R. S., Wood, R. P., Pillen, T. J. and Shaw, B. W. Jr. (1990) Hepatic failure associated with imipramine therapy. *Pharmacotherapy*, **10**, 66–69

Inborn errors of metabolism associated with disordered liver function or hepatomegaly

This chapter is assigned to inborn errors of metabolism in which disturbed liver function and structure and/or hepatomegaly or hepatosplenomegaly are an integral part of the disorder. The emphasis will be on features which assist in recognition, diagnosis and treatment with only sufficient biochemical details to assist in diagnosis and to provide a rationale for monitoring therapy. Many highlight the liver's key role in metabolism while glycogen storage diseases and disorders of fat oxidation highlight its capacity to provide energy required by other tissues. Numerically important metabolic disorders with a predominant liver presentation such as alpha-1 antitrypsin deficiency and Wilson's disease are considered elsewhere (see Chapters 17, 18).

All disorders are inherited in an autosomal recessive fashion unless stated otherwise. Prenatal diagnosis is possible for virtually all. For further biochemical, metabolic and genetic details Scriver *et al.* (1989) and Schaub *et al.* (1991) should be consulted. Bone marrow and liver transplantation (see Chapter 25) have revolutionized the outlook for some patients with particular metabolic disorders. With gene therapy in humans a reality, hepatic targeting of functioning genes in experimental animals already achieved and the determination of the DNA sequence of the human genome an achievable goal, the next decade will see exciting developments in the understanding of the pathophysiology and treatment of inherited metabolic disorders affecting the liver.

Presenting clinical and laboratory features

The presenting feature may be asymptomatic hepatomegaly or hepatosplenomegaly, with or with clinical and/or biochemical evidence of disturbed liver function or structure. Clinical syndromes include fetal or neonatal ascites (Table 15.1), hepatitis syndrome in infancy (Chapter 4), acute liver failure with or without early jaundice (Table 15.2 and Chapter 8), cirrhosis (Chapter 13) or neurological dysfunction (Chapters 8, 9). The rate of recovery from coma in response to intravenous glucose helps in differential diagnosis (Table 15.3).

Hypotonia, dysmorphic features or failure to thrive may be prominent features which assist in reaching the correct diagnosis. Acidosis frequently accompanies disorders starting in infancy. It may be due to organic acidaemias, renal tubular lesions or lactic acidosis.

Lactate is produced from glucose during glycolytic energy production and reconverted into glucose in the liver in the Cori cycle. Lactate is also metabolized by muscle and renal cortex. Excessive lactic acid production occurs in many non-genetic conditions which cause tissue hypoperfusion, asphyxia or liver disease as well as in many metabolic

Table 15.1 Metabolic disorders causing foetal or neonatal ascites

GM1 gangliosidosis
Mucopolysaccharidosis VII
Niemann-Pick type C
Gaucher's disease
Wolman's disease
Tyrosinaemia
Salla disease
Sialidosis
Carbohydrate-deficient glycoprotein syndrome

disorders. In identifying the cause the measurement of urinary organic acids by gas chromatography-mass spectrometry (GC-MS) is frequently diagnostic. Simultaneous measurement of blood pyruvate, glucose, ammonia, acetoacetate, 3-hydroxy-butyrate and urinary ketones will often allow a provisional diagnosis which can be confirmed by measuring enzymatic activity. A lactic acid/pyruvate ratio of <25 indicates defective pyruvate dehydrogenase or gluconeogenesis while a ratio of >35 suggests pyruvate carboxylase or a respiratory chain defect or a mitochondrial myopathy. The last two are also suggested by a 3-hydroxy-butyrate/acetoacetate ratio of >2:1.

Congenital or neonatal ascites

Intrauterine, congenital or neonatal ascites may be a presenting feature of metabolic disorders (Table 15.1). Ascites can be caused by haematological disorders, cardiac anomalies including arrhythmias, genitourinary or gastrointestinal malformations. It may occur as part of anasarca in feto-maternal or twin-twin transfusions and with placental anomalies. A metabolic cause is suspected by finding vacuolated lymphocytes in the peripheral blood, storage cells in the bone marrow or increased urinary excretion of

Table 15.2 Liver dysfunction with early jaundice

Galactosaemia
Fructosaemia
Tyrosinaemia
Alpha-1 antitrypsin deficiency
Niemann-Pick type C

Liver dysfunction but with neurological abnormalities occurring before jaundice

Urea cycle defects
Defects in mitochondrial oxidative phosphorylation
  Glutaric aciduria type 2
Deficiencies of:
  succinate:cytochrome reductase
  cytochrome c oxidase
  pyruvate carboxylase
  phosphoenolpyruvate carboxykinase

Table 15.3 Encephalopathy and hepatomegaly

Corrected by glucose infusion
  hyperinsulinism
  Glycogen storage disease I
  Glycogen storage disease III
  Fructose-1,6-diphosphatase deficiency

Not corrected by glucose infusion except in early stages
  Urea cycle defects
  Organic acidaemias
    methylmalonic acidaemia
    propionic acidaemia
    HMG-CoA lyase deficiency
    glutaric aciduria I and II
  Fatty acid oxidation defects

oligosaccharides or sialic acid. Diagnosis is established by lysosomal enzyme assay on peripheral blood leucocytes or cultured fibroblasts, or other specific investigations. The cause of the ascites in metabolic disorders is obscure. Ascites is not clearly related to the severity of liver damage. It may respond to restriction of fluid and salt intake or spironolactone. In severe cases death within the first month of life from pulmonary hypoplasia and ventilatory insufficiency is common.

Glycogen storage diseases

Definition

Glycogen storage diseases (GSD) are disorders in which the concentration and/or molecular structure of glycogen is abnormal in any tissue of the body. The estimated frequency is 1 in 50 000 births. Liver and skeletal muscle are the tissues most severely affected but heart, kidney, bones and brain may be involved. Each disease arises from a deficiency of an enzyme or a transporter involved in the degradation of glycogen by phosphorolysis or hydrolysis.

Classification

The type and severity of the deficiency define the GSD and determine the biochemical and pathological features, including the long-term prognosis and treatment (see Figure 15.1 and Table 15.4). A wide spectrum of clinical severity can occur within each type. The classification, that employed by Hers *et al.* (1989), is simpler than in earlier editions comprising types I to VII. Type VI now includes phosphorylase and phosphorylase kinase deficiencies. Seven different types of phosphorylase b kinase deficiency have been identified. Some were previously categorized as types IX to XII. Undoubtedly even greater genetic heterogeneity and distinct clinical variability will be found. All at present show sufficient similarity to be considered as one group for clinical management. On the other hand it is clear that there are important clinical differences between types Ia and types Ib and Ic. Insufficient patients with types Id and IaSP (stabilizing protein) have been described to assess important differences. In most of these disorders there is excess glycogen but deficient storage can occur. Data at present available indicate that these disorders are inherited in an autosomal recessive fashion, one variant (type III) being possibly X-linked. One form of type VI, in which only liver, leucocytes and erythrocytes are affected, muscle being spared, is inherited in an X-linked fashion.

Biochemistry

Glycogen is formed from glucose postprandially and is broken down during periods of fasting to maintain the blood glucose level within a strict range. The core of the glycogen molecule is glucose units linked in a 1--4 configuration, with branching side chains linked in a 1--6 fashion after every four, 1--4 linkages. A large molecule with a molecular weight of between 6 and 60 million with multiple branches is formed. Glycogen is stored in the cytoplasm primarily in hepatic and muscle cells. It is metabolized also in lysosomes. Liver glycogen is broken down to glucose. Muscle glycogen is metabolized locally as a glycolytic fuel to lactic acid or carbon dioxide and water.

Pathology

The hepatocytes have pale cytoplasm being distended by glycogen and excess fat. The sinusoids are compressed. There may be increased fibrosis and rarely cirrhotic change, particularly in type III GSD, but these changes can also occur in types I and VI. In these types adenomata develop particularly after puberty, especially in types I and III. These appear to be slow growing but can be associated with massive bleeding and alphafetoprotein positive malignant change. Focal glomerulonephritis associated with proteinuria, haematuria, renal calculi and renal failure may be detected from 2 years of age in type I GSD. In type IV GSD the abnormal glycogen is only partially soluble with diastase and there is severe fibrosis with death from cirrhosis or heart failure usually by 3 years of age. Over 80% may have polycystic ovaries.

Clinical and biochemical features

Glycogen storage disorders must be considered in any infant or child (and adult) who presents with hypoglycaemia and hepatomegaly, or with cardiac, muscular or neurological dysfunction. Symptoms may start in the first month of life but are often delayed until the frequency of feeding falls particularly between 1 and 12 months of age but this may be noted in later childhood or, as has been recently recognized, in early adult life (Pears *et*

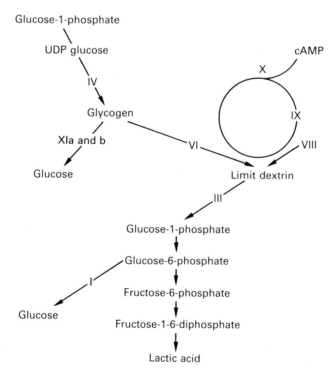

Figure 15.1 Metabolites in glycogen formation and glycolysis. Roman numbers indicate site of action of enzyme which is defective in that glycogenosis. VIII, IX and X represent activating enzymes for phosphorylase and XIa and b, identified disorders

Table 15.4 Hepatic involvement in glycogen storage disease

Type	Hepatomegaly	Splenomegaly	Biopsy	Fibrosis	Cirrhosis	Adenomata (prevalence at 10 years)
I a and b	+	30%	Uniform hepatocellular distension with glycogen except where interrupted by lipid vacuoles. Mosaic appearance due to cellular enlargement with collapse of sinusoids.	+ or −	0	28%
II	+	0	Liver cells are mildly distended with glycogen in membrane-bound vacuoles.	0	0	
III	+	10%	As in Type I.	+	+ or −	10%
IV	+	5%	Pale amphophilic hyaline material in cyotoplasm throughout lobule. It may have a fibrillary birefringent appearance. Cryostat sections stain blue with Lugol's iodine due to amylopectin content.	+	+	
V	0	0	Normal.	0	0	
VI	+	0–20%	Irregular sized hepatocytes with maximal distension by glycogen at periphery of hepatic lobule or as in Type I.	+	0	2%

al., 1992). Exceptionally the disorders occurring in partial form may not be recognized until the sixth decade.

Hypoglycaemia is complicated by hypoinsulinism, hyperglucagonaemia, hyper-cortisolism and raised growth hormone secretion. If it is severe or persistent, convulsions and mental retardation may occur. Virtually all patients have abdominal distension due to the large liver, which may extend to the iliac crest. The liver is typically smooth and may be so soft that it is not detected. There may be a minimal increase in firmness. Surprisingly 7 of 30 patients attending our service with types I, III or VI had splenomegaly. Adiposity with particularly fat cheeks and trunk but with poor muscle bulk in the limbs is a striking feature. From the age of 6 months short stature is evident. In mild cases hypoglycaemic episodes are not prominent and the child presents with abdominal distension and failure to thrive. Epistaxis is common due to platelet dysfunction caused by metabolic derangement. There may be evidence of renal tubular malfunction.

In *type I* glycogen storage diseases there is hepatic, renal, pancreatic or intestinal deficiency of the microsomal enzyme glucose-6-phosphatase (type Ia) or carrier proteins (type Ib: glucose-6-phosphate translocase; type Ic: phosphate/pyrophosphate translocase; or type Id: glucose translocase) or stabilizing protein (type IASP) all resulting in a similar clinical picture except as indicated below.

Clinical features are frequently more severe and persistent than in other predominantly hepatic forms since glucose cannot be formed by glycogenolysis or gluconeogenesis. A recent report has emphasized that sudden unexpected death may occur prior to diagnosis (Burchell *et al.*, 1989). Acidosis, vomiting and diarrhoea are major problems in some patients. Xanthoma may develop in association with high serum triglycerides and cholesterol. Gouty tophi with serum high uric acid are caused by excess production (via the pentose phosphate pathway and ATP depletion) and reduced excretion (competitively inhibited by lactate at the renal tubule). Hypoglycaemia becomes less troublesome with increasing age affecting only six of 41 patients over the age of 10 years in a recent report (Smit *et al.*, 1990) but blood concentrations of triglyceride, cholesterol and uric acid were elevated in 85, 82 and 54% of patients respectively. Serum transaminases at diagnosis are between two and 12 times normal but are within the normal range in 50% of adolescents. Forty-six percent were growth retarded and 97% had hepatomegaly while 28% had hepatic adenomata. Tumour rupture and haemorrhage are potential hazards. Eight of 32 reported cases had malignant change (Conti *et al.*, 1992). Significant renal problems have been emphasized in recent reports (Chen *et al.*, 1988; de Parscau *et al.*, 1989). Proteinuria with an increased glomerular filtration rate affecting 14 of 38 patients at ages ranging from 2 to 30 (median 15) years, leading to renal failure, hypertension, haematuria and renal stones have been reported. Osteoporosis, anaemia and pulmonary hypertension have been reported (Hamaoka *et al.*, 1990). Features of *type Ib* and *c* are similar but recurrent neutropaenia makes the patient very susceptible to bacterial infection. They may have an increased incidence of leukaemia, Crohn's disease or hyperpyrexia (Couper *et al.*, 1991).

In *type III* disease (amylo-1,6-glucosidase deficiency) features are similar to type I but in general less severe except that hepatic fibrosis is much more marked. Cirrhosis may develop. Serum transaminases at diagnosis are between 3 and 40 times normal but are within the normal range in 50% of in adolescents. Muscle involvement including cardiac muscle as evidenced by raised serum creatinine kinase is more prominent. Cardiac involvement is usually asymptomatic but failure and sudden death may occur. Growth retardation, hepatomegaly and hypercholesterolaemia decrease with increasing age. In a study of 50 patients over the age of 10 years 8% had hypoglycaemia, 68% hepatomegaly, 10% hepatic adenomata, with 36% still being growth retarded in spite of catch upgrowth in late childhood. Forty percent had hypercholesterolaemia (Smit *et al.*,1990).

Type IV disease (amylo-1,4 1,6-transglucosidase deficiency), a rarely recognized disorder, is characterized by features of cirrhosis with symptoms usually starting between 3 and 12 months of age, with or without evidence of cardiac or neurological involvement. Death by 3 years of age is usual. Variants with later onset have been reported; an atypical case identified in adult life. I have seen one well characterized case at the age of 12 years with no features except asymptomatic portal hypertension and splenomegaly secondary to cirrhosis. Hepatomegaly present in early infancy had resolved.

Type VI (phosphorylase/phosphorylase b kinase deficiency) is a heterogeneous group comprising at least seven different genetic defects. In general the features are milder than types I and III with normal serum lactate and uric acid. Growth retardation occurred in only four of 43 in the above study although 18 had hepatomegaly and 50% had hypercholesterolaemia. One to two percent develop adenomata and 1% cirrhosis (Hers *et al.*, 1989). Changes in transaminases are similar to those seen in type I.

Diagnosis

The diagnosis of glycogen storage disease is suspected on the basis of the clinical findings. Hypoglycaemia on fasting, lactic acidosis or hyperlipidaemia are supporting evidence. The response to glucagon, glucose or galactose loads may provide further support but since false positive and false negative results occur with all types it is essential to use more specific investigations of glycogen metabolism. In GSD types III and VI erythrocyte glycogen is increased. Specific enzyme defects may be demonstrated in leucocytes in types II, III, IV, and VI. If these investigations are not diagnostic percutaneous liver biopsy essential in type I GSD and possibly muscle biopsy is indicated to obtain tissues for enzymatic or biochemical studies.

The five types of type I are distinguished by kinetic analysis, with and without microsomal disruption, using 2 substrates for glucose-6-phosphatase (Burchell and Gibb, 1991). Prenatal diagnosis is not available for type 1.

Treatment

In all forms the aim of treatment is to maintain the blood sugar within the normal range. This controls symptoms, restores vigour, minimizes secondary metabolic problems and produces a more normal growth rate. Constant glucose absorption, increased at times of excessive utilization is the mainstay of management. This is achieved with small feeds 2–3 hourly, continuous nasogastric feeding at night or uncooked corn starch at 6-hourly intervals. The diet must contain sufficient calories and other nutrients. The intensity of treatment obviously will vary with the severity of the disorder and to some extent with the specific enzymatic defect.

At yearly intervals hepatic ultrasonography and serum alpha-fetoprotein should be performed to monitor for tumours, with urinalysis for renal involvement. Rarely liver (or renal) transplantation may be required.

In *type I* disease a high glucose/glucose polymer intake with continuous nasogastric feeding during sleep affords optimum control. There is a hazard with this mode of treatment in that patients become extremely carbohydrate dependent and have severe, even fatal, hypoglycaemic features at blood sugar concentrations which had previously been well tolerated, the brain having acquired the ability to utilize the high serum lactic acid. It is essential therefore to guarantee a continuous supply of glucose particularly during intercurrent infections with additional carbohydrates before vigorous exercise. It is considered that the blood lactate should be kept elevated at 4–6 mmol/litre to minimize the risk of brain damage. An equally effective and often preferred alternative to nocturnal continuous feeding is to give a 50% suspension of cold, uncooked corn starch in tap water in a dose of 2 g/kg at 4–6 hourly intervals.

Because it is slowly digested it will maintain the blood sugar within the normal range for up to 6 hours. It may produce diarrhoea particularly in infants. Galactose and fructose are omitted from the diet since they aggravate lactic acidaemia. Infants require 8–9 mg glucose/kg/min, toddlers and older children 5–7 mg glucose/kg/min during the day with 5 mg glucose/kg/min at night and adults 3–4 mg glucose/kg/min at night. This can often be achieved with a starch-containing meal late in the evening. It is uncertain what effect the management has on increased intrahepatic fibrosis or the development of adenoma or hepatocellular carcinoma or on renal complications, although with corn starch feeds abnormalities of proximal tubular function are reversed. Anecdotal reports suggest that adenomata do regress with strict dietary management. Allopurinol may occasionally be required for control of hyperuricacidaemia and bicarbonate for acidosis.

In *type III* glycogen storage disease frequent feeds, a high protein diet (since gluconeogenesis is unimpaired) with protein providing 25% of the calories and carbohydrates 50–55% partly in the form of corn starch, will improve hypoglycaemia, growth retardation, myopathic symptoms and reduce liver size. Severe disease may need nasogastric feeding. It is not clear if diet influences intrahepatic fibrosis.

Type IV requires similar but less rigorous treatment to type 1. Galactose and fructose are permitted. Cold, uncooked corn starch is a useful carbohydrate source, minimizing hypoglycaemia (Green *et al.*, 1988b)

In type VI treatment similar to that used in type I has a striking effect on hypotonia in infants and young children but how rigorous treatment needs to be in later childhood is unclear. Although nearly all children grow normally over 50% have hypercholesterolaemia.

Tumours   Strict dietary management should be instituted in all cases if symptomatic and accessible surgical removal is essential. *Liver transplantation* has been reported in types I and IV. In type I it corrects the disorder and promotes growth even in adults (Kirschner *et al.*, 1991). It should be considered in infants or children with very severe disease which cannot be controlled by diet or if there is suspected malignant disease confined to the liver. Its role in those with multiple adenomata, which may be stable for up to 5 years, has not been defined. The response in type IV disease is unpredictable as yet with an apparent beneficial effect on cardiac function in three cases (Selby *et al.*, 1991) but another child transplanted at 9 months of age died of cardiac involvement which became apparent only 6 months after transplantation (Sokal *et al.*, 1992).

Galactosaemia

Galactose derived largely from lactose is rapidly metabolized to glucose through the uridine nucleotide pathway. Several enzymatic steps are required (Figure 15.2). Deficiency of two of these causes a galactose toxicity syndrome with prominent hepatic features.

Galactose-1-phosphate uridyl transferase deficiency

This severe form of galactosaemia is characterized by a cellular deficiency of galactose-1-phosphate uridyl transferase which results, in the majority of patients, in an almost complete inability to metabolize galactose to carbon dioxide. The deficiency is life-long. Several variants have been described in which up to 10% of normal enzymatic activity is

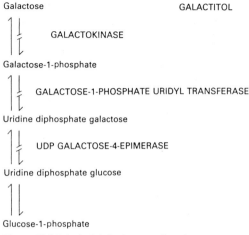

Figure 15.2 Principal defective steps in galactose metabolism (broken arrows) and enzymes deficient in galactosaemic syndromes. Galactitol is an abnormal metabolite produced in excess when galactose accumulates. Hepatic dysfunction occurs only in transferase deficiency

found in the liver and such patients may be able to metabolize limited amounts of galactose. Exposure to galactose causes galactose-1-phosphate accumulation in tissues with a severe toxicity syndrome characterized by inanition, vomiting, diarrhoea, liver disease, failure to thrive, cataracts and mental retardation. Patients die undiagnosed, of Gram-negative sepsis. The reported incidence is from 1 in 18 000 to 1 in 180 000 births. The gene locus is on chromosome 9 p13.

Hepatic pathology and pathogenesis of hepatic lesion

The changes in the liver are distinctive but not pathognomonic. The first feature is marked fatty change and periportal cholangiolar proliferation. By 6 weeks of age there is pseudoacinar transformation of hepatic plates, haemosiderosis with extramedullary haematopoiesis and increasing fibrosis leading to cirrhosis by 3–6 months of age if galactose intake continues. The exact mechanism of hepatic toxicity is unknown. Galactose-1-phosphate accumulates intracellularly restricting the availability of phosphate for high energy bonds. Adenosine 5'-triphosphate (ATP), guanosine 5'-triphosphate (GTP) and cytidine 5'-triphosphate (CTP) concentrations are reduced with severe metabolic derangement in the brain, liver and kidney. Galactose-1-phosphate uridyl transferase deficiency causes hypoglycaemia by decreasing glucose release from glycogen and inhibiting enzymes involved in gluconeogenesis. The high galactose-1-phosphate levels lead by alternate pathways to the production of potentially toxic galactitol, galactonate and galactonolactone. There is no evidence of galactosamine accumulation.

Clinical features

Death from septicaemia within a day or two of ingesting milk occurs in the most severe forms. In slightly less severely affected infants a marked unconjugated hyperbilirubinaemia with haemolysis occurs on the second or third day followed within 1–3 days by a conjugated hyperbilirubinaemia with clinical and biochemical evidence of acute liver failure with hepatomegaly, bleeding diathesis, ascites and renal tubular dysfunction. Increased intracranial pressure may be the presenting feature. The most common presentation is with prolonged neonatal jaundice with failure to thrive, vomiting and a less severe hepatitis. Cirrhosis develops if galactose ingestion continues. The mildest cases present with mental retardation and cataracts and are found to have firm hepatomegaly and abnormal biochemical tests of liver function. Cataracts may be seen on slit-lamp examination as early as 5 days of age. Irreversible brain damage may occur from the effects of hyperbilirubinaemia as well as from the effects of galactosaemia.

Laboratory investigations

Liver function tests are deranged, the blood galactose is elevated and there may be hyperchloraemic acidosis with albuminuria and hyperaminoaciduria. Hypoglycaemia is rare. Glycosuria may be detected for a short period after a galactose load.

Diagnosis

A presumptive diagnosis may be made if the urine gives a positive test with Clinitest tablets but is negative to the Clinistix which detects glucose only. Confirmation of the diagnosis is made by demonstrating absent or <10% of normal enzymatic activity in red blood cells. Transfused red cells may give falsely normal values for 3 months. A presumptive diagnosis may be supported by demonstrating heterozygote levels in the parents.

Treatment and prognosis

For the majority of patients with complete absence of enzymatic activity a galactose-free diet must be maintained for life. Following the institution of the diet there should be a rapid improvement in the infant's condition within 48 hours with regression of the jaundice, gastrointestinal symptoms, bleeding, renal abnormalities and cerebral features unless tissue damage is irreversible. In patients in whom cirrhosis is established it probably does not regress. The majority do improve and have no subsequent hepatic problems. Rarely, decompensated cirrhosis or hepatocellular carcinoma may develop. Cataracts are stabilized and may regress slightly. Brain damage is irreversible.

Dietary control is considered optimum if the erythrocyte galactose-1-phosphate is consistently below 3 mg/dl. Even with excellent control children frequently have lower IQs than their healthy siblings and require intensive teaching to overcome difficulties with language, visual perception and abstract thinking. Speech problems affected 56% of 243 aged more than 3 years (Waggoner *et al.*, 1990). It has been postulated that some of the neurological problems stem from intrauterine brain damage from maternal galactose crossing the placenta. Thus galactose restriction in carrier 'at risk' pregnancies has been advised although there is no evidence of its efficacy. However, a progressive decline in IQ between 3 and 16 years, worse in females, with 45% of 177 in one study being developmentally delayed, and hypotonia, tremor and ataxia developing in late childhood suggests a postnatal factor in the brain damage.

Hypergonadotrophic hypogonadism with high follicle stimulating hormone levels and amenorrhoea affects up to 75% of girls. Normal pregnancies may occur in the others. Growth failure in childhood is more marked in females than males. There is at present no evidence to incriminate age at diagnosis, poor dietary control or high galactose-1-phosphate levels for these complications. The incidence of ovarian dysfunction and neurodevelopmental abnormalities is similar in those diagnosed because of clinical problems or as a result of screening. It has been suggested on the basis of low red cell uridine diphosphate galactose in red cells of treated patients that deficiency of the enzyme product, may be critical but the validity of this observation has been challenged (Kirkman, 1992). Oral administration of uridine or its precursors has been advocated as a useful addition to management but its efficacy is as yet unproved.

Epimerase deficiency galactosaemia

This is a very rare recently recognized disorder. The majority of patients with epimerase deficiency galactosaemia are asymptomatic, being discovered during neonatal screening programmes which detect high blood galactose. In these uridine diphosphate-galactose-4-epimerase deficiency is limited to red blood cells. In a few families a generalized deficiency has been found giving the features of transferase deficiency galactosaemia. Galactose intake is limited to a level which keeps the red cell galactose-1-phosphate normal (1–2 g/day) aiming to provide sufficient galactose to avoid toxicity but enough for essential galactoprotein and galacto-lipid synthesis. There is insufficient experience to assess the efficacy of this therapy.

Fructosaemia

Fructose is widely distributed. The free monosaccharide and sucrose (glucose-fructose disaccharide) are important sources of dietary carbohydrate. Fructose is absorbed at half the rate of other monosaccharides and rapidly metabolized in the liver, small intestine and kidney. It is synthesized *in vivo* from glucose via sorbitol (Figure 15.3).

Three defects in fructose metabolism have been characterized:

(1) fructose-1-phosphate aldolase B deficiency causing hereditary fructose intolerance;
(2) fructose-1, 6-diphosphatase deficiency, a severe disorder of gluconeogenesis;
(3) hepatic fructokinase deficiency, an asymptomatic disorder, previously called benign or essential fructosaemia.

Hereditary fructose intolerance

This disorder is characterized by absence or severely reduced activity of fructose-1-phosphate aldolase B in liver, renal cortex and small intestinal mucosa. More than one genotype may be involved. Exposure to fructose causes vomiting, hepatic and renal dysfunction, neurological abnormalities and behaviour difficulties. The incidence has been estimated at 1:20000 in Switzerland. The disorder is probably underdiagnosed elsewhere.

Hepatic pathology

There may be complete hepatic necrosis. In the typical case biopsied after fructose withdrawal there is diffuse steatosis with necrosis of a few hepatocytes, some of which may show giant cell transformation. ·If fructose ingestion continues, periportal and intralobular fibrosis progresses to cirrhosis. Ultrastructural studies show polymorphic

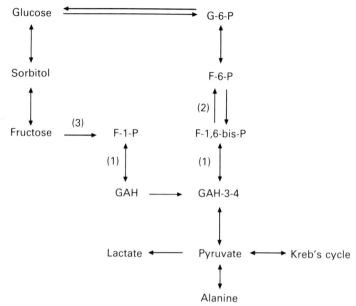

Figure 15.3 The main metabolic pathway of fructose and its interaction with glucose, pyruvate, alanine and the Krebs' cycle are shown. F-1-P = fructose-1-phosphate, F-6-P = fructose-6-phosphate; GAH = glyceraldehyde; GAH-3-4 = dehydroacetone phosphate; F-1,6-bis-P = fructose-1,6-bis-phosphate; G-6-P = glucose-6-phosphate. The numbers in parenthesis indicate the site of action of enzymes which may be deficient: (1) fructose-aldolase; (2) fructose-1,6-bis-phosphatase; (3) fructokinase

cytoplasmic inclusions in both hepatocytes and Kupffer cells. The pathological effects are all secondary to the accumulation of fructose-1-phosphate and ATP depletion. The latter causes high serum Mg^{2+} and uric acid concentrations.

Clinical features

Symptoms start as soon as fructose is ingested. Classically this occurs when breast milk is substituted by a milk containing fructose, sucrose or honey or on weaning. Vomiting is a particularly prominent feature. Poor feeding, failure to thrive, hepatomegaly and spontaneous bleeding are almost universally present in cases presenting in infancy. Many such infants also have pallor, jaundice, drowsiness, irritability, tremor with jerky limb movements and oedema. They may be critically ill with the syndrome of acute liver and renal failure. Convulsions may complicate hypoglycaemia which is typically short-lived. Death may occur.

Older infants and children may show a marked aversion to fructose-containing food but this is slowly learned, and continuous exposure to fructose causes hepatomegaly, abdominal distension and features suggesting a chronic hepatitis, storage disorder or cirrhosis. Behaviour may be very disturbed and development slow. Inadvertent ingestion of large doses of fructose causes acute symptoms such as drowsiness and vomiting and may precipitate fulminant hepatic failure. Thus, fructose intolerance presents as a disorder of extreme variability particularly in early infancy. Differential diagnosis includes pyloric stenosis, hiatus hernia, food intolerance, galactosaemia and other metabolic disorders affecting the liver.

Laboratory findings

Raised serum transaminases, prolonged prothrombin time, hyperaminoacidaemia, hyper-uricacidaemia, hypoalbuminaemia and jaundice occur in the majority of cases. Hypoglycaemia, if present, may be transient. Anaemia, acanthocytosis and thrombocytopenia are frequently present. Serum phosphate and potassium are low. A lactic acidosis is usual. Fructosuria, proteinuria, hyperaminoaciduria and organic aciduria are often found.

Diagnosis

The diagnosis is suggested by the above clinical features in an infant or child with a history of fructose intake. A detailed dietary history is therefore essential. Withdrawal of fructose from the diet causes regression of vomiting almost immediately and thereafter a gradual improvement in the other features unless fulminant liver and/or renal failure has occurred. The diagnosis is subsequently confirmed by demonstrating low enzymatic activity in liver or intestinal mucosal biopsy.

Treatment and prognosis

A fructose-, sucrose- and sorbitol-free diet must be maintained for life. Vitamin C supplements are required. For acute liver failure exchange transfusions, plasma and blood infusions and intravenous glucose may be essential. With the institution of a fructose-free diet hepatomegaly gradually regresses in 50%, liver function tests return to normal over the course of 1 or 2 years and hepatic fibrosis decreases. The hepatic steatosis diminishes but never completely clears. Two of 12 cases with cirrhosis at diagnosis died (Endres, 1988a and b). Hepatoma was reported in a possible adult case (See *et al.*, 1984). Patients or their parents should state their intolerance to fructose on any hospital admission since fructose given in infusion solutions or enterally may cause fatal fulminant hepatic failure.

The structure of the gene and its localization (chromosome 9 q 13–32) and the mutation have been defined in four patients suggesting that antenatal diagnosis should soon be possible. Subsequent siblings should be regarded as suffering from fructosaemia until the diagnosis has been excluded.

Fructose-1,6-diphosphatase deficiency

Fructose-1,6-diphosphatase deficiency is a disorder of gluconeogenesis caused by deficiency or absence of fructose-1,6-diphosphatase in liver, jejunum and kidney. The course is characterized by dramatic life threatening episodes of hypoglycaemia with ketosis. Although there is a degree of fructose intolerance, fasting and/or acute infections rather than fructose ingestion provoke attacks.

Hepatic pathology

The liver is enlarged. Light microscopy shows fatty infiltration with no increase in fibrosis.

Clinical features

Fifty percent of patients present in the newborn period with hypoglycaemia with irritability, convulsions and apnoea or hyperventilation due to severe acidosis. Hypotonia and hepatomegaly are prominent. In older children these may be the main features between episodic exacerbations which are precipitated by fasting, vomiting usually during intercurrent infections or fructose or sucrose ingestion. A similar pattern of features including coma, and convulsions may develop. There is no aversion to fructose-containing foods. Vomiting or failure to thrive is unusual.

Laboratory features

Hypoglycaemia associated with increased gluconeogenic precursors, lactate, ketones, glycerol and amino acids in the blood and urine are the characteristic abnormalities, although ketosis may occur without hypoglycaemia. Liver and renal function tests are normal.

Diagnosis

Diagnosis may be suspected on the basis of the history, the severe hypoglycaemia and ketoacidosis. The main differential diagnoses are other defects of gluconeogenesis or lactic acidosis. Diagnosis is confirmed by demonstrating the specific enzymatic deficiency in a liver biopsy specimen.

Treatment and prognosis

Dietary fructose and sucrose are severely reduced. Acute exacerbations are controlled by intravenous glucose and bicarbonate. Fasting must be avoided. If vomiting occurs, intravenous glucose should be given. Hepatomegaly and hypotonia gradually regress and normal growth and development should occur if there has been no brain damage due to hypoglycaemia. In the majority of case reports the mode of inheritance appears to be autosomal recessive but two families have been reported with parents and children affected. Antenatal diagnosis is at present not possible.

Diabetes mellitus

Hepatomegaly in diabetes occurs both as an acute phenomenon, for example in diabetic ketosis, and also as a chronic abnormality when diabetic control is persistently poor. In acute hyperglycaemia with diabetic ketosis the liver may enlarge so rapidly as to cause abdominal pain, usually attributed to stretching of the liver capsule.

Poor diabetic control and persistent hepatomegaly may be associated with growth retardation. In severe cases, a protuberant abdomen, moon-shaped face and fat deposition on the shoulders and abdomen complete the full *Mauriac syndrome*. With more satisfactory 24-hour-control of diabetes by dietary means and long-acting or twice-daily soluble insulin, this syndrome is now distinctly rare, but is unfortunately not extinct (see Figure 15.4).

It is unclear whether diabetes cause an increased incidence of chronic liver disease although chronic hepatitis may be more common in childhood diabetes (Lorenz and Barenweld, 1979). In adults with fatty infiltration a slowly progressive fibrosis leading to cirrhosis has been described (Nagore and Scheuer, 1988).

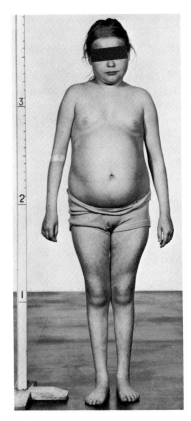

Figure 15.4 Clinical photograph of a patient aged 14 years with Mauriac syndrome. Diabetes mellitus developed at 20 months. Throughout childhood diabetic control had been very difficult with blood sugar levels of from 40 to 500 mg/dl within 24 hours. There is severe growth retardation, massive hepatomegaly (soft liver edge palpable 10 cm below costal margin) and marked obesity. Liver biopsy showed excessive glycogen in all hepatocytes but no other abnormality

Hypertyrosinaemia

Hypertyrosinaemia may occur secondary to acute and chronic liver disease. Neonatal tyrosinaemia is thought to be due to a relative deficiency of *p*-hydroxyphenylpyruvate oxidase. This transient abnormality causes lethargy, poor feeding and jaundice, disordered liver function or hepatomegaly. It may be followed by mental retardation in premature infants. The protein intake should be reduced to 2–3 g/kg/day. Some infants respond to ascorbic acid 100 mg, four times daily.

Two genetically determined forms of hypertyrosinaemia are currently recognized. Type I deficiency is associated with acute and chronic liver disease. The type II characterized deficiency of hepatic tyrosine aminotransferase activity causes corneal and dermal erosions, with hyperkeratosis but no liver disease.

Tyrosinaemia type I (fumaryl acetoacetate hydrolase deficiency, EC 3.7.1.2)

Hereditary tyrosinaemia is due to an inherited defect of fumaryl acetoacetate hydrolase (FAH). The gene has been mapped to chromosome 15 q23–25. Recent studies have shown that disease severity is wider than previously appreciated ranging from acute liver failure with a bleeding diathesis in the first weeks of life to asymptomatic hepatomegaly or rickets in the second decade (Kvittigen, 1991).

The diagnosis should be considered in any child with chronic liver disease or rickets.

Pathology

The liver is large. Hepatocytes show intense fatty infiltration and hepatocellular necrosis in the acute stage. There is gradually increasing intrahepatic fibrosis which progresses to cirrhosis with prominent regeneration nodules. Hepatoma develop in up to 33% of cases surviving beyond two years of age (Weinberg *et al.*, 1976).

Pathogenesis

The pathway of oxidative degradation of tyrosine and phenylalanine and the enzymes involved is given in Figure 15.5. Two tyrosine metabolites, succinylacetone or succinyl acetoacetate (SA) accumulate and are excreted at concentrations more than 100 times normal. The current hypothesis is that renal and liver damage is caused by the accumulation of succinylacetone and its immediate precursors. These metabolites inhibit renal tubular function and porphobilinogen synthetase. There is an increase in Δ-aminolaevulinic acid concentration, giving features of porphyria. Maleyl acetoacetate hydrolase may be decreased as well. There is some experimental evidence that these could cause direct effects on renal tubules and hepatic membranes by interacting with SH-containing compounds. Reduced glutathione reacts with succinyl acetone precursors decreasing glutathione and inhibiting glutathione-dependent detoxicating mechanisms and inhibiting cell growth. What causes the wide range in severity of tyrosinaemia disease is not clear.

Clinical features

The disorder is characterized by progressive hepatocellular damage, coagulopathy, renal tubular dysfunction and hypophosphataemic rickets. There may be a porphyria-like

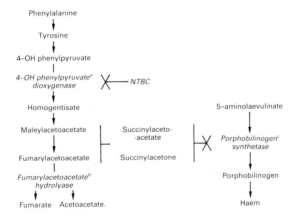

Figure 15.5 Key enzymes[a,b,c] and metabolites of phenylalanine and tyrosine degradation in hereditary tyrosinaemia type I, their interaction with porphyrin synthesis and the site of action of the enzyme inhibitor NTBC (see text). The primary defect is deficiency of enzyme[b], which causes accumulation of succinylacetoacetate and succinylacetone. These inhibit aspects of renal and hepatic metabolism and, by their action on[c], impair porphyrin synthesis which produces porphyric crises. NTBC by inhibiting enzyme[a] greatly reduces synthesis of these toxic products

syndrome, cardiomyopathy and glomerular failure. There is a high propensity to hepatocellular carcinoma.

The disorder has been divided into acute – presenting in the first 6 months of life, subacute – presenting from 6–12 months, and chronic thereafter (van Spronsen *et al.*, in press). Those presenting in the first 2 months of life have a particularly bad prognosis and should be considered separately (see below). The *acute* form presents with severe liver disease with hepatomegaly, oedema, ascites, splenomegaly and a bleeding diathesis with melaena and epistaxis. Jaundice occurs in about one-third of patients. There is failure to thrive, vomiting, diarrhoea and sometimes a cabbage-like odour. Episodes of acute abdominal pain, polyneuropathy and hypertension with intermittent porphyria-like biochemical abnormalities (*porphyria-like syndrome*) occur in up to one-third. Death occurs from liver failure, a bleeding diathesis, sepsis or respiratory failure as part of the porphyria-like syndrome.

The *chronic* form may continue from the acute form or present with features of cirrhosis, renal tubular dysfunction and hypophosphataemic rickets. Hypoglycaemia occurs in both forms of the illness. The Fanconi syndrome which may be severe and complicated by glomerular failure and hypoglycaemia occurs in both forms of the illness. Death in the subacute or chronic forms occurs from porphyria-like syndrome or hepatocellular carcinoma usually developing after 2 years of age. Both acute and chronic forms may occur in the same family.

Laboratory investigations

Standard biochemical tests of liver function are abnormal with decreased albumin and cholesterol and prolonged prothrombin time. Serum alpha-fetoprotein is raised to 1–10,000 times the upper limit of normal. There may be severe hypoglycaemia and hypophosphataemia. Both acidosis and alkalosis may occur. Haematuria, glycosuria and a generalized hyperaminoaciduria is present. Red cell glutathione and plasma cysteine are decreased. There may be a normochromic anaemia with leucocytosis.

Diagnosis

Excessive serum and urinary concentrations of succinylacetone or low activity of fumaryl acetoacetate hydrolase in lymphocytes, fibroblasts or tissues are diagnostic. In rare instances urinary succinylacetone is normal. Note that a sensitive GCMS method is required. It is unstable in urine and low levels are found in severe liver disease. Serum tyrosine may be normal. Note that a low FAH dominantly inherited pseudodeficiency state may be found in lymphocytes, amniocytes and chorionic cells. Plasma tyrosine and phenylalanine are increased with high methionine in the acute form. There is always excessive urinary excretion of other products of tyrosine degradation, of Δ-aminolaevulinic acid and catecholamines. Such changes are non-specific and not diagnostic.

Treatment and prognosis

Dietary restriction of phenylalanine, tyrosine and methionine and liver transplantation have been the mainstays of treatment until 1992. Preliminary results with an inhibitor of tyrosine metabolism proximal to the metabolic defect suggest that the prognosis may be radically improved, delaying the requirement for early transplantation. Oral administration of NTBC (2-(-2-nitro-4-trifluromethyl-benzoyl)-,3-cyclohexanedione) in a dose of 0.1 to 0.6 mg/kg/day in two or three divided doses stops tyrosine degradation by inhibition of the enzyme 4-hydroxy-phenylpyruvate dioxygenase (Lindstedt *et al.*, 1992). Succinylacetone cleared from the serum over a 3-month period. The effect was a marked improvement in liver function with a normalization of the prothrombin time and a fall in serum alpha-fetoprotein to values less than twice normal in four of five patients treated. There was a reduction in liver parenchymal heterogeneity on computed tomography. Renal tubular function improved and the control of rickets became easier. Neurological crises were averted. No side-effects were detected. Tyrosine levels should be between 0.5 and 1 mg/dl. Dietary control must be continued. At present it is too early to know what the full impact of NTBC therapy will be.

Rickets can be controlled by phosphate and vitamin D supplements. Hypoglycaemia, hypopotassaemia, acidosis, alkalosis, ascites and bleeding may all require symptomatic management. These measures improve wellbeing and promote growth for a time but it was not clear, prior to the introduction of NTBC, that they delayed the inevitable progression to liver failure in the acute forms or the development of hepatocellular carcinoma. Whether NTBC will prevent liver cell dysplasia and malignant change is unknown.

It has been suggested that monitoring urinary succinylacetone or Δ-aminolaevulinic acid may be useful in assessing efficacy of dietary treatment. If values are high, consideration should be given to the use of glutathione and drugs like penicillamine which promote inactivation of maleyl acetate and fumaryl acetoacetate.

With the improving results of liver transplantation this form of therapy must be considered for patients with the acute form. In a recent multicentre survey of 108 patients, 83 with acute onset, the risk of early death decreased as the age at onset increased. Of 39 presenting in the first 2 months of life the risk of death within 1 month was 18%, increasing to 31%, 45%, 60% and 70% at 2, 6, 12 and 24 months. Of the 44 presenting at 2–6 months the percentage dying at these ages were 5, 19, 23, 26 and 29. Only one, presenting after 6 months, died by 2 years of age. The authors concluded that in those presenting in the first 2 months liver transplantation should be considered as soon as possible. NTBC used for a minimum period of 3 months would appear to be the best initial treatment for these patients but further observations will be required to determine subsequent optimum management. In patients with a persistently raise alpha-fetoprotein after 3 months on NTBC early transplantation would seem to be desirable. For the chronic form porphyria-like syndrome and hepatocellular carcinoma are the main hazards.

Liver transplantation should be undertaken from 2 years onwards, being delayed only if there is no apparent tumour formation detected by ultrasonography or CT scanning performed at yearly intervals. It is essential that liver transplantation be performed before metastases develop. Note that alpha-fetoprotein levels and imaging appearances cannot distinguish between nodular formation and malignant change within the liver. Computed tomography showing large low attenuation areas was considered suggestive of malignancy in one small series. Hepatoma may occur with normal alpha-fetoprotein levels. Combined liver and renal transplantation (without removing the recipient's kidneys) may be necessary if there is a severe Fanconi syndrome or glomerular failure with a filtration rate of $<60 \, \text{ml/m}^2$.

Prenatal diagnosis   An increased concentration of succinylacetone in amniotic fluid is highly accurate and specific for the disorder. A normal fumaryl acetoacetate hydrolase activity in cultured amniotic cells excludes the diagnosis but a low level is not diagnostic.

Urea cycle disorders

The function of the urea cycle is twofold. It converts nitrogen not required for biosynthetic purposes into urea and thus avoids neurotoxicity due to ammonium and glutamine accumulation. The cycle is also responsible for the synthesis of arginine which becomes an essential amino acid in all defects of the cycle except arginase deficiency. Five enzymatic reactions occur almost exclusively in the liver. Four enzymes operate in a cyclic manner using ornithine as the substrate that is regenerated. A series of enzymatic reactions produce carbamyl phosphate which enters the cycle to combine with ornithine. The other nitrogen atom of urea is derived from aspartate which is condensed with citrulline. Substrates are formed in muscle, kidney, intestine and liver (Figure 15.6).

Neurotoxicity due to accumulation of ammonia and glutamine is the main clinical effect. Treatment of these disorders is now feasible but early diagnosis and effective management of hyperammonaemic episodes are essential to prevent brain damage.

Main urea cycle defects

Four well documented diseases are each caused by defective functioning of one of four enzymes in the urea cycle: deficiencies of carbamyl phosphate synthetase (CPSD), ornithine transcarbamylase (OTCD), argininosuccinic acid synthetase (ASD) and argininosuccinate lyase (ALD). The symptoms and signs of all four are sufficiently similar to be considered together. All show considerable genetic and phenotypic variability with a continuous spectrum of clinical expression. The treatment differs with the disorder and

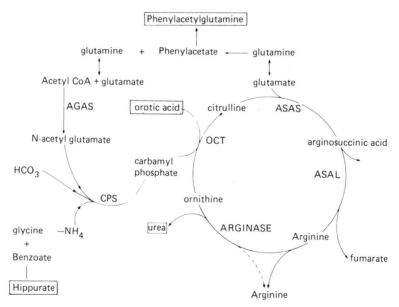

Figure 15.6 The urea cycle. Substrates, intermediates and co-factors required for urea synthesis. Excreted products are within the boxes. The excretion of hippurate and phenylacetylglutamine is increased by drug therapy. AGAS = acetyl glutamate synthetase; CPS = carbamyl phosphate synthetase; OCT = ornithine carbamyl transferase (also called ornithine transcarbamylase); ASAS = argininosuccinic acid synthetase; ASAL = argininosuccinic acid lyase (also called argininosuccinase)

its severity (Table 15.5). OTCD deficiency is inherited as an X-linked disorder. Females heterozygous for this condition have varying degrees of deficiency.

Pathology

The principal abnormalities at autopsy are cerebral, cercbellar and basal ganglia degeneration and atrophy. In experimental animals the initial changes in hyper-ammonaemia are in astrocytes which show swelling with pleomorphic mitochondria. These occur before there are any changes in neurons or their processes. The changes may be mediated by glutamine which is formed from ammonium in astrocytes. Glutamine levels in cerebrospinal fluid may be between 10 and 12 times higher than normal in hyperammonaemic coma. Serum glutamine levels may increase before the onset of coma. Because astrocyte processes are intimately related to cerebral capillaries it is believed that the astrocyte-induced changes in cerebral blood flow cause cerebral oedema and many secondary biochemical and pathological abnormalities. The liver is usually reported as being normal or showing a minimal increase in fat and glycogen with no other histological abnormality. Patients with CPSD or OTCD may have mild hepatic necrosis and portal inflammation. Portal fibrosis has been reported in OTCD and ALD; it is usually mild but may be severe with possible cirrhosis.

Clinical features

Symptoms may start with a lethal episode in the neonatal period or be delayed until late childhood or adult life. Irreversible hyperammonaemic coma may develop at any age but particularly around puberty. Hepatomegaly and raised transaminases indicate hepatic involvement.

The most dramatic presentation occurs in neonates. After appearing normal for 1 to 3 days they develop reluctance to feed, vomiting, lethargy which progresses to coma, often with seizures, hypo- or hyperthermia and hyperventilation. Increased intracranial pressure may be evident. Without ventilatory support cardiorespiratory arrest may occur. Severe hepatomegaly occurs in ALD. Pulmonary, intracranial and gastrointestinal haemorrhage may occur as a terminal event. There may be a history of consanguinity or neonatal deaths in the sibship or close male relatives.

The late onset group includes girls with OTCD in whom the mutant allele is expressed in the majority of hepatocytes. Symptoms may appear in later infancy, early childhood or even adult life. The onset may be related to intercurrent infection or high protein meal or may occur for no obvious reason. The classic features are episodic vomiting with neurological dysfunction. This may take the form of lethargy, irritability, agitation, combative behaviour, drowsiness, disorientation, bizarre conduct, slurred speech, visual defects, ataxia and coma. Seizures may occur. There may be features of increased intracranial pressure. Ataxia is particularly prominent in 2–5 year olds; language and behaviour problems at puberty and in adult life. There may be delayed physical growth and development. The patient may select a relatively low protein intake. The only phenotypic difference is that ALD and ASD may be associated with trichorexis nodosa.

Diagnosis

Hyperammonaemia is a characteristic feature of defects of the urea cycle. Contrary to earlier reports frequently there is no acidosis at presentation (Bachmann, 1992). Urinary organic acids should be measured to exclude organic acidurias. The degree of

Table 15.5 Urea cycle disorders

Disorder	Tissue diagnosis	Age at onset	Diet and drug therapy (g/kg/day)					
			Deitary protein	Essential amino acids	Citrulline	Arginine	Sodium benzoate	Sodium phenylacetate
N-acetyl glutamate synthetase deficiency	Liver	Neonatal	2.0[a]			0.7		
Carbamyl phosphate synthetase deficiency (CPSD)	Liver	Neonatal, Weaning	0.6	0.6	0.18	0.7	0.25	0.25
Ornithine carbamyl transferase deficiency (OTCD)	Liver	Neonatal (males), Infancy and childhood, Neonatal–9 years (females)	0.6	0.6	0.18	0.7	0.25	0.25
Argininsuccinic acid synthetase deficiency (ASD)	Fibroblasts	Neonatal, 1–12 months, 1–48 years	1.2–1.5			0.4–0.7	0.25	0.25
Argininsuccinate lyase deficiency (ALD)	Erythrocytes	Neonatal, 6 months–12 years	1.2–1.5			0.4–0.7		
Arginase deficiency	Erythrocytes		0.5				0.25	

[a] Carbamyl glutamate 1–3 mmol/kg/day

hyperammonaemia varies with the severity of the defect and with protein intake. Values of 20 to 30 times the upper limit are typical with neonatal onset; more than twice normal in the older infant and toddler and twice normal in older children.

Intercurrent infection, operations and anaesthesia may aggravate hyperammonaemia. Serum concentrations of ornithine, citrulline and arginosuccinic acid define the site of the defect in most cases. Citrulline levels exceed 1000 μmol/litre in ASD and are between 100–300 μmol/litre in ALD and are very low or undetectable in OTCD and CPSD (normal 10–20 μmol/litre) in cases with neonatal onset. With the late onset forms of OTCD and CPSD there may be no diagnostic amino acid abnormality. Arginosuccinic acid concentration is high in ALD. Orotic aciduria increases from diversion of carbamyl phosphate to pyrimidine in OTCD, ASD and ALD. The diagnosis may be confirmed, after the patient's clinical condition has been stabilized, by measuring the specific enzymatic activity in a percutaneous liver biopsy in CPSD and OTCD or in fibroblasts in the others.

Glutamine, alanine and aspartate concentrations in the serum may also be elevated. In neonates urea may be as low as 2 mmol/litre but usually urea concentration in blood and urinary urea excretion is normal, urea being produced by the accumulation of substrate proximal to the block and from arginine (except in arginase deficiency). Serum aminotransferase concentrations are usually high during acute episodes and may remain elevated between attacks. The prothrombin time may be markedly prolonged. Orotic acid excretion may be increased. Respiratory alkalosis is transiently present in acute exacerbations.

If hyperammoniaemia is recognised the main *differential diagnosis* in the newborn period is transient hyperammonaemia of the newborn which occurs particularly in premature infants due to a deficiency of intracellular ATP, and pyruvate dehydrogenase deficiency or glutaric acidaemia type II, methyl malonic acidaemia and propionic acidaemia.

With the late onset forms a wider differential diagnosis must be considered. This includes an increasing range of organic acidurias, e.g. fatty acid acyl CoA dehydrogenase deficiencies and isovaleric acidaemia. Lysinuric protein intolerance must also be considered. Acute hepatic necrosis or Reye's syndrome are to be suspected if there is a prolonged prothrombin time or hypoglycaemia.

In achieving a diagnosis it is often essential to obtain at presentation plasma and urine specimens in which to measure plasma pH, bicarbonate, amino acids, urinary orotic acid and organic acids by gas chromatography-mass spectroscopy.

Treatment

The aim of treatment is to allow normal growth and development while avoiding or rapidly controlling episodes of hyperammonaemic encephalopathy. The immediate objectives are to reduce concentrations of ammonia and glutamine to normal, to decrease the need for urea formation and to prevent arginine deficiency. Such treatment can only be achieved with rigorous dietetic control with careful monitoring of the concentrations of serum amino acids and ammonia. A normal plasma glutamine may be the best single indication of effective treatment since serum concentrations increase before ammonium levels. Urinary orotic acid excretion should be normal in OTCD heterozygotes.

Exact details of management will vary from case to case. The mainstay of chronic management is to provide just sufficient protein for growth and development and to promote excretion of waste nitrogen by alternate pathways. It may be necessary to restrict protein intake to essential amino acids only. Keto analogues of amino acids have been used in an effort to decrease further the protein load but are bitter and poorly tolerated. Sufficient calories must be provided in the form of carbohydrates. Two agents which cause increased urinary nitrogen excretion are helpful in controlling acute hyperammonaemic crises and in preventing hyperammonaemia. Sodium benzoate combines with glycine to form hippurate and phenylacetate combines with glutamate to form phenylacetylglutamine, both conjugates being excreted in the urine. The latter is the more efficient pathway provided the capacity of the liver and kidney to form phenylacetylglutamine is not exceeded. Both agents are potentially toxic and have to be used with care, particularly in the presence of renal failure. It is important to appreciate that as growth slows protein accretion declines, causing a decrease in protein tolerance.

Acute exacerbations with hyperammonaemic coma occur unpredictably as well as with intercurrent infections, surgery or anaesthesia. These are treated with infusions of glucose and lipids, arginine (10% in 10% glucose:2 ml/kg and (except in ALD) benzoate and phenylacetate (250 mg/kg of each in 35 ml 10% glucose over 90 minutes initially and then over 6 hours). If ammonia is greater than 400 μmol/litre removal of ammonia by haemodialysis or exchange transfusion is necessary. These are much more efficient than peritoneal dialysis or haemofiltration. Ventilatory support is usually necessary. With such management even severe cases may survive through the first year of life. Therapy is highly effective in ASD but in ALD brain damage may occur. With neonatal onset of OTCD and CPSD many infants are mentally retarded. Even with intensive prospective treatment in cases diagnosed antenatally, with no protein intake in the first 48 hours and measures as described above to prevent hyperammonaemia, six of 11 died, three with OTCD are well after liver transplantation at 1–4 years of age, while 2 with CPSD on medical treatment are handicapped (Maestri et al., 1991). Orthotopic liver transplantation (OLT) has been reported in OTCD (six), CPSD (two) and ASD (one) with six being well (Todo et al., 1992). OLT should be considered in the neonatal period in CPSD but medical therapy for 12–24 months may minimize its risk in OTCD. Cases of later onset have a better prognosis. In patients in whom dietary management proves ineffective liver transplantation should be considered. Note that following OLT serum amino acid concentrations may remain slightly abnormal but hyperammoniaemia ceases.

Arginase deficiency

Arginase deficiency is a rare disorder characterized by progressive spastic paraplegia, seizures and mental retardation. There is hyperammonaemia, hyperargininaemia, diaminoaciduria and orotic aciduria. Treatment with a reduced amino acid intake and diversion of nitrogen from urea genesis by sodium benzoate and phenylacetate may be beneficial.

N-Acetylglutamate synthetase deficiency

N-Acetylglutamate synthetase deficiency was described in a single asymptomatic neonate with hyperammonaemia. Two siblings had died in the neonatal period. Treatment with carbamyl glutamate controlled the hyperammonaemia.

Genetic counselling for urea cycle defects

Where enzyme deficiency can be detected in fibroblasts, antenatal diagnosis by amniocentesis has been achieved. Techniques for identification of distinct restriction fragment length polymorphism have been employed in the diagnosis of CPSD, OTCD and arginase deficiency. The prognosis is difficult to establish for female OTCD hetero-zygotes. Enzyme activity in fetal liver biopsies has given useful information in some families.

Rare disorders with hyperammonaemia and disturbed amino acid metabolism
(Table 15.6)

Familial protein intolerance (lysinuric protein intolerance)

This disorder appears to be due to a genetically determined defect in the transport of basic amino acids, lysine and arginine. There is both a defect in intestinal absorption and increased renal losses. The enzymatic abnormality underlying this defect has not been identified. There is a secondary failure of the urea cycle due to lack of essential substrate amino acids. Pathological changes are limited to the liver in which there is some lymphocyte and macrophage infiltrate in the portal tract with increased fibrosis. In the second decade this progresses to early cirrhosis.

Clinical features are vomiting and diarrhoea which start when protein intake increases when breast feeding is supplemented. An aversion to protein-rich foods develops around the age of 1 year. There is growth failure, hepatomegaly and splenomegaly, hypotonia and sparse hair. The limbs are very thin, the torso relatively stocky with adequate subcutaneous fat. There may be mental retardation. With high protein intakes there may be psychotic behaviour, abdominal pain and coma. Osteoporosis occurs due to lysine deficiency. Interstitial pneumonia may develop.

The blood ammonia is normal when fasting but increases to above normal with moderate amounts of protein. Urinary orotic acid is high reflecting urea cycle failure. The blood urea is typically low. Serum lysine, arginine and ornithine are low while alanine and citrulline are high. There is excessive lysine and arginine in the urine.

Treatment consists of a low protein intake (<1.5 g/kg in children, 0.8 g/kg in adults), with 2.5–8.5 g (14–48 mmol) as citrulline. The citrulline guarantees adequate urea cycle intermediates for urea formation. Hyperammonaemic crises require treatment with protein withdrawal and intravenous glucose.

Table 15.6 Disorders causing hyperammonaemia

Liver failure	Transient hyperammonaemia of the newborn
Reye's syndrome	Lysinuric protein intolerance
Urea cycle disorders	Hyperammonaemia ⎫
	Hyperornithinaemia ⎬ syndrome
	Hypercitrullinaemia ⎭
	Homocitrullinuria

+ *hypoglycaemia*

Pyruvate carboxylase deficiency
Multiple carboxylase deficiency
Methylmalonic acidaemia
Glutaric aciduria type I and II
HMG-CoA lyase deficiency
Proprionic acidaemia
Dicarboxylic acidurias
Carnitine deficiency
Glutaric aciduria Type II

Hyperornithinaemia, hyperammonaemia, homocitrullinuria syndrome

An enlarged liver with bizarre elongated mitochondria containing crystalloid structures has been described in patients with hyperornithinaemia, hyperammonaemia and homocitrullinuria syndrome.

The underlying defect(s) has not been identified. There is thought to be a defect in transport of ornithine into mitochondria. The syndrome which has a wide range of clinical severity is characterized by intermittent postprandial hyperammonaemia and mental retardation. Symptoms may start in the neonatal period or in adult life. Treatment is by dietary protein restriction.

Mitochondrial defects in fatty acid β-oxidation

Fatty acid oxidation in mitochondria is a major energy source during fasting. The process preserves glucose for tissue such as the brain for which it is an obligatory fuel. Fatty acids liberated from adipose tissues are taken from the circulation by the liver and metabolized in the cytoplasm to acyl-CoA esters. These cross the mitochondrial membrane as carnitine esters. Within the mitochondria nine enzymes have been identified as participating in their oxidation to carbon dioxide and ketones. In the last decade a series of disorders of the fatty acid beta-oxidation pathway have been described. These are characterized by hypoglycae-

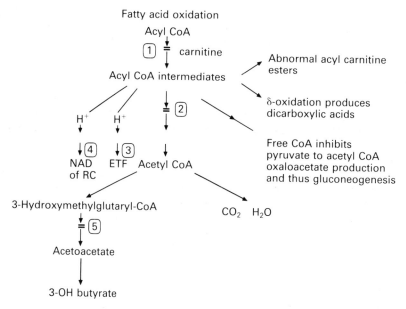

Figure 15.7 Diagrammatic representation of the major metabolic steps in the oxidation within mitochondria of fatty acids to carbon dioxide and ketones. The enzyme complexes in which function may be defective are indicated numerically. (1) Carnitine palmitoyl transferases I and II. (2) Defect of fatty acid chain-length-specific acyl-CoA dehydrogenase or enzymes of fatty acid oxidation spiral. (3) Electron transfer flavoprotein cycle. (4) NAD complexes in respiratory chain. (5) 3 hydroxy-3-methylglutaryl CoA lyase deficiency. Byproducts of major clinical or diagnostic importance which accumulate when oxidation is impaired are shown on the upper right

mia with inappropriately low ketone production during episodes of vomiting and lethargy or more severe coma. Hyperammonaemia, prolongation of the prothrombin time and raised serum transaminases are usual during these episodes. There is fat accumulation in hepatocytes and in some instances myopathy (Bartlett *et al.*, 1991).

Acyl-CoA dehydrogenase deficiencies

A series of chain-length specific acyl-CoA dehydrogenases are responsible for initiating a complex cycle of oxidative reactions which remove two carbon atoms from fatty acid acyl-CoA esters in mitochondria. Acetyl-CoA is produced and the chainshortened acyl-CoA re-enters the oxidation cycle. Electron transfer flavoproteins are necessary to complete this process, transferring electrons to the electron transport chain.

Three forms of Acyl-CoA dehydrogenase deficiency have been characterized with different but overlapping chain-length specificities; these are respectively long chain (LCAD), medium chain (MCAD), and short chain (SCAD). MCAD is the most common. Fatty acids proximal to the metabolic block accumulate and are excreted in the urine as their acylcarnitine derivatives, dicarboxylic acids, hydroxy acids and glycine conjugates. Excretion may be episodic. Deficiency of the electron transfer flavoproteins cause difficulties in metabolizing all chain lengths.

Pathology

Hepatic light microscopy findings are microvesicular or macrovesicular fatty infiltration. Minimal ultrastructural changes are seen in mitochondria. Cerebral oedema is found at post mortem in most cases. Cardiomegaly may be found in LCAD.

Clinical features

The clinical features are episodic. The onset is usually between 2 and 48 months of age, when the feeding frequency has decreased sufficiently for the infant to utilize fat stores. Precipitating factors are infection and starvation. The child presents with vomiting and lethargy which may proceed to coma. There may be a previous history of recurrent episodes of coma, convulsions or Reye's syndrome or a family history of sudden infant death syndrome or Reye's syndrome. The liver may be enlarged. There is a prompt response to intravenous 10% dextrose unless cerebral oedema has developed.

LCAD, SCAD and defects of electron transport flavoproteins usually present by 6 months of life with features like MCAD but in addition a chronic cardiomyopathy, muscle weakness and developmental delay are prominent features. Cardiorespiratory arrest may occur.

Laboratory findings

During acute episodes the blood sugar is usually low but may be at the lower end of the normal range. Urinary ketones are inappropriately low. Serum transaminase and blood ammonium values are raised up to five times normal. The prothrombin time may be prolonged. Plasma carnitine is low. The ratio of free fatty acids to 3-hydroxybutyrate is elevated. The serum creatinine phosphokinase is normal in MCAD but raised in the other disorders.

The diagnosis is suspected when acylcarnitine derivatives appropriate for the metabolic block are detected as dicarboxylic acids by gas-liquid chromatography–mass spectroscopy. It has to be emphasized that the excretion may only occur when the patient is symptomatic. Other disorders and ingestion of medium chain triglyceride supplements can give the same derivatives.

When the patient is well, high plasma concentrations of *cis*-4-decanoic acid support the diagnosis of MCAD deficiency; DNA analysis will detect the mutation causing the majority of cases. The diagnosis is confirmed by specific enzyme studies in fibroblasts.

Treatment

MCAD   Acute episodes require treatment with intravenous 15–20% glucose and the management of coma associated with increased intracranial pressure (Chapters 8, 9). To prevent recurrences it is essential to give glucose intravenously during episodes of vomiting or starvation. In most patients it is essential to take food more frequently than 8 hourly. The dietary fat should be restricted to 20% of the calorie requirements. Considerable clinical heterogeneity exist; some will need to feed more frequently, others will be able to fast for longer. Dietary supplements with medium chain triglycerides or intravenous fat emulsions must be avoided. Sodium valproate is contraindicated since it may further inhibit mitochondrial function. Carnitine supplements, 25 mg/kg, three to four times daily may help.

LCAD   The treatment is similar to MCAD but medium chain triglycerides can be a useful energy source. Nasogastric tube feeding may be required because of hypotonia.

SCAD   The management is as for MCAD. Infants with a defect in the flavoprotein electron transfer cycle respond to riboflavin in a dose of 100 mg twice daily and a low fat intake. Carnitine may exacerbate the disorder.

Carnitine palmitoyl transferase deficiency

Palmitoyl CoA combines with carnitine in the presence of carnitine palmitoyl transferase (CPT) allowing palmitoyl carnitine to traverse the mitochondrial membrane. CPT-1 deficiency is usually reported as presenting with features of Reye's syndrome with coma, moderate hepatomegaly and massive lipid accumulation in hepatocytes with or without hypoglycaemia. Free fatty acids are high. There is reduced ketone production. Serum carnitine levels may be elevated. Total hepatic carnitine concentration is normal. The transaminases may be elevated and a metabolic acidosis is usual. C10 and C12 dicarboxylic acids may be detected in urine. In one family the features were of hypotonia and progressive hepatic fibrosis and death from liver failure and alimentary bleeding by 5 years of age. CPT activity in liver and fibroblasts is undetectable. The onset is in the first year of life. A low fat diet with medium chain triglyceride supplements correct the metabolic consequences of this deficiency state.

Systemic carnitine deficiency

Systemic carnitine deficiency is characterized by low serum, urinary and tissue carnitine. It is associated with episodic hepatic and cerebral dysfunction, underdeveloped muscles and sometimes cardiomyopathy. Symptoms start between 2 months and 4 years.

Carnitine is synthesized predominantly in the liver. It is not known whether carnitine deficiency can result from a failure in synthesis. There is good evidence for a failure of renal reabsorption in this disorder with in one case excessive faecal losses suggesting a failure in intestinal transport (Sholte *et al.*, 1990). Secondary carnitine insufficiency which occurs in many organic acidurias, but usually is associated with an increased or normal excretion of acyl carnitine, is more common.

Hepatic features during acute exacerbations are those of Reye's syndrome with markedly elevated transaminases and blood ammonia, prolonged prothrombin time and hypoglycaemia with macrovesicular lipid accumulation in the hepatocytes. There is no ketosis but dicarboxylic acid excretion is increased. Diagnosis is indicated by a low free carnitine and decreased acyl carnitine concentrations in plasma and urine. Diagnosis is confirmed by a low carnitine concentration in liver and muscle tissue after some months of carnitine supplementation. Symptomatic episodes can be prevented by carnitine administration in a dose sufficient to prevent dicarboxylic aciduria. A dose of 1–4 g/day is usually required. Biotin 0.5 mg daily is also helpful.

Recurrent familial Reye-like syndrome

Five of 13 siblings suffered from recurrent Reye-like syndrome with abdominal pain. During these episodes there was evidence of an unusual disturbance of amino acid and organic acid metabolism as well as defective fatty acid oxidation (Elpeleg *et al.*, 1990).

Dicarboxylic aciduria with progressive liver disease

A few children with fatty infiltration and chronic active hepatitis progressing to cirrhosis have been found to excrete abnormal amounts of fatty acid metabolites particularly 3-hydroxysebacic acid. Some appear to have improved with a low fat diet (Pollitt *et al.*, 1987, and unpublished observations).

Defects in mitochondrial oxidative phosphorylation

Mitochondrial oxidative phosphorylation transfers energy from oxidation of fuel molecules into ATP. In this process the mitochondrial respiratory chain, a series of multi-protein complexes on the inner mitochondrial membrane, couples oxidative electron transport with the production of ATP. The complexes involved include flavoproteins, cytochromes, ubiquinone, iron-sulphur proteins and protein bound copper. Some of the proteins are encoded by nuclear genes others by mitochondrial genes. Genetic defects may cause any symptom in any organ at any age! (Munnich *et al.*, 1992). This includes fatal hepatocellular deficiency with panlobular fatty infiltration and lactic acidosis (Parrot-Roulaud *et al.*, 1991). Diagnostic clues are a lactate/pyruvate molar ratio >20 and ketoacidosis. Confirmation requires enzymatic activity estimation in tissues. Any mode of inheritance can be observed.

Glutaric acidaemia type II

Glutaric acidaemia type II, although the best characterized of these defects, has considerable clinical and genetic heterogeneity. In most cases there is a defect in a flavoprotein or a flavoprotein:ubiquinone oxidoreductase. The form with neonatal onset occurs with or without multiple congenital anomalies.

With neonatal onset hypotonia, hepatomegaly, severe hypoglycaemia, metabolic acidosis and a smell of sweaty feet are characteristic. There may be huge kidneys, facial dysmorphism, rocker bottom feet, genital anomalies and defects in the anterior abdominal wall. Most die in the first week of life but some may survive a few months to die of cardiomyopathy. With later onset there may be a history of neonatal hypoglycaemia, recurrent Reye's syndrome, proximal myopathy or features like glycogen storage disease type I.

Typical investigation findings are severe hypoglycaemia without ketonuria, mild or moderate hyperammonaemia, and metabolic acidosis in the neonatal period. In later life there are acute episodes with abnormal liver function tests, prolonged prothrombin time and cardiomyopathy. Plasma lactic acid is usually elevated. Renal cysts may be seen on ultrasound or CT. Gas chromatography-mass spectrometry demonstration of 2-hydroxy-glutaric in urine clinches the diagnosis. Deficiency of enzymes in fibroblasts, amniocytes or tissues can be demonstrated. High glutaric acid concentrations in amniotic fluid also allow prenatal diagnosis. Treatment of late onset or mild cases with a diet low in protein and fat, oral riboflavin (100–300 mg/day), oral carnitine (100–200 mg/kg/day in four doses) should be tried. In acute exacerbations intravenous carnitine 30 mg/kg as a bolus and repeated in 24 hours may help.

Rare disorders with no effective treatment as yet

Defective activity of succinate:cytochrome c reductase

A hepatitis syndrome with persistent vomiting, hypoglycaemia, coagulopathy, hyper-ammonaemia, lactic acidosis and renal insufficiency failure leading to death at 3 months of age has been described with defective activity of succinate:cytochrome c reductase (Vilaseca et al., 1991).

Cytochrome c oxidase deficiency

Cytochrome c oxidase deficiency may produce liver failure in infancy associated with recurrent apnoea and severe metabolic acidosis with ketosis. The diagnosis is suspected by demonstrating ketonuria with a lactate/pyruvate molar ratio of more than 20 and a 3-hydroxybutyrate/acetoacetate molar ratio of 2 or more. Liver biopsy shows a panlobular steatosis with no cytolysis, inflammation or fibrosis. Symptoms start immediately after birth. Death may occur by 4 months of age, although survival to 19 months and early childhood has been reported (Cormier et al., 1991).

Pyruvate carboxylase deficiency

Pyruvate carboxylase is an intramitochondrial enzyme with a key regulatory role in gluconeogenesis in the liver. In astrocytes it stimulates glutamine and gamma-aminobutyric acid synthesis while in neurons it stimulates myelin formation. It is totally acetyl CoA dependent. The deficiency may be limited to the brain causing Leigh's disease with lactic acidaemia but if generalized also causes hyperammonaemia, with high citrulline, lysine, alanine and proline. The liver is enlarged with lipid accumulation in hepatocytes, hyperplasia of the endoplasmic reticulum and abnormal mitochondria. Death by 3 months of age is usual. Prenatal diagnosis is possible.

Phosphoenolpyruvate carboxykinase deficiency

Phosphoenolpyruvate carboxykinase converts oxaloacetic acid formed from pyruvate to phosphoenolpyruvate from which glucose is formed. In the deficiency state lactic acidosis, hypotonia and failure to thrive are associated with hepatomegaly, hyperammonaemia and raised serum transaminases. There is hepatic steatosis which may be very marked. There may be hepatic fibrosis. The disorder is aggravated by fasting. An infant with progressive liver dysfunction leading to death from liver failure by 1 year of age is now thought to have had a more generalized defect of mitochondrial function (Clayton, 1991).

Defects in the metabolism of essential branched chain amino acids

These may give rise to episodic illnesses mimicking Reye's syndrome or chronic hepatic features.

3-Hydroxy-3-methylglutaryl-CoA lyase deficiency

3-Hydroxy-3-methylglutaric (HMG) aciduria is a disorder of leucine metabolism and ketone biosynthesis from fatty acid oxidation caused by HMG-CoA lyase deficiency. Severe acidosis, vomiting, lethargy and hypotonia occurring with periodic exacerbations are the main features: 90% are hypoglycaemic but not ketotic; 50% have hyperammoniaemia, hepatomegaly due to fatty infiltration and/or raised transaminases. Some have features of Reye's syndrome. Presentation is usually between 3 and 12 months but it may be in the first week of life or in the second year.

Diagnosis is established by finding high concentrations of 3-hydroxy-3-methylglutaric acid in the urine or demonstrating HMG-CoA lyase deficiency in white blood cells or fibroblasts.

Treatment   A high carbohydrate diet with fat providing only 25% of calories and protein restricted to <2 g/kg/day and intravenous glucose during periods of unavoidable fasting allows normal development. Prenatal diagnosis by chorionic villus biopsy is possible (Chalmers et al., 1989).

Mevalonic aciduria

Mevalonic aciduria is a recently described heterogeneous disorder due to deficiency of mevalonic acid 5-phosphate kinase. Hepatosplenomegaly, anaemia, enteropathy and failure to thrive are common features. The cholesterol may be low. Diagnosis is made by finding large amounts of mevalonic acid in the urine or by enzymatic analysis. There is no established treatment.

Disorders of propionate and methylmalonate metabolism

Disturbed acid-base balance and developmental failure are the main features of these disorders of catabolism of lipids and protein. Some have major hepatic features.

Propionic acidaemias

This is a heterogeneous group of related disorders caused by defective enzymatic carboxylation of propionyl-CoA, a product of catabolism of essential amino acids, odd-chain fatty acids and cholesterol. Biotin is a co-enzyme for the pathway. Patients usually present in the newborn period with severe metabolic acidosis, refusal to feed, vomiting, lethargy, hypotonia and hepatomegaly. Relapses are precipitated by intercurrent infection, excessive protein intake or constipation. Patients may present later with episodic ketoacidosis, developmental delay or seizures. Leucopenia and thrombocytopenia occur frequently. *Diagnosis* is established by high propionic acid concentrations in blood or urine or enzymatically in leucocytes or fibroblast.

Treatment   A diet low in propionic acid precursors and oral L-carnitine seems to be the best management but some disorders are helped by biotin. Constipation should be avoided.

Methylmalonic acidaemia

This disorder is caused by one of four genetic deficiencies of the mitochondrial matrix enzyme methylmalonyl coenzyme A (CoA) mutase which catalyses the conversion of methylmalonyl CoA to succinyl CoA. Adenosylcobalamin is an essential co-factor. *Clinical features* are failure to thrive, vomiting, acidosis (usually with ketosis), hypotonia, mental retardation, anaemia, leucopenia and thrombocytopenia starting in the neonatal period or infancy. There is an increased susceptibility to infection. *Hepatic manifestations* are rapid changes in liver size due to microvesicular fat accumulation, hyperammonaemia, hypoglycaemia and raised transaminases. The *diagnosis* is suspected on the basis of the clinical features and the presence of ketosis and acidosis. It is established by demonstrating the typical urinary methylmalonic excretion by gas-liquid chromatography and confirmed by specific enzyme determination in fibroblasts. The mainstays of *treatment* are protein restriction with L-carnitine supplements and intramuscular cyanocobalamin during hyperammonaemic crises. The response varies from early death to survival in health through to 14 years of age depending on the genetic type. Those with early onset need closely supervised care if mental impairment is to be avoided. Prenatal diagnosis by methylmalonic determination in amniotic fluid or enzyme levels in amniotic cells has been accomplished.

Defects in lysine oxidation

Glutaric acidaemia type I

This is a defect in lysine oxidation caused by deficiency of glutaryl-CoA dehydrogenase which is characterized clinically by dystonia, dyskinesia and acute attacks of Reye's syndrome features. Episodes of unexplained high fever are frequent. The onset is within the first 2 years of life with slow progression to death during the first decade.

   Diagnosis is established by low enzymatic activity in leucocytes of fibroblasts or the finding of 3-hydroxyglutaric acid in the urine during acute exacerbations. *Treatment* with a low protein diet, riboflavin 200–300 mg/day, and rapid correction of hypoglycaemia and acidosis during intercurrent infections may minimize the neurological features but there is no good evidence as yet that the eventual outcome is improved.

Bile salt metabolism

Bile acids are synthesized in the liver. The major pathway of primary bile acid synthesis involves at least twenty-nine different intermediates and more than 15 enzymes which modify the cholesterol nucleus or side chains. All of the reactions occur in liver mitochondria except for the steps after C26 hydroxylation which occur in peroxisomes and are thus defective in Zellweger's disease and related peroxisomal disorders. Clinically relevant intermediates and enzymatic steps are shown in Figure 15.7. The microsomal cholesterol 7α-hydroxylase responsible for the first reaction is subjected to a negative feedback regulation by primary bile acids, chenodeoxycholic acid and cholic acid, reabsorbed from the gut. In the adult it is considered that side chain oxidation and hydroxylation which reduces the steroid from a C27 sterol to a C24 bile acid occurs only after the nucleus has been modified.

In an alternative pathway 7α-hydroxy-4-cholesten-3-one may undergo 26 hydroxylation to form 7α,26-dihydroxy-4-cholesten-3-one, which can be metabolized to chenodeoxycholic acid. In another alternative pathway for side chain oxidation 5-cholestane-3α,7α, 12α triol may be 25-hydroxylated by a microsomal 25-hydroxylase to yield 5-cholestane-3α, 7α, 12α, 25-tetrol. This compound may be metabolized to cholic acid. This pathway is particularly active when there is a defect in 26-hydroxylation as occurs in the autosomal recessive disorder cerebrotendinous xanthomatosis.

Defects in bile acid synthesis

Defects in bile acid synthesis are thought to have two important pathophysiological sequelae: deficiency of primary bile acids which reduces bile production and flow and causes malabsorption; the putative toxic effect of metabolites of bile acid intermediates proximal to the defect. Their production is accelerated by loss of primary bile acid feedback inhibition of cholesterol 7α-hydrolase.

The application of quantitative gas chromatography-mass spectrometry fast atom bombardment mass spectrometry techniques to urine, plasma and bile has since 1987 defined two distinct inborn errors of bile acid metabolism associated with liver disease. Both can be helped with oral primary bile salts. More remain to be characterized (Clayton, 1991; Setchell et al., 1992).

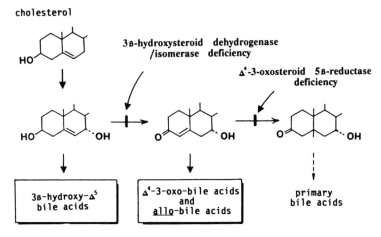

Figure 15.8 Diagrammatic representation of the effects of enzyme deficiencies on the conversion of cholesterol to primary bile acids. The AB-ring structure of the cholesterol steroid nucleus only is shown. The boxes highlight the atypical bile acids resulting from the specific enzyme deficiency. (Reproduced with permission from Setchell et al., 1992)

3β-Hydroxy-Δ-5 C27 steroid dehydrogenase deficiency

This disorder is characterized by very low or undetectable primary bile acids in plasma and large amounts of bile acid metabolites derived from 7 hydroxycholesterol in urine (Figure 15.8). The urine gives a deep purple colour with Lifschutz reagent (glacial acetic acid/conc H_2SO_4; 10/1 v/v).3β-Hydroxy-Δ-5 C27 steroid dehydrogenase activity is absent in cultured fibroblasts. All except one of the reported cases have presented with cholestatic liver disease in the neonatal period, often without pruritus and untreated have died of cirrhosis by 5 years. One patient was alive with liver disease at 12 years of age. Histologically there is a non-specific giant cell hepatitis which proceeds to a micronodular cirrhosis. Treatment with primary bile acids, chenodeoxycholic ± cholic acid or ursodeoxycholic acid in a total dose of 15 mg/kg/day causes a gradual improvement in clinical, laboratory and pathological features in all reported patients.

3-Oxo-Δ⁴-steroid 5β-reductase deficiency

This disorder is characterised by the almost exclusive presence of 3-oxo-Δ^4 bile acids and their derivatives in urine and virtual absence of primary bile acid derivatives. 3-oxo-Δ^4-steroid 5β-reductase is not expressed in fibroblasts. Immunoblotting techniques have shown absence of enzyme protein in the liver of four patients. Reported cases have presented with a severe hepatitis in the neonatal period; seven untreated cases died. Treatment with a combination of cholic acid and ursodeoxycholic acid appears efficacious. It should be noted that 3-oxo-Δ^4 bile acids may be present in excess in other forms of liver disease.

Defects of peroxisomal biogenesis

In Zellweger's syndrome and milder defects of peroxisomal function di- and trihydroxy-coprostanic acids, the precursors of cholic and chenodeoxycholic acids, abnormal C27 bile acids and a C29-dicarboxlic bile acid accumulate because of a generalized defect in peroxisomal beta-oxidation affecting the cholesterol side chain (see below). Bile acid therapy has no beneficial effect in Zellweger's syndrome.

Unidentified defects in peroxisomal bile acid metabolism

A number of patients with liver disease and incomplete forms of Zellweger's syndrome or with partial failure of peroxisomal function and abnormal bile acid metabolism have been described. In some the defect appears to be in uptake into peroxisomes. A specific defect in bile acid metabolism with the formation of excess trihydroxycoprostanic acid was described in two male siblings who died by 2 years of age with intrahepatic disease, including bile duct hypoplasia. A defect in side chain oxidation was considered responsible but no tests of peroxisomal integrity were performed (Clayton, 1991).

Cerebrotendinous xanthomatosis (hepatic mitochondrial 26-hydroxylase deficiency)

Cerebrotendinous xanthomatosis is caused by defective hydroxylation of C26 on the cholesterol side chain. Primary bile acids are not formed from cholesterol. Bile acid precursors which are synthesized into the bile alcohol, cholestanol which replaces cholesterol in the central nervous system and peripheral nerve myelin. The major clinical features are tendon xanthomata, cataracts, dementia, pyramidal paresis and cerebellar ataxia. The onset is usually between 10 and 20 years of age.

Hepatocytes contain golden brown amorphous electrondense material pigment. Diagnosis is based on the clinical features and confirmed by a plasma cholestanol level between three and 15 times normal. Long-term treatment with chenodeoxycholic acid, 75 mg/day reverses the metabolic abnormality and arrests progression of the disease.

Porphyrias

Porphyrias are inherited or acquired disorders in which there is partial deficiency of activity of one of seven enzymes involved in haem biosynthesis (Figure 15.9). Specific patterns of overproduction and excretion of haem precursors accompanies each disorder.

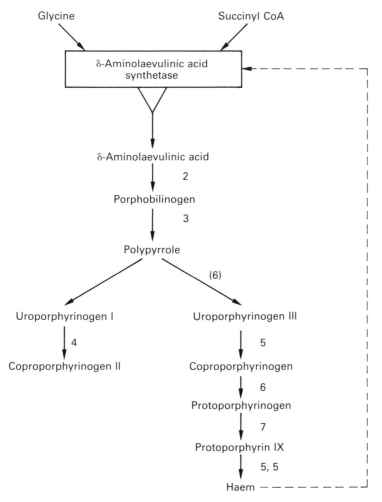

Figure 15.9 Diagrammatic representation of pathways of haem biosynthesis. Pathway is controlled by a feedback inhibition of this enzyme by haem. The numbers in the diagram show the site of action of the enzyme deficient in the porphyria summarized in Table 15.7

Porphyrias are generalized disorders but are classically designated as hepatic or erythropoietic depending on whether the main site of haem precursor accumulation is in the liver or bone marrow (Table 15.7). In protoporphyria and hepatoerythropoietic porphyria, either organ may overproduce porphyrins. The designation 'hepatic' does not necessarily indicate significant hepatic pathology. Conversely, marked hepatic changes can occur in erythropoietic porphyria. The genetic abnormality may be aggravated by drugs, toxins and neoplasms. Porphyria cutanea tarda may not be entirely genetic. An important factor in producing symptoms in porphyria is an uncontrolled, excessive activity of the enzyme Δ-aminolaevulinic acid synthetase. It is the rate-limiting enzyme for the synthesis of haem. Normally the activity of this enzyme is controlled by the amount of haem produced. The activity of the enzyme can be increased up to 40-fold by many exogenous and endogenous factors.

The most prominent clinical features in porphyria are cutaneous photosensitivity, acute neurological crises or abdominal pain and vomiting. The clinical features, mode of inheritance, and diagnostic features are outlined in Table 15.7. For detailed consideration of these disorders and possible pathophysiological mechanisms the reviews of Kappas *et al.* (1989) and Nordmann (1991) should be consulted.

Hepatic abnormalities in porphyria

Minor abnormalities of biochemical tests of liver function are almost universal in *porphyria cutanea tarda* but it is uncertain whether they indicate mild hepatic dysfunction which has caused decreased biliary clearance of porphyrin changing a latent disorder to clinically evident disease rather than being secondary to the porphyria. Liver biopsy findings in such patients include birefringent crystals in large vacuoles, fat deposition and haemosiderosis. Cirrhosis and hepatocellular carcinoma have been reported in this disorder. In *acute intermittent porphyria*, the histological findings are similar to porphyria cutanea tarda. In *congenital erythropoietic porphyria* hepatomegaly and haemosiderosis are common and cirrhosis has been described in an adult. Mild hepatitis is common in hepatoerythropoietic porphyria, another disorder in which cirrhosis has occurred.

Serious hepatic complications occur in *protoporphyria*. Cirrhosis has been described as early as 6 years of age with death from liver failure as early as 11 years. Histological examination of liver biopsies shows deposits of birefringent crystals in the lysosomes of Kupffer cells and in the cytoplasm of hepatocytes. When clinically evident liver disease is present the liver is nodular and brown in colour due to massive pigment accumulation in Kupffer cells, bile canaliculi and in portal tract macrophages. There is portal tract inflammation, features of chronic aggressive hepatitis and cirrhosis. Once clinical features of cirrhosis develop steady deterioration and death within 1 or 2 years is usual.

Diagnosis

The diagnosis of porphyrias is made on the basis of the pattern of excretion of porphyrins in the urine or stools. The specific enzyme defect associated with these may be identified in erythrocytes, skin fibroblasts or liver biopsy specimens.

Treatment

In patients with evidence of hepatic dysfunction there is anecdotal evidence that cholestyramine may have a beneficial effect. It is presumed to act by reducing the reabsorption of protoporphyrins from the intestine. Red cell transfusions may also reduce

Table 15.7 Summary of main clinical and biochemical features of porphyrias

Disorder	Enzyme defect	Clinical features	Age of onset	Main excretory products	
				Urine[a]	Stools
Hepatic porphyrias					
Acute intermittent porphyria (D)	Porphobilinogen deaminase (3)	Neurological and abdominal	Any	ALA and PBG	–
Hereditary coproporphyria (D)	Coproporphyrinogen oxidase (6)	Neurological Abdominal Photosensitivity Jaundice	Early childhood	ALA and PBG	Coproporphyrin iii
Porphyria variegata (D)	Protoporphyrinogen oxidase (7)	Photosensitivity Neurological Abdominal	Adult life	ALA and Coproporphyrin	Coproporphyrin
Deficiency of δ-ALA dehydrogenase (R)		Neurological	Late childhood	ALA and Coproporphyrin iii	–
Porphyria cutanea tarda (D)	Uroporphyrinogen decarboxylase (heterozygote) (5)	Photosensitivity Disturbed liver function	After puberty	Uroporphyrin	–
Erythropoietic porphyrias					
Congenital erythropoietic porphyrias (R)	Uroporphyrinogen synthase (4)	Photosensitivity Haemolytic anaemia Splenomegaly Gall stones	Late childhood	Uroporphyrin	–
Erythropoietic coproporphyria (D)	Ferrochelatase (8)	Progressive hepatic damage ± photosensitivity	Childhood	Uroporphyrin	Protoporphyrin
Hepatoerythropoietic porphyria (D)	Uroporphyrinogen decarboxylase (homozygous) (5,5)	Photosensivity Liver damage	First year	Uroporphyrin	–

[a] ALA = gamma-aminolaevulinc acid; PBG = porphobilinogen; D = dominant inheritance are recessive; R = recessive.
The numbers in parenthesis indicate the site of enzyme activity in haem biosynthesis depicted in Figure 15.9. Hepatoerythropoietic porphyria is the homozygous form of porphyria cutanea tarda.

protoporphyrin levels and lead to improved hepatic status. Splenectomy should be indicated if there is marked anaemia and splenomegaly. The cutaneous lesions are lessened by protection from direct sunlight. Beta-carotene in a dose of 120 mg/day maintaining a blood level of 600–800 μl lessens the severity of skin damage but takes 2–3 months to have any evident effect. The role of vitamin E as an antioxidant in this disorder is uncertain. Haematin, 3 mg/kg intravenously, is effective in aborting acute exacerbations. Liver transplantation has been performed for advanced liver disease due to protoporphyria but the disease recurs in the grafted organ.

Disorders of iron storage

Normal iron absorption transport and storage

A sensitive, finely controlled regulatory mechanism for iron absorption keeps body iron stores in equilibrium if dietary iron intake is sufficient. The precise factors regulating this function in enterocytes are still not completely understood. Iron is transported from the intestinal lumen into the mucosal cells as free iron or in haem by an energy dependent process. A rate-limiting step transfers this iron into the plasma in association with transferrin, a glycoprotein synthesized in the liver. It carries two atoms of ferric iron to the reticulo-endothelial system or tissue stores which express transferrin receptors, e.g. hepatocytes and Kupffer cells. The Kupffer cell is also involved in the recycling of iron from senescent erythrocytes. Transferrin concentrations fall if iron stores increase. Within the tissues iron is stored in a large protein, ferritin. In the adult liver iron stores account for 10% of total body iron. Haemosiderin, multiple aggregates of ferritin which stain blue with ferrocyanide, and ferritin are available for haemoglobin formation. Healthy full-term infants have high serum iron concentrations and high saturations of transferrin, hyperferritinaemia with high serum concentrations of cytoferritin, a low molecular weight iron-binding compound found mainly in cytoplasm.

Haemochromatosis

Haemochromatosis is characterized by tissue damage, e.g. cirrhosis or fibrosis in the liver, occurring with markedly increased iron stores (Table 15.8). Characteristic pathological and functional changes may occur also in the heart, pancreas and endocrine organs. The pattern of change is similar irrespective of the cause. Haemosiderosis (or siderosis) denotes an increase in tissue iron without tissue damage.

Table 15.8 Iron storage diseases with hepatic involvement

Congenital transferrin defect
Neonatal iron storage diseases
Zellweger's syndrome
Liver damage with hypermethioninaemia
Primary haemochromatosis
Haemochromatosis with chronic haemolytic anaemia
Dietary iron overload
Pancreatic exocrine insufficiency
Chronic haemodialysis

Pathology

The liver is enlarged and has a deep red/brown colour. There is cirrhosis with extensive deposition of iron as haemosiderin in parenchymal cells, Kupffer cells and bile duct cells. In haemochromatosis associated with chronic anaemia, iron first accumulates in Kupffer cells where it is associated with fibrosis on electron microscopic examination as early as 3–13 months of age. As the child grows older the Kupffer cells appear to become saturated with iron and iron appears in the parenchymal cells. Hepatocellular necrosis is often seen in association with this. Portal fibrosis is evident between 3 and 5 years of age. In a study of thalassaemic patients in Italy covering the years 1976–81, cirrhosis was present as early as seven years of age with 50% having cirrhosis by 11 years and all by 16 years (Moroni *et al.*, 1984). The liver iron content is increased to between five and ten times normal.

Pathogenesis

A combination of a defect in iron metabolism and a relatively positive iron balance is required to produce severe tissue damage. Iron-induced lipid peroxidation in mitochondria, microsomes and lysosomes or a direct stimulating effect on collagen biosynthesis have been proposed as a mechanism for liver injury. Whether there is increased liver avidity for iron or impaired biliary excretion in some forms is unclear. In haemochromatosis associated with chronic anaemia other hepatotoxic factors which have to be considered include chronic hypoxia, stasis due to cardiac involvement and nutritional deficiencies. Repeated blood transfusions expose the child to blood-borne viral infections, particularly hepatitis B and C (Mieli-Vergani *et al.*, 1984, see pages 103–120).

Clinical features

A firm enlarged liver, splenomegaly or features of cirrhosis are the principal hepatic features although hepatoma can develop. Skin pigmentation and diabetes mellitus are prominent in the idiopathic form; in that associated with chronic anaemia failure of endocrine organs and cardiac failure are particularly prominent. There may be a specific arthropathy with a joint distribution similar to rheumatoid arthritis.

The *congenital forms* present in the neonatal period or early infancy with hepatic failure and intense iron accumulation in non-reticulo-endothelial cells in the liver and other organs particularly the pancreas, heart and thyroid. Whether it represent a disorder(s) of iron metabolism, an unusual response to a form of liver injury or an abnormality of materno-fetal iron transport is unknown. Death in the first week is usual but may be delayed to 5 months of age (Witzleben and Uri, 1989). Familial cases have usually followed a similar course but in one family in which the proband died at 17 days of age a second sib who had liver failure with grade 4 siderosis at 3 days of age, gradually recovered and survived at 15 months of age. In one infant serum ferritin values were more than 10 times those in cord blood with cytoferritin values increase by more than 100-fold (Knisely *et al.*, 1989a). Transferrin-receptor and ferritin synthesis in fibroblasts from two affected siblings were normal (Knisely *et al.*, 1989b). No significant association with the HLA-A3 alloantigen was demonstrated in a study of 10 cases and their families (Hardy *et al.*, 1990). Exogenous iron overload (Bove *et al.*, 1991) and fetal liver disease may lead to similar extrahepatic siderosis (Hoogstraten *et al.*, 1990).

Haemochromatosis associated with chronic anaemia usually presents in late childhood or early adult life. Death usually occurs at between 16 and 24 years of age due to failure of heart, liver and endocrine organs. Intercurrent infection may cause death at an earlier age.

Hereditary haemochromatosis is inherited in an autosomal recessive fashion. The gene is closely associated with the HLA-A3 locus on chromosome 6. Relatives with similar HLA status to the proband are at high risk of developing haemochromatosis. The gene frequency is as high as 1:20. The gene product(s) remain unidentified. The age at onset is related to iron intake. Features usually appear between 40 and 60 years of age but exceptionally appear in childhood. Observations in transplanted patients confirm that the lesion is in the gut not the liver (Kowdley and Tavill, 1992). Whether the gene contributes to the development of haemochromatosis associated with chronic anaemia or the other disorders mentioned in Table 15.8 is at present unknown.

Diagnosis

The diagnosis of haemochromatosis is made on the basis of the classic clinical features, together with liver biopsy evidence of cirrhosis or widespread fibrosis and laboratory investigations indicative of excessive iron stores. A high serum iron concentration, saturation of the total iron-binding capacity and hepatic iron concentrations of more than $180\,\mu mol/g$ dry weight (normal $<36\,\mu mol/g$ dry weight) provide firm evidence for the diagnosis. CT scanning showing increased liver attenuation correlates closely with liver iron concentrations (Roudot-Thoraval *et al.*, 1983). Correlation is better than with serum ferritin which is sometimes taken as indicative of high body iron stores. Ferritin is increased in a number of other diseases, particularly hepatocellular disorders.

Treatment

The therapy of hereditary haemochromatosis is repeated venesection until the iron stores have been depleted. In haemochromatosis secondary to anaemia, the basis of treatment is to maintain the haemoglobin above a level at which excessive iron absorption will occur and to give desferrioxamine to increase iron excretion. In thalassaemia the haemoglobin should be maintained above 12 g/dl with infusions at 2–3-weekly intervals. Such therapy should be started as soon as the diagnosis is made. Desferrioxamine is commenced at the second transfusion given subcutaneously in a dose of 40–50 mg/kg over 8 hours, 5 days per week. Vitamin C supplements of 200 mg given with each injection double the iron excretion. Splenectomy is performed when the blood transfusion requirements exceed 500 ml/kg/year. It should be preceded by pneumococcal vaccination. Penicillin V 125 mg twice daily must be maintained for life. Hepatitis B vaccination at diagnosis is advised. Bone marrow transplantation is another possible therapy. There is no specific therapy for congenital forms.

Disorders in transport of unconjugated bilirubin (see Chapter 3)

Disorders in bilirubin glucuronide transport

The Dubin-Johnson syndrome

Definition This disorder is characterized by chronic benign conjugated hyperbilirubinaemia and the deposition of melanin-like pigment in the liver. Bromsulphophthalein (BSP) is cleared normally from plasma but the serum concentration rises between 45 and 90 minutes due to the defect in biliary secretion. There is an unexplained associated abnormality of coproporphyrin metabolism. The exact mode of inheritance is uncertain but recent research suggests autosomal recessive.

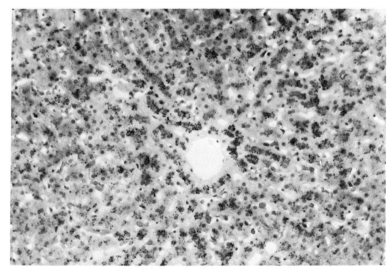

Figure 15.10 Dubin-Johnson syndrome. The liver architecture is normal. There are dark granules in the hepatocytes, particularly around the central vein. Cholestasis is not seen. There is no cellular infiltrate or fibrosis. (Percutaneous biopsy: haematoxylin and eosin; × 100, reduced to seven-eighths in reproduction)

Pathological features   The precise nature of the pigment which gives the liver its characteristic greenish-black appearance is controversial. It is found predominantly in the central lobular region as fine granules or globules associated with lysosomes. It has melanin-like properties and may be derived from noradrenaline or adrenaline (Figure 15.10). The characteristic histology but may not be apparent in early infancy. The pathogenesis is undetermined. There is deficient hepatic excretion of cholecystographic agents, bromsulphophthalein sodium, methylene blue and indocyanine green, but bile salts are excreted normally.

Clinical features   The apparent age of onset of jaundice is from birth to 40 years. It is often intermittent but may rise to levels as high as 450 µmol/litre (25 mg/dl) with between 25 and 75% of the bilirubin as diconjugates. Jaundice is exacerbated by trauma, surgery, pregnancy, oral contraceptives and anabolic steroids. There is no pruritus. There are no other features of liver disease but vague upper abdominal pain and nausea may occur. There is no hepatomegaly and standard tests of liver function are normal. Oral cholecystography fails to reveal the gall bladder. Bromsulphophthalein sodium retention in the serum at 45 minutes is generally between 10 and 20% but higher concentrations are found at 90 to 120 minutes. Coproporphyrin excretion in urine is normal but the coproporphyrin III to coproporphyrin I ratio in the urine changes from the normal 3:1 to 1:4.

   No treatment is required for this benign disorder. Drugs aggravating the jaundice should clearly be avoided.

Rotor syndrome

This is a rare benign familial disorder with predominantly conjugated hyperbilirubinaemia, similar to the Dubin-Johnson syndrome but without pigment deposition in the hepatocytes. The exact mode of inheritance is uncertain. In some families both the Dubin-Johnson syndrome and Rotor syndrome have been described.

Clinical features   There is lifelong mild conjugated hyperbilirubinaemia with bilirubin levels of around 80–100 μmol/litre (4–5 mg/dl) with 85% of the bilirubin conjugated mainly as monoconjugates. There are no clinical abnormalities, liver function tests are normal except for increased bromsulphophthalein sodium retention in the serum at levels of around 35% or 45 minutes after injection. No rise occurs in the bromsulphophthalein sodium concentration at 120 minutes. Urinary coproporphyrin excretion is increased two to five times, with coproporphyrin I comprising 65%. Cholecystography is normal, and the liver biopsy is often normal. Prognosis is excellent, no treatment is required.

Lethal familial pigmentary liver disease

Intrahepatic pigmentation with staining characteristics similar to the pigment found in the Dubin-Johnson syndrome has been reported in the livers of four male children in a family of North African descent who died within 3 months of birth. Arthrogryposis multiplex associated with rarefaction of the anterior horn cell, renal dysfunction with nephrocalcinosis and hepatomegaly with conjugated hyperbilirubinaemia and a haemorrhagic diathesis were the main features (Nezelof *et al.*, 1979).

Benign recurrent cholestasis

See Chapter 4.

Disorders of peroxisomal function

Zellweger's syndrome is the most common of the peroxisomal disorders which have been progressively characterized in the last decade. They are estimated to occur with a frequency of 1 in 25 000 to 1 in 50 000 births. Others are neonatal onset adrenoleucodystrophy, juvenile Refsum disease, hyperpipecolic acidaemia and one form of Leber congenital amaurosis.

Zellweger's syndrome (cerebro-hepato-renal syndrome)

Zellweger's syndrome is characterized by absence of peroxisomes and defective function of peroxisomal enzymes. At present it is not clear whether Zellweger syndrome arises from a structural defect in assembly of the peroxisomal membrane or a deficient receptor system necessary for the incorporation of enzymes into the membrane. Both phenotypic and genetic heterogeneity are reported. It is a multi-system disorder with profound abnormalities of neuronal migration and brain structure, hepatic malfunction, renal cortical cysts, abnormal calcification, retinal degeneration and multiple congenital anomalies. Diagnostic biochemical abnormalities include greatly diminished levels of plasmalogens, defects in bile acid synthesis with an increase in dihydroxy- and trihydroxy-coprostanic acid, defective oxidation and abnormal accumulation of very long chain fatty acids and of phytanic acid and increased pipecolic acid (a product of lysine degeneration). The recognition of milder incomplete forms with features shared with other disorders of peroxisomes will create diagnostic difficulty until the underlying pathogenesis is clarified.

Hepatic pathology

The histology of the liver varies from near normal to diffusely fibrotic or micronodular cirrhosis depending on the age of the patient. There is excessive hepatic iron in the first 5 to 18 weeks of life dropping to normal thereafter. In neonates in whom the biopsy looks normal there is frequently an irregular relationship between portal tracts and central veins. In the first few weeks of life abnormalities are limited to steatosis but there may be mild portal or perilobular fibrosis, cholestasis, intrahepatic bile duct hypoplasia or proliferation and giant cell transformation. By 8–10 weeks of age fibrosis is severe with distortion of the architecture and micronodular cirrhosis is established by 20 weeks of age. Ultrastructural studies show absence of peroxisomes and distortion of a small proportion of mitochondria.

Clinical features

Patients with 'classic' Zellweger's syndrome manifest profound hypotonia, hyporeflexia, severe psychomotor retardation, sometimes complicated by blindness and deafness and a typical craniofacial dysmorphism. The forehead is prominent with shallow orbital ridges, epicanthic folds and a broad nasal bridge. The sutures are abnormally open and the fontanelle large. There is micrognathia and the external ear is abnormal. Poor sucking and feeding difficulties are almost universal. Corneal clouding, cataract, glaucoma and nystagmus are frequently described.

Hepatomegaly is present at birth in approximately 40% of cases but develops in the first month in 80%. Sixty percent are jaundiced after 1 week of age. Cirrhosis has been documented in 40% of reported cases.

Laboratory investigations

Standard biochemical tests of liver function are abnormal. There may be hypoglycaemia, prolonged prothrombin time and high serum iron levels. X-rays show calcific stippling of the patella, acetabulum or greater trochanter. Increased pipecolic acid is found in serum and urine after 4 weeks of age. There is increased urinary excretion of dicarboxylic acids. Diagnostic investigation are given in the introduction. There are characteristic abnormalities of bile salt metabolism. 5-Cholestane-3,7,12-triol is oxidized to 3,7,12-trihydroxy-5β-cholestanoic acid, 5β-cholestane-3,7-diol to 3,7-dihydroxy-5β-cholestanoic acid. These are not metabolized to cholic acid or desoxycholic acid but accumulate and undergo either side chain elongation to form C29 bile acids or nuclear changes.

Treatment

There is no effective treatment. The administration of ether lipids and reduction of long chain fat and phytanic acid intake normalizes some of the biochemical abnormalities but have no clinical effects. Neither clofibrate, which markedly increases the number of peroxisomes in mammalian liver, nor bile acid supplements had any influence on clinical features.

Prenatal diagnosis

The following biochemical studies can be demonstrated in amniocytes: (1) a more than fivefold increase in very long-chain fatty acid concentrations; (2) defective dihydroxyacetone phosphate acyl transferase (first step in plasmalogen formation); (3) a reduced ratio of 1,4C-hexadecanol to 1-O-(9,10–3H) hexadecyl glycerol incorporation in plasmalogens (the former reduced in Zellweger's syndrome).

Hepatic aspects of other peroxisomal disorders.

Increased hepatic fibrosis occurs in *neonatal onset adrenoleucodystrophy* a disorder with a few peroxisomes and a similar but less severe phenotype than Zellweger's syndrome. The function of at least five different peroxisomal enzymes is impaired. There is impaired cortisol response to ACTH. Neonatal jaundice, hepatomegaly, abnormal biochemical tests of liver function and cirrhosis have been reported in *juvenile Refsum disease*. Cholesterol and lipoprotein concentrations are often low. In a third somewhat similar relatively mild disorder *hyperpipecolic acidaemia*, hepatomegaly and cirrhosis has been reported. Hepatomegaly is reported in *Leber congenital amaurosis*.

Disorders of lysosomal enzymes

Almost all disorders of lysosomal enzymes are caused by the deficiency of a specific enzyme required for the degradation of complex macromolecules. The exceptions are I-cell disease and pseudo-Hurler polydystrophy in which lysosomal enzymes are normally synthesized but are secreted into the extracellular matrix rather than being targeted to lysosomes. Undegraded molecules accumulate in the cytoplasm in these two disorders but in lysosomes in all others. Cellular, tissue or organ dysfunction results. Hepatomegaly usually with splenomegaly, abnormal facies, progressive mental deterioration, corneal clouding, ophthalmic abnormalities, skeletal changes, cardiac dysfunction, lung involvement and vacuolated lymphocytes manifest to varying degrees should prompt consideration of these conditions. Features of the main groups of such disorders are given in Tables 15.9, 15.10 and 15.11. There is considerable overlap. The lipid disorders with prominent hepatic features are considered in the text. Diagnosis (post- and prenatal) is by specific enzyme assay in leucocytes, fibroblasts or chorionic villi. The genetic basis of the considerable heterogeneity within each disorder is gradually being unravelled. Treatment is supportive. Early bone marrow transplantation from an HLA compatible donor may have a role in Gaucher's, mucopolysaccharidosis and Niemann-Pick group I disease but the mortality is 30% (Hobbs, 1992). Infusions of deglycosylated glucocerebrosidase which is preferentially accumulated in lysosomes of macrophages, given every 2 weeks, improve haematological abnormalities, reduce liver and spleen size and ameliorate skeletal features in Gaucher's disease. Their long-term role is unclear (Barton *et al.*, 1991).

Lipid storage disorders

Definition

Lipid storage disorders are disorders in which fatty acids, cholesterol or complex lipids are abnormally stored. Although hepatomegaly and/or splenomegaly are prominent features in lipid storage disorders, gastrointestinal symptoms and hepatic dysfunction are of little clinical significance in the majority of cases compared with features due to nervous system involvement. These disorders do require consideration in the differential diagnosis of hepatomegaly.

Table 15.9 Complex carbohydrate storage disorders causing hepatomegaly

Disorder	Material stored	Enzyme deficient	Age at onset	Splenomegaly	Other clinical features	Diagnostic investigations
Mucopolysaccharidosis I (Hurler)	Heparan and dermatan sulphates	Alpha-L-iduronidase	6–18 months	Moderate	Cloudy cornea, gibbus, joint deformity, respiratory infections, progressive mental deterioration	Dermatan and heparan sulphate in urine or enzyme deficiency in leucocytes
II (Hunter)	Heparan and dermatan sulphates	Sulpho-iduronate sulphatase	1–3 years	Moderate	As in Type I but no corneal clouding	Dermatan and heparan sulphate in urine
III (San Filippo)	Heparan sulphate	Four non-allelic disorders[a]	1–3 years	Minimal	As in Type I but mental regression is extremely marked	Heparan sulphate in urine
IV (Maroteaux–Lamy)	Dermatan sulphate	Arylsulphatase B	1–3 years	Minimal	Growth retardation, skeletal abnormalities, corneal opacities, normal intelligence	Dermatan sulphate in urine
VII (Sly)	Heparan and dermatan sulphate	β-glucoronidase	2 years	Moderate	Unusual facies, kyphosis, mental retardation, leucocyte inclusions	Deficient enzymatic activity in leucocytes, fibroblasts and amniocytes
I-Cell disease (Mucolipidosis II)	High lysosomal enzymes in serum	Defective enzyme location	Neonatal or at 4–5 years	Occasional	As in Hurler syndrome gingival hypertrophy, cardiomegaly and heart failure	10–20-fold elevation of acid hydrolases in serum (no excess of dermatan or heparan)
Pseudo–Hurler polydystrophy	High lysosomal enzymes in serum	Defective enzyme location	2–4 years	0	Slowly progressive mental retardation with survival to fourth decade	As immediately above

[a] Lysosomal enzymes deficient: Type A, heparan-N-sulphatase; Type B, N-acetyl-α-D-glucosaminidase; Type C, acetyl CoA:glucosaminide N-acetyltransferase; Type D, N-acetyl-α-D-glucosaminide-6-sulphatase

Table 15.10 Lipid storage disorders causing hepatomegaly

Disorder	Material stored	Enzyme deficient	Age at onset	Splenomegaly	Other clinical features	Diagnostic investigations
Tay-Sachs disease	Ganglioside G_{m2}	Ganglioside G_{m2}, hexosaminidase (hexosaminidase A)	1st year, 5–10 years, 10 years	Absent	Dementia, tetraplegia, cherry-red spot in macula	Enzyme deficient in serum, leucocytes and amniocytes
G_{m1} Gangliosidosis Type 1	Ganglioside G_{m1}	β Galactosidases	Infancy	Absent	Motor and mental retardation	Enzyme deficient in leucocytes and amniocytes
Gaucher's disease	Glucosyl ceramide	Glucosyl ceramide β glucosidase	Acute in infancy, chronic in later childhood	Marked	Skin pigmentation, bone and lung involvement, hypersplenism	Enzyme deficient in leucocytes, bone marrow, liver biopsy and amniocytes
Wolman's disease	Cholesterol esters and triglycerides	Acid esterase	Infancy	Moderate	Vomiting, diarrhoea, developmental delay, calcified adrenals	Enzyme deficient in leucocytes, liver biopsy and amniocytes
Cholesterol ester storage disease	Cholesterol esters and triglycerides	Acid esterase	Late childhood	Moderate	Malabsorption	Enzyme deficient in leucocytes and amniocytes
Abetalipoproteinaemia	Triglyceride	Defective synthesis of apo B	Birth	Absent (Hepatomegaly rare)	Malabsorption, acanthocytosis, hypocholesterolaemia, neuropathy due to vitamin E deficiency, cirrhosis? due to MCT	Clinical and laboratory features
Tangier disease	Cholesterol esters	Deficient formation apo A-1	1–5 years	Moderate	Large orange tonsils, peripheral neuropathy	Local cholesterol, high triglycerides, HDL absent
Sulphatide lipidosis	Galactosyl sulphatide	Arylsulphatase A	Infancy, 6–9 years ?	0	Small non-functioning gall bladder with many polyps.	??
Multiple sulphatase deficiencies	As above	Arylsulphatase A, B and C	Less than 1 year	Moderate	Unusual leucocyte abnormality and progression in 2nd year, death usually in 1st decade	Elevated arylsulphatide, enzyme deficiencies in leucocytes

Table 15.11 Disorders of glycoprotein degradation

Disorder	Material stored	Enzyme deficient	Age at onset	Splenomegaly	Other clinical features	Diagnostic investigations
Mannosidosis Type 1	Mannose-rich glycoproteins	Acidic α-A and B-mannosidase	3–12 months	Moderate	Psychomotor retardation, coarse facies, skeletal abnormalities, lens opacities, vacuolated lymphocytes	Deficient enzymatic activity in leucocytes, fibroblasts and amniocytes
Type II	Mannose-rich glycoproteins	Acidic α-A and B-mannosidase	1–4 years	Moderate	Synovitis, pancytopenia	As in Type I
Fucosidosis Type I	Fucose-containing glycolipids and polysaccharides	α-L-fucosidase	3–18 months	Moderate	Mental deterioration, cardiomyopathy, high sweat sodium, vacuolated lymphocytes	Enzyme deficient in leucocytes, fibroblasts and amniocytes
Type II	Fucose-containing glycolipids and polysaccharides	α-L-fucosidase	1–2 years	Moderate	Normal facies, skeletal abnormalities, mental deterioration, angiokeratomata	As in Type I
Sialidosis Type II	Sialyloligo-saccharides	α-neuraminidase	*In utero* 0–12 months 2–20 years		Hydrops, fetalis, still-births, neonatal ascites, renal involvement angiokeratomata. All show mental deterioration, coarse features dystosis multiplex, vacuolated lymphocytes	Enzyme deficient in leucocytes, fibroblasts and amniocytes
Aspartylglycosaminuria	Aspartyl-glycosamine	Aspartyl-glucosaminidase	1–5 years	Hepatomegaly and splenomegaly infrequent	Coarse facies, mental retardation, lens opacities, vacuolated lymphocytes	Enzyme deficiency in leucocytes, fibroblasts and amniocytes

Sphingomyelin-cholesterol lipidosis (The Niemann-Pick group of diseases)

The Niemann-Pick group of diseases are characterised by abnormal storage of sphingomyelin, cholesterol, glycosphingolipids and bis(monoacylglycero) phosphate which are seen as large 'foam' cells in the reticulo-endothelial system. In group I the metabolic defect is a decrease of more than 90% in the activity of sphingomyelinase, which degrades sphingomyelin to ceramide and phosphocholine. The metabolic basis of the three categories considered below is unknown. In group II sphingomyelinase activity is normal except in cultured fibroblasts in which it may be normal or decreased to as little as 15% of normal.

Niemann-Pick type II disease   Within this group a large number of the patients have been shown to have in cultured fibroblasts a unique abnormality in the translocation of exogenous cholesterol (Vanier *et al.*, 1991). Whether all group II patients have this abnormality is unclear. Cholesterol is retained in lysosomes in an unesterified form rather than transferred to the endoplasmic reticulum or plasma membrane. In approximately 15% of cases of later onset the severity of the defect as assessed by the degree of cholesterol esterification is less severe. Endogenous cholesterol is apparently metabolized in a normal fashion. What relation these abnormalities have to the primary deficit is unknown. They are important in diagnosis particularly prenatally. In the absence of better metabolic definition of these heterogeneous conditions further classification is arbitrary and not very satisfactory. It is now proposed that both types I and II be divided into three categories depending on the age at onset of features of central nervous system involvement:

A (acute) – onset *in utero* – 2 years; death <5 years in group I, <8 years in group II.
S (subacute) – onset at 0–3 years in group I and 0–18 years in group II; age at death uncertain.
C (chronic) – onset at >20 years; age at death uncertain.

In both groups I and II categories S and C have sea-blue histiocytes in reticuloendothelial cells.

The clinical features common to all forms are hepatosplenomegaly and central nervous system involvement. In *Niemann-Pick type II disease* at least 55% present in early infancy with jaundice as part of a hepatitis syndrome. A few present with fetal ascites (MacConachie *et al.*, 1989). Approximately 30% of these patients die of liver disease within the first 6 months of life. In the remainder features of hepatitis regress, liver functions test return to normal but modest hepatomegaly or splenomegaly persists. There may be progression to cirrhosis but symptomatic liver disease is rare. Clinical features of neurological involvement may occur as early as 2 years of age but may still be absent at 20 years. Supranuclear vertical ophthalmoplegia, a typical finding, is detected after 7 years of age. Death from bulbar involvement may occur as early as 7 years. Epilepsy develops in 75% around 10 years of age. The remaining cases come to medical attention when hepatomegaly and/or splenomegaly is detected or because of neurological abnormalities, psychomotor retardation or psychiatric features developing as late as the sixth decade.

The diagnosis is established by the normal sphingomyelinase activity in leucocytes, the presence of typical Sudan black positive PAS negative storage cells in bone marrow and in nerve cells in a rectal biopsy. Note that storage cells can be overlooked in liver biopsies from cholestatic infants. In cultured fibroblasts decreased exogenous cholesterol esterification can be demonstrated in >85% of cases, the remainder showing defective translocation.

There is no effective treatment for this condition. A low cholesterol diet and cholesterol lowering drugs are subjects of ongoing trials. Liver transplantation does not arrest the progression of the neurological disease. Bone marrow transplantation has not been reported.

Sulphatide Lipidosis

Metachromatic leucodystrophy is caused by the accumulation of galactosyl sulphatide due to deficiency of arylsulphatase A (EC 3.1.6.1). Tissues with an excretory function such as bile duct cells contain metachromatic material but such material is also found in periportal hepatocytes and Kupffer cells. The gall bladder is particularly affected being small, fibrotic with polyploid masses and non-functioning. There are usually no clinical features of hepatobiliary involvement.

Acid esterase deficiency

Wolman's disease

Wolman's disease is due to a total deficiency of lysosomal acid esterase resulting in an accumulation of cholesterol esters and triglycerides in many organs, particularly the liver and the intestinal mucosa. The liver is large, firm and yellow in colour. The parenchymal cells are engorged by membrane-lined vacuoles of different size. Foamy histiocytes with similar vacuoles are found in clumps, both in the portal areas and between parenchymal cells. There is an increase in portal fibrosis and cirrhosis may develop. The disease commonly presents in the first few weeks of life with vomiting, abdominal distension, diarrhoea, hepatosplenomegaly, steatorrhoea and failure to thrive.

Standard tests of liver function are abnormal. Radiology will show adrenal calcification in over 90% of cases. There is decreased adrenal endocrine activity. The diagnosis is confirmed by the low esterase concentration in leucocytes. Prenatal diagnosis in amniocytes has been accomplished. There is no specific treatment. Bone marrow transplantation corrected metabolic features in one patient who died of aspergillosis 80 days after grafting.

The clinical course is of progressive deterioration with anaemia, massive hepato-splenomegaly and death usually by 6 months of age. In some cases there is very severe liver involvement with jaundice prior to death.

Hepatic cholesterol ester storage disease

Hepatic cholesterol ester storage disease is associated with acid esterase activity in the liver decreased to values between 10% and 30% of normal. The liver shows similar lipid accumulation to that of Wolman's Disease with 50% of cases having increased fibrosis.

The clinical presentation is usually asymptomatic hepatomegaly noticed at a median age of 3 years (range: birth to 23 years). One-third of patients develop splenomegaly and variceal bleeding has been recorded. Hypertriglyceridaemia and hypercholesterolaemia are found in the majority. Standard biochemical tests of liver function are usually mildly abnormal. The long-term prognosis is uncertain, but death from liver failure has occurred at 18 years of age and one patient underwent liver transplantation for hepatic failure at 14 years of age. Suppression of cholesterol and apolipoprotein B synthesis by HMG-CoA reductase inhibitors (simvastatin) may be beneficial.

Gaucher's disease (glucosylceramide lipidosis)

Gaucher's disease in which glucosylceramide accumulates because of deficiency of glucocerebrosidase, is the most prevalent lysosomal storage disease. It takes three main forms:

(1) Type 1 a chronic non-neuropathic disorder starting at any time between birth and old age with very variable but frequently slow progression.
(2) Type 2 (acute neuropathic) starts in the first 6 months of life and leads to a neurological death by the age of 2 years.
(3) Type 3 (subacute neuropathic) presents with visceral features but neurological features develop usually in the first 5 years of life and are gradually progressive thereafter. Death usually occurs in the third decade.

Hepatic pathology

Groups of Gaucher cells – large, multinucleated cells with a reticular pale-staining cytoplasm – surround the central hepatic veins and obstruct the sinusoids. The liver architecture is often deranged and hepatic fibrosis may be severe. This may be complicated by portal hypertension and ascites in all three types of the disease. Chronic active hepatitis has been described. Death from liver failure is rare.

Liver function tests are frequently abnormal but there is no specific pattern. Hypersplenism eventually occurs in nearly all patients with type I or type III disease. It may be aggravated by an associated haemolytic anaemia or by displacement of erythrocyte precursors from the bone marrow by Gaucher's cells. Bone marrow transplantation immediately following splenectomy produces some regression in the clinical features with a decrease in bone pain and a reduction in liver size but intrahepatic fibrosis may progress. Enzyme replacement may have a role (see p. 286).

Mucopolysaccharidosis

The mucopolysaccharidoses are a group of related chronic, progressive, multi-system disorders caused by deficiency of lysosomal enzymes needed to degrade glycosaminoglycans (mucopolysaccharides). These accumulate in lysosomes and/or are excreted in the urine. Visceral enlargement, skeletal changes and abnormal facies are manifest to varying degrees. Progressive mental deterioration, impaired cardiovascular function, vision and hearing may occur. The main disease groups causing hepatomegaly are shown in Table 15.12. All are inherited in an autosomal recessive fashion, except for Hunter's syndrome which is inherited in an X-linked fashion.

Bone marrow transplantation has arrested progression and produced short-term biochemical and clinical improvement in types I, II and VI but the mortality is 30% even with HLA identical donors (Hobbs and Riches, 1992).

'Mucopolysaccharidosis'-like conditions

I-cell disease and pseudo-Hurler polydystrophy are mucolipidoses that have many clinical features in common with the mucopolysaccharidoses, but splenomegaly is minimal. They are not true lysosomal storage diseases arising as they do from abnormal lysosomal enzyme transport which produces abnormal inclusions in cytoplasm. Diagnosis is established by the clinical features and high serum concentration of lysosomal enzymes. There is no treatment.

Table 15.12 Disorders causing hepatomegaly/hepatic dysfunction and frequently neurological abnormalities or development delay

Chronic hepatic encephalopathy	
Fulminant hepatic failure	
Reye's syndrome	
Infective disorders	
Intrauterine	eg. rubella, CMV, syphilis, toxoplasmosis
Neonatal	eg. listeriosis, herpes simplex virus infection
Childhood	eg. Weil's disease
Inborn errors of metabolism	
Carbohydrate	Galactosaemia
	Fructosaemia
	Glycogen storage disease (Table 15.4)
Amino acids	Urea cycle disorders
	Hyperammonaemias
	Homocystinuria
	Tyrosinaemia
Lipids	A-beta lipoprotein deficiency
	Alpha-lipoprotein deficiency
Lysosomal storage disorders	(see Tables 15.9, 15.10, 15.11)
Haem metabolism	Crigler-Najjar syndrome
	Porphyria
Mineral disorders	Wilson's disease
	Haemochromatosis
Peroxisomal disorders	Zellweger's syndrome
Rare disorders of uncertain cause	Biliary hypoplasia with characteristic phenotype (Alagille's syndrome)
	Leigh's encephalopathy
	Progressive neural degeneration of childhood liver disease
	Lissencephaly syndrome
	Lipodystrophy
	Familial haemophagocytic reticulosis
	Congenital hepatic fibrosis and polycystic disease of the kidneys and brain malformation
	Shwachmann's syndrome
	Fetal alcohol syndrome
	Carbohydrate-deficient glycoprotein disorder

Disorders of glycoprotein degradation

Glycoproteins comprise oligosaccharide chains covalently linked to serine, threonine or asparagine in a peptide backbone. They too share many features of mucopolysaccharidoses. Vacuolation can usually be found in lymphocytes (Table 15.11).

Lysosomal transport disorders

Cystinosis

Cystinosis is due to defective carrier-mediated transport of the amino acid cystine. Cystine accumulates in lysosomes in most tissues. The major clinical manifestation is nephropathy presenting by 12 months of age and leading to renal failure in the first decade. With the natural history being modified by dialysis and renal transplantation, hepatic involvement is emerging as a potential problem; over 40% of patients aged 10 or older have hepatomegaly. Liver function tests become slightly abnormal. Hepatic storage of cysteine is noted as early as 22 weeks' gestation. Histological examination in childhood shows hypertrophied Kupffer cells, fatty change in central areas and mild to moderate portal fibrosis. Portal hypertension may cause alimentary bleeding requiring injection sclerotherapy.

Free sialic acid storage disorders

Defective carrier-mediated transport of sialic acid causing increased tissue and urinary concentrations of sialic acid results in psychomotor retardation which is progressive in the *infantile form*. In this form hepatosplenomegaly and coarse features are prominent. Ascites may develop *in utero* or postnatally.

Carbohydrate deficient glycoprotein syndrome (olivopontocerebellar atrophy of neonatal onset; disialotransferrin developmental deficiency syndrome)

This disorder is a familial disorder of unknown cause characterized biochemically by abnormal glycosylation of serum glycoproteins such as transferrin and caeruloplasmin. As well as the specific nature of the brain atrophy, retinitis pigmentosa, renal microcysts, skeletal and hepatic steatosis and fibrosis are typical pathological features. In some patients cirrhosis may develop. Hepatomegaly, ascites, oedema with low serum albumin and raised transaminases are the main hepatic features. In patients surviving beyond 2 years of age hepatic features are less prominent or absent.

Abetalipoproteinaemia

Abetalipoproteinaemia is a genetic disorder in which the major defect is absence of plasma beta-lipoprotein and complete inability to produce chylomicrons and very low density lipoproteins. There is severe fat malabsorption. Triglycerides accumulate in enterocytes and liver. Cirrhosis has been reported in patients treated with medium chain triglycerides. Degenerative lesions of the spinal cord and brain are due to vitamin E deficiency.

Clinical features   The disease is characterized by steatorrhoea, starting in the first months of life, acanthocytosis and fat-soluble vitamin deficiency. Progressive ataxia, and retinitis pigmentosa becomes detectable after the fifth year of life.

Diagnosis   The diagnosis may be suspected by the finding of acanthocytosis in a fresh, wet, peripheral blood film. Serum cholesterol phospholipid and triglyceride levels are extremely low. Electrophoretic demonstration of lack of beta-lipoprotein confirms the diagnosis.

Treatment   This takes the form of a low triglyceride diet and fat soluble vitamin supplements. Medium chain triglycerides have been used to improve fat absorption but should be used sparingly because their use has been linked with the development of cirrhosis.

Progressive neuronal degeneration of childhood with liver disease (Alpers Disease)

This familial disorder is characterized by a distinctive pattern of cortical neuronal loss and latent liver disease leading to cirrhosis (Harding *et al.*, 1986). There is cortical atrophy affecting particularly the occipital area. Neuronal loss and astrocytosis is associated with pigment-laden macrophages which give a distinctive dark-brown discoloration to the cortical ribbon. Before clinical features of liver involvement appear histological changes are limited to microvesicular steatosis, periportal inflammation and sparse hepatocellular necrosis. At autopsy the liver shows a subacute hepatitis comprising massive fatty degeneration, hepatocyte loss, bile duct proliferation, bridging necrosis and micronodular cirrhosis. Twenty-four cases have been reported from 16 kindreds suggesting an autosomal recessive inherited metabolic defect.

Clinical and laboratory features

Early development is normal but between 1 month and 3 years of age developmental arrest, intractable epilepsy, hypotonia, vomiting or failure to thrive develop. Long-track and cranial nerve signs may appear. The majority die of status epilepticus by 3 years of age. There are frequently no clinical features of liver involvement until the last 2 to 8 weeks of life when hepatomegaly, ascites or jaundice may develop and test of hepatic synthetic function are abnormal. Death from liver failure occurs at 1 to 8 years of age. Typical high voltage slow waves with polyspikes are seen on EEG may allow a diagnosis in life. The visual evoked response is absent or disorganized. Two to fivefold increases in aspartate aminotransferase values are first noted at 4 to 80 months of age.

Familial haemophagocytic lymphohistiocytosis

This disorder appears to be inherited in an autosomal recessive fashion. It is characterized by progressive visceral, central nervous system and bone marrow infiltration with lymphocytes and large erythrophagocytic histiocytes. A constitutional impairment of lymphocytotoxic mechanisms has been reported (Arico *et al.*, 1988). The clinical features are fever, irritability, pallor, oedema, hepatosplenomegaly, jaundice, skin rash, usually starting in the first year of life. Pancytopenia, liver dysfunction, coagulopathy with prevalent *hypofibrinogenaemia, a lymphohistiocytic meningitis and hypertriglycer- idaemia* are the main laboratory features. The diagnosis is established by the bone marrow findings or liver or brain biopsy. The main differential diagnosis is virus-associated haemophagocytic syndrome. Treatment with etoposide, steroids and intrathecal metho- trexate with cranial irradiation may prevent a fatal outcome (Fischer *et al.*, 1985).

Disorders causing hepatomegaly or hepatic dysfunction and neurological abnormalities or developmental delay

Many acquired or genetically determined disorders affect both the liver and the nervous system. The purpose of this section is simply to bring together the range of such disorders. These include various forms of hepatic encephalopathies, infective disorders affecting both the liver and brain and well-defined inborn errors of metabolism. In addition, miscellaneous rare disorders with a putative familial or genetic basis and distinct clinical or pathological features are added. [The list (see Table 15.12) aims to be comprehensive but with already over 5000 separate genetic disorders described, I apologize in advance for inevitable oversights at the time of writing and for inadequacies before the book came to press.]

Neurological syndromes range from delayed neurological development, gradual progressive global loss of brain function, acute coma to specific syndromes such as the extrapyramidal lesion in Wilson's disease or acute peripheral neuropathy in porphyria.

Chronic hepatic encephalopathy (page 222), fulminant hepatic failure (Chapter 8) and Reye's syndrome (Chapter 9) have been described in detail earlier. The diagnosis and management of the treatable inborn errors of metabolism, galactosaemia, fructosaemia, tyrosinaemia (pp. 251–261), glycogen storage diseases (page 246), and Wilson's disease (Chapter 17) have been considered in detail elsewhere.

Other rare but currently untreatable disorders such as Zellweger's syndrome which introduced new ideas on pathogenesis of liver disease, and have been the subject of many recent research reports, are dealt with elsewhere in this chapter. The remaining disorders are indicated by name only but the references chosen do provide useful further reading.

Bibliography and references

General

Arias, I. M, Jakoby, W. B., Popper, H., Schachter, D. and Shafritz, D. A. (1987) *The liver: biology and pathobiology*, 2nd edn, Raven Press, New York
Clayton, P. T. (1991) Diagnosis of metabolic liver disease in infancy. *Curr. Paediatr.*, **1**, 224–227.
Hobbs, J. R. (1992) Bone marrow transplantation in genetic diseases. *Eur. J. Pediatr.*, **151**, S44–S49.
Schaub, J., Van Hoof, F. and Vis, H. L. (eds) (1991) *Inborn Errors of Metabolism*, Raven Press, New York
Scriver, C. R., Beaudet, A. L., Sly, W. S. and Valle, D. (eds). (1989) *The Metabolic Basis of Inherited Disorders*, 6th edn, McGraw-Hill, New York
Touraine, J.-L. (1991) The place of fetal liver transplantation in the treatment of inborn errors of metabolism. *J. Inher. Metab. Dis.*, **14**, 619–626.
Wu, G. Y., Wilson, J. M. and Wu, C. H. (1988) Targeting genes: delivery and expression of a foreign gene driven by an albumen promoter in vivo. *Hepatology*, **8**, 1251

Neonatal ascites

Gillan, E., Lauden, J. A., Gaskin, K. and Cutz, E. (1984) Congenital ascites as a presenting sign of lysosomal storage disease. *J. Pediatr.*, **104**, 225
Maconochie, I. K., Chong, S., Mieli-Vergani, G. *et al.* (1989) Fetal ascites: an usual presentation of Niemann-Pick disease type C. *Arch. Dis. Child.*, **10**, 1391–1393.
Renlund, M. (1984) Clinical and laboratory diagnosis of Sella disease in infancy and childhood. *J. Pediatr.*, **104**, 232

Glycogen storage disease

Burchell, A., Bell, J. E., Busuttil, A. and Hume, R. (1989) Hepatic microsomal glucose-6-phosphatase system and sudden infant death syndrome. *Lancet*, **ii**, 291–294
Burchell, A. and Waddell, I. D. (1990) Diagnosis of a novel glycogen storage disease: type 1aSP. *J. Inher. Metab. Dis.*, **13**, 247–249.
Burchell, A. and Gibb, L. (1991) Diagnosis of Type 1b and 1c glycogen storage disease. *J Inher. Metab. Dis.*, **14**, 305–307.
Calcado, A., Trivedi, P., Portmann, B. and Mowat, A. P. (1991) Serum concentrations of extracellular matrix components: novel markers of metabolic control and hepatic pathology in glycogen storage disease. *J. Ped. Gastroenterol. Nutr.*, **13**, 1–9
Chen, Y. T., Coleman, R. A., Scheinman, J. I., Kolbeck, P. C. and Sidbury, J. B. (1988) Renal disease in type 1 glycogen storage disease. *N. Engl. J. Med.*, **18**, 7–11
Chen, Y. T., Scheinman, J. I., Coleman, R. A. and Roe, C. R. (1990) Amelioration of proximal renal tubular dysfunction in type I glycogen storage disease with dietary therapy. *New Engl. J. Med.*, **323**, 590–603
Conti, J. A. and Kemeny, N. (1992) Type Ia glycogenosis associated with hepatocellular carcinoma. *Cancer*, **69**, 1320–1332.

Couper, R., Kapelshnik, J. and Griffiths, A. M. (1991) Neutrophil dysfunction in glycogen storage disease 1b: association with Crohn, S-like colitis. *Gastroenterology*, **100**, 549–554

de Parscau, L., Guibaud, P., Labourne, P. and Odievre, M. (1989) Long term outcome of hepatic glycogen storage disease: the French experience. Abstracts of the Society for the study of inborn errors of metabolism, **27**, 001

Fernandes, J., Leonard, J. V., Moses, S. W. *et al.* (1988) Glycogen storage disease: recommendations for treatment. *Eur. J. Pediatr.*, **147**, 226–228

Fink, A., Apelman, H. D. and Thompson, M. W. (1985) Haemorrhage into a hepatic adenoma and Type 1A glycogen storage disease. A case report and review of the literature. *Surgery*, **97**, 117

Green, H. L., Brown, B. I., McClenathan, D. T., Agostini, R. M. and Taylor, S. R. (1988a) A new variant of type IV glycogenosis: deficiency of branching enzymatic activity without apparent progressive liver disease. *Hepatology*, **8**, 302–306

Greene, H. L., Ghishan, F. K., Brown, B., McClenathan, D. T. and Freese, D. (1988b) Hypoglycemia in type IV glycogenosis: hepatic improvement in two patients with nutritional management. *J Pediatr.*, **112**, 55–58

Guerra, A. S., van Diggelen, O. P., Carneiro. F., Tsou, R. M., Simoes, S. and Santos, N. T. (1986) A juvenile variant of glycogenosis IV (Andersen disease). *Eur. J. Pediatr.*, **145**, 179–181

Hamaoka, K., Nakagawa, M., Furukawa, N. and Sawada, T. (1990) Pulmonary hypertension in type 1b glycogen storage disease. *Ped. Cardiol.*, **11**, 54–56

Hers, H.-G., Hoof, F. V. and de Barsy, T. (1989) Glycogen storage diseases. In *Metabolic Basis of Inherited Disorders*, (eds. Scriver, C. R., Beaudet, A. L., Sly, W. S. and Valle, D.). 6th edn, McGraw-Hill, New York, 1989, pp. 425–452

Kirschner, B. S., Baker, A. L. and Thorp, F. K. (1991) Growth in adulthood after liver transplant for glycogen storage disease type I. *Gastroenterology*, **101**, 238–241.

Maire, I. and Mathieu, M. (1986) Possible prenatal diagnosis of type III glycogenosis. *J. Inher. Metab. Dis.*, **9**, 89–91.

Maire, I., Baussan, C., Moatti, N., Mathieu, M. and Lemonnier, A. (1991) Biochemical diagnosis of hepatic glycogen storage diseases: years French experience. *Clin. Biochem.*, **24**, 169–178

Nagai, T., Matsuo, N., Tsuchiya, Y., Cho, H., Hasegawa, Y. and Igarashi, Y. (1988) Proximal renal tubular acidosis associated with glycogen storage disease type 9: case report. *Acta Paediatr. Scand.*, **77**, 460–463

Olshan, J. S., McKenzie, S. E., Stanley, C. A. and Baker, L. (1991) Anaemia in glycogen storage disease type 1 (GSD-1). *Ped. Research*, **29**, 197A: p. 1167

Park, H. K., Kahler, S. G. and Chen, Y.-T. (1991) Brain abscess in glycogen storage disease type lb. *Acta Paediatr. Scand.*, **80**, 1103–1106

Pears, J. S., Jung, R. T., Hopwood, D., Waddell, I. D. and Burchell, A. (1992) Glycogen storage disease diagnosed in adults. *Q. J. Med.*, **82**, 207–222

Roe, T. F., Coates, T. D., Thomas, D. W., Miller, J. H. and Gilsanz, V. (1992) Brief report: Treatment of chronic inflammatory bowel disease in glycogen storage disease 1b with colony stimulating factors. *NEJM*, **326**, 1666–1669

Sanderson, I. R., Bisset, W. M., Milla, P. J. and Leonard, J. V. (1991) Chronic inflammatory bowel disease (Crohn's) in glycogen storage type 1b. *J. Inher. Metab. Dis.*, **14**, 771–776

Schmidt, H., Ullrich, K., von Lengerke H.-J. and Peters, P. E. (1991) Peliosis hepatitis with type 1 glycogen storage disease. *J. Inher. Metab. Dis.*, **14**, 691–697

Selby, R., Starzyl, T., Yunis, E., Brown, B. I., Kendall, R. S. and Tzakis, A. (1991) Liver Transplantation for type IV glycogen storage disease. *N. Engl. J. Med.*, **324**, 126–128

Shin, Y. S. (1990) The diagnosis of glycogen storage disease. *J. Inher. Metab. Dis.*, **13**, 419–434

Smit, G. P. A., Fernandes, J., Leonard, J. V. *et al.* (1990) The long term outcome of patients with glycogen storage diseases. *J. Inher. Metab. Dis.*, **13**, 411–418

Sokal, E. M., Hoof, F. V., Alberti, D., de Ville de Goyet, J., de Barsy, T. and Otte, J. B. (1992) Progressive cardiac failure following orthotopic liver transplantation for type IV glycogenosis. *Eur. J. Pediatr.*, **151**, 200–203

van den Berg, I. E. T. and Berger, R. (1990) Phosphorylase b kinase deficiency in man: a review. *J. Inher. Metab. Dis.*, **13**, 442–451

Wolfsdorf, J. I., Keller, R. J., Landy, H. and Crigler, J. F. (1990) Glucose therapy for glycogenosis type 1 in infants: comparison of intermittent uncooked cornstarch and continuous overnight glucose feedings. *J. Pediatr.*, **117**, 384–391

Carbohydrate disorders

Disorders of galactose metabolism

Otto, G., Herfarth, C., Senninger, N. and Feist, G. (1989) Post Gmelin K Hepatic transplantation in Galactosaemia. *Transplantation*, **47**, 902–903

Segal, S. (1989) Disorders of galactose metabolism. In *The metabolic basis of inherited disease*, 6th edn., (eds. Scriver, C. R., Beautt, A. L., Sly, W. S. and Valle, D.). McGraw-Hill, New York, pp. 453–480

Waggoner, D. D., Buist. N. and Donnell, D. (1990) Long-term prognosis in galactosaemia: results of a survey of 350 cases. *J. Inher. Metab. Dis.*, **13**, 802–818

Fructosaemia

Hereditary fructose intolerance

Bender, S. W., Vieweg, B., Posselt, H.-J. *et al.* (1982) Hereditary fructose intolerance. *Monatsschr. Kinderheilkd.*, **130**, 21

Endres, W. (1988a) Die hereditare fruktose intoleranz: ubersicht und kritische auseinandersetzung mit persistierenden problemen. *Akt. Endokr. Stoffw.*, **9**, 140–145

Endres, W., Sierck, T. and Shin, Y. S. (1988b) Clinical course of hereditary fructose intolerance in 56 patients, *Acta Paediatr. Jpn.*, **30**, 452–456

Gitzelmann, R., Steinmann, B. and van den Berghe, G. (1989) Disorders of fructose metabolism. In: *The metabolic basis of inherited disease*, 6th edn. (eds Scriver, C. R., Beautt, A. L., Sly, W. S. and Valle, D.). McGraw-Hill, New York, pp. 481–499

Odievre, M., Gentil, C., Gautier, M. and Alagille, D. (1978) Hereditary fructose intolerance in childhood. *Am. J. Dis. Child.*, **132**, 605

See, G., Marcha, G. and Odievre, M. (1984) Hepatocarcinome chez un adulte suspect d'une intolerance hereditaire au fructose, Ann. Pediatr., **31**, 49–51

Steinmann, B. and Gitzelmann, R. (1981) Diagnosis of hereditary fructose intolerance. *Helv. Pediatr. Acta*, **36**, 297

Streb, H., Possalt, H. G., Woolter, K. and Bender, S. W. (1981) Aldolase activity in the small intestinal mucosa in malabsorption states and hereditary fructose intolerance. *Eur. J. Pediatr.*, **137**, 5

Fructose-1, 6-diphosphatase deficiency

Corbeal, L., Eggermont, E., Eeckels, R. *et al.* (1976). Recurrent attacks of ketoacidosis associated with fructose-1, 6-diphosphatase deficiency. *Acta Paediatr. Belg.*, **29**, 29

Largilliere, C., Adedee-Manesme, O., Marsak, C. *et al.* (1984). Unusual features in a case of hepatic fructose-1. 6-diphosphatase deficiency. *Arch. Fr. Pediatr.*, **41**, 421

Diabetes mellitus

Lorenz, G. and Barenweld, G. (1979). Histological and electronmicroscopic liver change in diabetic children. *Acta Hepato-Gastroenterol.*, **26**, 435

Nagore, N. and Scheuer, P. (1988) Pathology of Diabetes mellitus. J. Path., **156**, 155–160.

Tyrosinaemia

Almedia, I. T., Leandro, P. P., Silva, M. F. B. *et al.* (1990) Tyrosinaemia type I with normal levels of plasma tyrinosine. *J. Inher Metab. Dis.*, **13**, 305–307

Coskun, T., Ozalp, I., Kocak, N., Yuce, A., Caglar, M. and Berger, R. (1991) Type hereditary tyrosinaemia: presentation of 11 cases. *J. Inher. Metab. Dis.*, **14**, 765–770

Dehner, L. P., Snover, T. C., Sharp, H. L., Ascher, N., Nakhleh, R. and Day, D. L. (1989) Hereditary tyrosinaemia (chronic form): pathological findings in the liver. *Human Path.*, **20**, 149–158

Elpeleg, O. N., Christensen, E., Hurvitz, H. and Branski, D. (1990) Recurrent, familial Reye-like syndrome with a new complex amino and organic acifuria. *Eur. J. Pediatr.*, **149**, 709–712

Flye, M. W., Riely, C. A., Hainline, B. E. *et al.* (1990) The effects of early treatment of hereditary tyrosinaemia type 1 in infancy by orthotopic liver transplantation. *Transplantation*, **49**, 916–921

Gilbert-Barness, E., Barness, L. A. and Meisner, L. F. (1990) Chromosomal instability in hereditary tyrosinaemia type 1. *Pediatr. Pathol.*, **10**, 243–252

Goldsmith, G. A. and Leberge, C. (1989) Tyrosinemia and related disorders. In: *The metabolic basis of inherited disease*, 6th edn (eds Scriver, C. R., Beautt, A. L., Sly, W. S. and Valle, D.). McGraw-Hill, New York, pp. 547–562

Kvittigen, E. A., Talseth, T., Halvorsen, S., Jacobs, C. and Hovig, T. (1991) Renal failure in adult patients with hereditary tyrosinaemia type 1. *J. Inher. Metab. Dis.*, **14**, 53–62

Kvittigen, E. A. (1991) Tyrosinaemia type 1 – an update. *J. Inher. Metab. Dis.*, **14**, 554–562

Kvittigen, E. A. (1986) Hereditary tyrosinaemia type I: An overview. *Scand. J. Clin. Lab. Invest.*, **46**, 27–34

Lindstedt, S., Holme, E., Lock, E. A., Hjalmarson, O. and Strandvik, B. (1992) Treatment of hereditary tyrosinaemia by inhibition of 4-hydroxyphenylpyruvate dioxygenase. *Lancet*, **340**, 813–817

Macvicar, D., Dicks-Mireaux, C., Leonard, J. V. and Wight, D. G. D. (1990) Hepatic imaging with computed tomography of chronic tyrosinaemia type 1. *Br. J. Radiol.*, **63**, 605–608

Nakajima, M., Ishii, S., Mito, T. *et al.* (1988) Clinical, biochemical and ultrastructural study of the pathogenesis of the hyperornithinaemia, hyperammonaemia, homocitrullinuria syndrome. *Brain Dev.*, **10**, 181–185

Paradis, K., Weber, A., Seidman, E. G. *et al.* (1990) Liver transplantation for hereditary tyrosinaemia: The Quebec experience. *Am. J. Hum. Gen.*, **47**, 338–342

Riudor, E., Ribes, A., Lloret, J. *et al.* (1991) Liver transplantation in two children with hereditary tyrosinaemia type 1: Biochemical aspects. *J. Inher. Metab. Dis.*, **14**, 281–284

Sharp, H. L., Lindahl, J. A., Freese, D. K. *et al.* (1988) A new Hepatico-pancreato-renal disorder resembling tyrosinaemia involving neuropathy and abnormal metabolism of polyunsaturated fatty acids. *J. Ped. Gastro. Nutr.*, **7**, 167

Spronsen, F. J., Berger, R., Smit, G. P. A. *et al.* (1989) Tyrosinaemia type I: Orthotopic liver transplantation as the only definitive treatment to a metabolic as well as an oncological problem. *J. Inher. Metab. Dis.*, **13**, S2 339–342

van Spronsen, F. J., Thomasse, Y., Smith, G. P. A., Leonard, J. V., Clayton, P. T., Fidler, V., Berger, R. and Heymans. H. S. A. Prognosis of hereditary tyrosinaemia type 1 with guidelines for timing of liver transplantation. *J. Pediatr.* (in press)

Weinberg, A. G., Mize, C. E. and Worthen, H. G. (1976) The occurrence of hepatoma in the chronic form of hereditary tyrosinaemia. *J. Pediatr.* **88**, 434

Other amino acid disorders

Kekomaki, M. P., Visakorpi, J. K., Perhanentypa, J. and Salen, L. (1967) Familial protein intolerance with deficient transport of basic amino acids. *Acta Pediatr. Scand.*, **56**, 617

Rajantie, J., Simell, O., Rapola, J. and Perheentupa, J. (1980) Lysinuric protein intolerance – a two year trial of dietary supplementation therapy with citrulline and lysine. *J. Pediatr.*, **97**, 927

Urea cycle defects and related disorders

Bachmann, C. (1992) Ornithine carbamoyl transferase deficiency; findings, models and problems. *J. Inher. Metab. Dis.*, **15**, 578–591

Brusilow, S. W., Danney, M., Webber, L. J. *et al.* (1984) Treatment of episodic hyperammonaemia in children with inborn errors of urea synthesis. *New Engl. J. Med.*, **310**, 1630

Brusilow, S. W and Horwich, A. L. (1989) Urea cycle enzymes. In: *The metabolic basis of inherited disease*, 6th edn (eds Scriver, C. R., Beautt, A. L., Sly, W. S. and Valle, D.). McGraw-Hill, New York, pp. 629–663

Drogeri, E. and Leonard, J. V. (1988) Late onset ornithine carbamoyl transferase deficiency in males. *Arch. Dis. Child.*, **63**, 1363–1367

Largilliere, C., Houssin, D., Gottrand, F. *et al.* (1989) Liver transplantation for ornithine transcarbamylase deficiency in a girl. *J. Pediatr.*, **115**, 415–417

Maestri, N. E., Hauser, E. R., Batholomew, D. and Brusilow, S. W. (1991) Prospective treatment of urea cycle disorders. *J. Pediatr.*, **119**, 923–928

Msall, M., Batshaw, M. L., Suss, R. *et al.* (1984) Neurological outcome in children with inborn errors of urea synthesis. *New Engl. J. Med.*, **310**, 1500

Ohtani, Y., Ohyanagi, K., Yamamoto, S. and Matsuda, I. (1988) Secondary carnitine deficiency in hyperammonemic attacks of ornithine transcarbamylase deficiency. *J. Pediatr.*, **112**, 409–414

Rabier, D., Narcy, C., Bardet, J., Parvy, P., Saudubray, J. M. and Kamoun, P. (1991) Arginine remains an essential amino acid after liver transplantation in urea cycle disorders. *J. Inher. Metab. Dis.*, **14**, 277–280

Todo, S., Starzl, T. E., Tzakis, A. *et al.* (1992) Orthotopic liver transplantation for urea cycle enzyme deficiency. *Hepatology*, **15**, 419–422

Tokatli, A., Coskun, T., Cataltepe, S. and Ozalp, I. (1991) Valproate-induced lethal hyperammonaemic coma in a carrier of ornithine carbomyltransferase deficiency. *J. Inher. Metab. Dis.*, **14**, 836–837

Tuchman, M., Tsaik, M. Y., Holznecht, R. A. and Brusilow, S. W. (1989) Carbamyl phosphate synthetase and ornithine transcarbamylase activities in enzyme-deficient human liver measured by radiochromatography and correlated with outcome. *Pediatr. Res.*, **26**, 77–82

Tuchman, M. (1989) Persistent acitrullinaemia after liver transplantation for carbamylphosphate synthetase deficiency. *N. Engl. J. Med.*, **320**, 1498–1499

Zimmermann, A., Bachmann, C. and Baumgartner, R. (1986) Severe liver fibrosis in argininosucciniaciduria. *Arch. Pathol. Lab. Med.*, **110**, 136

Mitochondrial disorders

Bartlett, K., Aynsley-Green, A., Leonard, J. V. and Turnbull, D. M. (1991) Inherited disorders of mitochondrial beta-oxidation. In: *Inborn Errors of Metabolism* (eds Schaub, J., Van Hoof, F. and Vis, H. L.). Raven Press, New York, pp. 19–41

Chalmers, R. A., Mistry, J., Penketh, R. and McFadyen, I. R. (1989) First trimester prenatal diagnosis of 3-Hydroxy-3-methylglutaric aciduria. *J. Inher. Metab. Dis.*, **12**, 283–285

Clayton, P. T., Hyland, K., Brand, M. and Leonard, J. V. (1986) Mitochondrial phosphoenolpyruvate carboxykinase deficiency. *Eur. J. Pediatr.*, **145**, 46–49

Cormier, V., Rustin, P., Bonnefont, J.-P. *et al.* (1991) Hepatic failure in disorders of oxidative phosphorylation with neonatal onset. *J Pediatr.*, **119**, 951–954

Demaugre, F., Bonnefont, J. P., Mitchell, G. *et al.* (1988) Hepatic and muscular presentations of carnitine palmitoyl transferase deficiency: two distinct entities. *Pediatr. Res.*, **24**, 308–311

Elpeleg, O. N., Christensen, E., Hurvitz, H. and Branski, D. (1990) Recurrent, familial Reye-like syndrome with a new complex amino and organic aciduria. *Eur. J. Pediatr.* **149**, 709–712

Elpeleg, O. N., Joseph, A., Branski, D. *et al.* (1993) Profound carnitine palmitoyltransferase II deficiency. (Submitted for publication)

Green, A., Preece, M. A., De Sousa, C. and Pollitt, R. J. (1991) Possible deleterious effect of l-carnitine in a patient with mild multiple acyl-Coa dehydrogenation deficiency (ethylmalonic-adipic aciduria). *J. Inher. Metab. Dis.*, **14**, 691–697

Munnich, A., Rustin, P., Rotig, A. *et al.* (1992) Clinical aspects of mitochondrial disorders. *J. Inher. Metab. Dis.*, **15**, 448–454

Ohtani, Y., Ohyanagi, K., Yamamoto, S. and Matsuda, I. (1988) Secondary carnitine deficiency in hyperammonemic attacks of ornithine transcarbamylase deficiency. *J. Pediatr.*, **112**, 409–414

Pandya, A. L., Koch, R., Hommes, F. A. and Williams, J. C. (1991) N-acetylglutamate synthetase deficiency: clinical and laboratory observations. *J. Inher. Metab. Dis.*, **14**, 685–690

Parrot-Roulaud, F., Carre, M., Lamirau, T. *et al.* (1991) Fatal neonatal hepatocellular deficiency with lactic acidosis: a defect in the respiratory chain. *J. Inher. Metab. Dis.*, **14**, 289–292

Pollitt, R. J., Losty, H. and Westwood, A. (1987) 3-hydroxydicarboxylic aciduria: a distinctive type of intermittent dicarboxylic aciduria of possible diagnostic significance. *J. Inher. Metab. Dis.* **10**, (suppl 2): 266–269

Scholte, H. R., Rereira, R. R., de Jonge, P. C., Luyt-Houwen, I. E. M., Verduin, M. H. M. and Ross, J. D. (1990) Primary carnitine deficiency. *J. Clin. Chem. Clin. Biochem.*, **28**, 351–357

Scholte, H. R., Ross, J. D., Blom, W. *et al.* (1992) Assessment of deficiencies of fatty acyl-CoA dehydrogenases in fibroblasts, muscle and liver. *J. Inher. Metab. Dis.*, **15**, 342–346

Touma, E. H. and Charpentier, C. (1992) Medium acyl-CoA dehydrogenase deficiency. *Arch. Dis. Childh.*, **67**, 142–145

Vilaseca, M. A., Briones, P., Ribes, A., Carreras, E., Llacer, A. and Querol, J. (1991) Fatal hepatic failure with lactic acidaemia, Fanconi syndrome and defective activity of succinate:cytochrome c reductase. *J. Inher. Metab. Dis.*, **14**, 285–288

Bile acid disorders

Clayton, P. T. (1991) Inborn errors of bile acid metabolism. *J. Inher. Met. Dis.*, **14**, 478–496

Hanson, R. F., Isenberg, J. N., Williams, G. C. *et al.* (1975) The metabolism of 3, 7, 12, trihydroxy-5βcholestan-26-oic acid in two siblings with cholestasis due to intrahepatic bile duct anomalies. *J. Clin. Invest.*, **56**, 577

Ichimiya, H., Nazer, H., Gunasekaren, T. *et al.* (1990) Treatment of chronic liver disease caused by 3beta-hydroxy delta-C_{27}-steroid dehydrogenase deficiency with chenodeoxycholic acid. *Arch. Dis. Childh.*, **65**, 112–114

Setchell, K. D. R., Suchy, F. J., Welsh, M. B. *et al.* (1988) Delta[4]-3-oxosteroid 5beta-reductase deficiency described in identical twins with neonatal hepatitis. A new inborn error of metabolism. *J. Clin. Invest.*, **82**, 2148–2157

Setchell, K. D. R., Piccoli, D., Heubi, J. and Balistreri, W. F. (1992) Inborn errors of bile acid metabolism. In: *Paediatric Cholestasis. Novel approaches to treatment* (eds Lentz, M. J. and Reichen, J.). Kluwer, London, p. 153

Haem metabolism

Porphyria

Bonkowsky, H. L. and Schnedd, A. R. (1986) Fatal liver failure in protoporphyria. *Gastroenterology*, **90**, 191

Herbert, A., Corbin, D., Williams, A., Thompson, D., Buckels, J. and Elias, E. (1991) Erythropoietic protoporphyria: Unusual skin and neurological problems after liver transplantation. *Gastroenterology*, **100**, 1753–1757

Nordmann, Y. (1991) Human hereditary porphyrias. In *Oxford Textbook of Clinical Hepatology* (eds. N. McIntyre, J.-P. Benhanou, J. Bricher, M. Rizzetto and J. Rodes). Oxford Medical Publications, Oxford. p. 974–985

Haemochromatosis

Bove, K. E., Wong, R., Kagen, H., Balistreri, W. and Tabor, M. W. (1991) Exogenous iron overload in perinatal hemochromatosis: a case report. *Pediatr. Pathol.*, **11**, 389–397

Hardy, L., Hansen, J. L., Kushner, J. P. and Knisely, A. S. (1990) Neonatal Haemochromatosis. Genetic analysis of Transferrin-receptor, H-apoferritin, and L-apoferritin Loci and of the human leucocyte antigen Class 1 region. *Am. J. Path.*, **137**, 149–153

Hoogstraten, J., de Sa, D. J. and Knisely, A. S. (1990) Fetal liver disease may precede extrahepatic siderosis in neonatal hemochromatosis. *Gastroenterology*, **98**, 1699–1701

Jean, G., Terzoli, S., Mauri, R. *et al.* (1984) Cirrhosis associated with multiple transfusions in thalassaemia. *Arch. Dis. Childh.*, **59**, 67

Knisely, A. S., Grady, R. W., Kramer, E. E. and Jones, R. L. (1989a) Cytoferrin, maternofetal iron transport and neonatal hemochromatosis. *Am. J. Clin. Pathol.*, **92**, 755–759

Knisely, A. S., Harford, J. B., Klausner, R. D. and Taylor, S. R. (1989b) Neonatal haemochromatosis. The regulation of transferrin-receptor and ferritin synthesis by iron in cultured fibroblastic-line cells. *Am. J. Pathol.*, **134**, 439–445

Kowdley, K. V. and Tavill, A. S. (1992) An 'ironic' case of mistaken identity. *Hepatology*, **16**, 500–501

Mieli-Vergani, G., Vergani, D., White, Y. *et al.* (1984) Hepatitis B virus infection in thalassaemia major treated in London and Athens. *Br. Med. J.*, **288**, 1804

Moroni, G. A., Piacentini, G., Terzoli, S., Jean, G. and Masera, G. (1984) Hepatitis B or non-A, non-B virus infection in multi-transfused thalassaemic patients. *Arch. Dis. Childh.*, **59**, 1127–1129

Roudot-Thoraval, F., Halphen, M., Larde, D. *et al.* (1983) Evaluation of liver iron content by computed tomography: its value in the follow-up of treatment in patients with idiopathic haemachromatosis. *Hepatology*, **3**, 974–977

Witzleben C. L. and Uri, A. (1989) Perinatal Hemochromatosis: Entity or end result? *Human Pathol.*, **20**, 335–340

Conjugated hyperbilirubinaemia

Bar-Meir, S., Baron, J., Saligson, E. U. *et al.* (1982) ^{99Tcm}-HIDA cholescintigraphy in Dubin-Johnson and Rotor syndromes. *Radiology*, **142**, 473

Kando, T., Yagi, R. and Kuchiba, K. (1975) Dubin-Johnson syndrome in a neonate. *New Engl. J. Med.*, **292**, 1029

Nezelof, C., Dupart, M. C., Jaubart, F. and Eliachar, E. (1979) A lethal familial syndrome associating arthrogryposis multiplex congenita, renal dysfunction and a cholestatic and pigmentary liver disease. *J. Pediatr.*, **94**, 258

Saymour, C. A., Neale, G. and Peters, T. J. (1977) Lysosomal changes in liver tissue from patients with the Dubin-Johnson-Sprinz syndrome. *Clin. Sci. Molec. Med.*, **52**, 281

Shimizu, Y., Naruto, H., Ida, S. *et al.* (1981) Urinary coproporphyrin isomers in Rotor's syndrome: a study in 8 families. *Hepatology*, **1**, 173

Peroxisomal disorders

Lazarow, P. B. and Moser, H. W. (1989) Disorders of peroxisome biogenesis. In: *The metabolic basis of inherited disease*, 6th edn (eds. Scriver, C. R., Beautt, A. L., Sly, W. S. and Valle, D. McGraw-Hill, New York, pp. 1479–1509

Mieli-Vergani, G. and Mowat, A. P. (1987) Peroxisomal disorders. In *Liver Annual Volume 6* (eds Arias, I. M., Frankel, M. and Wilson, J. H. P.). Elsevier, Amsterdam, pp. 429–433

Roels, F., Espeel, M. and De Craemer, D. (1991) Liver Pathology and Immunocytochemistry in congenital peroxisomal diseases: a review. *J. Inher. Metab. Dis.*, **14**, 853–875

Wanders, R. J. A., van Roermund, C. W. T., Schutgens, R. B. H. *et al.* (1990) The inborn errors of peroxisomal beta-oxidation: a review. *J. Inher. Metab. Dis.*, **13**, 4–34

Wilson, G. N., Holmes, R. D. and Hajraa, A. K. (1988) Peroxisomal Disorders: Clinical Commentary and Future Prospects. *Am. J. Med. Genet.* **30**, 771–792

Lysosomal disorders

Barton, N. W., Furbish, F., Murray, G. J., Garfield, M., O'Brady (1990) Therapeutic response to intravenous infusions of glucocerebrosidase in a patient with Gaucher disease. *Proc. Natl. Acad. Sci. USA*, **87**, 1913–1916

Barton, N. W., O'Brady, R., Dambrosia, J. M. *et al.* (1991) Replacement therapy for inherited enzyme deficiency-macrophage targeted glucocerebrosidase for Gaucher's Disease. *New Engl. J. Med.*, **324**,

1464–1470

Ferry, G. D., Whisennand, H. H., Finegold, M. J., Alpert, E. and Glombicki, A. (1991) Liver transplantation for cholesteryl ester storage disease. *J. Ped. Gastroenter. Nutr.*, **12**, 376–378

Gal, A., Beck, M., Sewell, A. C., Schwinger, E. and Hopwood, J. J. (1992) Gene diagnosis and carrier detection in Hunter Syndrome by the iduronate-2-sulphatase cDNA probe. *J. Inher. Metab. Dis.*, 342–346

Gartner, J. C., Bergman, I., Malatack, J. J., Zitelli, B. J. and Jaffe, R. (1987) Progression of neurovisceral storage with supraocular ophthalmoplegia following liver transplantation. *Pediatrics*, **77**, 104–106

Henderson, J. M., Gilinsky, N. H., Lee, E. Y. and Greenwood, M. F. (1991) Gaucher's disease complicated by bleeding esophageal varices and colonic infiltration by Gaucher cells. *Am. J. Gastroenterol.*, **86**, 346–348

Hobbs, J. R. and Riches, P. G. (eds) (1992) *Correction of Certain Genetic Diseases by Transplantation.* Cogent Trust, London

Hoeg, J. M., Demonsky, S. J., Pescovitz, O. A. and Brewer, H. B. (1984) Cholesterol ester storage disease and Wolman's Disease; Phenotypic variants of lysosomal acid cholesteryl ester hydrolase deficiency. *Am. J. Human Genet.*, **36**, 1190–11197

Horslen, S. P., Clayton, P. T., Harding, B. N., Hall, N. A., Keir, G. and Winchester, B. (1991) Olivopontocerebellar atrophy of neonatal onset and disialotransferrin developmental deficiency syndrome. *Arch. Dis. Childh.*, **66**, 1027–1032

Jones, D. R., Hoffman, J., Downie, R. and Haqqani, M. (1991) Massive gastrointestinal haemorrhage associated with ileal lymphoid hyperplasia in Gaucher's disease. *Postgrad. Med. J.*, **67**, 479–481.

Maconochie, I. K., Chong, S., Mieli-Vergani, G. *et al.* (1989) Fetal ascites: an usual presentation of Niemann-Pick disease type C. *Arch. Dis. Childh.*, **64**, 1391–1393

Patel, S. C., Davis, G. L. and Barranger, J. A. (1986) Gaucher's disease in a patient with chronic active hepatitis. *Am. J. Med.* **80**, 523–525

Tassoni, J. P., Fawaz, K. A. and Johnston, D. E. (1991) Cirrhosis and portal hypertension in patient with adult Niemann-Pick disease. *Gastroenterology*, **100**, 567–569

Tsai, P., Lipton, J. M., Sahdev, I. *et al.* (1992) Allogenic bone marrow transplantation in severe Gaucher disease. *Pediatr. Res.*, **31**, 503–507

Vanier, M. T., Wenger, D. A., Cowley, M. E., Rousson, R., Brady, R. O. and Pentchev, P. G. (1988) Niemann-Pick disease type C: clinical variability and diagnosis based on defective cholesterol esterification. A collaborative study based on seventy patients. *Clin. Genet.*, **33**, 331–338

Vanier, M. T., Pentchev, P., Rodriguez-Lafrasse, C. and Rousson, R. (1991) Niemann-Pick disease type C: an update. *I.J. Inher. Metabol. Dis.*, **14**, 580–594

Wilson, J. A. P. and Raufman, J. P. (1986) Case report: hepatic failure in adult Niemann-Pick disease. *Am. J. Med. Sci.*, **292**, 168–172

Progressive neuronal degeneration with liver disease

Alpers, B. J. (1931) Diffuse progressive degeneration of the grey-matter of the cerebrum. *Arch. Neurol. Psychiat.*, **25**, 469

Harding, B. N., Egger, J., Portmann, B. and Erdohazi, M. (1986) Progressive neuronal degeneration of childhood with liver disease. *Brain*, **109**, 181

Huttenlocher, P. R., Solitaire, G. B. and Adams, G. (1976) Infantile diffuse cerebral degeneration with hepatic cirrhosis. *Arch. Neurol.*, **33**, 186

Narkewicz, M. R., Sokal, R. J., Beckwith, B., Sondheimer, J. and Silverman, A. (1991) Liver involvement in Alpers disease. *J. Pediatr.*, **119**, 260–267

Familial erythrophagocytic lymphohistiocytosis

Arico, M., Nespoli, L., Maccario, R. *et al.* (1988) Natural cytotoxicity impairment in familial haemophagocytic lymphohistiocytosis. *Arch. Dis. Childh.*, **63**, 292–296

Fischer, A., Virelizter, J. L., Arenzana-Seisdedos, F. *et al.* (1985) Treatment of four patients with erythrophagocytic lymphohistiocytosis by a combination of epipodophyllotoxin, steroids, intrathecal methotrexate and cranial irradiation. *Pediatrics*, **76**, 263

Galactosaemia

Kirkman, H. N. (1992) Short report: Estimates of uridine diphosphate glucose in human erythrocytes. *J. Inher. Metab. Dis.* **15**, 940–941

Chapter 16

Genetic and familial structural abnormalities of the liver and biliary system

Hereditary fibropolycystic disorders

Hereditary cystic disorders of the liver and biliary system comprise a heterogeneous group of disorders in which there is increased intrahepatic fibrosis occurring in association with cysts lined by biliary epithelium. The amount of fibrous tissue gradually increases with age as does the severity of portal hypertension. Cholangitis occurs particularly if the cysts communicate with the biliary system. There is usually little or no impairment of liver function but it can occur even in the absence of cholangitis. Cysts may be microscopic or so large they function as space-occupying lesions. In adults, they may be the site of carcinomatous change (Summerfield *et al.*, 1986). During hepatic development a two-cell thick ductal plate in the form of a sheath is formed around portal vein branches. The ductal plate is progressively remodelled to form ever smaller segments of bile duct as gestation proceeds.

Abnormalities of portal vein development and or arrest of this remodelling process are suggested as a possible explanation for the vascular and bile duct changes seen in congenital disorders of the intrahepatic bile ducts. Cysts associated with fibrosis may occur in other organs, particularly in the kidneys, leading to renal failure. In such patients hypertension and renal failure are the main clinical problems. With renal transplantation modifying the natural history of these disorders, long-term hepatic complications may become more common. Although described below as distinct entities they frequently co-exist in various combinations and may occur in association with choledochal cysts (see Chapter 24).

Autosomal recessive polycystic disease of the kidneys and liver

Autosomal recessive polycystic disease (ARPD) of the kidneys and liver is characterized by renal and hepatic enlargement due to replacement of the renal parenchyma by cysts and fibrous tissue, and periportal hepatic fibrosis with dilatation of bile ductules. The designation ARPD replaces infantile polycystic disease of the kidneys and liver since the disorder may be seen in adults. The disorder may cause death *in utero* or present in infancy or in late childhood (Blyth and Ockenden, 1971).

Pathology

In the kidney, the essential lesion appears to be cystic transformation of the terminal collecting tubules, while in the liver the lesion is at the level of the junction of the canals of Hering and adjacent intralobular bile ducts. What causes these lesions is not known. Both are associated with a marked increase in fibrous tissue. In the kidney, there is also a loss of functioning nephrons.

The renal weight and size may be increased to as much as ten times normal but the shape is usually preserved. Cysts lined by cuboidal or cylindrical epithelium are distributed radially in both cortex and medulla. In infancy these tend to be less than 1 cm in size but with increasing age the cysts tend to become larger, up to 2 cm. The interstices around the cysts contain much fibrous tissue, immature in infancy, but mature later in childhood (Figure 16.1). It is only late in childhood that enlarged cysts and increasing fibrosis start to deform the capsule and compress the calyces. With age there is increasing fibrous tissue and loss of renal parenchyma. In the majority of cases renal failure develops early in infancy. The secondary pathological effects are those of renal failure and systemic hypertension. In early infancy abdominal distension and pulmonary oedema cause marked respiratory distress. Pneumonia is a frequent complication.

The liver is enlarged but to a much lesser extent than the kidneys. There are no macroscopic abnormalities. The microscopic lesions are in the portal tracts which are enlarged due to increased fibrous tissue. At the periphery of the portal tracts are irregularly-shaped, interconnected biliary channels lined by cuboidal epithelium. They may represent partially remodelled embryonic ductal plates. Normal bile ducts may be absent in these portal tracts but the abnormal channels may be in continuity with the

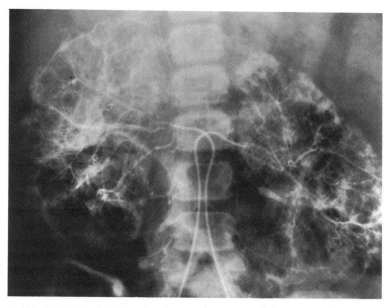

Figure 16.1 Bilateral selective renal angiogram showing large kidneys containing a multitude of cysts which are less than 1 cm in size. There is a considerable reduction in functioning renal tissue. The appearances are typical of polycystic disease at this age

biliary system at other levels. Portal vein branches are distorted. Whether this is an integral part of the malformation or secondary to it is not clear. The intrahepatic fibrosis increases progressively with age causing portal hypertension. The hepatic lobular architecture is unchanged and the liver cells are normal.

In individual cases there is considerable variability in the degree of renal and hepatic involvement. In some instances, renal involvement appears to be focal rather than diffuse. Because of the different ages of presentation of cases in individual families, Blyth and Ockenden (1971) have suggested that four or even five distinct phenotypic varieties of ARPD may exist. However, no unique pathological differences have as yet been discerned in these groups.

Clinical features

In the perinatal period, ARPD may present as a difficulty in delivery because of marked abdominal distension caused by the gross enlargement of the kidneys. There are no features of liver involvement. Death may occur within a few hours due to pulmonary insufficiency or soon afterwards from renal failure.

In the neonatal period and early infancy the clinical features are those of renal involvement (Table 16.1). There is marked abdominal distension often causing respiratory embarrassment. Renal failure, systemic hypertension, congestive cardiac failure, respiratory tract infection and failure to thrive are the main problems.

Table 16.1 Features of autosomal recessive polycystic disease of the kidneys and liver

Fetal	Neonatal	Infancy	Childhood
Oligohydramnios	Marked abdominal distension	Renal failure	Splenomegaly
Potter's facies	Bilateral renal enlargement	Failure to thrive	Hypersplenism
Dystocia	Renal failure	Hepatomegaly	Alimentary bleeding
	Hypertension	Splenomegaly	Abnormal IVP
	Congestive cardiac failure		Late onset renal failure
	Respiratory distress		
	Histological evidence of liver involvement		

The diagnosis may be suspected by the finding of bilateral huge renal masses with or without hepatomegaly and splenomegaly. Death often occurs from pneumonia or congestive cardiac failure. If congestive cardiac failure can be controlled, however, this feature gradually settles with increasing age and it is often possible to stop digitalization around the age of 2 years. Relapse may occur with intercurrent infection.

Where renal cyst formation is less widespread, the disease may not present until later infancy or early childhood, with features of renal failure such as polyuria and failure to thrive. In both groups features of progressive renal failure inevitably occur, often requiring support by dialysis or renal transplantation by the age of 5–10 years. In cases presenting in later childhood the hepatic lesion predominates. The features are those of congenital hepatic fibrosis (see below).

Investigative findings

Tests of liver function are typically normal although occasionally the alkaline phosphatase may be elevated. There is evidence of renal impairment such as polyuria, decreased urinary osmolarity, raised blood urea and creatinine and reduced creatinine clearance tests. The most useful investigation is plain radiography of the abdomen and excretory urography (Table 16.2). The typical findings are illustrated in Figure 16.2. If the blood urea is too high to permit excretory urography, ultrasonic scanning of the kidneys may be helpful in excluding large cysts or obstructive nephropathy.

In rare instances it will be necessary to perform kidney or liver biopsy so that firm genetic guidance can be given. If alimentary bleeding has occurred, endoscopy or barium meal may be necessary to demonstrate varices. Table 16.3 lists the investigative procedures for suspected polycystic disease of the liver and kidneys.

Table 16.2 IVP abnormalities in autosomal recessive polycystic disease of the kidneys and liver

Bilateral, massively enlarged kidneys
Alternating radiodense-radiotransluscent streaks on the nephrogram
Homogeneous nephrogram
A persistent nephrogram (hours or days)
Blunted, shortened, indistinct calyces
Rarely, collections of contrast medium in renal papillae indistinguishable from medullary sponge kidney

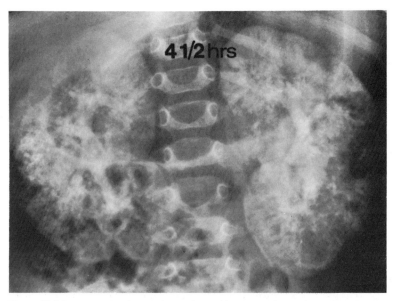

Figure 16.2 Intravenous pyelogram in a patient with autosomal recessive polycystic disease of the kidneys and liver. Four and a half hours after injection of Urografin a clear nephrogram persists. The kidneys are massively enlarged. There are alternating radiodense and radiolucent streaks in the cortex. The main calyces are normal but the extremities are blunted and indistinct

Table 16.3 Investigations of suspected polycystic disease in liver and kidneys

Excretory urography	Full blood count
Ultrasonic scan of kidneys and liver	Standard tests of liver function
Renal function tests (blood urea, serum	Chest radiography
creatinine, creatinine clearance tests)	Barium meal
Endoscopy	Liver scintiscan
In selected cases:	
Aortoportography	Kidney biopsy
Splenic venography	ECG
Liver biopsy	Radiology of wrists and hands to
	exclude renal osteodystrophy

Treatment and prognosis

Death in infancy usually arises from renal failure, fluid retention or bronchopneumonia. In later childhood death is likely to arise from progressive renal failure. In late childhood or adult life the features of portal hypertension may become more important. Complications described under congenital hepatic fibrosis develop.

Treatment is limited to dietary measures to combat the renal failure, drug treatment of systemic hypertension, renal dialysis and transplantation. Aspirin should be avoided since it may provoke alimentary bleeding. Portacaval shunting has been employed in patients who have bled from oesophageal varices, being well tolerated in the short term.

Congenital hepatic fibrosis

Definition

Congenital hepatic fibrosis (CHF) is a condition defined pathologically by the presence within the liver of bands of fibrous tissue which often contain linear or circular spaces lined by bile duct epithelial cells. The bands of fibrous tissue join all portal tracts. It is commonly associated with intrahepatic portal hypertension but hepatocellular function is almost always preserved. It is not a single entity but in clinical usage the term is usually reserved for a syndrome in which portal hypertension occurs without significant impairment of renal or hepatic function. Pathologically it is most commonly associated with significant renal disease, such as ARPD. It must be distinguished from cirrhosis and other causes of portal hypertension in childhood since management and prognosis are different.

Pathology

The liver is enlarged, smooth and hard. The unique pathological feature of this condition is the presence throughout the liver of bands of fibrous tissue which are clearly demarcated from hepatic parenchyma (Figure 16.3). Portal tracts are widened. All are linked by these bands of fibrous tissue. The width of the bands varies from case to case, and may increase with age. Most frequently the bands contain many irregularly shaped narrow, elongated spaces lined by bile duct epithelial cells. In some biopsies these channels are very rare. In others they are prominent and may be dilated and almost circular. It is uncertain whether these two varieties are different disease entities. Portal vein branches are small and sparse. There is sparse inflammatory cell infiltrate except in

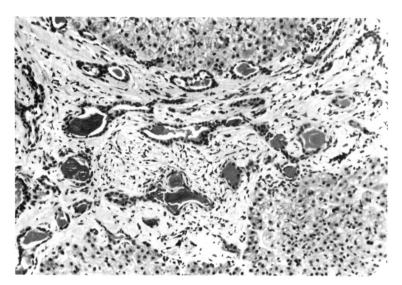

Figure 16.3 Congenital hepatic fibrosis. A wide band of fibrous tissue is seen
separating two areas of hepatic parenchyma. Within the fibrous tissue a conspicuous
feature is the variously shaped spaces lined by bile duct epithelial cells. Some spaces
contain densely staining material. No portal vein branches can be seen. There is no
inflammatory cell infiltrate. The hepatic parenchyma is normal (percutaneous liver
biopsy: haematoxylin and eosin × 100, reduced to seven-eighths in reproduction)

cases complicated by cholangitis in which numerous neutrophils are present in and around
the biliary spaces. Micro-abscesses may form. Hepatic parenchyma is almost always
normal. The histological changes within the liver may be indistinguishable from those
seen in ARPD. Outside the liver there is splenomegaly and other features of portal
hypertension.

Associated disorders

Conditions associated with congenital hepatic fibrosis are as follows:

(1) Autosomal recessive polycystic disease of the kidneys and liver. In some children
    with this syndrome only 10% of the renal tubules may be involved. Renal failure and
    hypertension occur late by which time the effects of hepatic fibrosis are manifest. In
    many reports on congenital hepatic fibrosis cases of infantile polycystic disease are
    excluded since the renal manifestations of this disorder are so prominent.
(2) Ivemark's familial dysplasia. This is a familial disorder characterized by hep-
    atomegaly with features of congenital hepatic fibrosis and localized renal dysplasia
    with primitive collecting tubules and much interstitial fibrosis. Renal changes often
    lead to renal failure in infancy. Increased fibrosis and cystic change is seen also in
    the pancreas (Ivemark *et al.*, 1959; Nathan and Batsakis, 1969).
(3) Meckel's syndrome. This is a disorder in which encephalocele, or anencephaly, cysts
    in the kidney, polydactyly, and other anomalies may occur. General hepatic fibrosis
    may also be present (Fried *et al.*, 1971; Rapola and Salonen, 1985).

(4) Adult type polycystic disease.
(5) Without renal disease, rarely (Murray-Lyon *et al.*, 1973).
(6) Jeune's syndrome.
(7) Nephronophthisis. These are familial disorders inherited in an X-linked or autosomal recessive fashion and characterized by numerous glomerular cysts, marked periglomerular fibrosis, tubular dilatation and interstitial fibrosis. All lead to renal failure at varying ages but have differing degrees of hepatic fibrosis (Landing *et al.*, 1990).
(8) Medullary cystic disease has similar features but presents in adult life and is inherited in an autosomal dominant fashion.
(9) A syndrome comprising nephronophthisis, pigmentary retinopathy, with or without cone-shaped epiphysis usually presents with features of renal impairment at 6–10 years of age rather than with those of CHF. It is presumed to represent a number of disorders inherited in an autosomal recessive fashion (Fernandez-Rodriguez *et al.*, 1990).
(10) Cortical and medullary renal cysts. Lieberman *et al.* (1971) described five cases of congenital hepatic fibrosis in which the renal parenchyma contains cysts within the cortex and medulla apparently arising in the distal and collecting tubules. The cysts were not radially orientated but were lined by columnar epithelium unlike ARPD: four out of the five patients described had renal impairment.
(11) Medullary sponge kidney (Kerr *et al.*, 1962).
(12) Intestinal lymphangiectasia with secondary diarrhoea and protein-losing enteropathy (Pelletier *et al.*, 1986).

Clinical features

The principal clinical features are abdominal distension, firm hepatomegaly which may lead to consideration of malignancy, splenomegaly, hypersplenism and haematemesis or melaena due to alimentary bleeding secondary to portal hypertension. Only rarely is the liver not enlarged. Other features include: abdominal pain, which in some instances may be very prominent; fever due to cholangitis in dilated bile ductules; the hepatitis syndrome of infancy; ascites; and features of associated conditions, particularly the renal disorders (Table 16.4)

This is a disorder of childhood or early adult life. Where congenital hepatic fibrosis does not complicate infantile polycystic disease, or the other rare syndromes described above, it usually presents at the age of 1 to 2 years with abdominal distension or with asymptomatic hepatosplenomegaly in early childhood. In later childhood and in adult life, the typical presentation is alimentary bleeding. The time of initial bleed, however, has varied from 8 months to 60 years. It is in late childhood and adult life that abdominal pain and cholangitis most frequently occur. Another cause for abdominal pain is splenic infarction.

Hypersplenism is rarely a problem in early infancy but may be evident by the age of 5 years. Liver function is well preserved but we have observed end-stage liver disease requiring liver transplantation in a girl of 14 years with ARPD and good renal function.

Diagnosis

Alkaline phosphatase and gamma-glutamyl transpeptidase may be slightly elevated but other standard tests of liver function are typically normal. Even if there is no urea retention

Table 16.4 Features of commoner renal lesions associated with congenital hepatic fibrosis (CHF)

	ADPD	ARPD	Medullary sponge kidney	Medullary cystic kidney (or nephronophthisis)
Inheritance	Autosomal dominant	Autosomal recessive	Uncertain (occasionally autosomal recessive)	Variable (or autosomal recessive)
Age of onset	Early childhood to late adulthood	0–10 years	Late childhood or adulthood	Early childhood to about 30 years
Symptoms	Abdominal pain Haematuria Slow onset of uraemia	Uraemia of variable progression	Haematuria Renal calculi Often asymptomatic	Salt wasting leading to progressive uraemia
Associations	Polycystic liver and pancreas Aneurysms of circle of Willis	CHF	CHF uncommon	Retinitis pigmentosa CHF occasionally
Radiology	Grossly enlarged kidneys with large patchily distributed cysts	Slightly enlarged kidneys Multiple cysts Blunted calyces	Normal sized kidneys Multiple calculi Visualization of dilated tubules by contrast	Small lobulated contracted kidneys Thinned cortices
Grey scale ultrasound	Large irregular echoes	Poorly defined echoes throughout	Irregular widened central echoes	Well defined cysts or pelvicalyceal echoes
Histology	Entire nephron involved	Multiple small cysts in both cortex and medulla	Small less numerous cysts at apices of renal pyramids	Glomerular sclerosis Interstitial fibrosis Cysts confined to corticomedullary junction

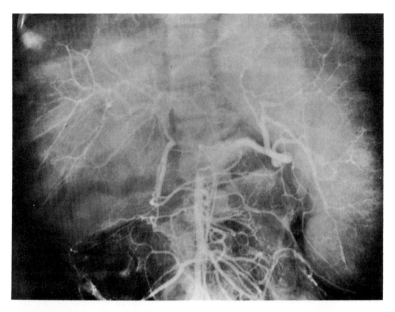

(a)

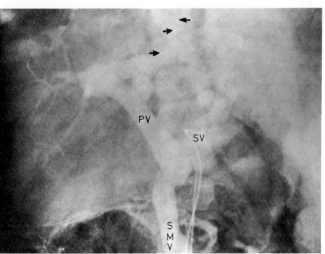

(b)

Figure 16.4 Selective splenic and superior mesenteric angiograms in a patient aged 13 years with autosomal recessive polycystic disease of the kidneys and liver and congenital hepatic fibrosis. Symptoms had started at the age of 4 years with alimentary bleeding due to portal hypertension. This had never been a severe problem, however, but hypersplenism now is marked. For the last 4 years she has had significant urea retention. Angiography has been performed by placing a catheter through the femoral artery into the splenic and superior mesenteric artery. (a) Showing marked splenomegaly with numerous small aneurysms in the branches of the splenic artery. (b) The portal (PV) and superior mesenteric (SMV) veins are large and patent. The splenic vein (SV) is not well shown. Much of the splenic outflow appears to run into large gastric and oesophageal collateral veins (→). The right branch of the portal vein and its intrahepatic branches are small. The left portal vein is large and its branches probably normal, suggesting that the right lobe of the liver is more affected than the left. In the capillary and venous phase it is seen that the hepatogram is slightly mottled but there are no clear filling defects

or elevation of the blood pressure, the intravenous pyelogram may be abnormal in up to 30% of cases, showing renal enlargement or distortion of the calyces. Barium meal or endoscopy may show varices. Ultrasonography confirms organomegaly, portal vein patency and may show features of portal hypertension. The kidneys may be abnormal. The diagnosis is confirmed by percutaneous liver biopsy provided an adequate specimen is obtained.

Treatment

The main problem in clinical management is portal hypertension causing alimentary bleeding. This can usually be controlled by injection sclerotherapy. Surgical portosystemic shunts should be considered if this fails or for patients living in circumstances where skilled injection sclerotherapy is not available. A further indication may be the child or adolescent who has hypersplenism, has had alimentary bleeding and develops features of progressive renal failure. Prophylactic shunting with splenectomy facilitates renal transplantation (McGonigle *et al.*, 1981). If the shunt procedure includes splenectomy there is an increased risk of severe bacterial infection. If it is followed by thrombosis of the shunt other parts of the portal venous system may also thrombose (Figure 16.4). Abdominal pain should be treated with analgesics. Cholangitis requires vigorous treatment with systemic antibiotics such as kanamycin or gentamicin with, however, regular checks on serum levels since there may be renal impairment. Cholangiography and surgery on the biliary tree should be avoided but may have to be considered if calculi develop. Partial hepatectomy with resection of focal dilatation of bile ducts may be indicated.

Autosomal dominant polycystic disease (adult type)

This condition, which is inherited in an autosomal dominant fashion with high penetrance is characterized by the occurrence of multiple cysts in the liver and kidney and occasionally in other organs. The defective gene on chromosome 16 has not been identified. Although most commonly diagnosed in adult life it may present in infancy.

Pathology

Cysts may be distributed diffusely through the liver or restricted to one area, usually the left lobe. They vary in size from less than 1 mm to more than 12 cm in diameter. They are lined by cuboidal or columnar epithelium and contain clear, colourless or light yellow fluid. Typically the cysts do not communicate with the biliary system although they appear to be related to bile ducts and the portal area. They are surrounded by a narrow band of dense fibrous tissue. They may be associated with discrete round complexes containing bile ductules in a dense fibrous stroma (Von Meyenberg complexes). These micro-hamartoma have been reported to undergo malignant transformation.

Clinical and laboratory features

Hepatic involvement is frequently asymptomatic and morbidity and mortality are largely due to renal involvement. Clinical features are those of a hepatic mass causing hepatomegaly. It may be associated with upper abdominal discomfort and occasionally nausea, vomiting and fever. Portal hypertension is a rare complication. Large cysts may cause obstruction to bile flow. Liver function is usually normal. The cyst are demonstrated on ultrasonography or computed tomography. Diagnosis is made on the basis of the liver histology and the demonstration of lesions in liver and kidney in a parent.

Treatment

Treatment is rarely required but patients with severe pain, portal hypertension or obstructive jaundice may benefit from draining the cysts into the peritoneal cavity or from resection if possible.

Focal dilatation of intrahepatic bile ducts (Caroli's syndrome)

This very rare condition is characterized by a non-obstructive dilatation of intrahepatic bile ducts. Only a portion or the whole of the liver may be involved. Saccular or cylindrical dilatations of the main right and left hepatic ducts and of the common hepatic duct may also occur. Diverticulae may arise from the right and left hepatic ducts. Bile duct dilatation predisposes to recurrent cholangitis, liver abscess, intraductal lithiasis, fatal sepsis and 7% develop carcinoma. The hepatic parenchyma is normal apart from inflammation and fibrosis around dilated segments which have become infected.

The condition may occur as a single isolated abnormality (Caroli's disease) or with congenital hepatic fibrosis. The latter produces portal hypertension and its problems. It also occurs in association with choledochal cysts. Renal cysts, tubular ectasia, medullary sponge kidney and adult polycystic kidney disease are occasional associations.

Clinical and laboratory features

Patients present with abdominal pain, fever and jaundice due to cholangitis or with features of Gram-negative septicaemia. The clinical picture may suggest cholecystitis or cholangitis. There may biliary colic if calculi develop. If the lesion is associated with congenital hepatic fibrosis, portal hypertension is likely to be present. Symptoms may occur at any time in life but frequently start in childhood or following surgery or invasive investigation of the biliary tree.

The diagnosis is suspected by the demonstration of cystic formations within the liver by ultrasonic scanning or computed tomography. A central dot sign thought to represent portal vein branches surrounded by dilated ducts is typically found (Inui *et al.*, 1992). Hepatobiliary excretion scans may show 'cold' areas in the early phase with concentration and retention of isotope in dilated ducts later. Invasive techniques such as percutaneous cholangiography or operative cholangiography, must be avoided unless cholangitis has occurred and there are strong grounds for suspecting the presence of biliary calculi. Most surgical procedures are liable to be followed by an exacerbation of the cholangitis.

Treatment

Treatment consists of antibiotics to control cholangitis, but it is rarely possible to produce complete sterility of the bile. Since there is no mechanical obstruction bile duct surgery is contraindicated unless there is very clear evidence of secondary bile duct obstruction due to calculi. Left lobe hepatectomy or partial resection of the right lobe with removal of calculi may be helpful, particularly if the disease is localized. For diffuse disease liver transplantation should be considered.

Hereditary haemorrhagic telangiectasis (Osler-Rendu-Weber disease)

Hereditary haemorrhagic telangiectasia is characterized by the presence of multiple telangiectasia of the skin and mucous membrane. Inheritance is autosomal dominant. Hepatic involvement occurs in almost every case. The liver may look macroscopically nodular or cirrhotic with telangiectasia on the surface. Microscopically there may be a honeycomb network of dilated sinusoidal channels lined by epithelial cells, tortuous thick-walled veins flanked by numerous wide calibre arteries or enlarged portal tracts with numerous dilated vessels. These vascular arrangements may interfere with the nutrition of liver cells. Arteriovenous fistulae lead to portal hypertension, variceal haemorrhages and high output heart failure. Haemobilia may occur.

The diagnosis is made on the basis of the clinical features, the family history and angiography or CT scanning.

Hepatic involvement in rare malformation syndromes

Increased portal tract fibrosis with prominent bile ducts occurs in such syndromes as Elis-Van Creveld, Jeune, Laurence-Moon-Biedl, Backet's, tuberous sclerosis, medullary cystic disease and Meckel's. The pathological severity ranges from an apparent isolated hamartomatous transformation to features reminiscent of ARPD. In some disorders there is prominent pancreatic and renal fibrosis. In all these disorders the hepatic features, which take the form of hepatomegaly or portal hypertension, are usually of secondary clinical importance except in instances when the natural history of the disease has been changed as for example following renal transplantation in the Laurence-Moon-Biedl syndrome. Macroscopic cysts occur in the lethal Meckel's syndrome. In Jeune's syndrome dilatation of intrahepatic and extrahepatic bile ducts occurs with cholestasis and periportal fibrosis leading to cirrhosis which may happen by 12 months of age (Hudgins *et al.*, 1992).

Mulibrey (muscle, liver, brain, eye) nanism is an autosomal recessive syndrome characterized by growth failure, a triangular face with a hydrocephalic skull, hypotonia and venous congestion caused by pericardial constriction. Hepatomegaly is a constant feature. The majority are lost by abortion or neonatal and infantile death but less severely affected cases survive to adult life.

Bibliography and references

General

Benhamou, J.-P. and Menu, Y. (1991) Non-parasitic cystic disease of the liver and intrahepatic biliary tree. In: *Oxford Textbook of Clinical Hepatology* (eds McIntyre, N., Benhamou, J.-P., Bricher, J., Rizzetto and Rodes, J). Oxford Medical Publications, Oxford, pp. 520–525

Desmet, V. J. (1992) Congenital diseases of intrahepatic bile ducts: variations on the theme 'ductal plate malformation'. *Hepatology*, **16**, 1069–1083

Landing, B. H., Wells, T. R., Lipsey, A. I. and Oyemade, O. A. (1990) Morphometric studies of cystic and tubulointerstitial kidney disease with hepatic fibrosis in children. *Pediatr. Pathol.*, **10**, 959–972

Summerfield, J. A., Nagafuchi, Y., Sherlock, S. *et al.* (1986) Hepatobiliary fibropolycystic disease: A clinical and histological review of 51 patients. *J. Hepatol.*, **2**, 141

Witzleben, C. L. (1990) Cystic diseases of the liver. In: *Hepatology. A textbook of liver disease*, 2nd edn (eds Zakim, D. and Boyer, T. D.). W. B. Saunders, Philadelphia, pp. 1395–1411

Autosomal recessive polycystic disease of the kidneys and liver

Annand, S. K., Alon, U., Chan, J. C. M. *et al.* (1984) Cystic diseases of the kidney in children. *Adv. Pediatr.*, **31**, 371

Blyth, H. and Ockenden, B. G. (1971) Polycystic disease in the kidneys and liver presenting in childhood. *J. Med. Genet.*, **8**, 257

Breuing MH, Devoto, M. and Romeo, G. (1992) Polycystic kidney disease. In: *Contributions to Nephrology.* Karger, Basel, p. 97

Gabow, P. A., Ikle, D. W., Holmes, J. H. *et al.* (1984) Polycystic kidney disease: Prospective analysis of non-azotaemic patients and family members. *Ann. Intern. Med.*, **101**, 238

Lieberman, E., Salihnas-Madrigal, L., Gwinn, J. L. *et al.* (1971) Infantile polycystic disease in kidneys and liver. *Medicine (Baltimore)*, **50**, 277

Premkumar, A., Berdon, W. E., Levy, J., Amodio, J., Abramson, S. J. and Newhouse, J. H. (1988) The emergence of hepatic fibrosis and portal hypertension in infants and children with autosomal recessive polycystic kidney disease. *Pediatr. Radiol.*, **18**, 123–129

Congenital hepatic fibrosis

Alvarez, F., Bernard, O., Brunel, F. *et al.* (1981) Congenital hepatic fibrosis in children. *J. Pediatr.*, **99**, 370

Alvarez, E., Hadchouel, M. and Bernard, O. (1982) Latent chronic cholangitis in congenital hepatic fibrosis. *Eur. J. Pediatr.*, **139**, 203

Blyth, H. and Ockenden, B. G. (1971) Polycystic disease in the kidneys and liver presenting in childhood. *J. Med. Genet.*, **8**, 257

Bodaghi, E., Zaman, T. and Kheradpir, M. H. (1980) Familial nephropathy associated with congenital hepatic fibrosis, degenerative retinitis and cone-shaped epiphyses. *Int. J. Pediatr. Nephrol.*, **1**, 153

Caine, Y., Deckelbaum, R. J., Weizmann, Z. *et al.* (1984) Congenital hepatic fibrosis, unusual presentation. *Arch. Dis. Childh.*, **59**, 1094

Fernandez-Rodriguez, R., Morales, J. M., Lizasoain, M. *et al.* (1990) Senior-Loken syndrome (nephronophthisis and pigmentary retinopathy) associated to liver fibrosis: a family study. *Nephron*, **55**, 74–77

Fried, K., Liban, E., Lurie, M. *et al.* (1971) Polycystic kidneys associated with malformation of the brain, polydactyly and other birth defects. *J. Med. Genet.*, **8**, 285

Inue, A., Fujisawa, T., Suemitsu, Y., *et al.* (1992) A case of Caroli's disease with special reference to hepatic CT and US findings. *J. Pediatr. Gastroenterol. Nutr.*, **14**, 463–466

Ivemark, B. I., Oldfeldt, V. and Zetterstrom, R. I. (1959) Familial dysplasia of kidneys, liver and pancreas, A probably genetically determined syndrome. *Acta Paediatr. Scand.*, **48**, 1

Kerr, D. N. S., Warrick, C. K. and Hart-Mercer, J. (1962) A lesion resembling medullary sponge kidney in patients with congenital hepatic fibrosis. *Clin. Radiol.*, **13**, 85

Lieberman, E., Salinas-Madrigal, L., Gwinn, J. L. *et al.* (1971) Infantile polycystic disease in kidneys and liver. *Medicine (Baltimore)*, **50**, 277

McGonigle, R. J. S., Mowat, A. P., Bewick, M. *et al.* (1981) Congenital hepatic fibrosis and IPCD: Role of portacaval shunting and transplantation in 3 patients. *Q. J. Med.*, **199**, 269

Murray-Lyon, I. M., Ockenden, B. G. and Williams, R. (1973) Congenital hepatic fibrosis – is a single clinical entity? *Gastroenterology*, **64**, 653

Nathan, M. and Batsakis, J. O. (1969) Congenital hepatic fibrosis. *Surg. Gynecol. Obstet.*, **128**, 1033

Odievre, M., Chaumont, P. and Oiry, P. (1976) Roentgenographic abnormalities of the intrahepatic portal system in congenital hepatic fibrosis. *Radiology*, **122**, 427

Patterson, M., Gonzalez-Vitale, J. C. and Fagin, J. C. (1982) Polycystic liver disease: A study of cyst fluid constituents. *Hepatology*, **2**, 475

Pelletier, V. A., Saleano, N., Brocho, P. *et al.* (1986) Secretory diarrhoea with protein-losing enteropathy, intestinal lymphangiectasia and congenital hepatic fibrosis. *J. Pediatr.*, **108**, 61

Sokhi, O. S., Morrice, G. J., McGee, J. and Blumgart, L. (1975) Congenital hepatic fibrosis: aspects of diagnosis and surgical managemen t. *Br. J. Surg.*, **62**, 621

Witzleben, C. L. and Sharp, A. R. (1982) Nephronophthisis – congenital hepatic fibrosis. *Hum. Pathol.*, **13**, 728

Adult polycystic disease

Grunfeld, J. P., Albouze, G., Jungers, P. *et al.* (1985) Liver changes and complications in adult polycystic kidney disease. *Adv. Nephrol.*, **14**, 1

Kaplan, B. S., Rabin, J. and Drummond, K. M. (1977) Autosomal dominant polycystic renal disease in children. *J. Pediatr.*, **90**, 782

Mulutinovic, J., Failkow, P. J., Rudd, T. G. *et al.* (1980) Liver cysts in patients with autosomal dominant polycystic kidney disease. *Am. J. Med.*, **68**, 741

Shokeir, M. H. K. (1978) Expression of 'adult' polycystic renal disease in the fetus and new born. *Clin. Genet.*, **14**, 61

Intrahepatic bite duct dilatation

Caroli, J. and Corcos, V. (1964) La dilatation congenitale des voies biliaires intra-hepatiques. *Rev. Med. Chir. Mal. du Foie*, **39**, 1

Hermansen, M. C., Starshak, R. J. and Werlin, S. L. (1979) Caroli disease: the diagnostic approach. *J. Pediatr.*, **94**, 879

Jordan, D., Harpaz, N. and Thung, S. N. (1989) Caroli's disease and adult polycystic disease: a rarely recognised association. *Liver*, **9**, 30–35

Murray-Lyon, I. M., Shilkin, K. B., Laws, J. W., Illing, R. C. and Williams, R. (1972) Non-obstructive dilatation of intrahepatic biliary tree with cholangitis. *Q. J. Med.*, **41**, 477

Nagasue, N. (1984) Successful treatment of Caroli's disease by hepatic resection. *Ann. Surg.*, **200**, 718

Hereditary haemorrhagic telangiectasia (Osler-Rendu-Weber disease)

Daly, J. J. and Schiller, A. L. (1976) The liver in hereditary haemorrhagic telangiectasia. *Am. J. Med.*, **60**, 723

Henderson, J. M., Liechity, E. J. and Jahnke, R. W. (1981) Liver involvement in hereditary haemorrhagic telangiectasia. *J. Comput. Assist. Tomogr.*, **5**, 733

Rare malformation syndromes

Bohm, N., Feduca, M., Staudt, R. *et al.* (1978) Chondroectodermal dysplasia (Ellis-Van Creveld syndrome) with dysplasia of renal medulla and bile ducts. *Histopathology*, **2**, 267

Carles, D., Serville, F., Duberq, J. P. and Gonnet, J. M. (1988) Renal, pancreatic and hepatic dysplasia sequence. *Eur. J. Pediatr.*, **147**, 431–432

Hudgins, L., Rosengren, S., Treem, W. and Hyams, J. (1992) Early cirrhosis in survivors with Jeune thoracic dystrophy. *J. Pediatr.*, **120**, 754–756

Landing, B. H., Wells, T. R. and Claireaux, A. E. (1980) Morphometric analysis of liver lesions in cystic diseases of childhood. *Hum. Pathol. (Suppl.)*, **11**, 549

Perheentopa, J., Autio, F., Leisti, S. *et al.* (1975) Mulibrey nanism. A review of 23 cases. *Birth Defects, Original Article Series*, **11**, 3

Rapola, J. and Salonen, R. (1985) Visceral anomalies in the Meckel syndrome. *Teratology*, **31**, 193

Roussel, B., Leroux, B., Gaillard, D. and Faudre, G. (1985) Chronic diffuse tubulo-interstitial nephritis and hepatic involvement in the Laurence-Moon-Bardet. Biedl Syndrome. *Helv. Paediatr. Acta*, **40**, 405

Chapter 17

Wilson's disease

Wilson's disease in childhood may mimic any form of parenchymal hepatic disorder. More than 50% of cases present before puberty with no neurological abnormality. Without treatment there is progressive damage to the liver and/or brain, and premature death. Early treatment is relatively free from side-effects and very effective. Wilson's disease with all its protean presentations must be considered in all children with unexplained hepatic disorders, deteriorating school performance, acquired neurological abnormalities or general ill-health. Equally important is the recognition and treatment of asymptomatic siblings and cousins of probands.

Definition

Wilson's disease is an inborn error of metabolism characterized by defective biliary copper excretion and the effects of accumulation of toxic amounts of copper in liver, brain, kidney and cornea. Rarely, there may be evidence of skeletal and endocrine involvement. The disorder is inherited in an autosomal recessive fashion. The basic genetic defect is unknown but genetic linkage analysis has located the site of the mutant gene to a 50-kilobase section of the long arm of chromosome 13(q14.2–14.3).

Epidemiology

The disorder occurs worldwide in all races with an estimated prevalence of 1:30 000 to 1:100 000 subjects. In socially isolated communities with consanguineous mating the prevalence can be much higher. Clinical disease is not recognized before 5 years of age. The onset may be delayed to the sixth decade. Whether the onset is earlier with excessive copper intake is unknown.

Pathogenesis

An abnormality in the transport and storage of copper resulting in copper accumulation is thought to be important in pathogenesis. The liver in health plays a major role in copper homeostasis. Ingested copper on absorption in the small intestine may be retained in enterocytes, bound to metallothionein. Some passes into the portal system and is carried to the liver bound to albumin or to a copper-binding protein called transcuprein. In the liver it is incorporated into essential metalloenzymes or caeruloplasmin, stored or excreted in bile in a form which is not reabsorbable. The biliary excretion matches absorption. Two major abnormalities in copper metabolism occur in Wilson's disease: diminished biliary excretion of copper and impaired incorporation of copper into caeruloplasmin. A persistently positive copper balance is present in patients with Wilson's disease in spite of increased urinary copper excretion. Intestinal absorption of copper is normal, as is hepatic clearance of albumin-bound absorbed copper early in the disease. Liver copper concentrations rise to values up to 50 times the normal mean in the presymptomatic stage of the disease. In Wilson's disease the concentration is increased in the cytoplasm and in the mitochondria early in the disease. How it is sequestrated is unclear. As the liver copper-binding sites become saturated there is, first, slowing down of hepatic uptake followed by biochemical and histological evidence of liver damage. Copper can then be seen in lysosomes. With hepatocellular injury there is release of copper which causes further liver damage and release of copper into the circulation. The non-caeruloplasmin serum copper rises and copper accumulates in and damages other tissues. A characteristic pattern of brain damage develops. Manifestations of renal tubular injury usually appear simultaneously.

High concentrations of copper are found in the liver, brain, corneas and renal tubules in patients dying with this disease. Very rapid copper release is thought to cause the haemolytic anaemia sometimes seen early in the clinical course of Wilson's disease. Recent suggestions for pathogenesis include the synthesis of an abnormal copper binding protein in the hepatic cytoplasm, defective lysosomal processing and thus biliary excretion or the lack of a copper-binding protein in bile, the absence of which would facilitate copper reabsorption (Ivengar *et al.*, 1988).

Caeruloplasmin is a blue, copper-containing serum alpha-2 globulin glycoprotein of uncertain physiological function which is synthesized in the liver. In adult life, serum caeruloplasmin levels are relatively constant at between 0.2 and 0.45 g/litre. In cord blood the levels are much lower, usually being less than 0.1 g/litre. By the age of 2 months, adult levels are reached and early in infancy the levels are often higher, declining to the adult range by the age of 10–12 years. The newborn liver has a much higher concentration of copper than the adult, the concentrations varying up to 63 µg/g dry weight, as opposed to the usual adult range of 15–50 µg/g dry weight. In the newborn 60% of the copper is located in the lysosomes in the form of metallothionein.

Copper incorporation into caeruloplasmin is deficient in Wilson's disease. An abnormally low serum concentration of caeruloplasmin is found in over 90% of patients in reported series but this prevalence may be spuriously high if a low serum concentration of caeruloplasmin is an essential criterion for diagnosis. How the abnormalities of caeruloplasmin metabolism contribute to pathogenesis is unclear. Similarly, low caeruloplasmin values are found with no pathological effects in some heterozygotes and in genetic hypocaeruloplasminaemia. Note that the gene for caeruloplasmin is on chromosome 3 and for metallothioneins on chromosome 16. The similarities in copper status of newborn and in Wilson's disease has given rise to the hypothesis that Wilson's disease may be caused by a defect in a control gene determining the switch to the adult form of copper metabolism rather than to a defect in a structural gene.

The contribution of environmental factors such as cumulative copper intake and intercurrent viral hepatitis in the pathogenesis of liver damage is unclear. Note that identical twins may present at different ages and with different features, one with mainly hepatic features and the other neurological.

Pathology

Hepatic   From asymptomatic patients investigated because of an affected relative, some knowledge of the early hepatic pathology is available. By electron microscopy hepatic

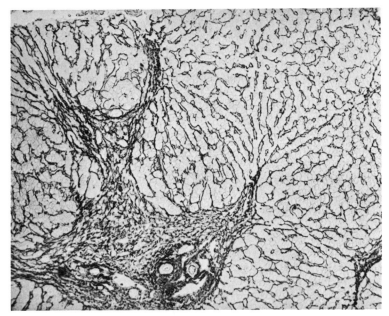

Figure 17.1 Wilson's disease. Percutaneous liver biopsy (reticulin × 150, reduced to seven-tenths in reproduction) from a girl aged 9 years. It shows extensive fibrosis around an enlarged portal tract with wide fibrous septa extending out into the hepatic parenchyma. The reticulin framework for the hepatocytes within the hepatic parenchyma is normally orientated. A hepatic vein branch is seen in the upper right-hand corner. The patient presented 5 months previously with malaise and tiredness. The mucosae were pale but there were no other abnormalities on examination. The haemoglobin was 8.0 g/dl with slightly hypochromic red cells. The reticulocyte count ranged from 7 to 14%. There was no ocult blood loss and extensive investigations uncovered no cause for haemolysis. Because the serum aminotransferase level was elevated on one occasion, she was referred for further hepatic investigations. There were no clinical features of liver disease. Wilson's disease was diagnosed on the basis of Keyser–Fleischer rings, very low serum caeruloplasmin, high urinary copper and high copper content in the liver biopsy. A low copper diet, penicillamine and pyridoxine were recommended. Liver function tests have remained normal, the patient is no longer anaemic. There have been no neurological abnormalities

mitochondria are seen to be pleomorphic with electron dense vacuoles which sometimes contain granular or crystalloid material. Peroxisomes may be enlarged and dense. The earliest histological change is microvesicular (sometimes macro-) fatty infiltration of hepatocytes, often with prominent glycogen-containing vacuoles in the nuclei. Such changes are associated with a mesenchymal reaction with increased fibrosis and eventually cirrhosis (see Figure 17.1). In symptomatic patients the liver may be enlarged but is commonly normal in size or even shrunken due to macronodular cirrhosis. In addition features of a 'toxic' hepatitis, chronic aggressive hepatitis, varying degrees of hepatocellular necrosis with multinucleated large hepatocytes and Mallory's cytoplasmic hyalin, as seen in alcoholic liver disease, may also be present. In advanced disease the appearances are those of cirrhosis with no specific features although a few hepatocytes may show fatty change and glycogen-containing nuclei. Pigmented granules are frequent. There are commonly features of secondary portal hypertension and often of hypersplenism. Hepatocellular carcinoma is a rare complication.

Early in the disease specific stains for copper using rubeanic acid are negative, even though the liver copper determined chemically is between three and 30 times normal. Rubeanic acid stains for copper are positive when there is liver damage although liver copper concentration may be lower than in the early stages of the disease. Focal orcein staining of copper-associated protein is seen when liver damage is present.

Cerebral   The cerebral changes are found mainly in the corpus striatum which shows shrinkage, cavitation, decrease in the number of neurons and in myelinated nerve fibres and increased astrocytosis. Similar, but less severe changes are seen in the cerebellum, the thalamus and the cortex.

Other sites   Copper is found deposited also in the deep layers of the cornea just within the limbus, extending in a ring around the cornea. It may be deposited also in the lens to give a 'sunflower' cataract. Copper can be found in renal tubular cells.

Clinical features

The initial symptoms in children with Wilson's disease are unfortunately relatively non-specific, such as lethargy, anorexia, pallor, abdominal pain, vomiting, weight loss and epistaxis. Evidence of hepatic involvement is the most frequent presentation in pre-pubertal patients but four of seven children with a predominantly neurological presentation had no clinical evidence of liver disease, although all had abnormal biochemical tests of liver function (Lingham *et al.*, 1987). Liver damage in Wilson's disease may mimic any form of liver disease in childhood (Table 17.1). A deterioration in school performance or behaviour was present in one-fifth of those presenting in our unit with liver disease. The diagnosis is usually unsuspected until evidence of hepatic, neurological and/or renal disease and/or haemolysis emerges (see also Table 14.2). Pancreatitis may be a presenting feature. The majority are diagnosed between 8 and 10 years.

The neurological abnormalities associated with Wilson's disease in childhood include deteriorating school performance with particular difficulties in writing and speaking, behaviour problems, clumsiness, slurring of speech and difficulties with fine movements. The classic form of the disease, progressive lenticular degeneration with tremor, increasing muscular rigidity, psychiatric features and asymptomatic cirrhosis is infre-

Table 17.1 Hepatic presentations of Wilson's disease

Asymptomatic hepatomegaly
Hepatosplenomegaly with vague gastrointestinal symptoms
Jaundice with oedema and ascites
Subacute hepatitis (non-A, non-B hepatitis)
Fulminant hepatitis
Chronic aggressive hepatitis
Asymptomatic cirrhosis
Gastrointestinal haemorrhage due to portal hypertension
? Cholestatic liver disease of infancy

Table 17.2 Non-hepatic presentations in Wilson's disease

Neurological disorders
Deteriorating school performance
Deteriorating behaviour
Personality changes
Massive albuminuria
Renal tubular abnormalities
Renal rickets
Acute haemolysis
Recurrent abdominal pain
Arthralgia
Fever
Kayser–Fleischer rings
Melanin hyperpigmentation of legs and scars

quently found in childhood. Occasionally convulsions and hemiparesis may be features (Table 17.2).

Renal involvement may take the form of massive albuminuria with peripheral oedema and ascites mimicking a nephrotic syndrome. Renal rickets and a full-blown Fanconi syndrome may also be the first indication of disease. Acute haemolysis is another presentation. Some patients are diagnosed by finding Kayser-Fleischer rings on routine ophthalmic examination in which a slit-lamp has been used or following the finding of asymptomatic hepatosplenomegaly.

Laboratory findings

Liver function tests indicate a variable degree of hepatocellular necrosis with or without hypoalbuminaemia and hypoprothrombinaemia. Although jaundice due to haemolytic anaemia is usually transient a significant rise in reticulocyte count may persist. There may be features of hypersplenism (Figure 17.2). Urinary abnormalities secondary to excess copper deposition may include haematuria, proteinuria, glycosuria, hyperaminoaciduria and renal tubular acidosis. Phosphaturia and uricosuria may cause low serum concentrations of phosphate and uric acid.

Serum immunoglobulin concentrations may be elevated and significant titres of non-organ-specific autoantibody may be found mimicking autoimmune chronic active hepatitis. Cranial CT scanning or nuclear magnetic resonance scanning may reveal dilated ventricles and abnormalities in lenticular, thalamic, caudate and dentate nuclei even in patients with no neurological abnormalities. Positron emission tomography indicates a loss of dopamine presynaptic and postsynaptic receptors with dopamine synthesis preserved.

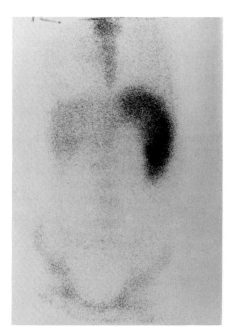

Figure 17.2 Technetium-99m colloid in a boy of 10 years with compensated cirrhosis due to Wilson's disease. There is intense imaging over the spleen, a marked increase in bone marrow uptake and very poor uptake in the liver although at the time of the study the serum albumin was 34 g/litre and the prothrombin time prolonged by only 5 seconds. The serum bilirubin was 50 mmol/litre and the aspartate aminotransferase 350 IU/litre. The disproportionate decrease in liver uptake is a typical but non-specific finding in some patients with Wilson's disease. With penicillamine therapy the biochemical tests of liver function have returned to normal

Course

The course of untreated Wilson's disease is variable. Usually there is gradual progression of the hepatic disease with involvement of other systems. There may be spontaneous remission of symptoms with exacerbation of intercurrent infection. Jaundice due to haemolytic episodes may recur over 1 to 2 years to be followed by an asymptomatic period of some years before features of liver insufficiency appear. There may be rapid hepatic deterioration giving acute liver failure or the gradual development of decompensated cirrhosis and hepatic encephalopathy with death usually in a few years. Neurological features may never appear but when they do, they may be mistaken for those of portosystemic shunting. In others liver damage is asymptomatic and cirrhosis with or without abnormalities of transaminases is found in a patient with neurological features.

Diagnosis

Its clinical features are non-specific in the early stages. It is essential to exclude Wilson's disease in any child with clinical or laboratory evidence of liver disease which is unexplained or if the course of acute hepatitis is unusual. Consanguinity of parents unexplained liver or neurological disease in siblings, previous history of haemolytic anaemia or clinical evidence of neurological abnormality should be additional prompts to exclude this disorder by the following investigations.

Ophthalmoscopic examination by slit-lamp

Kayser-Fleischer rings must be sought by an experienced examiner using a slit-lamp. They appear as brown or greenish-brown deposits of copper just within the limbus. They are always bilateral and usually complete but occasionally they may be absent at the medial and lateral aspects. They may be seen by the naked eye especially if viewed with a light directed from the side, but most frequently they can only be demonstrated with a slit-lamp. Such rings are rarely found below the age of 7. Their absence therefore does not exclude the diagnosis. This sign is pathognomonic of Wilson's disease except in children with chronic cholestasis in whom it may occur on rare occasions.

Serum caeruloplasmin determination

A low caeruloplasmin of less than 20 mg/dl (1.25 μmol/litre) is suggestive of Wilson's disease, in the absence of nephrotic syndrome, severe malabsorption or protein-losing enteropathy. In most forms of liver disease the caeruloplasmin is high, but in fulminant hepatitis, chronic active hepatitis and tyrosinaemia low values may be obtained. Low values are unfortunately found also in 10–20% of heterozygotes who have no evidence of disease.

   Between 4% and 20% of patients with Wilson's disease have a normal caeruloplasmin. In some the concentration falls as the liver disease comes under control with therapy. Pregnancy, oestrogens and oral contraceptives cause elevation of caeruloplasmin, even when it is genetically low.

Urinary copper determination before and after penicillamine

This is an essential diagnostic investigation in patients without Kayser-Fleischer rings. Two consecutive complete 24-hour urine collections are made into copper-free containers.

D-Penicillamine in a dose of 500 mg was given orally at the beginning of the second 24-hour collection and repeated after 12 hours. In a comparative study of copper estimations in 17 patients with Wilson's disease and 58 with other liver disorders in our unit the 24-hour urinary copper excretion after penicillamine challenge proved the most accurate single diagnostic test, levels of >25 μmol/24 hours being present in 15 of 17 patients with Wilson's disease, but in only one other child (who had acute liver failure) out of the 58 with other disorders (da Costa *et al.*, 1992). Values ranged from 20.3 to 70 μmol/ 24 hours (median 34.2) in Wilson's disease. Normal individuals, and heterozygotes for Wilson's disease, excrete less than 800 μg (10 μmol) per day. Urinary copper excretion without penicillamine ranged from 1.8 to 34.1 μmol (median 8.2) compared with less than 40 μg (0.6 μmol) per day in health. In six children with Wilson's disease urinary copper excretion was just above the upper limit of normal, overlapping with values obtained in 10 children with other liver disorders. In this study borderline increases in pre-penicillamine urinary copper values in Wilson's disease became massive with penicillamine. Excretion exceeded 20 μmol/24 hours after penicillamine in six patients with other chronic disorders but all had normal urinary copper excretion prior to penicillamine. The two estimations thus complement one another.

Total serum copper determinations are not helpful in the diagnosis of Wilson's disease since very low, normal or high values may be found. In the above study only six with Wilson's disease had free copper concentrations above those in other disorders while five had no detectable free copper. Caeruloplasmin concentration was above the cut-off value in three with Wilson's disease and below it in three with other disorders.

Copper content of liver biopsy

The normal liver copper concentration is usually between 20 and 40 μg/g dry weight and levels of greater than 40 μg are unusual. In Wilson's disease the liver copper is commonly greater than 250 μg/g dry weight, although levels as low as 90 μg may be found in some patients. In the above study liver copper concentration was less than the cut-off in three of 12 with Wilson's disease (range 64–2636, median 580 μg/g/dry weight) and above it in three of 11 (range 25–1450,median 2000 μg/g/dry weight) anicteric patients with other disorders. Heterozygotes have levels of between 40 and 210 μg/g dry weight. Very high liver coppers may be found in chronic cholestatic states and in Indian childhood cirrhosis (see Chapter 18).

Radioactive copper studies

Studies using radioactive isotopes of copper are rarely necessary for diagnosis. In patients with equivocal copper studies, in whom liver biopsy is contraindicated, the rate of copper incorporation into caeruloplasmin may help in the diagnosis. This test involves the intravenous injection of copper-64 (half-life 12.8 hours) or copper-67 (half-life 68 hours) followed by the determination of total serum copper and that bound to caeruloplasmin at 12-hourly intervals in the subsequent 3 days.

In Wilson's disease, practically no copper is incorporated into caeruloplasmin but it does occur to an appreciable extent in heterozygotes and in patients with other forms of liver disease causing hypocaeruloplasminaemia and occurs to a greater extent in normal individuals. Such investigations should only be undertaken in referral units with the necessary expertise.

Differential diagnosis

Although the clinical presentation is very variable and may be compatible with a wide range of hepatic disorders laboratory diagnosis presents no difficulties if the above investigations are performed except in patients with fulminant hepatic failure in whom no Kayser-Fleischer rings are present and in whom liver biopsy is contraindicated because of deranged clotting. In patients with idiopathic (non-A, non-B) fulminant hepatic failure, the serum caeruloplasmin and urinary copper concentrations are similar to those found in Wilson's disease. Serum copper concentrations may be discriminatory being high in Wilson's disease but low or low/normal in other causes of fulminant hepatic failure. A high bilirubin (>six times normal) and a relatively low aspartate transaminase (<four times normal) or a low alkaline phosphatase has been claimed to be indicative of Wilson's disease but it is not so in every case (Sallie *et al.*, 1992).

Treatment

Untreated Wilson's disease is invariably fatal. Oral chelating agents or liver transplantation are the two main therapies. Oral chelating agents which increase urinary copper excretion will arrest hepatocellular injury except in advanced disease. Such therapy is accompanied by a low copper diet, with restricted salt and water if there is oedema or ascites. In advanced disease liver transplantation gives the only prospect of survival. It corrects all features of the disease unless brain damage is severe.

Diet

Chocolate, nuts, mushrooms, cocoa, broccoli, liver and shellfish should be avoided. This will give less than 0.6 mg copper/day as opposed to the normal dietary copper of 1–5 mg/day and may help to minimize positive copper balance.

Chelating agents

D-Penicillamine, introduced in 1956, is the most effective agent available at present for diminishing copper stores. Its efficacy has been confirmed in many patients. If therapy is started in the pre-symptomatic phase, the development of disease can be prevented. If given sufficiently early in the presence of hepatic disease there is gradual clinical improvement over the course of 1–6 months, with laboratory test of liver function returning to normal over the course of up 4 years. A fall in the prothrombin time, usually occurring after 2–6 weeks of therapy is the first significant change in laboratory investigation in the patient who is responding. The cirrhosis remains stable, compensated and has a good long-term prognosis, if therapy continues. Neuropsychiatric abnormalities may go on improving over 3–4 years, with up to 30% deterioration initially including some with no pretreatment problems. If there is neuron loss or advanced sclerosis permanent sequelae will remain. Before starting treatment a full peripheral blood count and urinalysis should be performed. Therapy should start with a dose of 10 mg/kg/day given in divided doses just before meals. If there is no proteinuria or depression of the peripheral blood count the dose is increased to 20 mg/kg after two weeks.

Toxicity from penicillamine takes the form of an acquired epidermolysis bullosa and penicillamine dermopathy and pyridoxine deficiency, both of which appear to be more frequent with prolonged usage and high dosage. Up to 30% develop proteinuria which is partially dose-related. Urinalysis should be performed weekly at first but the interval may be gradually lengthened. Bone marrow depression is also a risk. Full blood counts should

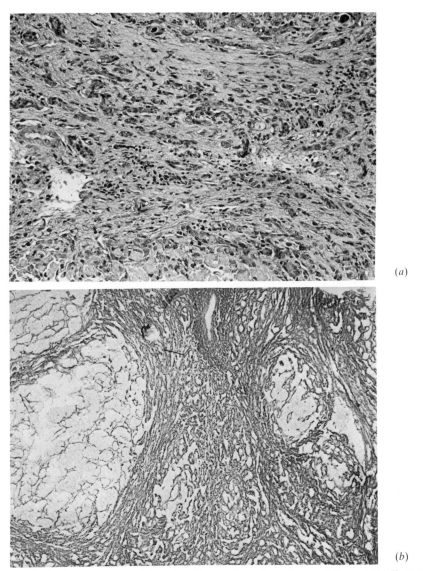

(a)

(b)

Figure 17.3 Wilson's disease. Postmortem liver specimen from a boy aged 11 years ((a) Haematoxylin and eosin, × 150; (b) Reticulin, × 150, both reduced to seven-tenths in reproduction.) The features are those of cirrhosis. (a) Showing an area of fibrous tissue with many bile ducts, presumably due to collapse of hepatic lobules. There is much fibrous tissue but little inflammatory cell reaction. (b) Showing regenerative nodules with hepatocytes of varying size surrounded by dense bands of fibrous tissue. Twelve months previously the parents had become concerned because of deteriorating school performance and lethargy. After 7 months some abdominal discomfort and abdominal distension was noted. Liver disease was suspected 9 weeks before his death when he became anorexic, vomited, and developed jaundice. A clinical diagnosis of infectious hepatitis was made at that time but when it was found the prothrombin time was prolonged by 15 seconds and albumin 24 g/litre, chronic underlying liver disease was suspected. The serum caeruloplasmin was 10 mg/dl, slit-lamp examination of the cornea showed typical Kayser–Fleischer rings. Purpura and alimentary haemorrhage, generalized oedema, ascites, and encephalopathy rapidly developed. Penicillamine and steroids as well as full supportive therapy as for fulminant hepatitis, did not arrest the downhill course. Unfortunately, the patient is just one of a number of children and young adults in whom the diagnosis of Wilson's disease had not been made until decompensated cirrhosis was present. In none has therapy arrested the progression of the disease

be carried out weekly in the first 8 weeks of therapy and in the weeks after any increase in dose.

Serious unpredictable toxic effects include immunologically-induced lesions such as systemic lupus erythematosus, immune complex nephritis, pemphigus, buccal ulceration and Goodpasture's syndrome. Urticaria, fever and lymph gland enlargement may also occur early in therapy. The onset of these side-effects is an indication for stopping treatment. It may be possible to re-introduce it gradually starting with a dose of 1 mg/kg. On occasions this may be achieved successfully while patients take antihistamines or corticosteroids.

If penicillamine has to be stopped after the serum albumin has returned to normal and liver function has markedly improved oral zinc may be substituted. If a substitute is required earlier trientine (triethylene tetra-amine) is an effective alternative. Experience with the drug is limited. A dose of 25 mg/kg/day given in three doses before a meal is effective. Some patients are reported to have developed lupus nephritis, neutropenia, sideroblastic anaemia and possible myopathy. Dyspepsia and allergic skin reaction are the only other adverse reactions reported. Occasionally, patients have been treated with unithiol and tetrathiomolybdate (Walshe, 1984).

Zinc

There has been a recent revival of interest in utilizing the antagonistic action of zinc on copper absorption as a mode of therapy in patients intolerant of penicillamine. Zinc induces an increase in copper excretion in the stools thought to be due to copper retention in metallothionein in enterocytes which are shed from intestinal villi. Two published reports show that zinc sulphate, 100 mg three times a day, maintains a negative copper balance and reversal of abnormal biochemical and pathological features in patients who have already received penicillamine (Alexiou et al., 1985; Caillie-Bertrend et al., 1985b). In three of seven adult patients deteriorating neurological features prompted a return to penicillamine. A number of adults presenting with neurological disease and one child with symptomatic liver disease have been treated with zinc alone. It may be important to ensure that sufficient zinc is taken to reduce copper absorption as assessed by the appearance of orally administered radiocopper in serum.

We have used zinc and penicillamine alternatively at 6-hourly intervals in 13 patients without adverse effects and have seen four recover in whom the hepatic prognostic index (see below) suggested that early death was likely.

The degree of decoppering should be ascertained by periodic measurements of 24-hour urinary excretion of copper. If the excretion falls below 800 μg (12.5 μmol) per day treatment should be interrupted for a few days and then a standard dose of penicillamine 0.5 g given at 12-hourly intervals. When successfully decoppered the baseline urinary copper excretion is usually less than 80 μg (1.25 μmol) per day and with penicillamine increases to less than 800 μg (12.5 μmol) per day. Alternatively a free serum copper of <1.6 μmol/litre (10 μg/dl) may be used as evidence of adequate decoppering.

Symptomatic therapy may be required for complications of cirrhosis. Surgical procedures are poorly tolerated. Portosystemic shunts should not be performed since these almost invariably are followed by progressive hepatic encephalopathy.

Liver transplantation

Liver transplantation is the only measure which will save patients presenting with encephalopathy with acute hepatic failure or those who develop liver failure with

Table 17.3 Assessment of hepatic prognosis of Wilson's disease at diagnosis

Bilirubin (μmol/litre)	Aspartate aminotransferase (IU/litre)	Prothrombin time prolongation (s)	Prognostic score
N< 20	N< 40	N< 4	
<100	<100	4	0
101–150	101–150	4– 8	1
151–200	151–200	9–12	2
201–300	201–300	13–20	3
>300	>300	>20	4

If total score is <6 a satisfactory response to chelation and dietary therapy is to be expected.

haemolysis after unwisely stopping therapy. Based on the severity of abnormality of serum aspartate aminotransferase, bilirubin and prothrombin time at diagnosis in 27 cases, we derived a prognostic index (Table 17.3) which proved useful in predicting the response to treatment in a subsequent nine cases (Nazer et al., 1986). We have recently reviewed our experience with the index in a further 20 symptomatic children. If the prognostic index remained less than 6 all recovered completely with chelation, with or without zinc. One with an initial index of 6 died with spontaneous peritonitis occurring as the index climbed at weekly intervals to 11. If the index is greater than 9 death within a week is likely (although one survived for 23 days) and urgent transplantation is essential (Figure 17.3). Patients with a scored of 6 to 9 should be listed for transplantation and treated with alternating zinc and penicillamine (see above). Transplantation can be deferred if no complications occur and the index is falling when a liver becomes available. As yet no deaths have occurred after 60 days of drug therapy. The results of liver transplantation reported in 57 patients followed for a mean of 2.7 years in 18 centres are similar to those in other conditions (Schilsky et al., 1992). The 1 year survival was 72%, with 4 requiring retransplantation. Surprisingly, 20 of 27 with fulminant liver failure survived, a better outcome following transplantation than in any other category of liver failure.

Investigation of siblings of patients with Wilson's disease

Siblings of a patient have a 1:4 chance of having the disease. It is estimated that if the proband and both parents are investigated using sophisticated genetic linkage analysis techniques it should be possible to identify affected individuals or heterozygotes with 99% accuracy in 90% of families. Absence of symptoms or abnormalities on clinical examination do not exclude the possibility that the individual is affected by the disease. Appropriate treatment before clinical features are evident prevent the development of the disease.

Even if such studies are confidently reported it would be prudent to carry out procedures 1–5 listed in Table 17.4. If genetic linkage analysis is impossible such investigations are mandatory. If these are normal, it may be presumed that the individual does not have Wilson's disease. If they show any abnormality, the usual course would be to proceed to percutaneous liver biopsy for determination of the copper content. This should establish the presence or absence of Wilson's disease. If liver biopsy is

Table 17.4 Investigation of siblings of patients with Wilson's disease

(1) Clinical examination for evidence of hepatic or neural disease
(2) Ophthalmic examination for Kayser–Fleischer rings
(3) Biochemical studies for evidence of liver or renal disease
(4) Serum caeruloplasmin determination
(5) Urinary copper determination with and without penicillamine 0.5 g twice a day
(6) If not contraindicated, percutaneous liver biopsy for copper determination and routine histological examination
(7) If biopsy is not indicated and investigations 2–5 are not diagnostic, intravenous radioactive infusion followed by determination of total and caeruloplasmin bound copper over 3 days

haemolysis after unwisely stopping therapy. Based on the severity of abnormality of serum aspartate aminotransferase, bilirubin and prothrombin time at diagnosis in 27 cases, we derived a prognostic index (Table 17.3) which proved useful in predicting the response to treatment in a subsequent nine cases (Nazer *et al.*, 1986). We have recently reviewed our experience with the index in a further 20 symptomatic children. If the prognostic index remained less than 6 all recovered completely with chelation, with or without zinc. One

Bibliography and references

Aisen, A. M., Martel, W., Gabrielsen, T. O. *et al.* (1985) Wilson's disease of the brain: MR imaging. *Radiology*, **157**, 137

Alexiou, D., Hatsis, T. and Koutselinis, A. (1985) Oral zinc therapy as a long-term treatment of Wilson's disease. *Arch. Fr. Pediatr.*, **42**, 447

Berman, D. H., Leventhal, R. I., Gavaler, J. S., Cadoff, E. M. and Van Thiel, D. H. (1991) Clinical differentiation of fulminant Wilsonian hepatitis from other causes of hepatic failure. *Gastroenterology*, **100**, 1129–1134

Brewer, G. J., Yuzbasiyan-Gurcan, V. and Young, A. B. (1987) Treatment of Wilson's disease. *Semin. Neurol.*, **7**, 209–220

Caillie-Bertrend, M. V., Gegenhert, H. J., Luijendijk, I. *et al.* (1985a) Wilson's disease: assessment of D-penicillamine treatment. *Arch. Dis. Childh.*, **60**, 652

Caillie-Bertrend, M. V., Gegenhert, H. J., Visser, H. K. A. *et al.* (1985b) Oral zinc sulphate for Wilson's disease. *Arch. Dis. Childh.*, **60**, 656

da Costa, C. M., Baldwin, D., Portmann, B, Lolin, Y., Mowat, A. P. and Mieli-Vergani, G. (1992) The value of urinary copper excretion after penicillamine challenge in the diagnosis of Wilson's disease. *Hepatology*, **15**, 609–615

Danks, D. M. (1989) Disorders of copper transport. In: *The metabolic basis of inherited disorders* (eds Scriver, C. R., Beaudet, A. L., Sly, W. S. and Valle, D.). McGraw-Hill, New York, pp. 1411–1431

Davies, S. E., Williams, R. and Portmann, B. (1989) Hepatic morphology and histochemistry of Wilson's disease presenting as fulminant hepatic failure: a study of 11 cases. *Histopathology*, **15**, 385–394

Ede, R. J. and Mowat, A. P. (1984) Wilson's disease: a 1984 perspective. *Compr. Ther.*, **10**, 40

Frydman, M., Bonne-Tamir, B., Farrer, L. A. *et al.* (1985) Assignment of the gene for Wilson disease to chromosome 13. *Proc. Natl. Acad. Sci. USA*, **82**, 1819–1921

Gaffney, D., Walker, J. L., O'Donnell, J. G. *et al.* (1992) DNA-based Presymptomatic Diagnosis of Wilson Disease. *J. Inher. Metab. Dis.*, **15**, 161–170

Gottrand, F., Razemon, M., Otte, J. B., Vigier, J. E., Farriaux, J. P. (1988) Indications de la transplantation hepatique au cours d'une maladie de Wilson. *Arch. Fr. Pediatr.*, **45**, 187–188

Hoogenraad, T. U., Van Hattum, J. and Van den Hamer, C. J. A. (1987) Management of Wilson's disease with zinc sulphate. *J. Neurol. Sci.*, **77**, 137–146

Ivengar, V., Brewer, G. J., Dick, R. D., Owyang, C. (1988) Studies of cholestokinin-stimulated biliary secretions reveal a high molecular weight copper binding substance in normal subjects that is absent in patients with Wilson's Disease. *J. Lab. Clin. Med.*, **111**, 267

Kraut, I. R. and Yogev, R. (1984) Fatal fulminant hepatitis with haemolysis in Wilson's disease. *Clin. Pediatr.*, **23**, 637

Lingham, S., Naser, H., Mowat, A. P. and Wilson, J. (1987) Neurological abnormalities in Wilson's disease are reversible. *Neuropediatrics*, **18**, 11

McCollough, A. G., Fleming, C. R., Thistle, I. L. *et al.* (1983) Diagnosis of Wilson's disease presenting as fulminant hepatic failure. *Gastroenterology*, **84**, 161

Marsden, C. D. (1987) Wilson's disease. *Quart. J. Med, New Series*, **65**, 959–966

Melendez, M. G., Williams, D. M., Batty, B. and Cartwright, G. E. (1980) Clinical studies of a large family with Wilson's disease. *South Med. J.*, **73**, 607

Milanino, R., Marrella, M., Moretti, U. *et al.* (1989) Oral zinc sulphate as primary therapeutic intervention in a child with Wilson disease. *Eur. J. Pediatr.*, **148**, 654–655

Milanino, R., Dangenello, A., Marrella, M. *et al.* (1992) Oral zinc as initial therapy in Wilson's disease: two years in a 10 year old child. *Acta Paediatr.*, **81**, 163–166

Nazer, H., Ede, R. I., Mowat, A. P. and Williams, R. (1983) Wilson's disease in childhood – variability of clinical expression. *Clin. Pediatr.*, **22**, 755

Nazer, H., Ede, R. J., Mowat, A. P. and Williams, R. (1986) Wilson's disease: Clinical presentation and use of prognostic index. *Gut*, **27**, 1377

Polson, R. J., Rolles, K., Calne, R. Y., Williams, R. and Marsden, D. (1987) Reversal of severe neurological manifestations of Wilson's Disease following orthotopic liver transplantation. *Q. J. Med.*, **64**, 685–691

Rakela, I., Kurtz, S. B., McCarthy, J. T. *et al.* (1986) Fulminant Wilson's disease treated with post dilutional haemofiltration and orthotopic liver transplantation. *Gastroenterology*, **90**, 2004

Ramadori, G., Keidl, E., Hutteroth, T. H. *et al.* (1985) Oral zinc therapy in Wilson's Disease – An alternative to D-penicillamine. *Z. Gastroenterol.*, **23**, 25

Ritland, S., Steinnes, E. and Skrede, S. (1977) Hepatic copper content, urinary copper excretion and serum caeruloplasmin in Wilson's disease. *Scand. J. Gastroenterol.*, **12**, 81

Sallie, R., Katsiyiannakis, L., Baldwin, D. *et al.* (1992) Failure of simple biochemical indices to reliably differentiate fulminant Wilson's Disease from other causes of fulminant liver failure. *Hepatology*, **16**, 1206–1211

Sass-Korstak, A. (1975) Wilson's disease – a treatable liver disease in children. *Pediatr. Clin. North Am.*, **22**, 693

Scheingerg, I. H. and Sternlieb, I. (1984) *Wilson's disease*, Saunders, Philadelphia

Schilsky, M. L., Scheingerg, I. H. and Sternlieb, I. (1992) Hepatic transplantation for Wilson's disease: indications and outcome. *Hepatology*, **16**, 50a

Shaver, W. A., Bhatt, H. and Combes, B. (1986) Low serum alkaline phosphatase activity in Wilson's disease. *Hepatology*, **6**, 859–863

Stampfl, D. A., Munoz, S. J., Moritz, M. J. *et al.* (1990) Heterotopic liver transplantation for fulminant Wilson's disease. *Gastroenterology*, **99**, 1834–1836

Sternlieb, I. and Scheinberg, I. H. (1968) Prevention of Wilson's disease in asymptomatic patients. *New Engl. J. Med.*, **278**, 352

Sternlieb, I. (1988) Wilson's disease: transplantation when all else has failed. *Hepatology*, **8**, 975–976

Sternlieb, I. (1990) Perspectives on Wilson's disease. *Hepatology*, **12**, 1234–1239

Walshe, J. M. (1984) Copper: its role in the pathogenesis of liver disease. *Sem. Liver Dis.*, **4**, 252

Weizman, Z., Picard, E., Barki, Y. and Moses, S. (1988) Wilson's Disease associated with Pancreatitis. *J. Paediatr. Gastroenterol. Nutr.*, **7**, 931–933

Yuzbasiyan-gurkan, V., Brewer, G. J., Boerwinkle, E. and Venta, P. J. (1988) Linkage of the Wilson's Disease gene to chromosome 13 in North-American pedigrees. *Am. J. Hum. Genet.*, **42**, 825–829

Chapter 18

Indian childhood cirrhosis and copper toxicity or copper storage disorders

Indian childhood cirrhosis and other idiopathic copper storage disorders are considered together since they have high liver copper concentrations and similar unique histological and clinical features. Recent observations suggest that Indian childhood cirrhosis can be prevented by limiting copper ingestion and confirmed that liver damage can be dramatically arrested if treatment with penicillamine is commenced early. Whether such therapy would be effective in other copper storage disorders is unknown.

Indian childhood cirrhosis

Pathology

The four classic histological features of this disorder are: accumulation of hyaline within necrotic hepatocytes, distinctive coarse brown aggregates of orcein-stained copper-associated protein in hepatocytes, marked pericellular fibrous tissue accumulation isolating single groups of liver cells producing a micro-micronodular cirrhosis, and a striking lack of regeneration nodules. These may develop later in survivors.

Early in the disease there is swelling and vacuolation of hepatocytes with focal polymorphonuclear inflammatory cell infiltrate around necrotic cells. There is minimal infiltration and inflammation of the portal tracts. Hepatocytes contain Mallory's hyalin bodies which are distinct reddish-purple bodies with smooth or irregular outlines seen in the perinuclear region of hepatocytes when stained with haematoxylin and eosin. Electron microscopy shows that the hyalin is composed of loose bundles of thin, actin-like cytoplasmic filaments enclosing and surrounded by many free ribosomes. When the disease is fully established the hepatocytes become more swollen and contain more marked hyalin accumulations. Hepatocytes appear to merge into large cells and in 10% of cases giant cell transformation is seen. There is marked glycogen depletion but no fatty infiltration. The nuclei may be normal or pale and in some instances have very prominent nucleoli giving the so-called 'bird's-eye' appearance. Kupffer cells are prominent, containing much iron and lipofuscin. There is a marked aggressive mesenchymal reaction with fibroblasts proliferating throughout the hepatic lobules, isolating small clumps of hepatocytes which become surrounded by bands of active, fibrous tissue. This severe mesenchymal reaction is associated with increased serum levels of the procollagen III N-peptide reflecting increased fibrogenesis or decreased endothelial cell clearance. There is a striking lack of regeneration, although the final picture may be not unlike micronodular cirrhosis, with marked distortion of the liver architecture. In the late stages

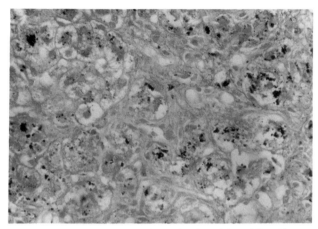

Figure 18.1 Indian childhood cirrhosis. Orcein staining of liver biopsy shows distinctive coarse black staining copper-associated protein within swollen hepatocytes. Note the vacuolation of hepatocytes caused by fat and the intense fibrosis seen encircling small aggregates of necrotic liver cells (magnification × 340, reduced to one-half in reproduction)

there may be hyperplasia of bile ducts with lymphocytic and polymorphonuclear neutrophil leucocyte infiltration in the portal tracts. Eosinophil and plasma cell infiltration is rarely seen.

In 1978 Portmann *et al.* deduced that the orcein-stained deposits of distinctive coarse dark-brown aggregates within the hepatocytes represented copper-associated protein (Figure 18.1). This has been confirmed in subsequent studies which have demonstrated that the aggregates are of a sulphur-containing protein to which copper is attached. The liver copper concentration is extremely high (Tanner *et al.*, 1979). Liver copper values have ranged from between 15 and 150 times the upper limit of normal (Bhave *et al.*, 1982). The copper is concentrated in lysosomes. The severity of histological abnormality correlates poorly with the liver copper concentration (Talbot *et al.*, 1985). A high copper concentration is found in renal tissue.

Prevalence and epidemiology

Indian childhood cirrhosis is a significant cause of mortality in the pre-school child in India and was the fourth most common cause of death in large paediatric centres and the most common chronic liver disease in children in that country. An incidence of around 1 in 4000 live births was calculated in one rural area (Tanner, 1989). Boys are affected more often than girls. A positive family history is found in 30% of cases. Several successive siblings may be affected, or unaffected siblings may intervene. Maximum incidence is at the ages of 1 to 3 years (median 18 months) but it can present between 2 weeks and 10 years. It occurs less commonly in urban areas. It seems to be more common in middle income families, i.e. the less poor, in a country with a per capita income of only $450 per annum in 1990. The incidence of referred cases seems to be falling in some parts of India in the past few years. Indian childhood cirrhosis occurs in Pakistan, Sri Lanka, Burma and in Indian immigrants in Malaysia. It is very rare in Indians living in East Africa or in the United Kingdom.

Clinical features

In approximately 75% of cases the course moves insidiously through three stages. The early stage is characterized by irritability, anorexia and low grade fever. On examination there is abdominal distension with an enlarged smooth liver with a sharp 'leaf-like' edge, palpable up to 7 cm below the right costal margin. When cirrhosis is fully established the liver becomes hard, splenomegaly develops with progressive ascites, distension of subcutaneous portosystemic venous shunts and malnutrition. The gall bladder may be palpable. Once jaundice develops the condition rapidly progresses with gastrointestinal bleeding, repeated infection, often pulmonary, peripheral oedema, and hepatic encephalopathy.

The remainder have a more rapid course similar to that of subacute hepatitis with fever, abdominal distension and jaundice from the onset. Death occurs 3–4 months after the onset.

In a report of 85 cases, 45% died within 4 weeks of presentation, 74% within 8 weeks and 86% within 6 months. Three survived in good health 13–20 months after presentation (Bhave et al., 1982). The long-term survival of these few children did raise the possibility that survival might be improved with therapy and that older children with cryptogenic cirrhosis may have had unrecognized Indian childhood cirrhosis earlier in life.

Laboratory abnormalities

Standard tests of liver function show changes compatible with hepatocellular necrosis. There is a generalized amino aciduria, glycosuria and frequently other features of a renal tubular lesion. The serum albumin concentration gradually falls and the albumin/globulin ratio is reversed. Concentrations of serum immunoglobulins IgA, IgG, and IgM are elevated. Smooth muscle antibodies have been found in up to 45% of cases. In children less than 2 years of age serum alpha-fetoprotein is frequently elevated. Levels of the serum complement components C3 and Clq are very low. Cell mediated immunity is depressed as assessed by both the phytohaemagglutinin response of lymphocytes *in vitro* and also by depressed cutaneous hypersensitivity.

Studies of copper metabolism and environmental copper

Liver copper concentrations are higher even than in presymptomatic patients with Wilson's disease. Serum caeruloplasmin levels are normal or high except in end-stage disease. Urinary copper excretion is high. Patel et al. (1988) found copper concentrations of from 1200–9500 mg/g creatinine rising to 2220–42 800 mg/g after a single dose of penicillamine (20 mg/kg) in early cases. They concluded that a post-penicillamine urinary copper: creatinine ratio of >10 000 mg/g was supportive of the diagnosis. In jaundiced patients values were as high as 100 000 mg/g.

Tanner et al. (1983) have shown that boiled animal milk stored in copper pots has a very high copper concentration. When they compared the use of brass pots for storage of milk in families with Indian childhood cirrhosis with neighbouring control families a similarly high frequency was found in both groups. The feeding patterns were different, however, in that those with Indian childhood cirrhosis were rarely entirely breast fed, started animal milk supplements earlier and stopped breast feeding earlier, suggesting greater exposure to a high copper intake in stored animal milk. Asymptomatic siblings of cases have been found to have mild to moderate accumulations of copper and copper-associated protein but have no biochemical or pathological evidence of liver dysfunction. At present the relation of excessive copper accumulation to the pathogenesis of the liver injury is uncertain. There is good evidence of excessive accumulation of copper in the livers of children with Indian childhood cirrhosis. Some patients at least have a high copper intake starting early in infancy. It is unclear whether copper accumulation occurs in the presence of a genetic factor or is aggravated by environmental factors which may limit copper excretion, or whether copper accumulation occurs in the presence of liver damage initiated in some other fashion. Tanner and Mattocks (1987) have reviewed experimental evidence which supports the hypothesis that a wide range of plant and fungal derived toxins can be secreted in milk and could increase hepatic copper concentration and thus act synergistically with excess copper ingestion to cause Indian childhood cirrhosis. Neither quantitative nor qualitative malnutrition has been implicated. Aflatoxin has been suggested as a possible cause but this has not been supported by epidemiological or toxicological studies. Hepatitis A and B, Epstein-Barr virus and cytomegalovirus have not been implicated in its aetiology.

Prevention

On the assumption that copper can be hepatotoxic and could contribute to the pathogenesis a large educational programme was started in Pune in India to limit copper intake in infants at risk. It was followed by the virtual disappearance of the disease. In other centres in India there has been a marked fall in incidence possibly attributable to the substitution of aluminium, steel or plastic containers for the traditional copper containing ones.

Treatment

Further exposure to possible sources of dietary copper should be halted. In patients identified before jaundice or ascites occurs, treatment with penicillamine (20 mg/kg/day) prolongs survival and in over 50% of cases appears to arrest disease progression. The clinical features gradually resolve but hepatomegaly and splenomegaly persist for up to 2 years (Tanner et al., 1987). The classic histological features clear. After 20 months residual changes ranged from micro- and macronodular cirrhosis to a histologically normal liver (Bhusnurmath et al., 1991). Penicillamine has no beneficial effect in more severely affected children. The role, if any, of oral zinc is unclear (see Chapter 17).

Copper toxicity or idiopathic copper storage disorders

In the past two decades there have been case reports from Australia, North America and Europe of children with liver disease with histological features similar to those of Indian childhood cirrhosis. Serum caeruloplasmin concentrations were normal or elevated and abnormalities of copper metabolism were those of Indian childhood cirrhosis rather than Wilson's disease. In some cases the copper toxicity has been attributed to a high copper concentration in the drinking water (Weiss et al., 1989). In one family four siblings were affected. The majority have presented with liver disease by 2 years of age and have died of liver failure. Jaundice has been a late feature in most cases. Penicillamine given late in the course was ineffective (Adamson et al., 1992). Given its efficacy in Indian childhood cirrhosis earlier penicillamine therapy and interruption of copper exposure, with or without zinc, might arrest progression of the disorder.

Bibliography and references

Bhave, S. A., Pandit, A. N., Pradhan, A. M. *et al.* (1982) Liver disease in India. *Arch. Dis. Childh.*, **57**, 922

Bhusnurmath, S. R., Walia, B. N. S., Singh, S., Parkash, D., Radotra, B. D. and Nath, R. (1991) Sequential Histopathological Alterations in Indian Childhood cirrhosis treated with d-penicillamine. *Human Pathol.*, **22**, 653–658

Nayak, N. C. and Mawan, M. (1980) Excess hepatic copper and Indian childhood cirrhosis: Is there a cause-effect relationship? *Hepatology*, **4**, 9

Nayak, N. C. and Ramalingaswami, V. (1975) Indian childhood cirrhosis. *Clin. Gastroenterol.*, **4**, 333

Patel, H. R., Bhave, S. A., Pandit, A. N. and Tanner, M. S. (1988) Copper in urine and hair in Indian childhood cirrhosis. *Arch. Dis. Childh.*, **63**, 970–972

Popper, N., Goldfischer, S., Sternleib, I., Nayak, N. C. and Madnavn, T. V. (1979) Cytoplasmic copper and its toxic effects: studies in Indian childhood cirrhosis. *Lancet*, **i**, 1205

Portmann, B., Tanner, M. S., Mowat, A. P. and Williams, R. (1978) Orcein positive liver deposits in Indian childhood cirrhosis. *Lancet*, **i**, 1338

Sharda, B. and Bhandari, B. (1983) Oral zinc therapy in Indian childhood cirrhosis. *Clin. Pediatr.*, **22**, 514

Sharma, U., Saxena, S., Mahta, J. B. and Sharma, M. E. (1975) Indian childhood cirrhosis. A clinicopathological study of 50 cases. *Arch. Chld. Hlth. Calcutta*, **17**, 56

Talbot, J. C., Tanner, M. S. and Pradhan, A. M. (1985) Liver copper content correlates poorly with the severity of histological abnormality in Indian childhood cirrhosis. *Gut*, **25**, 1138

Tanner, M. S. and Mattocks, A. R. (1987) Hypothesis: plant and fungal biocides, copper and Indian childhood cirrhosis. *Ann. Trop. Paediatr.*, **7**, 264–269

Tanner, M. S. (1989) *Indian Childhood Cirrhosis*. Churchill Livingstone, Edinburgh, pp. 214–217

Tanner, M. S., Bhave, S. A., Kantarjian, A. J. and Pandit, A. N. (1983) Early introduction of copper-contaminated animal milk feeds as a possible cause of Indian childhood cirrhosis. *Lancet*, **ii**, 992

Tanner, M. S., Bhave, S. A., Pradnan, A. M. and Pandit, A. N. (1987) Clinical trials of D-penicillamine in Indian childhood cirrhosis. *Arch. Dis. Childh.*, **62**, 1118–1124

Tanner, M. S., Portmann, B., Mowat, A. P. *et al.* (1979) Increased hepatic copper concentration in Indian childhood cirrhosis. *Lancet*, **i**, 1203

Trivedi, P., Risteli, J., Risteli, L., Tanner, M. S., Bhave, S., Pandit, A. and Mowat, A. P. (1987) Serum Type III procollagen and basement membrane proteins as non-invasive markers of hepatic pathology in Indian Childhood Cirrhosis. *Hepatology*, **7**, 1249–1253

Copper toxicity or storage disorders

Adamson, M., Reiner, B., Olson, J. L. *et al.* (1992) Indian childhood cirrhosis in an American child. *Gastroenterology*, **102**, 1771–1177

Lefkowitch, J., Honig, C. L., King, M. E. and Hagstrom, J. W. C. (1982) Hepatic copper overload and features of Indian childhood cirrhosis in an American sibship. *N. Engl. J. Med.*, **307**, 271–277

Maggiore, G., Giacomo, C. D., Sessa, F. and Burgio, G. R. (1987) Idiopathic Hepatic copper toxicosis in a child. *J. Pediatr. Gastroenter. Nutr.*, **6**, 980–983

Walker-Smith, J. A. and Blomfield, J. (1973) Wilson's disease or chronic copper poisoning. *Arch. Dis. Childh.*, **48**, 476–479

Weiss, M., Muller-Hocker, J., Wiebecke, B. and Belohradsky, B. H. (1989) First description of "Indian childhood cirrhosis" in a non-Indian infant in Europe. *Acta Paediatr. Scand.*, **78**, 152–156

Chapter 19

Alpha-1 antitrypsin deficiency (PIZZ) and other glycoprotein storage diseases

Alpha-1 antitrypsin deficiency (PIZZ), first identified in two brothers with cirrhosis by Freier *et al.* in 1968, is a codominantly inherited disease which predisposes to liver disease, usually starting in early infancy, and emphysema starting in adult life. Alpha-1 antitrypsin is a small monomeric glycoprotein (molecular weight 52 kDa) with almost 80 known allelic variants. The deficiency state associated with the allelic variant PIZZ (PI = protease inhibitor, genotype ZZ) is by far the most common hereditary cause of liver disease. In infants with hepatitis syndrome it is the second most frequent single diagnosis after biliary atresia in populations of European descent. The clinical, laboratory and pathological features may be indistinguishable from biliary atresia. The prognosis is much worse than that of idiopathic hepatitis of infancy. Although less frequently presenting in later childhood it must be excluded in any child or adult presenting with chronic liver disease (Eriksson and Carlson, 1991; Hussain *et al.*, 1991). Liver disease associated with the PIZZ phenotype accounts for 8% of patients attending the paediatric liver service at King's College Hospital. It is the most common metabolic disease for which liver transplantation is performed (Mowat, 1992). The phenotype changes following liver transplantation confirming that the plasma glycoprotein is made in the liver.

Genetics, biosynthesis and physiology of alpha-1 antitrypsin

Alpha-1 antitrypsin is coded for by a single structural gene, the PI locus 10.2 kb in length, on chromosome 14q31–32.3. The inheritance of alpha-1 antitrypsin is codominant, with each allele functioning separately. The common phenotype is PIMM of which there are four subtypes. The PIMM subject and many other variants have normal serum concentrations of 20–50 µmol/litre. Two relatively frequent phenotypes, PIS and Z produce low serum concentrations: PIS homozygotes about 60% and PIZ homozygotes about 15% of levels in PIM homozygotes. Other rare alleles such as PIM_{malton} and PIZ_{tun} (Whitehouse *et al.*, 1989) have similarly low levels. PI null produces no detectable serum levels.

Serum alpha-1 antitrypsin has a single polypeptide core of 394 residues which is synthesized and glycosylated, by an asparaginyl link, with three complex carbohydrate sidechains in the endoplasmic reticulum of the liver. It is folded into its three-dimensional structure, translocated to the Golgi and secreted after modification of the side chains. It readily diffuses into tissue fluids. It is also synthesized but at a much slower rate in other tissues, particularly the gastrointestinal tract, and in macrophages (Perlmutter *et al.*, 1989, Cox, 1989).

Allelic variation is produced primarily by an amino acid substitution in the polypeptide core which produces secondary changes in the side chains. The PIZ allele arises from a point mutation at codon 342 which results in the replacement of glutamic acid of the PIM allele by lysine. The Z polypeptide is synthesized at normal rates but there is deficient secretion of the glycoprotein from the endoplasmic reticulum, the rate being approximately 15% of that of the M variant.

Alpha-1 antitrypsin inhibits a wide range of serine proteases. Its principal target is thought to be neutrophil elastase. This enzyme, stored in granules in neutrophils, functions as an extracellular protease. Its prime substrate is elastin but it also attacks many other proteins including a variety of proteins in the coagulation and complement cascades, *Escherichia coli* cell wall components and all major components of extracellular matrix. The increased degree of complement activation (C3d/C3 ratio) found in PIZZ children with liver disease, particularly if the disease is severe, may be secondary to diminished protease inhibition. Polymorphonuclear leucocytes stimulated by opsonized zymosan release proteases which directly damage liver cells *in vitro*. Hepatocyte cytotoxicity is decreased 75% by alpha-1 antitrypsin (Mavier *et al.*, 1988). Both polymorphonuclear leucocytes and monocytes from PIZZ subjects show enhanced activation, mediated via membrane-bound serine esterases, compared with those from PIMM subjects. The active centre of antitrypsin (methionine 358–serine 359) is easily inactivated by oxidants, for example by myeloperoxidase from activated neutrophils. Inactivation can also occur if the exposed molecular loop between amino acids 342 and 358 is cleaved by enzymes from such common organisms as *Pseudomonas aeruginosa*. If proteases are uninhibited tissue damage may be severe. Free neutrophil elastase causes inactivation of antithrombin and C1-inhibitor. A catastrophic increase in intravascular coagulation, complement activation and kallikrein-catalysed kinin release can then occur. The PIZ variant is a much slower inhibitor of neutrophil elastase. Within the liver these actions could have profound functional and structural sequelae.

Alpha-1 antitrypsin is thus thought to inhibit a wide range of tissue-damaging effects of proteases. The rise in serum alpha-1 antitrypsin levels in common with other acute phase reactants, during inflammation or tissue injury is assumed to preserve the balance between released proteases and proteases inhibitors.

Clinical implications

The clinically important variant is PIZ, with a homozygote frequency of between 1 in 1660 to 1 in 7000 newborns of European descent. The PIZZ individual is at risk of gradually developing *emphysema* evident in adult life, particularly if a heavy cigarette smoker. The mean age of onset is in the 30s in smokers and around 50 years in nonsmokers. Up to 60% may be affected. The risk of emphysema is also great in the rare null homozygote. There are isolated reports of emphysema in PISZ subjects. In emphysema the process of gradual destruction of alveolar wall occurs over the course of many years which makes direct study of the pathogenesis very difficult. There is much indirect evidence implicating protease-antiprotease imbalance in pathogenesis, in particular ineffective inhibition of neutrophil elastase by alpha-1 antitrypsin. The pathological change appears to develop in the centriacinar area where macrophages accumulate and release elastase (Wewers, 1989).

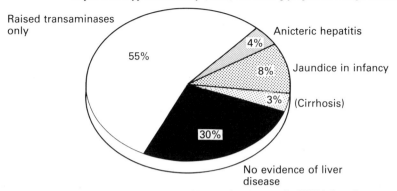

Figure 19.1 Diagrammatic representation of hepatic involvement in PIZZ infants from data of Sveger (1988)

Epidemiology of Liver Disease

Sveger and co-workers (1988) have been responsible for a remarkable epidemiological study of 120 PIZZ infants identified initially in a cohort of 200 000 Swedish newborn infants screened for low serum concentrations of alpha-1 antitrypsin. In the first 6 months of life up to 70% of infants had biochemical evidence of hepatitis (i.e. inflammation of the liver) with at least 2–3% progressing to a cirrhosis. In this cohort 11% had an icteric hepatitis (equivalent to 1/15 384 live births). A further 4% had clinical features of anicteric hepatitis (Figure 19.1).

In an epidemiological study in south-east England of infants identified by having a conjugated hyperbilirubinaemia lasting at least 2 weeks the incidence of PIZZ associated disease was remarkably similar at 1/19 200 live births (Dick and Mowat, 1985). The PIZZ frequency in England is estimated at 1 in 3400 live births (Psacharopoulos and Mowat, 1979). There appears to be a statistically significant increased risk of cirrhosis and primary hepatoma in males over the age of 50 (Eriksson *et al.*, 1986).

Liver disease with other PI phenotypes

Although liver disease has been reported in both infants and adults with phenotype SZ, SS and FZ (Kelly *et al.*, 1989) and an increased prevalence of MZ has been found in adult patients with cirrhosis and chronic active hepatitis, these may be chance observations (Cox, 1989). In Sveger's study 13 of 54 asymptomatic PISZ infants had raised alanine aminotransferase values at 6 months of age as did one at 4 to 12 years. A confounding factor is that the PIZZ genotype may give a SZ-like appearance on electrophoretic separation in the presence of liver disease. In our experience of almost 2000 infants and children with chronic liver disease PIZZ is the only phenotype more commonly represented than in the healthy population. PIM_{malton} and PIM_{duarte}, respectively 100 and 200 times rarer than PIZ, produce low concentrations of serum alpha-1 antitrypsin due to a defect in secretion from the liver. Too few have been reported to assess the risk of liver disease. Liver disease has been reported in an adult with PIM_{malton}.

Diagnosis

Alpha-1 antitrypsin phenotyping, preferably by isoelectric focusing, is required for diagnosis. It is an essential investigation in infants with hepatitis syndrome or suspected biliary atresia and in older children with chronic liver disease. The phenotype of both parents should be determined for genetic counselling. It is essential to do this also if a PISZ state is reported since some ZZ sera give a PISZ pattern in the presence of liver disease. Genotyping is necessary if prenatal diagnosis is planned for further pregnancies.

The deficiency state may be suspected by visual scanning of serum protein electrophoretic strips if no alpha-1 globulin is seen or by the typical appearance on liver biopsy after 12 weeks of age (see below). Since serum levels, measured by immunological techniques, may be increased or decreased by associated diseases or drugs these are unreliable in making a diagnosis (Cox 1989).

Pathological features

Liver biopsy in early infancy shows an acute hepatitis of variable severity, indistinguishable from the cryptogenic form except that giant cell transformation is rarely prominent. There may be conspicuous fatty infiltration around the portal tracts. The histological features may be very similar to those of extrahepatic biliary atresia. Fibrous tissue may be prominent in the portal tracts and linking portal tracts and/or hepatic venules. Cirrhosis may be evident as early as 8 weeks of age. It may be macronodular, micronodular or take a so-called biliary form.

Gradually the cholestasis, hepatocellular necrosis and inflammation settle and by 12 to 24 months of age the inflammatory cell infiltrate is largely limited to widened portal tracts, bands of fibrous tissue and to the immediately adjacent hepatocytes. If there is marked bile duct proliferation and portal tract fibrosis in early infancy, cirrhosis is likely to supervene in the first decade. In contrast, where there is little portal tract fibrosis or paucity of the interlobular bile ducts in the initial biopsy cirrhosis is less likely. Hepatocellular carcinoma may develop in adults both with and without cirrhosis. Cholangiocarcinoma has also been reported in two PIZZ siblings (Parham et al., 1989).

A distinctive pathological feature is the presence of diastase-resistant, PAS positive, magenta-coloured globules 2–20 nm in diameter seen most prominently in the periportal hepatocytes. These globules appear to correspond to the amorphous material which on electron microscopy is seen to distend the endoplasmic reticulum of some hepatocytes. Other intracellular organelles are normal. The material reacts with the specific fluorescein-tagged antibody to alpha-1 antitrypsin giving a bright fluorescence not seen in the hepatocytes of non-PIZ subjects. The accumulation of this material, which is antigenically similar to normal (PIM) serum alpha-1 antitrypsin occurs in PIZ subjects whether liver disease is present or not. It can be detected as early as 19 weeks' gestation (Malone et al., 1990). It is thought to represent the PIZ alpha1-antitrypsin which cannot be secreted from the endoplasmic reticulum. Note that the PAS positive, magenta-coloured globules are seen only after 12 weeks of age and therefore are of no diagnostic value at earlier ages.

The pathogenesis of liver damage and progressive liver disease

The physiological role of alpha-1 antitrypsin and the suspected pathogenesis of emphysema have been considered above. The cause of liver damage and progressive liver disease is unknown. The similarity in severity of liver disease in up to 80% of siblings suggests a second genetic factor may contribute to liver disease (Psacharopoulos et al., 1983). Among possible genetically influenced mechanisms which may be implicated in pathogenesis are defects in chemotaxis (Cox, 1989) and liver specific autoimmune reactions. This can be demonstrated *in vitro* as increased antibody-dependent lymphocyte induced hepatocyte cytotoxicity. The cytotoxicity can be inhibited by the addition of a purified liver membrane lipoprotein preparation suggesting that an immune reaction to liver membrane antigens may be involved in the pathogenesis of liver injury (Mondelli *et al.*, 1984). In a study of HLA phenotypes and class II (HLA-DR) gene polymorphism in 140 PIZZ subjects, 92 with liver disease, the class II DR3B gene was associated with liver disease while DR4 was apparently protective (Doherty *et al.*, 1990). The associations were weak, however, and other factors must be implicated. Serum concentrations of complement components C3 and C4 are low and measures of complement activation increased in children with liver disease suggesting that complement activation may have a role in pathogenesis (Littleton *et al.*, 1991).

We have observed two sets of identical twins in whom the liver disease ran a disparate course. One proband died of cirrhosis at 10 years of age, while his brother now aged 20 has no clinical or biochemical evidence of liver disease and had only slightly increased hepatic fibrosis on liver biopsy at 8 years of age. In the other set the proband had cirrhosis at 3 years of age while her sister has minor derangement of standard liver function tests only. Clearly environmental factors have a role. What these might be remains a matter for speculation. The relatively high frequency of low birth weight suggests that some factor may be operating *in utero*. Postnatally the absorption of macromolecules which are trapped in the Kupffer cells may initiate liver damage by stimulating protease release. Breast feeding has been associated with a lower incidence of severe liver disease in some but not all studies. The concentration of alpha-1 antitrypsin in breast milk is 30–40% that of serum. A poorer prognosis in males has also been suggested but this too is not consistent in all series (Labrune *et al.*, 1989).

Two hypotheses are currently being considered in pathogenesis. The first considers that accumulation of alpha-1 antitrypsin in the hepatocyte causes the process(es) that lead to severe liver damage. Against this is the observation that only 70% of PIZZ infants have abnormal liver function tests and at most 20–40% develop, in the course of a lifetime, clinically significant liver disease despite accumulation occurring in PIZZ subjects. Furthermore accumulations are least conspicuous early in infancy when disease activity appears to be greatest. It is conceivable that in certain circumstances these intracellular accumulations could produce cell surface changes which would initiate an immune attack on the hepatocyte or cause hepatocellular necrosis. Since abnormally folded proteins within cells can increase the synthesis of proteins induced by thermal or chemical stress (so-called heat-shock/stress proteins) a possible mechanism underlying liver damage might be the accumulation of such proteins. It has recently been shown that peripheral blood monocytes from PIZZ individuals with liver disease have enhanced synthesis of proteins in the heat shock/stress or chaperone gene family (SP90, SP70). These modulate the state of folding of proteins in cells. Synthesis is further increased by heat (42°C) and endotoxin. This change did not occur PIZZ subjects with emphysema and no liver disease or in PIMM individuals with advanced liver disease. The rate of polymerization of the Z protein *in vitro* increases if the temperature rises from 37°C to 41°C leading to the suggestion that when febrile not only is the rate of formation increased but so is the rate of aggregation (Lomas *et al.*, 1992). From the above it seems that alpha-1 antitrypsin accumulation may initiate changes which when associated with an unexplained increased synthesis of stress proteins may cause liver damage. Hepatocyte heterogeneity may explain why all hepatocytes are not equally affected (Sokal *et al.*, 1990). The synthesis of ubiquitin, which is conjugated with proteins during degradation in liver, was also significantly increased in PIZZ livers removed at grafting compared with MZ or MM livers (Perlmutter *et al.*, 1989).

Further studies will be required to determine whether these changes are due to a separate genetic defect(s) related to the metabolism of stress proteins or alpha-1 antitrypsin transport from the cell. Equally extrinsic factors may influence the metabolism of either or both.

The evidence stated in favour of the accumulation hypothesis is that while liver disease occurs in the other rare phenotypes with low serum levels and accumulation of alpha-1 antitrypsin, e.g. PIM$_{malton}$, no liver disease occurs in PIQ0 homozygotes who have no PAS positive globules in the liver. In fact studies of the liver histology in either the exceedingly rare and genetically pleomorphic PIQ0 or in PIM$_{malton}$ are limited to only one or two cases (Cox, 1989, Curiel et al., 1989). The evidence from the effect of the transfer of the Z gene to transgenic mice is inconclusive. The Z genes cause glycoprotein accumulation and infiltration with inflammatory cells, but no increase in hepatic fibrosis occurs (see Figure 19.2).

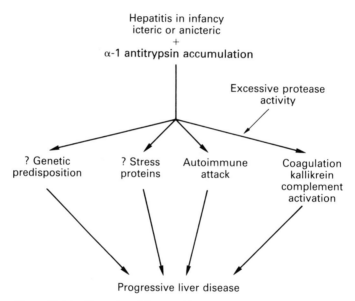

Figure 19.2 An illustration of factors which may be involved in perpetuating inflammation and stimulating the accumulation of components of the extracellular matrix, leading to increased intrahepatic fibrosis, cirrhosis and possible malignancy. (Reproduced with permission from Hussain et al., 1991)

The second hypothesis, protease–antiprotease imbalance, generally considered the cause of emphysema, has also been extended to the liver damage although it is difficult to obtain direct evidence of what may be happening in the hepatic microenvironment. With 1 g of elastase and 1 g of collagenase being produced daily, uninhibited action of such enzymes could cause disastrous tissue destruction and inflammation. Poly-morphonuclear leucocytes, stimulated by opsonized zymosan, release proteases which directly damage liver cells *in vitro* but cytotoxicity is decreased 75% by alpha-1 antitrypsin (Mavier et al., 1988). Both polymorphonuclear leucocytes and monocytes from PIZZ subjects show enhanced activation, mediated via membrane-bound serine esterases, compared with those from PIMM subjects. Proteases could also damage extracellular matrix components. These are now known to be much more than structural macromolecules. They interact with parenchymal cells through specific receptors and thus influence cell function. They also interact with inflammatory cells (Ruoslahti and Pierschbacher, 1988). The increased degree of complement activation (C3d/C3 ratio) found in children with liver disease, particularly if severe, may be associated with diminished protease inhibition. It has yet to be shown that complement activation causes liver damage in this disorder. The evidence quoted against this hypothesis is the absence of liver disease in the PIQ0 variant (see above). In favour is the observation that 23% of PISZ infants have increased serum transaminases. These subjects do not have significant hepatic accumulation but do have low serum levels. By 12 years of age only 2% had elevated transaminase levels. This time course of return to normal of serum transaminase mirrors that seen in the PIZZ subject (Sveger, 1988) and emphasizes the susceptibility of the newborn to liver dysfunction.

Any hypothesis should account for the fact that most liver disease starts in the first weeks of life. Many aspects of liver function and structure (e.g. liver cells two cells thick) are relatively immature or inefficient in the first months of life which may account for the high frequency of liver disease presenting at this time. The hepatic extracellular matrix may be particularly susceptible in early infancy when many metabolites of matrix components are present in high concentration in serum (Trivedi, 1989). Udall (1985) suggested that the developmental leakiness of the newborn gut could allow foreign proteins into the portal circulation. When trapped in the liver they might stimulate protease release and induce hepatitis which could become progressive if there were insufficient protease inhibitors present to inactivate the proteases. Bacterial colonization of the gut at this time could also increase the protease load coming to the liver. Viral infection in the liver, as evidenced by the demonstration of alpha interferon in Kupffer cells and inflammatory cells, is particularly common at this age which could cause monocyte elastase production. In early infancy the liver is clearly at its most vulnerable.

Clinical features of liver disease

Presenting features

Hepatitis syndrome in infancy

The most common presentation is as an acute icteric hepatitis which follows directly from neonatal physiological jaundice. It is suspected when the hyperbilirubinaemia is noted to be conjugated. The first sign is a change in the urine colour. It becomes distinctly yellow and is never colourless. The onset of jaundice may be at any time in the first 4 months of life. The mean age at recognition is between 2 and 3 weeks. Jaundice lasts on average for 3 months but may persist for as long as a year. It is most severe in the first 2 weeks of life when maximum serum bilirubin concentrations ranging from 60 to 360 μmol/litre may occur. The stools may contain no yellow or green pigment mimicking biliary atresia. The infants, the majority of whom will have been of low birth weight for gestational age, commonly have slow weight gain and some may show irritability or lethargy. They are at risk of septicaemia which can cause a devastating deterioration in liver function with marked prolongation of the prothrombin time. All have hepatomegaly and approximately 50% have splenomegaly (Mowat, 1984; Psacharopoulos and Mowat, 1979; Cox, 1989).

**Table 19.1 Presenting features of liver disease.
Experience at King's College Hospital, paediatric
liver service, 1971–89**

Neonatal ascites	0
Hepatitis of infancy	
Conjugated jaundice	178
Spontaneous bleeding	7
Complications of cirrhosis	
Ascites	1
Bleeding varices	2
Hepatosplenomegaly	3
Jaundice	1
Total	192

Rarely the presentation is with ascites in the newborn period (Ghisham *et al.*, 1983) (Table 19.1).

Bleeding diathesis in the first two months of life

(1) In approximately 5% the presenting feature is a bleeding episode at 2–6 weeks of age, the onset being later in infants who had received oral or parenteral vitamin K at delivery.
(2) The infant who is breast fed is at increased risk.
(3) Minor spontaneous bleeding from the nose, umbilicus or superficial injury is often disregarded.
(4) There may be exsanguinating bleeding from the umbilicus.
(5) Intracranial bleeding may be followed by long-term neurological abnormality with mental retardation and spasticity. Frequently such children require ventriculo-peritoneal shunts for the relief of hydrocephalus (Hope *et al.*, 1982; Psacharopoulos *et al.*, 1983). Invariably in these infants, there is clinical evidence of liver disease, including jaundice. Liver function tests are abnormal. In such children the prothrombin time (prothrombin ratio) is greatly prolonged. It reverts to normal within 6 hours with intravenous vitamin K. Such bleeding may be prevented by early recognition of the presence of liver disease and the administration of oral vitamin K.

Cirrhosis in later childhood

Less commonly children present with asymptomatic hepatosplenomegaly or with complications of cirrhosis such as ascites or haematemesis, with no prior history of jaundice in infancy. We have recently seen a 9 month old boy present with an apparent liver tumour which was a massive cirrhotic nodule.

Cirrhosis and hepatoma in later life

There is an increased risk of cirrhosis and primary hepatoma in adult life which is statistically significant in males over the age of 50 (Eriksson *et al.*, 1986). Few have a history of prolonged jaundice in infancy. The reported risk of cirrhosis is from 15–50%, with hepatoma developing in 15–30%. Hepatoma can occur in the absence of cirrhosis (Cox, 1989). Alpha-fetoprotein, usually elevated in hepatoma, is infrequently elevated in the PIZZ subject with this tumour. Interestingly the PIZZ infant with hepatitis has only minor elevations of alpha-fetoprotein concentrations in contrast to the very high values found in PIMM infants with a similar severity of liver damage (Johnston *et al.*, 1976).

Subsequent course of liver disease

Of the 15 infants with jaundice in Sveger's study (1988) two have died from cirrhosis which was found also in a four-year-old with aplastic anaemia and in a four-year-old killed by accident, although there had been no biochemical or clinical evidence of liver disease during life. The percentage with raised transaminases fell gradually throughout childhood from 70% at 6 months of age. At 12 years of age 3/15 with hepatitis in infancy and 14/102 with anicteric disease still had raised transaminases. None of the latter had developed clinical evidence of liver disease.

Three of the seven infants in the south-east of England study died of cirrhosis by the age of 3 years and one of the survivors now aged 20 years is asymptomatic but has cirrhosis. Two have no evidence of liver disease (Dick and Mowat, 1985).

Further information on the progression of liver disease can be derived from the reported experience of approximately 200 referred cases. It is impossible to assess the size of the referral population or what factors determined referral.

The course of the liver disease is similar irrespective of the mode of presentation in infancy. About 5% remain jaundiced, progress to decompensated cirrhosis and die in the first year of life. In the remainder the acute hepatitis settles, jaundice clears and the rate of growth and weight gain improves. A period of well-being ensues. Clinical examination in the majority, however, will show persistent hepatomegaly with or without splenomegaly. Standard biochemical tests of liver function such as aspartate and alanine aminotransferase, gamma-glutamyl transpeptidase and alkaline phosphatase remain elevated.

The subsequent evolution of the liver disease has followed four main patterns. In approximately 25% clinical and biochemical abnormalities gradually improve and results are in the normal range at ages by 3 to 10 years. The liver is not hard and there is no splenomegaly. Liver changes as seen on biopsy are limited to slight widening of portal

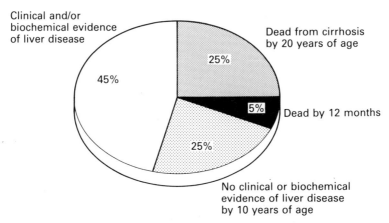

Figure 19.3 Diagrammatic representation of severity of liver damage and prognosis in PIZZ infants presenting with icteric hepatitis syndrome in infancy at King's College Hospital

Table 19.2 Age at death from cirrhosis. Experience at King's College hospital, 1971–89

Mean: 6.1 years (27 deaths)	
Less than 1 year	7
1 to 3 years	5
3 to 12 years	14
17 years	1

(excludes patients receiving liver grafts)

tracts and minimal increase in hepatic fibrosis. These patients have sufficient liver reserves to lead normal lives. Survival into the third decade without features of cirrhosis has been recorded in such patients (Figure 19.3). A further 25% have died from complications of cirrhosis at ages ranging from 6 months to 17 years (Table 19.2).

These patients will have had clinical and biopsy evidence of cirrhosis with a hard liver and splenomegaly. The majority will have some years of normal activities. Others may have slow growth rates and less than normal vigour. After a period ranging from a few months to 13 years hepatic decompensation occurred, as evidenced by ascites with hypoalbuminaemia, hyponatraemia, recurrence of jaundice, haematemesis or severe failure to thrive. Haematuria and/or albuminuria due to glomerular lesions is an infrequently reported complication (Levy, 1986) in such patients. It may predispose to severe systemic hypertension after transplantation (Noble-Jamieson et al., 1990). Without transplantation, death from liver disease occurred within 2 months to 4 years of the onset of hepatic decompensation.

The remainder are well through the first decade with persistently abnormal liver function tests although half have histologically confirmed cirrhosis. In those without clinical abnormalities or cirrhosis liver function tests may eventually become normal. In the remainder liver transplantation may be required.

Prognostic features in early infancy.

In general the prognosis of liver disease in childhood is related to the severity and duration of the acute hepatic dysfunction in early infancy, but in the individual patient liver biopsy is the more reliable guide to prognosis. In those who will die or develop cirrhosis in the first decade, liver biopsies in the first 6 months of life show marked portal tract and 'bridging' fibrosis or established cirrhosis. Intrahepatic bile duct hypoplasia has been associated with a good prognosis. Although children with liver disease have increased lung volumes (Hird et al., 1991) early progression to emphysema is unusual (Wall et al., 1990).

Management

The management is that of chronic cholestasis and of cirrhosis. There is no specific treatment for liver disease associated with alpha-1 antitrypsin deficiency short of liver transplantation.

Indications for liver transplantation

Liver transplantation should be planned as soon as cirrhosis decompensates. This can occur in early infancy. In the child in whom jaundice has cleared and there has been a period of wellbeing, increasing abdominal distension with loss of muscle bulk, ascites with hypoalbuminaemia, hyponatraemia and recurrence of jaundice are the main indications. Rarely severe failure to thrive may prompt transplantation. The onset of haematuria and/ or albuminuria due to glomerular lesions is another indication, as are complications of cirrhosis, such as recurrent variceal bleeding not readily prevented by injection therapy. The results are similar to those in other forms of cirrhosis except that hypertension may be more frequent. The longest follow-up is only 16 years making it too early to determine whether transplantation will prevent emphysema (Starzl *et al.*, 1989).

There is no evidence that the course of the disease is influenced by phenobarbitone given as an enzyme inducer or corticosteroids or penicillamine given as anti-inflammatory agents. Other agents which theoretically might limit the disease include aprotinin derivatives, polypeptides, and cephalosporin derivatives with broad spectrum protease inhibitory activity, vitamin E as an antioxidant and colchicine because of its inhibitory action on leucocyte metabolism and collagen formation. There is no evidence confirming the efficacy of any of these. It seems prudent to maintain serum vitamin E levels in the normal range. We are conducting a double-blind, 3 year, controlled trial of colchicine in infants with marked hepatic fibrosis.

In adults with emphysema it has been possible to bring plasma alpha-1 antitrypsin levels up to normal values with infusions of plasma derived alpha-1-antitrypsin. This has not been shown to modify the emphysema. Nor did it decrease to normal levels the elevated serum transaminases values found in a few patients who were treated in this fashion (Crystal *et al.*, 1989). Using recombinant DNA techniques, synthetic alpha-1 antitrypsin has been produced in bacteria and yeasts. The present material has a very short half-life since it is not fully glycosylated. Alpha-1 antitrypsin purified from the milk of transgenic sheep may prove to have a half-life equivalent to the plasma derived product (Cheras, 1992). It should be safer and perhaps cheaper.

Direct gene targeting to the liver *in vivo* is another possibility having been used successfully to stimulate albumin production in analbuminaemic rats (Wu *et al.*, 1989). The gene was contained in a plasmid which is targeted to the hepatocyte-specific asialoglycoprotein receptor and carried into the hepatocyte by pinocytosis. In this way the PIMZ state would be created. Another theoretical possibility is the correction of the hepatic secretory problem by insertion of another gene which makes a complementary change in the polypeptide allowing it to assume normal tertiary configuration which may facilitate secretion (Schwarzenberg and Sharp, 1990; Birrer *et al.*, 1991). Modifications to alpha-1 antitrypsin can be produced which make it more resistant to oxidative inactivation (George *et al.*, 1984). Perhaps more immediately practicable and attractive, to paediatric hepatologists if not to pulmonary physicians, would be a trial of exogenous serum-derived alpha-1 antitrypsin given intravenously at 1–4 weekly intervals, as is being used in emphysema but commencing as soon as significant liver damage is identified, perhaps in conjunction with a neonatal screening programme. It should be possible to construct a trial of therapy lasting 6–12 months which in the course of at most a decade, and perhaps much shorter, would indicate whether such therapy was efficacious.

Genetic counselling

For parents who are PIZ heterozygotes each fetus has a 25% chance of being a PIZ homozygote; if one parent is homozygote each fetus has a 50% chance of being homozygote. This state could formerly only be detected by fetal blood sampling from the umbilical vessels at 16 weeks' gestation. In families in whom a previously affected child has had severe liver disease the chances are 75% that a second PIZZ child will follow a similar course. In these circumstances families will frequently opt for termination of pregnancy. Earlier antenatal diagnosis is now possible by examining the DNA of chorionic villus samples using synthetic oligonucleotide probes specific for the M and Z gene or by restriction fragment length polymorphism. With the polymerase chain reaction results can be made available within a few days of sampling at 11 weeks' gestation. Preliminary studies confirm the validity of such techniques (Povey, 1990).

Hereditary fibrinogen deficiency

Hereditary fibrinogen deficiency is an autosomal dominant disorder characterized by plasma fibrinogen levels of 20–40 mg/100 ml (normal 200–400 mg/ml) and abnormal storage of fibrinogen in dilated cisternae of the endoplasmic reticulum. Its molecular basis is unknown. In some families immunoreactive fibrinogen level have been up to three times higher than thrombin clottable fibrinogen suggesting a dysfunctional molecule. Pale eosinophilic, weakly PAS-positive inclusions are demonstrated by direct immuno-fluorescence with fibrinogen antibody in the cytoplasm of some hepatocytes. The inclusions are not circumscribed and affect hepatocytes in a mosaic pattern throughout the lobule.

Reported patients have had chronic liver disease which has varied in severity from asymptomatic abnormalities of liver function tests to cirrhosis. No marked bleeding tendency has been noted. The diagnosis is to be suspected in patients with liver disease with no evidence of disseminated coagulation in whom the prothrombin time is disproportionately prolonged for the severity of liver damage. The thrombin-clottable fibrinogen levels are less than half normal values.

Alpha-1 antichymotrypsin deficiency

A familial deficiency of alpha-1 antichymotrypsin has been described with affected heterozygotes (prevalence 1/200–300 in Sweden) having an increase incidence of liver (and lung) disease of varying severity. Some hepatocytes adjacent to portal tracts and fibrous bands exhibit immunoreactive alpha-1 antichymotrypsin inclusions. Electron microscopy shows dilated endoplasmic reticulum but abnormal accumulation has not yet been reported. PAS-diastase staining shows faintly positive granules.

Bibliography and references

Birrer, P., McElvaney, N. G., Chang-Stroman, L. M. and Crystal, R. G. (1991) Alpha 1-antitrypsin deficiency and liver disease. *J. Inher. Metab. Dis.*, **14**, 512–525

Brantly, M., Nukiwa, T. and Crystal, R. G. (1988) Molecular basis of alpha-1-antitrypsin deficiency. *Am. J. Med.*, **84**, 13–31

Brantly, M., Courtney, M. and Crystal, R. G. (1988) Repair of the secretion defect in the Z form of alpha$_1$-antitrypsin by the addition of a Second Mutation. *Science*, **242**, 1700–1702

Carrell, R. W. (1986) Alpha-1-antitrypsin: molecular pathology, leukocytes and tissue damage. *J. Clin. Invest.*, **78**, 1427–1431.

Cheras, J. (1992) Sheep to produce alpha1-antitrypsin. *Br. Med. J.*, 304, 527

Cohen, A., O'Grady, J., Mowat, A. P. and Williams, R. (1989) Liver transplantation for metabolic disorders. In: *Bailliere's Clinical Gastroenterology*, **3**, 767–786

Corney, G., Whitehouse, D. B., Hopkinson, D. A. *et al.* (1987) Prenatal diagnosis of alpha-1-antitrypsin deficiency by fetal blood sampling. *Prenatal Diagnosis*, **7**, 101–108

Cox, D. W. (1989) Alpha-1-antitrypsin deficiency. In: *The metabolic basis of inherited disease*, 6th edn (eds Scriver, C. R., Beautt, A. L., Sly, W. S. and Valle, D.). McGraw-Hill, New York, pp. 2409–2437

Crystal, R. G., Brantly, M. L., Hubbard, R. C., Curiel, D. T., States, D. J. and Holmes, M. D. (1989) The alpha$_1$-antitrypsin gene and its mutations. Clinical consequences and strategies for therapy. *Chest*, **95**, 196–208

Crystal, R. G. (1990) Alpha$_1$-antitrypsin deficiency, emphysema and liver disease. Genetic basis and strategies for therapy. *J. Clin. Invest.*, **85**, 1343–1351

Curiel, D. T., Holmes, M. D., Okayama, H. *et al.* (1989) Molecular basis of the live rand lung disease associated with alpha-1-antitrypsin deficiency allele M_{malton}. *J. Biol. Chem.*, **264**, 13938–13945

Dick, M. C. and Mowat, A. P. (1985) Hepatitis syndrome in infancy. An epidemiological survey with 10-year follow up. *Arch. Dis. Child.*, **60**, 512–516

Doherty, D. G., Donaldson, P. T., Whitehouse, D. B. *et al.* (1990) HLA phenotypes and gene polymorphism in juvenile liver disease associated with alpha-1-antitrypsin deficiency. *Hepatology*, **12**, 218–223

Eriksson, S. and Carlson, J. (1991) Alpha-antitrypsin deficiency and related disorders. In N. McIntyre, J.-P. Benhamou, J. Bricher, M. Rizzetto and J. Rodes (eds) *Oxford Textbook of Clinical Hepatology*. Oxford Medical Publications, Oxford. p. 958–967.

Eriksson, S., Carlson, J. and Velez, R. (1986) The risk of cirrhosis and primary liver cancer in alpha-1-antitrypsin deficiency. *New Engl. J. Med.*, **314**, 736–739

Freier, E., Sharp, H. L. and Bridges, R. A. (1968) Alpha-1-antitrypsin deficiency associated with familial infantile liver disease. *Clin. Chem.*, **14**, 782

George, P. M., Travis, J., Vissers, M. C. M., Winterbourn, C. C. and Carrell, R. W. (1984) A genetically engineered mutant of alpha-1-antitrypsin protects connective tissue from neutrophil damage and may be useful in lung disease. *Lancet*, **2**, 1426–1428

Ghishan, F. K. and Greene, H. L. (1988) Liver disease in children with PIZZ alpha-1-antitrypsin deficiency. *Hepatology*, **8**, 307–310

Ghishan, F. X., Gray, G. F. and Greene, H. L. (1983) Alpha-1 antitrypsin deficiency presenting with ascites and cirrhosis in the neonatal period. *Gastroenterology*, **85**, 435–439

Greenough, A., Pool, J. B., Ball, C., Mieli-Vergani, G. and Mowat, A. P. (1988) Functional residual capacity related to hepatitic disease. *Arch. Dis. Child.*, **63**, 850–882

Hird, M. F., Greenough, A., Mieli-Vergani, G. and Mowat, A. P. (1991) Hyperinflation in children with liver disease due to Alpha-1-antitrypsin deficiency. *Pediatr. Pulmonol.*, **11**, 212–216

Hope, P. L., Hall, M. A., Millward-Sadler, G. H. and Normand, I. C. S. (1982) Alpha-1 antitrypsin deficiency presenting as a bleeding diathesis in the newborn. *Arch. Dis. Child.*, **57**, 68–70

Hussain, M., Mieli-Vergani, G. and Mowat, A. P. (1991) Alpha-1-antitrypsin Deficiency and Liver Disease: Clinical presentation, diagnosis and treatment. *J. Inher. Metabol. Dis.*, **14**, 497–511

Ibarguen, E., Gross, C., Savik, S. K. and Sharp, H. L. (1990) Liver disease in alpha-1-antitrypsin deficiency: Prognostic Indicators. *J. Pediatr.*, **117**, 864–870

Johnston, D. I., Mowat, A. P., Orr, H. and Kohn, J. (1976) Serum alpha-fetoprotein levels in extrahepatic biliary atresia, idiopathic neonatal hepatitis and alpha1-antitrypsin PIZZ. *Acta Paediatr. Scand.*, **65**, 623–628

Kelly, C. P., Tyrell, D. N. M., McDonald, G. S. A., Whitehouse, D. B. and Prichard, J. S. (1989) Heterozygous FZ alpha-1-antitrypsin deficiency associated with severe emphysema and hepatic disease: case report and family study. *Thorax*, **44**, 758–759

Krivit, W., Miller, J., Nowicki, M. and Freier, E. (1988) Contribution of monocyte-macrophage system to serum alpha-1-antitrypsin. *J. Lab. Clin. Med.*, **112**, 437–442

Labrune, P., Odievre, M. and Alagille, D. (1989) Influence of sex and breastfeeding on liver disease in alpha-1-antitrypsin deficiency. *Hepatology*, **10**, 122

Levy, M. (1986) Severe deficiency of alpha-1-antitrypsin associated with cutaneous vasculitis, rapidly progressive glomerular nephritis and colitis. *Am. J. Med.*, **81**, 363

Lomas, D. A., Evans, D. L., Finch, J. T. and Carrell, R. W. (1992) The mechanism of Z alpha₁-antitrypsin accumulation in the liver. *Nature*, **357**, 605–607

Littleton, E. T., Bevis, L., Hensen, L. J. *et al.* (1991) Alpha-1-antitrypsin deficiency, complement activation and chronic liver disease. *J. Clin. Pathol.*, **44**, 855–858

Malone, M., Mieli-Vergani, G., Mowat, A. P. and Portmann, B. (1989) The fetal liver in PiZZ Alpha-1-antitrypsin Deficiency: A Report of 5 Cases. *Pediatr. Pathol.*, **9**, 623–631

Mavier, P., Preaux, A.-M., Guigul, B., Lescs, M.-C., Zafarani, E.-S. and Dhumeaux, D. (1988) *In vitro* toxicity of polymorphonuclear neutrophils to hepatocytes: evidence for a proteinase-mediated mechanism. *Hepatology*, **8**, 254–256

Mondelli, M., Mieli-Vergani, G., Eddleston, A. L. W. F., Williams, R. and Mowat, A. P. (1984) Lymphocyte cytotoxicity to autologous hepatocytes in Alpha1-antitrypsin deficiency. *Gut*, **25**, 1044–1049

Mowat, A. P. (1984) Alpha-1-antitrypsin deficiency in liver disease. In: *Gastroenterology* Volume 4, 1 (eds Butterworths International Medical Reviews). Butterworths, London, pp. 52–75

Mowat, A. P. (1992) Liver transplantation in the management of metabolic disorders. *European Journal of Paediatrics*, **151**, S32–S38

Nebbia, G., Hadchouel, M. and Alagille, D. (1983) Early assessment of evolution of liver disease associated with alpha-1 antitrypsin deficiency in childhood. *Pediatrics* **102**, 661–668

Noble-Jamieson, G., Mowat, A. P., Thiru, S. and Barnes, N. (1990) Severe hypertension after liver transplantation in children with alpha-1-antitrypsin deficiency. *Arch. Dis. Child*, **65**, 1217–1219.

Parham, D. M., Paterson, J. R., Gunn, A. and Guthrie, W. (1989) Cholangiocarcinoma in two siblings with emphysema and alpha-1-antitrypsin deficiency. *Q. J. Med.*, **71**, 359–367

Perlmutter, D. H., Schlesinger, M. J., Pierce, J. A., Punsal, P. I. and Schwartz, A. L. (1989) Synthesis of stress proteins is increased in Individuals with PIZZ alpha-1-antitrypsin deficiency and liver disease. *J. Clin. Invest.*, **84**, 1551–1561

Peters, R. L. (1983) Early development of the liver: a review. In: *Paediatric liver disorders* (eds Fischer, M. and Roy, C. C.). Plenum Press, New York, pp. 1–19

Povey, S. (1990) The genetics of alpha-1-antitrypsin deficiency in relation to neonatal liver disease. *Molecular Biology and Medicine*, **7**, 161–172

Psacharopoulos, H. T. and Mowat, A. P. (1979) Incidence and early history of obstructive jaundice in infancy in SE England. In: *Neonatal Hepatitis and Biliary Atresia*. DHEW Publication (NIH) 79; 1296, Washington, US Government Printing Office, pp. 167–171

Psacharopoulos, H. T., Mowat, A. P., Cooke, P. J. L., Carlile, P. A., Portmann, B. and Rodeck, C. H. (1983) Outcome of liver disease associated with alpha-1 antitrypsin deficiency. Implications for genetic counselling and antenatal diagnosis. *Arch. Dis. Childh.*, **58**, 882–887

Ruoslahti, E. and Pierschbacher, M. D. (1987) Molecular Basis of Cell-Extracellular Matrix interactions. In: *The Liver Biology and Pathobiology*, 2nd edn (eds Arias, I. M., Jakoby, W. P., Popper, H., Schachter, D. and Shafritz, D. A.). Raven Press, New York, pp. 739–745

Schroeder, W. T., Miller, M. T. E., Woo, S. L. C. and Saunders, G. F. (1985) Chromosomal localisation of the human alpha-1-antitrypsin gene (Pi) to 14 Q31-32. *Am. J. Human Genet.*, **37**, 868–872

Schwarzenberg, S. J. and Sharp, H. L. (1990) Pathogenesis of alpha-1-antitrypsin deficiency associated liver disease. *J. Pediatr. Gastroenterol. Nutr.*, **10**, 5–12

Sharp, H. L., Bridges, R. A., Krivit, W. and Friere, E. R. (1969) Cirrhosis associated with alpha-1-antitrypsin deficiency: a previously unrecognised disorder. *J. Lab. Clin. Med.*, **73**, 934–939

Sokal, E., Trivedi, P., Portmann, B. and Mowat, A. P. (1989) Developmental changes ian the intra-acinar distribution of succinate dehydrogenase, glutamate dehydrogenase, glucose 6 phosphatase and NADPH dehydrogenase in rat liver. *J. Pediatr. Gastro. Nutr.*, **8**, 522–527

Starzl, T. E., Demetris, J. and Van Thiel, D. (1989) Medical progress: liver transplantation. *New Engl. J. Med.*, **321**, 1014–1022, 1092–1099

Strife, C. F., Hug, G., Chuck, G., McAdams, A. J., Davis, C. A. and Kline, J. J. (1983) Membranoproliferative glomerulonephritis and alpha-1-antitrypsin deficiency in children. *Pediatrics*, **71**, 88–92

Sveger, T. (1988) The natural history of liver disease in alpha-1-antitrypsin deficient children. *Acta Paediatr. Scand.*, **77**, 847–851

Talbot, I. C. and Mowat, A. P. (1975) Liver Disease in Infancy: Histological features in relationship to Alpha-1-antitrypsin phenotype. *J. Clin. Path.*, **28**, 559–563

Travis, J. (1988) Structure, function and control of neutrophil proteinases. *Am. J. Med.*, **84**, 37–42

Trivedi, P., Hindmarsh, P., Risetli, J., Risteli, L., Mowat, A. P. and Brook, C. G. D. (1989) Growth velocity, growth hormone therapy and serum concentrations of the aminoterminal propeptide of type III procollagen. *J. Pediatr.*, **114**, 225–230

Udall, I. N., Dixon, M., Newman, A. P., Wright, J. A., James, B. and Bloch, K. I. (1985) Liver disease in alpha-1 antitrypsin deficiency. A retrospective analysis of the influence of early breast versus bottle feeding. *J. Am. Med. Assoc.*, **253**, 2679–2682

Wall, M., Moe, E., Eisenberg, J., Powers, M., Buist, N. and Buist, S. (1990) Long-term follow-up of a cohort of children with alpha-1-antitrypsin deficiency. *J. pediatr.*, **116**, 248–251

Wewers, M. (1989) Pathogenesis of emphysema. *Chest*, **95**, 190–195

Whitehouse, D., B., Abbott, C. M., Lovegrove, J. U. *et al.* (1989) Genetic studies on a new deficiency gene (PI* Ztun) at the PI locus. *J. Med. Genet.*, **26**, 744–797

Whitehouse, D. B., Lovegrove, J. U., Mieli-Vergani, G., Mowat, A. P. and Hopkinson, D. A. "SZ like" alpha-1-antitrypsin phenotypes in PIZZ children with cirrhosis. (Submitted for publication)

Wu, W. J., Wilson, J. M. and Wu, Ch. (1989) Targeting genes: detection of targeted human albumin gene expression in genetically analbuminaemic rats. *Hepatology*, **10**, 618

Hypofibrinogenaemia

Callea, F., Lucinini, L., Torchio, B. and Kojima, T. (1988) Cryptogenic chronic liver disease in patients with hypofibrinogenaemia and hepatic storage of fibrinogen. *J. Hepatology*, **7**, S16

Deficiency of alpha-1-antichymotrypsin

Lindmark, B. and Eriksson, S. (1991) Partial deficiency of deficiency of alpha-1-antichymotrypsin is associated with chronic cryptogenic liver disease. *Scand. J. Gastroenterol.*, **26**, 508–512

Chapter 20

Hepatobiliary lesions in cystic fibrosis

Introduction

Cystic fibrosis (CF) is the most common lethal genetic disease in Caucasian populations with an estimated prevalence of 1:2000 live births. It is a generalized disorder of exocrine glands, inherited in an autosomal recessive pattern. The defective gene located on the middle of the long arm of chromosome 7 at 7q31 was isolated in 1989. Already more than 200 different defective mutations have been identified. The delta F508 mutation is present on 70% of CF chromosomes in northern Europe and North America, but rather less in other communities. The mutant genes produce a faulty transmembrane conductance regulator (TMCR) which controls chloride channels in epithelial membranes. The effect is impaired Cl⁻ reabsorption and increased sodium and chloride concentrations in the secretions of serous glands, such as sweat or saliva. There is no convincing evidence of an abnormality in macromolecular secretion. The abnormally tenacious viscid secretion of mucus-producing glands is secondary. Both abnormalities contribute to the pathological effects of the disorder. An unexplained feature of the condition is the variable severity of pathological change in different organs. Although a number of genotype/phenotype correlations have been claimed these require confirmation. Principal changes occur in the respiratory system, intestine and pancreas. Affected males are usually sterile due to absence of the vas deferens. Nasal polyps are common. Heat prostration due to salt loss occurs in warm environments.

Full consideration of the pathological and clinical effects of involvement of these organs would be inappropriate in this text. Pancreatic exocrine insufficiency can largely be corrected by oral pancreatic supplements.

Prognosis of cystic fibrosis

The course of the disease is very variable from patient to patient. Respiratory involvement accounts for more than 90% of the morbidity and mortality. With earlier diagnosis, the introduction of comprehensive treatment of pulmonary problems prior to the onset of irreversible lung damage and better nutritional care, there has been a steadily improving prognosis in the last 40 years. In 1950 survival beyond infancy was unusual. Median survival in the USA has increased from 14 years in 1969 to 21 years in 1978 and 27 years in 1990. In the UK in 1985 60% of males and 50% of females were alive at 20 years. With prolonged survival it is now evident that 5–10% of adolescents with cystic fibrosis have cirrhosis and its complications.

Pathology and pathogenesis

Among the 48 cases of cystic fibrosis described by Anderson in 1938, there were three instances of biliary cirrhosis and fatty infiltration of the liver was a frequent finding in the remainder. In subsequent reports various clinical and pathological abnormalities of the liver and biliary tract have emerged. Some are thought to be specific for cystic fibrosis, such as focal biliary cirrhosis and the small gall bladder; others, such as cholelithiasis, occur with a higher frequency than normal. Some appear to be secondary to involvement in other organs such as the heart and pancreas.

Why particular subjects with cystic fibrosis develop hepatobiliary complications remains unknown. The possible pathological factors or mechanisms contributing to liver disease in cystic fibrosis are summarized in Table 20.1.

Table 20.1 Possible pathological factors or pathogenic mechanisms contributing to liver disease in cystic fibrosis

Bile duct obstruction by abnormal mucus causing focal biliary fibrosis
    and eventual cirrhosis
Nutritional and gastrointestinal factors causing fatty liver
Abnormally small malfunctioning gall bladder and gall-stones
Abnormal bile salt metabolism
Cardiac cirrhosis
Hepatic injury caused by:
    Hepatotrophic viruses
    Products of bacterial infection
    Drug toxicity
Abnormal immune response to liver membrane antigen

Focal biliary fibrosis (cirrhosis)   The characteristic hepatic lesion in cystic fibrosis is usually termed 'focal biliary cirrhosis' although in fact it starts as a focal biliary fibrosis without derangement of hepatic architecture or nodular regeneration. There is accumulation in the intrahepatic ducts of amorphous eosinophilic PAS-positive diastase-resistant material which on electron microscopy is shown to contain lipid and bile pigment and to have a filamentous structure. This material obstructs some intrahepatic bile ducts. The portal tracts draining to these develop oedema, chronic inflammatory cell infiltrate, bile duct proliferation and increased fibrosis.

With increasing age the frequency and severity of portal tract fibrosis increases, focal biliary fibrosis being present at post mortem in 11% at 3 months of age, 27% at 1 year and in 72% of those age over 24 years. It is not clear what abnormality(ies) within or around the biliary system causes these changes in only a proportion of cystic fibrosis subjects and or causes, over a period of months or years, cirrhosis with regenerative nodules to appear in up to 30% of patients. Canalicular bile, formed by highly specialized areas of adjoining liver cells, is modified by secretion and absorption in the intrahepatic bile ducts with some substances thought to undergo a cholehepatic recirculation. The larger intrahepatic and the extrahepatic ducts have two diametrically opposed rows of glands which produce both serous and mucous secretions.

Hyperviscid secretions of these glands must be a factor. TMCR has been demonstrated in bile ductules and bile ducts but not in canaliculi. There is no evidence of a more severe degree of involvement in the peribiliary mucus-producing glands in patients with liver disease. *Stenosis of the distal common bile duct* appeared to be an important contributory factor in one study using percutaneous cholangiography to investigate the biliary system but another study using endoscopic cholangiography did not confirm the association. No significant difference in the frequencies of the delta F508, G551 or R553X *cystic fibrosis gene mutations* are found in those with and without liver involvement. A low familial concordance for liver disease suggests that genes outside the cystic fibrosis locus or environmental factors may be involved in pathogenesis. Cirrhosis at post mortem has been associated with meconium ileus or meconium ileus equivalent. An unexpected preponderance of affected adolescent males (3:1) were found in a recent large study (Scott-Jupp *et al.*, 1991). *Sensitization against liver membrane antigens*, whether arising primarily or secondarily to some other injurious lesion, may contribute to the progression of liver damage. An *HLA-associated genetic factor* controlling such immune responses may contribute to liver damage. HLA antigens A2, B7, DR2(DRw15) and DQw6 are present in an increased frequency in those with liver disease, probably due to the increased frequency of the HLA A2-B7-DR2-DQw6 haplotype. The relative risk for chronic liver disease increases from HLA2 to DQ suggesting that a disease-associated allele may lie near the DQB locus (Duthie *et al.*, in press). Lymphocytes have a key role in stimulating via cytokines, the production of collagen and other macromolecules of the extracellular matrix during fibrogenesis.

Abnormalities of the gall bladder and gall-stones Pathological, radiological and ultrasonic investigations indicate that up to one-third of patients with cystic fibrosis have small or hypoplastic gall bladders which do not concentrate cholecystographic agents. Gall-stones are found on ultrasonography in up to 12% of cases with a further 12% having sludge in the gall bladder. Intrahepatic calculi have also been described.

Abnormalities of bile salt metabolism Whether abnormalities of bile salt metabolism secondary to excessive faecal loss of primary and secondary bile acids contribute to gall-stone formation or liver disease by producing a tenacious or lithogenic bile remains conjectural (Angelico *et al.*, 1991). The improvement in both biliary excretion and biochemical tests of liver function with ursodeoxycholic acid administration provides support for this hypothesis although it has yet to be shown that this agent slows the development of chronic liver disease.

Cardiac cirrhosis Although cor pulmonale is a common terminal event in patients with severe chronic lung involvement, frank cardiac decompensation with peripheral oedema is unusual. There is no evidence that it contributes to cirrhosis.

Fatty liver Excessive accumulation in hepatocytes is an almost constant feature in liver biopsies in cystic fibrosis. The cause of fat accumulation is uncertain. Neither excessive fat accumulation in hepatocytes nor essential fatty acid deficiency have been shown to contribute to chronic liver disease.

Hepatic damage due to hepatotrophic viruses, bacteria or drugs There is no evidence of an increased predisposition to severe liver disease with viral hepatitis type A or B. Endotoxaemia associated with bacterial infections may cause acute impairment of hepatic function but whether it contributes to chronic liver disease in cystic fibrosis is unclear. Drug-induced hepatitis caused by isoniazid, ethionamide, ethambutol and/or rifampicin has been reported in patients with cystic fibrosis. Thus, cystic fibrosis patients are normally susceptible to a hepatic reaction to drugs and since they take a large number of drugs which may be potentially hepatotoxic, the possibility of drug-induced liver damage must be constantly considered. There is, as yet, no evidence that such drugs contribute to chronic liver disease.

Clinical syndromes

Prolonged conjugated hyperbilirubinaemia in infancy

This is a rare complication of cystic fibrosis, only 20 instances having been reported in the English literature. It may be a presenting feature of cystic fibrosis. The aetiology of the jaundice in the majority of these infants is unclear. Some have clinical and pathological features identical to those of cryptogenic giant cell hepatitis of infancy. Others have a variable degree of bile plugging in the portal tracts with excessive mucus in the intrahepatic bile ducts, bile duct hyperplasia and portal tract fibrosis. Others have tenacious mucus in the extrahepatic bile ducts at laparotomy.

Clinical features

Jaundice associated with dark urine and pale, even acholic, stools or haemorrhage due to vitamin K malabsorption are the presenting feature. In up to 50% of reported cases there is a history of meconium ileus. Hepatomegaly without splenomegaly is commonly found. Standard biochemical tests of liver function show a conjugated hyperbilirubinaemia with a moderate elevation of aspartate aminotransferase to between two and three times normal with the alkaline phosphatase level near the upper limit of normal for the child's age. The prothrombin time may be prolonged in the absence of parenteral vitamin K.

The diagnosis is suspected from a history of meconium ileus, previous cystic fibrosis in the family or by the detection of albumin in meconium or a raised serum immunoreactive trypsin. Until a satisfactory sweat sample is obtained the features have to be distinguished from other forms of hepatitis in infancy or extrahepatic bile duct obstruction, such as biliary atresia (Furuya et al., 1991).

Management

Like all infants with reduced bile flow, these infants require fat-soluble vitamin supplements, particularly K and D. Medium chain triglyceride supplements added to feeds and Maxijul may improve nutrition. Pancreatic supplements are required. Mild cases resolve spontaneously. In patients with completely acholic stools laparotomy should be undertaken to exclude other abnormalities such as biliary atresia, and if necessary to remove by irrigation inspissated material in the biliary system. Irrigation may have to be continued via a tube left in the gall bladder or biliary system following surgery (Evans et al., 1991). Liver disease may resolve completely and not recur at follow-up through 20 years of age.

Massive hepatic steatosis (fatty liver) in infancy

Massive hepatomegaly due to severe fatty infiltration of the liver may be an initial feature of cystic fibrosis. In some infants such hepatomegaly may occur as an isolated abnormality with raised serum transaminases as the only abnormality on laboratory investigations. In others it occurs in association with oedema, ascites and severe hypoalbuminaemia in part due to protein malabsorption. These features and hepatomegaly usually reverse when pancreatic supplements are given and nutrition improves. Carnitine deficiency may occur. Cirrhosis has not been reported as a sequel.

Cirrhosis

In its early stages focal biliary cirrhosis gives rise to no clinical manifestation or laboratory evidence of hepatic involvement. As more and more portal tracts become involved the liver increases in size and becomes palpable more than 3 cm below the costal margin in the right mid-clavicular line. The liver edge is firm and not tender. Nodules may be discerned on its edge or on the anterior surface. As fibrosis becomes more severe, the right lobe of the liver becomes shrunken, its edge recedes above the right costal margin and hepatic dullness is reduced to a small area on the right central lateral chest wall. At the same time the left lobe enlarges in the epigastrium.

Clinically significant hepatic involvement (Figure 20.1)

With increasing hepatic fibrosis the spleen progressively enlarges. An enlarged spleen is the single most important sign of portal hypertension but the size of the spleen bears little relation to the portal pressure or the risk of alimentary bleeding. Most patients are asymptomatic but some patients complain of pain over the spleen due to perisplenitis associated with infarction or of increasing abdominal distension, tiredness and listlessness. In others, the first sign of hepatic involvement is alimentary bleeding from oesophageal varices. Examination may reveal other features of cirrhosis such as portosystemic collaterals, spider angiomata, palmar erythema and gynaecomastia. In advanced cirrhosis jaundice, ascites or encephalopathy may occur.

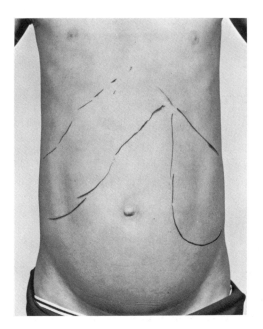

Figure 20.1 A girl aged 8 years who had been found to have cystic fibrosis at the age of 3 years, when a sibling was born with a meconium ileus. The patient had mild respiratory symptoms. Hepatomegaly became evident by the age of 5 years and splenomegaly by 6 years. The spleen and liver have subsequently become larger. There are no other clinical features of liver disease. The liver function tests are normal other than the transaminase, elevated at 58 IU/litre. There is moderate hypersplenism, with a platelet count of between 50 and 90 × 10^9/l

Laboratory assessment of hepatic involvement

In patients with clinical features of cirrhosis, the prothrombin time is frequently prolonged by more than 4 seconds and the albumin may be low. In a recent study (Scott-Jupp et al., 1991) abnormal liver function tests were seen in 12.9% of those in whom they were measured, but correlated poorly with clinical evidence of liver disease. Thus six of 46 patients with hepatosplenomegaly had normal serum enzyme activities while 50 of 524 with no clinical evidence of liver disease had raise enzymatic activity. There may be haematological features of hypersplenism.

If portal hypertension is present oesophageal varices can be detected at endoscopy or by barium studies. Their presence may be suspected by abnormal subhepatic collaterals detected on ultrasound. Ultrasonic examination of the liver may show increased echogenicity but this is as likely to be due to fat as increased intrahepatic fibrosis. Changes in blood flow velocity in the portal vein, hepatic vein or artery may suggest hepatic fibrosis. Ultrasonography is invaluable in identifying gall-stones and bile duct dilatation. Liver biopsy may show a well established cirrhosis but may give a totally misleading indication of the amount of fibrous tissue or persisting hepatic parenchyma because of the focal nature of the hepatic lesions. In patients in whom liver function tests are still normal, a hepatic excretory scintiscan may show diminished hepatic uptake, delayed excretion and prolonged retention in the biliary system.

Differential diagnosis

The child with cystic fibrosis is susceptible to all other forms of chronic liver disease in childhood. It is particularly important to consider the possibility of correctable disorders such as Wilson's disease, choledochal cyst and constrictive pericarditis. The coexistence of autoimmune chronic active hepatitis has also to be considered. Other genetic causes of liver disease must also be excluded because of their importance in prognosis and to other family members.

Epidemiology of cirrhosis in cystic fibrosis

Postmortem data suggest that the incidence of liver disease rises steadily with age, from 10.8% in infants less than 3 months of age, to 15.3% in those 3 months to 1 year, and to 26.8% in those over 1 year. The frequency of cirrhosis with portal hypertension in studies from CF centres has ranged from 0.5% to 8% in children and from 5% to 35% in adolescents and young adults (Sinaasappel, 1989). Cirrhosis may be recognized in early infancy but the prevalence of clinically evident liver disease rises in most studies with increasing age from 3.5–10% in the first decade to between 7 and 35% in the second decade (Nagel et al., 1989; Sinaasapel, 1989). In a large recent survey of 1100 patients with an overall prevalence rate of 4.4%, it rose from 0.3% in the 0 to 5 year age group, to a peak of 8.7% in those aged 16 to 20 years. It fell to only 4.1% in those aged more than 20 years (Scott-Jupp et al., 1991). Liver disease affected 5.4% of males and 2.6% of females. Between 11 and 15 years three times as many boys as girls were affected. Haemorrhage from oesophageal varices had occurred in six patients (0.5%). Varices, seen at endoscopy in 11 of 34 examined never occurred in the absence of splenomegaly. A further prospective study in the same patient population (Scott-Jupp et al., unpublished) revealed considerable under-recognition of liver disease. Bleeding from oesophageal varices occurs in only a small proportion of those with overt disease in Sinaasapel's study (1989).

Management of complications of cirrhosis

Complications and management of cirrhosis in cystic fibrosis are similar to those of other causes of cirrhosis and portal hypertension in childhood as discussed in Chapters 15 and 19. Only problems particular to cystic fibrosis are considered below.

Nutrition   As in all patients energy intake should be dictated by assessing total daily energy expenditure. It is likely to be between 120 and 150% of recommended requirements for height. Adequate and non-toxic amounts of fat soluble vitamins D, E and K should be given with appropriate monitoring since there may be increased requirements in the presence of liver disease. The role of vitamin A supplements is problematical. Clinical and biochemical evidence of vitamin A deficiency occurs, but liver concentration of vitamin A may be high possibly as a result of failure of retinol binding protein synthesis. Vitamin A administration in a malnourished adult and in a newly diagnosed infant with cystic fibrosis caused toxicity (Eid *et al.*, 1990). Susceptibility to vitamin A hepatoxicity may be familial (Sarles *et al.*, 1990). Much of the hepatic metabolism of both vitamin A and retinol takes place in the fat-storing (Ito) cells which are converted into myofibroblasts during hepatic fibrogenesis. Retinol is released during activation and may modulate collagen production by these cells (Davis *et al.*, 1987). Vitamin A supplementation might contribute to liver injury.

Ursodeoxycholic acid   Ursodeoxycholic acid (UDCA), the major bile acid in the bear, appears to be a promising agent for patients with liver disease associated with cystic fibrosis. UDCA accounts for a small proportion of bile acids in humans. UDCA competitively inhibits the absorption of the major primary bile acid, cholic acid, in the terminal ileum. After administration of UDCA for a few months it becomes the major bile acid in serum and bile. In the last 15 years it has been shown to be a safe and relatively effective therapy for the dissolution of small cholesterol gall-stones. A dose of 15–25 mg/kg/day causes an improvement in biochemical tests of liver function in patients with cirrhosis and CF. These improvements reverses when the drug is withdrawn. UDCA also improves biliary excretion (Colombo *et al.*, 1992). Large long-term randomised controlled studies will be required to demonstrate an effect of UDCA administration on hepatic fibrosis, portal hypertension, morbidity or mortality.

Portal hypertension

Injection sclerotherapy is as effective in this as in other forms of portal hypertension. Complications are no less frequent. Pulmonary function tests do deteriorate following this procedure in spite of vigorous physiotherapy. Nevertheless, in experienced hands the morbidity is much less than with other surgical procedures.

Portosystemic shunts or devascularization procedures are effective in controlling portal hypertension but should be limited to patients in whom injection sclerotherapy has failed or transplantation is inappropriate. Unexpected, rapid deterioration in liver function leading to death within 3 months of shunt surgery has been reported in a patient with good hepatic function (Alagille and Odievre, 1979). Shunts are also followed by an increased incidence of hepatic encephalopathy. This is true even when modified shunts such as the Warren procedure have been used in an effort to preserve blood flow to the liver. These procedures and other intra-abdominal operations make liver transplantation more difficult.

Massive splenic enlargement and hypersplenism

Massive splenomegaly, extending across the midline into the right iliac fossa is an occasional complication of portal hypertension in cystic fibrosis. Marked abdominal distension, respiratory embarrassment and recurrent abdominal pain localized over the spleen, sometimes with the presence of a splenic rub, are the main clinical features (Figure 20.2). These may be sufficiently troublesome for splenectomy to be considered. If it is to be performed the question arises, should the patient have a portacaval or splenorenal shunt at the same time. The majority of surgeons would favour this course probably proceeding to a splenorenal shunt but it must be remembered that splenectomy may be followed by

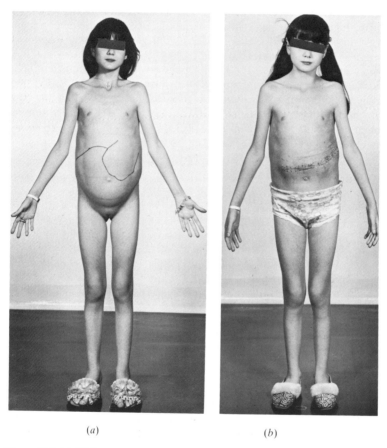

(a)   (b)

Figure 20.2 (a) Clinical photograph of a girl aged 11 years with distended abdomen due to massive splenomegaly and moderate hepatomegaly. Finger clubbing is present. She had three major alimentary bleeds from oesophageal varices during the preceding 18 months. She had only moderate respiratory symptoms having a Schwachman score of 78. Serum albumin was 38 g/litre, aspartate transaminase 57 IU/litre, prothrombin time was prolonged by 4 seconds. The haemoglobin was 10 g/100 ml, white count 3.8 × 10⁹/l and the platelet count 50 × 10⁹/l. (b) Following intensive physiotherapy, a splenectomy and lieno-renal anastomosis were performed. She made an uneventful recovery from surgery. Varices, assessed by barium meal, had disappeared within 4 months. For 3 years she had increased exercise tolerance and was more active than previously. Persistent *Pseudomonas* infection led to death from respiratory failure 4½ years after surgery

a marked rise in platelet count and a hypercoagulable state which may lead not only to thrombosis in the shunt but also to thrombosis in other parts of the portal-venous system. Shunting also carries the risk of encephalopathy. As in other disorders the patient has an increased risk of septicaemia and requires life-long penicillin prophylaxis. Splenectomy, therefore, is rarely undertaken.

Ascites

Ascites complicating cystic fibrosis may in part be due to impaired protein absorption. The management is as in other forms of cirrhosis but sodium restriction must be undertaken with care since in areas of high environmental temperatures the patient may lose a great deal of salt in the sweat. Sodium restriction must therefore be monitored by estimating the urinary sodium.

Hepatic encephalopathy

Since there is usually nothing that can be done to improve hepatic function the management is directed at preventing factors that contribute to the encephalopathy. It is important to remember that CNS depression in cystic fibrosis may in part be due to hypercapnia, hypoxia or vitamin E deficiency. Systemic infection, potassium depletion, sepsis and constipation are also important aggravating factors.

Gall-stones and bile duct obstruction

Symptoms of gall bladder disease develop in up to 4% of patients (Stern et al., 1986). Abdominal pain localized to the right upper quadrant with fever, leucocytosis, raised serum bilirubin and alkaline phosphatase suggest cholecystitis. There may be ultrasonic features of bile duct obstruction. Endoscopic, laparoscopic or surgical management is required for symptomatic patients. At present the trend is towards endoscopic and laparoscopic procedures because of the decrease in morbidity achieved if an upper abdominal operation can be avoided.

Laparoscopic cholecystectomy would appear to have advantages in those with poor respiratory reserve but it can have lethal complications and should only be performed in circumstances in which it is possible to proceed rapidly to laparotomy if necessary (Peters et al., 1991). Clearly sphincterotomy and gall-stone extraction, with or without biliary lavage and stent insertion performed endoscopically will cause less respiratory difficulties than major upper abdominal surgery.

Distal bile duct dilatation performed endoscopically would appear to be better than surgical diversion for distal bile duct obstruction but as in other disorders with common bile duct strictures and chronic pancreatitis the precise indications remain controversial. These problems are best managed in units with the full range of therapeutic options and suitably experienced staff.

Liver transplantation

Orthotopic liver transplantation (OLT) is a therapeutic option which is being used increasingly in the treatment of monogenetic liver-based metabolic disorders. The role of OLT in cystic fibrosis is at present less well defined than in other genetic forms of cirrhosis with less multi-system involvement. Disseminated aspergillosis or other fungal infections are contraindications. Liver transplantation has been reported in approximately

35 patients with 50% surviving with a very good quality of life. The oral dose of cyclosporin A needs to be larger than usual. There were major pulmonary difficulties initially. In the longer term (less than 4 years) pulmonary infections have proved less troublesome than anticipated, and in some patients lung function has improved significantly. Whether this is due to better chest movement following abdominal decompression, the effects of immunosuppressives or from protective effects of a normally functioning new liver is unknown. Combined liver-heart-lung transplant has been performed successfully in a few patients with symptomatic liver disease and severe lung disease. The precise indications for primary liver or heart-lung transplantation to be followed possibly by transplantation of the other as opposed to primary triple organ transplantation in patients with moderate/severe involvement of both lungs and liver are problematical.

The impact of liver disease in cystic fibrosis

The emergence of liver disease in the older child or adolescent with cystic fibrosis, often with only mild pulmonary involvement, causes great despondency in the family and their attendants. It must be emphasized that liver disease in cystic fibrosis is frequently only slowly progressive and that effective treatment for its main complication, portal hypertension, is available. Its detection therefore is not necessarily a harbinger of early death. The complications of cirrhosis, however, do have serious consequences and their optimum care requires the skill and resources available at centres specializing in the management of liver disorders. In cirrhosis with portosystemic shunting portal blood bypasses not only hepatocytes but phagocytic Kupffer cells, highly absorptive hepatic endothelial cells and fat storage cells. Particulate matter, endotoxin, cytokines, hormones, lipids, glycoproteins and many enzymes normally cleared in the liver are delivered directly into the systemic venous return to the right atrium and hence to the lung. To what extent this accelerates deterioration in lung function is unknown.

Research is urgently required to identify the factors that initiate liver disease and perpetuate liver damage in a proportion of those with cystic fibrosis. The results of genetic studies and the very variable frequency of cirrhosis in different centres suggests environmental factors may have a role in causing symptomatic liver disease.

Bibliography and references

Ahmed, F., Ellis, J., Murphy, J., Wootton, S. and Jackson, A. A. (1990) Excessive faecal losses of vitamin A (retinol) in cystic fibrosis. *Arch. Dis. Childh.*, **65**, 589–593

Alagille, D. and Odievre, N. (1979) *Liver and Biliary Disease in Children*. John Wiley, New York, p. 293

Anderson, D. N. (1938) Cystic fibrosis of pancreas and its relation to coeliac disease. *Am. J. Dis. Child.*, **56**, 344

Angelico, M., Gandin, C., Canuzzi, P. *et al.* (1991) Gallstones in cystic fibrosis: a critical reappraisal. *Hepatology*, **14**, 768–775.

Bilton, D., Fox, R., Webb, AK, Lawler, W., McMahon, R. F. T. and Howat, J. M. T. (1990) Pathology of common bile duct stenosis in cystic fibrosis. *Gut*, **31**, 236–238

British Paediatric Association Working party on Cystic Fibrosis (1988) Cystic Fibrosis in the United Kingdom 1977–85; an improving picture. *Br. Med. J.*, **297**, 1599–1602.

Burns, W. T. (1981) Gray Scale Ultrasonography: The liver and biliary tract in cystic fibrosis. In: *1000 Years of Cystic Fibrosis – Collected Papers* (ed. Warwick, W. J.). University of Minnesota, St Paul, p. 129

Busuttil, R. W., Seu, P., Millis, J. M. *et al.* (1991) Liver transplantation in children. *Annals of Surgery*, **213**, 48–57

Colombo, C., Roda, A., Roda, E. *et al.* (1984) Bile acid malabsorption in cystic fibrosis with and without pancreatic insufficiency. *J. Pediatr. Gastroneterol. Nutr.*, **3**, 556

Colombo, C., Setchell, K. D. R., Poda, M. *et al.* (1990) Effects of ursodeoxycholic acid therapy for liver disease associated with cystic fibrosis. *J. Pediatr.*, **117**, 482–489

Colombo, C., Crosignani, A., Assaisso, M. *et al.* (1992) Ursodeoxycholic acid therapy in cystic fibrosis-associated liver disease: a dose-response study. *Hepatology*, **16**, 924–930

Colombo, C., Castellani, M. T., Balistreri, W. F., Segerni, E., Assaiso, M. L. and Giunta, A. (1992) Scintigraphic documentation of an improvement in hepatobiliary excretory function after treatment with ursodeoxycholic acid in patients with cystic fibrosis and associated liver disease. *Hepatology*, **15**, 677–684

Cotting, J., Dufour, J. F., Lentze, M. J., Paumgartner, G. and Reichen, J. (1992) Ursodeoxycholate in the treatment of cholestasis in cystic fibrosis – a 2 year experience and review of the literature. In: *Paediatric Cholestasis. Novel Approaches to treatment* (eds Lentze, M. J. and Reichen, J.). Kluwer, London, p. 345

Davis, H. B., Pratt, B. M. and Madri, J. A. (1987) Retinol and extracellular collagen matrices modulate hepatic Ito cell phenotype and cellular retinol binding protein levels. *J. Biol. Chem.*, **262**, 1280–1286

Duthie, A., Doherty, D. G., Williams, C. *et al.* (1992) Genotype Analysis for F508, G551D, R553X mutations in children and young adults with cystic fibrosis with and without liver disease. *Hepatology*, **15**, 660–664

Duthie, A., Doherty, D. G., Mieli-Vergani, G., Mowat, A. P. and Vergani, D. Immunological abnormalities in cystic fibrosis. (Submitted for publication)

Eid, N. S., Shoemaker, L. R. and Samiec, T. D. (1990) Vitamin A in cystic fibrosis: case report and review of the literature. *Journal of Pediatric Gastroenterology and Nutrition*, **10**, 265–269

Evans, J. S., George, D. E. and Molit, D. (1991) Biliary infusion therapy in the inspissated bile syndrome of cystic fibrosis. *J. Pediatr. Gastroenterol. Nutr.*, **12**, 131–135

Furuya, K. N., Roberts, E. A., Canny, G. J. and Philips, M. J. (1991) Neonatal hepatitis syndrome with paucity of interlobular bile ducts in cystic fibrosis. *J. Pediatr. Gastroenterol. Nutr.*, **12**, 127–130

Gaskin, K. J., Water, D. L. M., Howman-Giles, R. N. *et al.* (1988) Liver disease and common-bile-duct stenosis in cystic fibrosis. *N. Engl. J. Med.*, **318**, 340–346

Gressner, A. M. and Bachem, M. G. (1990) Cellular sources of noncollagenous matrix proteins: Role of fat-storing cells in fibrogenesis. *Sem. Liver Dis.*, **10**, 30–46

Kearns, G. L., Mallory, G. B., Crom, W. R. and Evans, W. E. (1990) Enhanced hepatic drug clearance in patients with cystic fibrosis. *J. Pediatr.*, **117**, 972–979

Kerem, E., Reisman, J., Corey, M., Canny, G. J. and Levison, H. (1992) Prediction of mortality in patients with cystic fibrosis. *N. Engl. J. Med.*, **326**, 1187–1191

Lampert, C. R., Cole, M., Crozier, D. M. and Cannon, J. J. (1981) Intrahepatic common bile duct compression causing jaundice in an adult with cystic fibrosis. *Gastroenterology*, **80**, 169

Lloyd-Still, J. D. (1990) Cystic Fibrosis, Crohn's Disease, Biliary Abnormalities and Cancer. *J. Pediatr. Gastroenterol. Nutr.*, **11**, 434–437

Lloyd-Still, J. D. (1991) Impact of orthotopic liver transplantation on mortality from pediatric liver disease. *J. Pediatr. Gastroenterol. Nutr.*, **12**, 305–309

McHugo, J. M., McKeown, C., Brown, M. T., Weller, P. and Shah, K. J. (1987) Ultrasound findings in children with cystic fibrosis. *Br. J. Radiol.*, **60**, 137–141

Maurage, C., Lenaerts, C., Weber, A., Brochu, P., Ibrahim, Y. and Roy, C. C. (1989) Meconium ileus and its equivalent as a risk factor for the development of cirrhosis: An autopsy study in cystic fibrosis. *J. Pediatr. Gastroenterol. Nutr.*, **9**, 17–20

Mieles, L., Orenstein, D., Teperman, L., Podesta, L., Koneru, B. and Starzl, T. E. (1989) Liver transplantation in cystic fibrosis. *Lancet*, **1**, 1073–1078

Modson, M. E. Combined heart and lung transplantation in children. *Eur. J. Pediatr.* (in press)

Mondelli, M. (1987) Evidence against antibody-dependent cell-mediated immunity as a possible mechanism of liver cell injury in cystic fibrosis. *Boll. Ist. Sieroter Milan*, **66**, 66–69

Mondelli, M., Donaldson, P. T. and Mowat, A. P. (1984) Human leucocyte antigens (HLA) and haplotypes in cystic fibrosis patients. Possible increase of HLA B8 in those with liver disease. In *Cystic Fibrosis: Horizons* (ed. D. Lawson). John Wiley, Chichester, p. 183

Mowat, A. P. (1992) Orthotopic liver transplantation for liver-based metabolic disorders. *Eur. J. pediatr.*, **151**, S32–S38

Nagel, R. A., Westaby, D., Javaid, A. *et al.* (1989) Liver disease and bile duct abnormalities in adults with cystic fibrosis. *Lancet*, **2**, 1422–1425

Nawagawa, G., Colombo, C. and Setchell, K. D. R. (1990) Comprehensive study of the biliary bile acid composition of patients with cystic fibrosis and associated disease before and after ursodeoxycholic acid administration. *Hepatology*, **12**, 322–324

Penketh, A. R. L., Wise, A., Mearns, M. E., Hodson, and Batten, J. C. (1987) Cystic fibrosis in adolescents and adults. *Thorax*, **42**, 526–532

Perkins, W. G., Klein, G. L. and Beckerman, R. C. (1985) Cystic fibrosis mistaken for idiopathic biliary atresia. *Clin. Pediatr.*, **24**, 107

Peters, J. H., Gibbons, G. D., Innes, J. T. *et al.* (1991) Complications of laparoscopic cholecystectomy. *Surgery*, **110**, 769–778

Psacharopoulos, H. T., Howard, E. R., Portmann, B., Mowat, A. P. and Williams, R. (1981). Hepatic complications of cystic fibrosis. *lancet*, **ii**, 78

Psacharopoulos, N. T. and Mowat, A. P. (1983) The liver and biliary system. In: *Cystic Fibrosis* (eds Hodson, M. E., Norman, A. P. and Batten, J. C.). Bailliere Tindall, London, p. 164

Rayner, R. J., Tyrell, J. C., Hiller, E. J. *et al.* (1989) Night blindness and conjunctival xerosis caused by vitamin A deficiency in patients with cystic fibrosis. *Arch. Dis. Childh.*, **64**, 1151–1156

Resti, M., Adami Lami, C., Tucci, F. *et al.* (1990) False diagnosis of non-A/non-B hepatitis hiding two cases of cystic fibrosis. *Eur. J. Pediatr.*, **150**, 97–99

Rich, D. R., Anderson, M. P., Gregory, R. J. *et al.* (1990) Expression of transmembrane conductance regulator corrects defective chloride channel regulation in cystic fibrosis airway epithelial cells. *Nature*, **347**, 358–363

Richardson, V. F., Robertson, C., Mowat, A. P., Howard, E. R. and Price. J. (1984) Deterioration in Lung function after general anaesthesia in patients with cystic fibrosis. *Acta Paediatr. Scand.*, **73**, 75–79

Roy, C. C., Wenar, A. N., Morin, C. L. *et al.* (1982) Hepatobiliary disease in cystic fibrosis: A survey of current issues and concepts. *J. Pediatr. Gastroenterol. Nutr.*, **1**, 469

Sarles, J., Scheiner, C., Sarran, M. and Giraud, F. (1990) Hepatic hypervitaminosis A; a familial observation. *J. Pediatr. Gastroenterol. Nutr.*, **10**, 71–76

Scott-Jupp, R., Lama, M. and Tanner, M. S. (1991) Prevalence of liver disease in cystic fibrosis. *Arch. Dis. Childh.*, **66**, 698–701

Sinaasappel, M. (1989) Hepatobiliary pathology in patients with Cystic Fibrosis. *Acta Paediatr. Scand. (Suppl.)*, **363**, 45–51

Sokol, R. J., Reardon, M. C., Accurso, F. J. *et al.* (1989) Fat-soluble-vitamin status during the first year of life in infants with cystic fibrosis identified by screening of newborns. *Am. J. Clin. Nutr.*, **50**, 1064–1071

Stern, R. C., Rothstein, F. X. and Boersnuk, C. F. (1986) Treatment and prognosis of symptomatic gallbladder disease in patients with cystic fibrosis. *J. Pediatr. Gastroenterol. Nutr.*, **5**, 35

Tanner, M. S. (1986) Current clinical management of hepatic problems in cystic fibrosis. *J. Roy. Soc. Med. Suppl.*, **79**, 38–43

Treem, W. R. and Stanley, C. A. (1989) Massive hepatomegaly, steatosis and secondary carnitine deficiency in an infant with cystic fibrosis. *pediatrics*, **83**, 993–997

Vergani, G., Psacharopoulos, H. T., Nicholson, A. N. *et al.* (1980). Immune response to liver membrane antigens in patients with cystic fibrosis and liver disease. *Arch. Dis. Childh.*, **55**, 696

Vergesslich, K. A., Gotz, M., Mostbeck, G., Sommer, G. and Ponhold, W. (1989) Portal venous blood flow in cystic fibrosis: assessment by Duplex Doppler sonography. *Pediatr. Radiol.* **19**, 371–374

Vitulo, B., Rochon, L., Seemayer, T. A., Breadmore, N. and Debelle, R. (1978) Intrapancreatic compression of the common bile duct in cystic fibrosis. *J. Pediatr.*, **93**, 1060

Wainwright, B. J., Scrambler, P. J., Schmidike, S. R. *et al.* (1985) Localisation of cystic fibrosis locus to human chromosome 7, cen-q 22. *Nature*, **318**, 384

Warner, J. O. (ed.) (1992) Cystic fibrosis. *Br. Med. Bull.*, **48**, 717–978

Westaby, D. (ed.) (1992) *Management of Variceal Bleeding*. W. B. Saunders, Philadelphia

Whitington, P. F. and Balistreri, F. (1991) Liver transplantation in pediatrics: Indications, contraindications, and pretransplant management. *J. Pediatr.*, **118**, 169–177

Chapter 21

Liver and gall bladder disease in sickle cell anaemia

Introduction

Sickle cell anaemia is a severe chronic haemolytic anaemia caused by a genetically determined abnormality at position 6 in the beta polypeptide chain of haemoglobin. A valine molecule is substituted for a glutamic acid molecule. In affected individuals between 80 and 100% of haemoglobin is of the S variety, the remainder being haemoglobin F. The red cell life is limited to 15–25 days and bilirubin production increases sixfold.

In states of low oxygen saturation haemoglobin S molecules polymerize to arrange themselves in long, slightly rotated tubular structures which damage the red cell membrane leading to water loss and development of the typical crescent-shaped sickle cell. These rigid, fragile cells cause a marked increase in viscosity and adhere abnormally to endothelial cells thus blocking capillaries. Any circumstance which could lead to an increase in the degree of oxygen desaturation sets in train a vicious cycle of events of sickling, increased viscosity, stasis, more hypoxia, more sickling, cell death and organ damage. There is a great variability in the degree and severity of organ involvement. Infection, fluid and electrolyte loss and disorders causing hypoxia are major contributory factors.

Clinical features of sickle cell anaemia

The signs and symptoms of sickle cell anaemia are those of a haemolytic anaemia with, in addition, splenomegaly developing at 4–6 months of age being prominent in the first 3 to 5 years of life but by 6–8 years of age the spleen is reduced in size by repeated infarction and is rarely palpable after the age of 10 years. In 10–15% of children, however, there is persistent splenomegaly and hypersplenism.

Hepatomegaly is present in nearly all infants and children and becomes more marked during sickle cell crises, in which occlusion of blood vessels by masses of sickling cells leads to tissue hypoxia. Both liver and spleen may rapidly enlarge in so-called sequestration crises in which there is sudden entrapment of red blood cells in these organs causing acute, sometimes fatal, anaemia. Other crises take the form of sudden haemolysis or bone marrow hypoplasia, usually induced by parvovirus infection.

Infection is a serious problem in children with sickle cell disease. Functional abnormalities in the reticulo-endothelial system include diminished opsonization, inefficient phagocytosis and impaired chemotaxis of polymorphonuclear neutrophil leucocytes. Patients have an unusually high incidence of severe pneumococcal, *Haemophilus influenzae* and *Salmonella* infections.

Hepatic pathology in sickle cell disease

Patients with sickle cell anaemia do have an increased incidence of both liver and gall bladder disease. In three autopsy series comprising 132 cases, portal fibrosis was present in 15–30% with cirrhosis occurring in 16–29%, the incidence of both abnormalities increasing with age. Four of 24 with cirrhosis had massive increase in iron overload. By 10 years of age, 14% had gall-stones, the incidence increasing to 80% in adult life. Since abnormal tests of liver function are more prevalent with increasing age in this disorder, it has been suggested that there is a progressive hepatopathy to which the following factors may contribute:

(1) Anoxic necrosis of hepatocytes due to stasis in hepatic sinusoids.
(2) Hepatic infarcts caused by sickling in hepatic artery branches.
(3) Abnormal gall bladder function, cholelithiasis and choledocholithiasis.
(4) Viral hepatitis.
(5) Haemosiderosis.
(6) Congestive changes secondary to poor cardiac function.

Disorders considered to be due to vascular stasis

Portal vein blood during digestion has a low oxygen saturation. Hepatic cells extract more oxygen as the blood traverses the sinusoids. Sickling of red cells occurs within the sinusoids, particularly towards the central vein, and more so during sickling crises. Few sickled red cells are found in the hepatic veins, being trapped with platelets and fibrin within the dilated sinusoids. These aggregates are ingested by Kupffer cells which swell and appear to distort sinusoids. In addition, there is, within the space of Disse, deposition of collagen and basement membrane thickening. Anaemia and local circulatory effects due to these cellular changes may further damage hepatocytes. Hepatocytes around the central vein become enlarged and stain less intensely with haematoxylin and eosin.

The cells become depleted of glycogen. Electron microscopy shows that the rough endoplasmic reticulum occupies less volume, mitochondria become distorted and vary greatly in shape and size. There will be focal hepatocyte death. Within a few days of remission of the crisis, these hepatocellular changes become less marked and revert to near normal within 10–14 days. Kupffer cell hyperplasia persists. Hepatic infarction may occur due to sickling in the vasa vasorum of hepatic artery branches.

Hepatic features

Clinical and laboratory features

In the asymptomatic patient with sickle cell disease, hepatomegaly is usual and the serum bilirubin concentration is rarely within the normal range. With increasing age the serum bilirubin rises further. The aspartate transaminase and alkaline phosphatase are frequently elevated, particularly if the reticulocyte count is raised and the haemoglobin is low. The gamma-glutamyl transpeptidase is often normal in the first years of life but after 10 years of age the concentration rises and the prothrombin times are frequently prolonged by a few seconds. During sickle cell crises these clinical signs and biochemical abnormalities frequently become more abnormal.

Hepatic crisis characterized by tender hepatomegaly with a further rise in serum bilirubin up to concentrations of 30 mg/dl (560 µmol/litre) with over 60% conjugated and aspartate transaminase elevation up to six times normal are likely to be due to sinusoidal occlusion. A number of recent studies have suggested that patients with sickle disease appear to have a high prevalence of symptomatic *acute hepatitis A* with considerable morbidity. In acute hepatitis A serum bilirubin values may be in the same range or lower but aspartate aminotransferase levels are likely to be more than 10 times normal. Episodes of *extreme hyperbilirubinaemia* with serum bilirubin concentrations ranging up to 60 mg/dl (1000 µmol/litre) may occur. In some instances these have been shown to be due to acute hepatitis A. In a study of 47 hospitalized children with acute hepatitis, only three (of 34 with type A) developed *fulminant liver failure*. Two of these three were the only children with sickle cell disease, suggesting it predisposes to an increased mortality.

Zinc deficiency which in sickle cell disease has been associated with elevated blood ammonia levels, corrected when the zinc deficiency is corrected, has been suggested as a possible contributory factor to the hepatic failure.

Cholelithiasis

The persistent high level of bilirubin excretion and a degree of bile retention in the gall bladder (Everson *et al.*, 1989) may contribute to the formation of gall-stones. These are typically of the pigment type and are not radio-opaque. Many identified stones, however, do contain much calcium bilirubinate and in some reports up to 50% of identified stones are radio-opaque. Detection usually requires ultrasonography or cholecystography. The prevalence of gall-stones is at least 14% in those below 10 years of age rising to over 30% in patients aged 10–20 years, and to over 80% after 30 years of age (Bond *et al.*, 1987). With the exception of malignancy, all possible complications of gall-stones have been reported in this condition. Choledocholithiasis, perforation of the gall bladder, necrosis of the gall bladder and cholecystitis have all been documented in childhood.

Diagnosis

A major clinical problem is to try to distinguish symptoms and signs due to gall-stones from those due to an abdominal crisis and associated intrahepatic stasis. In both conditions there may be ill-localized upper abdominal pain and tenderness, perhaps more marked on the right side. The serum bilirubin is likely to be elevated to values up to between 6 and 10 mg/100 ml (100–170 µmol/litre) with 50% of the bilirubin conjugated. Modest rises of serum alkaline phosphatase to levels 50% above the upper limit of normal and of serum transaminases to three or four times normal, occur in both disorders. The diagnosis rests on radiological studies. As explained elsewhere, plain X-ray of the abdomen and ultrasonography identify cholelithiasis in the gall bladder but not cholecystitis (Figure 21.1). Hepatobiliary scanning with technetium-99m iminodiacetic acid derivatives (IDA) such as methyl bromo-IDA are useful in that in cholecystitis these are not concentrated in the gall bladder. If jaundice persists a percutaneous cholangiogram may be required.

If gall-stones are confirmed, it is still difficult to ascribe symptoms to them. The possible risk of stones in the gall bladder must be weighed against the risks of their surgical removal by cholecystectomy (Figure 21.1). This operation is not without its risk in any child, but carries an even greater risk in sickle cell disease without careful preoperative management. This entails replacement of the patient's haemoglobin S blood

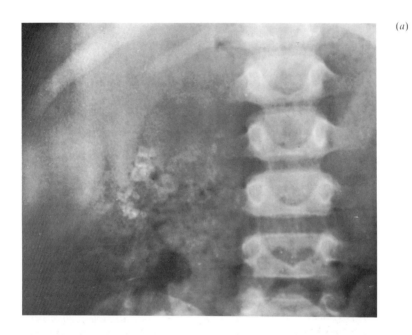

(a)

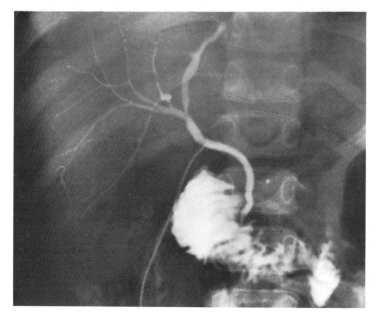

(b)

Figure 21.1 The patient was diagnosed as having sickle cell anaemia at the age of 18 months. She was admitted to hospital with a respiratory tract infection. The haemoglobin was 8.4 g/dl with a reticulocyte count of 38%. Haemoglobin electrophoresis showed haemoglobin S and A2. In the subsequent year she was admitted to hospital on a number of occasions with respiratory tract infections, sometimes complicated by severe anaemia with haemoglobins as low as 3.9 g/dl being recorded. Blood transfusion was required on four occasions. Between the age of 5 and 8 years she had episodes of intermittent jaundice associated with anorexia, nausea and right hypochondrial pain. Radiology of the abdomen (a) showed ring shadows in the gall bladder area indicative of gall-stones. Her jaundice had never been severe, the highest recorded level being 6.3 mg/dl (108 μmol/litre) but during some of these episodes the serum transaminases had been as elevated as 160 IU/litre (upper limit of normal 40). The case was unusual in that at the age of 8 years she had marked splenomegaly, the splenic edge being palpable 6 cm below the costal margin. Because her haemoglobin was lower than it had been earlier in life, it was elected to remove her spleen and gall bladder in one operation. When the decision to operate was taken the cells in the peripheral blood showing sickling was 79%. Over a 6 week period she awas transfused with 8 units of blood which resulted in the percentage of sickle cells falling to 9%. At laparotomy she was found to have an enlarged gall bladder which contained 10 black pigmented stones up to 0.8 cm in diameter. The epithelium of the gall bladder was ulcerated in some areas, the cystic duct was cannulated and through the cannula an operative cholangiogram showed free flow into the duodenum with no filling defects and no dilatation of the common bile duct or hepatic ducts. (b) The postoperative course was uneventful. A liver biopsy taken at laparotomy showed no abnormality. Since the operation the patient has continued to be anaemic but has had no further attacks of jaundice

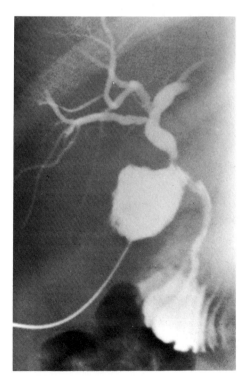

Figure 21.2 Showing the percutaneous cholangiogram of another child with sickle cell anaemia, diagnosed at the age of 3 years. One year before referral he had had two episodes of jaundice accompanied by abdominal pain. Cholecystectomy, which had been followed by an attempt to place a T-tube in the bile duct, had been followed by an increase in jaundice and persistence of abdominal pain. During the 8 month period between this operation and referral, jaundice had occurred on five occasions. For 6 weeks prior to referral, he had had pruritis and abdominal distension. The urine was dark, but the stool colour was normal. On examination there was jaundice, hepatomegaly and ascites. The haemoglobin was 8 g/dl, the total bilirubin 620 μmol/litre, the conjugated bilirubin 420 μmol/litre. Transfusion with compatible blood without sickle cell haemoglobin was given to reduce the percentage of sickled cells in peripheral blood to less than 30%. The percutaneous cholangiogram shows dilatation of the intrahepatic bile ducts with a marked stricture at the level of the portohepatis. At laparotomy a fibrotic mass was found in the portohepatis. A duct remnant was found within this and an end-to-side choledocho-jejunostomy was performed over a silastic splint. A Roux-en-Y loop of jejunum was fashioned. Following surgery the serum bilirubin fell to 102 μmol/litre, but the long-term prognosis must be very guarded

in a series of transfusions of group-compatible haemoglobin A blood, sufficient to reduce the percentage of haemoglobin S in the blood to less than 40%. A series of 1–2 unit transfusions at weekly intervals will usually produce this effect over 3 to 4 weeks. It is vital to prevent hypoxia during and after surgery.

Indications for cholecystectomy

At present cholecystectomy is recommended for gall-stones in children with sickle cell disease who have had complications of their gall-stones, or in patients who have repeated abdominal crises which are indistinguishable from gall bladder disease without invasive investigations. In these, it is clearly preferable to perform elective surgery for cholecystectomy than to be faced with the risk of subjecting a patient to surgery when the symptoms are due to a sickle cell crisis. Laparoscopic cholecystectomy may be possible.

Choledocholithiasis

This is a dangerous complication of cholelithiasis causing marked impairment of hepatic function and increased intrahepatic fibrosis (Figure 21.2).

Clinically there is commonly abdominal pain with fever, though in some instances severe jaundice and pruritus may be the only features. Ultrasonography may demonstrate stones in the common bile duct but such stones are notoriously difficult to identify by ultrasonography and CT scanning may be more satisfactory. If ultrasonography shows dilated bile ducts, percutaneous transhepatic cholangiography or endoscopic retrograde cholangiography are required to confirm the presence of stones. Such investigations may occasionally be justified in patients with persistent, unexplained severe jaundice. Pigment stones may pass spontaneously. Endoscopic sphincterotomy may allow larger stones to pass. This should be followed by elective cholecystectomy to prevent recurrence.

Haemosiderosis

A further factor causing possible liver damage is iron deposition within the liver. This arises from both increased iron absorption and from transfusions. Although iron accumulation in the liver in childhood in sickle cell disease is significant, evidence that this causes liver damage is at present tenuous.

Secondary hypersplenism

Very rarely, the spleen remains persistently large in patients with sickle cell disease. Hypersplenism becomes suspected when there is a progressive fall in haemoglobin concentration in the absence of crisis in a patient who previously maintained a constant low haemoglobin. It may be demonstrated more exactly by the reduced survival of normal erythrocytes in the patient's circulation. In such instances, splenectomy will remove the extracellular factor and allow the haemoglobin to return to a higher compensated level.

Treatment

No treatment is available which modifies the underlying defect. The value of blood transfusion in preparing the patient for surgery has already been emphasized. It has a place also in any severe complicating illness, such as severe hepatitis. Exchange transfusion has been used in the treatment of severe intrahepatic cholestasis (Sheehy *et al.*, 1980). Hypoxia and acidosis should be prevented. Patients with sickle cell disease are unduly prone to bacterial infection, particularly pneumococcal and *Haemophilus influenzae*. Immunization and prophylactic antibiotics are indicated.

Bibliography and references

Banerjee, A. K., Layton, D. M., Rennie, J. A. and Bellington, A. J. (1991) Safe surgery in sickle cell Disease. *Br. J. Surg.*, **78**, 516–517

Bauer, T. W., Moore, G. W. and Hutchins, J. M. (1980) The liver in sickle cell disease. A clinico-pathological study of 70 patients. *Am. J. Med.*, **69**, 833

Bond, L. R., Hatty, S. R., Horn, M. E. C., Dick, M., Meire, H. B. and Bellingham, A. J. (1987) Gallstones in sickle cell disease in the United Kingdom. *Br. Med. J.*, **295**, 234–236

Everson, G. T., Nemeth, A., Kourourian, S. *et al.* (1989) Gallbladder Function is altered in sickle hemoglobinopathy. *Gastroenterology*, **96**, 1307–1316

Johnson, C. S., Omata, M., Tong, M. J. *et al.* (1985) Liver involvement in sickle cell disease. *Medicine*, **64**, 349

Mallough, A. A. and Asha, M. I. (1988) Acute cholestatic jaundice in children with sickle cell disease: hepatic crises or hepatitis? *Pediatr. Infec. Dis. J.*, **7**, 689–692

Malone, B. S. and Werlin, S. L. (1988) Cholescystectomy and cholelithiasis in Sickle Cell Anaemia. *Am. J. Dis. Child.*, **142**, 799–800

Markowitz, R. J., Harcke, H. T., Ritchie, W. G. and Hough, D. S. (1980) Focal nodular hyperplasia of the liver in a child with sickle cell anaemia. *Am. J. Radiol.*, **134**, 594

Middleton, J. P. and Wolper, J. C. (1984) Hepatic biloma complicating sickle cell disease. *Gastroenterology*, **86**, 743

Nation, C. S. R., Bonch, C. and Weatherall, D. J. (1985) Hepatic sequestration in sickle cell anaemia. *Br. Med. J.*, **290**, 744

Prasad, A. S. and Cossach, Z. T. (1984) Zinc supplementation in sickle cell diseases. *Ann. Intern. Med.*, **100**, 367

Schubert, T. T. (1986) Hepatobiliary system in sickle cell disease. *Gastroenterology*, **90**, 2013

Serfani, A. N., Spolianski, G., Sfakianakis, G. N., Montalvo, B. and Jensen, W. N. (1987) Diagnostic studies in patients with sickle cell anaemia and acute abdominal pain. *Arch. Intern. Med.*, **147**, 1061–1062

Sheeny, T. W. (1977) Sickle cell hepatopathy. *South Med. J.*, **70**, 533

Sheeny, T. W., Law, D. E. and Wade, B. H. (1980) Exchange transfusion for sickle cell intra-hepatic cholestasis. *Arch. Intern. Med.*, **140**, 136

Ware, R., Filston, H. C., Schultz, W. H. and Kinney Tr. (1988) Elective cholecystectomy in children with sickle cell disease: successful outcome with preoperative transfusion regimen. *Ann. Surg.*, **208**, 17–22

Webb, D. K., Darby, J. S., Dunn, D. T., Terry, S. I. and Sargeant, G. R. (1989) Gallstones in Jamaican children with homozygous sickle cell disease. *Arch. Dis. Childh.*, **64**, 693–696

Yohannan, M. D., Arif, M. and Ramia, S. (1990) Aetiology of icteric hepatitis and fulminant hepatic failure in children and the possible predisposition to hepatic failure by sickle cell disease. *Acta Paediatr. Scand.*, **79**, 201–205

Chapter 22

Disorders of the portal and hepatic venous systems

Portal hypertension is the major feature of disorders of the portal and hepatic venous systems. Hepatic vein lesions also cause acute or chronic liver failure. A range of surgical, endoscopic or drug treatments has been developed to deal with these life-threatening complications. Precise diagnosis is essential in choosing the most appropriate management. Careful appraisal of acute and long-term effects of surgical therapy is very important since liver transplantation may be required for some disorders.

Anatomy of the portal vein

The portal venous system carries blood to the liver from the stomach, intestine, spleen, pancreas and gall bladder. The superior mesenteric and splenic veins join to form the portal vein. At the hilum of the liver it divides into two major trunks supplying the right and left lobes of the liver. These trunks undergo a series of divisions which supply segments of the liver (Chapter 1) and terminate in small branches which eventually pierce the limiting plate of the portal tract and enter adjacent sinusoids through short channels.

The main branches of the portal vein and tributaries are shown in Figure 22.1. The superior mesenteric vein is formed from vessels draining the small intestine, head of pancreas, colon and stomach. The splenic vein carries blood from the spleen, pancreas, left side of the colon, rectum and stomach via the short gastric vessels.

Portal hypertension

Portal hypertension exists when the pressure in the portal venous system rises above 10–12 mmHg. The normal value depends on the mode of measurement but is generally around 7 mmHg. Portal hypertension may arise due to prehepatic, intrahepatic, or posthepatic obstruction of blood flow to and through the liver. The intrahepatic block may be presinusoidal, sinusoidal or postsinusoidal. Rarely, portal hypertension results from increased blood flow to the liver from arteriovenous anastomosis. Sometimes only part of the portal system is affected.

Portal pressure may be measured directly at laparotomy or by means of percutaneously placed needles in the liver, spleen or major vessels. In sinusoidal forms the portal pressure is the same as the wedged hepatic vein pressure. The hepatic venous pressure gradient is the difference between that pressure and the free (unwedged) hepatic vein pressure.

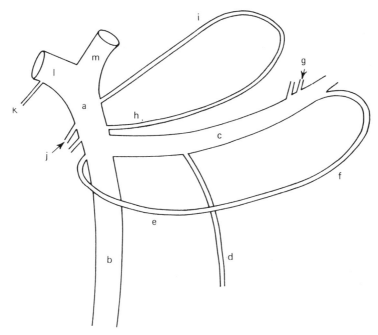

Figure 22.1 The portal vein and its tributaries

(a) portal vein
(b) superior mesenteric vein
(c) splenic vein
(d) inferior mesenteric vein
(e) right gastro-epiploic vein
(f) left gastro-epiploic vein
(g) short gastric veins

(h) right gastric vein
(i) left gastric vein
(j) pancreatico-duodenal vein
(k) cystic vein
(l) right branch of portal vein
(m) left branch of portal vein

The mode of presentation of each of these categories may be similar but the complications, naturally history and therapy can be very different. *Precise diagnosis is essential* if appropriate management is to be offered. The possible causes include intrahepatic disorders such as chronic active hepatitis and Wilson's disease, for which there are specific treatments. Intrahepatic disorders can be greatly aggravated by inappropriate surgery. Intra-abdominal surgery must therefore be delayed until a complete anatomical and pathological diagnosis is established. Iatrogenic factors frequently contribute to the morbidity and mortality of this disorder.

Pathology

Because of reduced portal vein flow the liver becomes dependent on the hepatic artery for oxygen and nutrition. In extrahepatic block particularly, the total liver bulk and individual liver cells are reduced in size, especially if there is a large collateral circulation. Portal tract fibrosis is present in more than two-thirds of cases. Perilobular fibrosis and steatosis are also frequently found. The other hepatic changes in intrahepatic or posthepatic causes are those of the primary disorder. The spleen becomes enlarged with a thickened capsule and increased reticulum around its dilated sinusoids. Histiocytes proliferate in the sinusoids. Erythrophagocytosis may be prominent. The splenic artery is enlarged and tortuous, and frequently there are aneurysms along its length or within the splenic substance. If the splenic vein and portal vein are patent they may also be enlarged, tortuous and occasionally calcified.

A major pathological effect is the development of collateral vessels which carry blood from the portal venous system to the systemic circulation, accounting for much of the symptoms and signs of this disorder. Collateral vessels develop: (a) where absorptive epithelium joins stratified epithelium in the oesophagus or rectum; (b) in the falciform ligament; (c) on the posterior abdominal wall, draining into the inferior vena cava; (d) draining to the left kidney; and (e) rarely, into the pulmonary vein. In extrahepatic obstruction there are, in addition, collaterals which attempt to carry blood around the blocked portal vein into the liver. They are also found in the suspensory ligaments of the liver and may include venae communicans of the portal vein and hepatic artery. Only the submucosal collaterals, especially those in the oesophagus, stomach and rectum, rarely those in the duodenum, jejunum, ileum or colon, are associated with alimentary bleeding. These ectopic varices are ten times more common in patients with extensive portal vein thrombosis but occur frequently at sites of abdominal or pelvic surgery. In biliary atresia brisk bleeding may come from stoma, jejunal conduit and at sites of bowel to bowel anastomosis. *Portal hypertensive gastropathy*, characterized by mucosal hyperaemia with dilated submucosal veins and capillaries, develops particularly in patients with advanced cirrhosis and gastric varices. The mucosa bleeds easily causing significant blood loss. With long standing disease collaterals may become more and more numerous, the portal pressure may fall and the risk of haemorrhage decrease. Portal hypertension may be complicated by ascites and by considerable oedema of the mucosa of the small intestine, which may lead to malabsorption.

An important complication in patients with large portosystemic shunts is hepatic encephalopathy. Septicaemia caused by Gram-negative intestinal organisms is an important cause of morbidity. A cause for failure to thrive may be bypassing of the liver by both absorbed food material and enteric hormones, such as insulin and glucagon. These pass directly to the systemic circulation where their metabolic effects are quite different from those which would have occurred had they been metabolized initially in the liver.

Clinical features

Cirrhosis, portal vein obstruction, congenital hepatic fibrosis and hepatic vein outflow obstruction are the main causes of portal hypertension in children. Portal hypertension may present with any of the features listed in Table 22.1. It may also present with features of the underlying hepatic disease of which it is a complication. Clinical examination may

Table 22.1 Clinical features of portal hypertension

Splenomegaly	Small liver or hepatomegaly
Haematemesis	Hypersplenism
Melaena	Ascites
Oesophageal varices	Malabsorption
Cutaneous portosystemic shunts	Protein losing enteropathy
Caput medusae	Failure to thrive
Venous hum above umbilicus	Hepatic encephalopathy
Internal haemorrhoids	

show jaundice or the stigmata of cirrhosis, such as vascular spiders, palmar erythema or xanthelasma. The patient may be anaemic, and there may be features of hepatic encephalopathy in intrahepatic disease.

An important clinical sign is dilated cutaneous collateral vessels carrying blood from the portal to the systemic circulation. These are seen carrying blood away from the umbilicus towards the tributaries of the superior vena caval system. In inferior vena caval obstruction blood flows from the inguinal region upwards over the abdominal wall. Bleeding from varices or asymptomatic splenomegaly is commonly the first indication of portal vein obstruction or congenital hepatic fibrosis. If there are no clinical or biochemical features of liver disease and the liver is small, portal vein obstruction is the most likely diagnosis although cirrhosis could be present. If the liver is large congenital hepatic fibrosis should be suspected.

Portal vein obstruction (extrahepatic portal hypertension)

In portal vein obstruction the main portal vein or splenic vein is obstructed somewhere along its course, between the hilum of the spleen and the portahepatis. The portal vein may be replaced by a fibrous remnant, a sheaf of small channels usually described as cavernous transformation, or contain an organized blood clot, web or diaphragm or be compressed from outside. The term extrahepatic is misleading in that the main intrahepatic branches of the portal vein are frequently occluded.

Aetiology

Many causes of extrahepatic portal hypertension are given in Table 22.2. In most series over 50% of cases have no evident cause. It has been inferred that a developmental defect may be responsible for some of the idiopathic cases. Congenital abnormalities in the heart, major blood vessels, biliary tree and renal system were found in 40% of cases (Odievre *et al.*, 1977).

Clinical features

The patients usually present with asymptomatic splenomegaly or with alimentary haemorrhage from oesophageal varices. Less commonly, they may present with ascites or failure to thrive. Signs may appear at any time from birth to the age of 15 years. Where

Table 22.2 Extrahepatic causes of portal hypertension

Obstruction of portal or splenic vein

Idiopathic	Septicaemia
Congenital	Cholangitis
Structural lesions	Trauma
Oomphalitis	Duodenal ulcer
Umbilical vein catheterization	Pancreatitis
Portal pyelophlebitis	Malignant disease
Intra-abdominal sepsis	Lymph gland enlargement
Surgery near the portahepatis	Choledochal cyst

Increased blood flow

Arteriovenous fistulae	Tropical splenomegaly

alimentary bleeding is the presenting feature, this most commonly occurs by the age of 7 years. Asymptomatic splenomegaly is more frequently a feature between the ages of 5 and 15 years.

Splenomegaly

Patients presenting with splenomegaly as the only feature are frequently well grown. There is no history of liver disease although a history of umbilical infection, catheterization or intra-abdominal problems early in life may be elicited. On clinical examination there is no jaundice or other evidence of chronic liver disease, generalized hyperplasia of the reticulo-endothelial system, bleeding diathesis, or intra-abdominal abnormality other than splenomegaly and, rarely, ascites. Dilated superficial portosystemic collaterals on the anterior abdominal wall are very rarely seen in extrahepatic portal hypertension, partly because the thrombosis frequently involves vessels draining into the falciform ligament.

A full history and clinical evaluation will often exclude the many infectiously acquired causes of splenomegaly, such as infectious mononucleosis, respiratory tract infection or metabolic storage disorders such as Gaucher's disease. Confirmatory investigations must be considered (see Table 22.5).

Alimentary bleeding

Extrahepatic portal hypertension may present with haematemesis or melaena. This typically occurs in a child who has previously been well, but complains of an acute onset of abdominal pain. Shortly thereafter the child is notably pale and vomits blood and/or has a melaena. This may be a life-threatening complication leading to rapid exsanguination and is said to be a contributory factor to early death in up to 12% of patients. It may occur at any age. Upper respiratory tract infections, especially if treated with aspirin, are frequent antecedents. The alimentary bleeding usually stops spontaneously. Bleeding, however, recurs at irregular intervals but becomes less frequent if collaterals develop in areas other than those immediately below the alimentary mucosal endothelium. Encephalopathy rarely complicates the alimentary bleeding. Some patients with portal vein obstruction never bleed. On clinical evaluation, no clue to the cause for bleeding is found other than the splenomegaly, and even this may not be evident if there has been much blood loss and the spleen has contracted. Collateral blood vessels are rarely present. The diagnosis of the cause of the bleeding is best made by emergency endoscopy. Barium contrast studies may be negative because the vascular volume is reduced and the varices are not distended.

Ascites

Ascites may occur around the time of onset of the portal hypertension. It can also occur following brisk intestinal haemorrhage. It is thought that this causes a degree of hepatic decompensation since the serum albumin level falls at the same time. If there is no further bleeding, ascites usually clears over the course of 2 to 3 weeks.

Rarely, *steatorrhoea* and *protein-losing enteropathy* may occur as part of the portal hypertension. Hepatic encephalopathy is distinctly uncommon. Minor features consistent with hepatic encephalopathy have been found in some children following portal systemic shunts. Where the main portal vein has been blocked, some deterioration of hepatic parenchymal function does occur in adult life and features of liver failure including encephalopathy may develop.

Diagnosis

Portal vein obstruction may be strongly suspected if an experienced ultrasonographer is unable to demonstrate a patent portal vein in a patient with the above features and biochemical tests of liver function are normal. In portal vein obstruction the prothrombin time is typically prolonged by 3–5 seconds. The serum albumin may be temporarily low following a bleed.

Splenic vein obstruction

This usually occurs in association with pancreatic disorders but any cause of portal vein obstruction may be responsible. The splenic flow bypasses the obstruction passing via the left gastric veins to the systemic circulation producing fundal and, rarely, lower oesophageal varices. Diagnosis is established by ultrasonography and/or angiography.

Arteriovenous fistulae

Congenital, traumatic or neoplastic fistulae linking the hepatic artery to the portal venous system causes portal hypertension with a marked increase in portal vein blood flow. The direction of blood flow may be reversed if the lesion is within the liver substance. There may be an associated increase in intrahepatic fibrosis. The patient may present with any of the features of portal hypertension including malabsorption, abdominal pain or a mass. Diagnosis may be suspected in the presence of portal hypertension if a systolic bruit is heard over the lesion. It is confirmed on angiography.

Intrahepatic portal hypertension

The features of many causes of intrahepatic portal hypertension given in Table 22.3 are considered in other chapters. Some aspects related to the management of portal hypertension in the more common ones are considered below.

Cirrhosis

Cirrhosis from whatever cause is almost always associated with portal hypertension. In many instances, symptoms and signs of hepatic disease have been present for years before portal hypertension is manifest. In others, the portal hypertension is found to be present when symptoms and signs first appear, while in some it is the first sign of liver disease.

Clinical features

The clinical features are those of the underlying liver disease. Physical examination in the majority will show cutaneous stigmata of chronic liver disease as well as a hard liver and splenomegaly. Periumbilical venous shunts may be present as well as signs of portal hypertension similar to those in portal vein obstruction. Hypersplenism with low haemoglobin concentrations, low total white count and thrombocytopenia are more frequently found. Some patients may have remarkably few signs and look well nourished. When gastrointestinal bleeding occurs, there may be a rapid deterioration in hepatic function and features of hepatic encephalopathy frequently occur.

Table 22.3 Intrahepatic causes of portal hypertension

Presinusoidal	Acute and chronic hepatitis
	Cirrhosis
	Congenital hepatic fibrosis
	Schistosomiasis
	Portal tract infiltration
	Granulomata
	Haemangiomata
	Vitamin A intoxication
	Hepatoportal sclerosis
	Idiopathic
Parasinusoidal	Cirrhosis
	Acute and chronic hepatitis
	Fatty liver
	Focal nodular hyperplasia
	Nodular regenerative hyperplasia
Postsinusoidal	Cirrhosis
	Metastatic malignancy
	Veno-occlusive disease
	Hepatic vein thrombosis

Congenital hepatic fibrosis

The clinical features are very similar to those of extrahepatic portal hypertension except that the liver is usually large and hard. The child is without stigmata of chronic liver disease. Splenomegaly, alimentary bleeding or ascites may be the presenting features. There may be a family history of liver, renal or vascular disease. On examination there are no features indicative of chronic liver disease. Kidneys may be enlarged and palpable if they are polycystic. The blood pressure may be elevated. Growth may have been slow. Parenchymal liver function is usually normal

Investigations will show normal liver function tests other than the serum alkaline phosphatase which may be elevated. Serum urea and creatinine may be elevated. Ultrasonography or intravenous pyelography shows features of renal involvement (see Chapter 16).

Hepatoportal sclerosis (non-cirrhotic portal fibrosis)

This poorly understood entity is characterized by portal hypertension with distinct changes in the branches of the portal vein as assessed on angiography but without distortion of hepatic architecture. Portal vein branches develop subendothelial thickening and sclerosis. Perisinusoidal fibrosis may be demonstrated by electron microscopy. Liver histology by light microscopy is normal initially but portal tract fibrosis subsequently develops. Rarely it may progress to cirrhosis. Causes include chronic arsenic ingestion, exposure to vinyl chloride monomers and treatment with methotrexate, azathioprine and 6-mercaptopurine. Clinical features are those of portal hypertension. Symptoms may start during infancy or childhood. The diagnosis requires angiographic demonstration of 'a withered tree' appearance of the portal vein branches and liver biopsy. Biochemical tests of liver function are normal.

Schistosomiasis

See Chapter 7.

Arterio–venous fistulae

See above (p. 373).

Posthepatic portal hypertension

Budd–Chiari syndrome (hepatic vein occlusion)

This syndrome is produced by obstruction of the hepatic veins occurring anywhere between the efferent hepatic venules and the entry of the inferior vena cava into the right atrium. Similar intrahepatic changes may occur complicating constrictive pericarditis or severe congestive cardiac failure.

Pathology

Thrombosis of the hepatic veins with total or partial occlusion occurs at some point in their course. The thrombus may contain malignant cells or polymorphs depending on the initial cause. In chronic cases the hepatic vein wall may be thickened, the lumen completely occluded, or replaced by a fibrous strand. There may be extensive fine collaterals.

The liver is enlarged and smooth. Around the central venule there is marked venous congestion with dilatation of the sinusoids, hepatocyte necrosis and increased fibrosis. Gradually this process extends across the lobule. Periportal areas are spared initially but marked fibrosis eventually develops in the parenchyma. Lymphatics may be dilated. Surviving liver cells are very similar to regenerating cells in cirrhosis. They often contain bile plugs. The caudate lobe may be spared if its hepatic veins, which often drain directly into the inferior vena cava, are not involved in the primary cause. It may undergo hypertrophy and compress the inferior vena cava. Ascites is present in virtually all patients and mild jaundice in most patients. The spleen enlarges and portosystemic collaterals develop.

Aetiology

In the vast majority of cases no cause can be found. It may be associated with thrombosis complicating polycythaemia, leukaemia, neoplasms (particularly hepatomas and hyper-nephromas), paroxysmal nocturnal haemoglobinuria, systemic lupus erythematosus or lupus anticoagulant, infection and trauma. In adolescents it may complicate the use of oral contraceptives. Antithrombin III, protein C or protein S deficiency must be excluded but differentiation from secondary deficiency due to liver failure may be difficult. Behçet's disease, liver abscesses, sarcoidosis and other granulomata may be responsible. It may arise secondary to a membranous obstruction in the inferior vena cava. We have seen one case in which it complicated intrahepatic haemangiomata. In adults the most common cause is latent or established myeloproliferative disorders (see Table 22.4).

Table 22.4 Posthepatic causes of portal hypertension

Congestive cardiac failure
Constrictive pericarditis
Budd–Chiari syndrome
  Polycythaemia
    Neoplasm
    Trauma
Inferior vena caval webs

Clinical features

In the acute form there is severe abdominal pain with vomiting, marked hepatomegaly, mild jaundice and the rapid onset of ascites which may be blood-stained. There may be features of the underlying disorder. Renal failure is usual. Diarrhoea is a frequent complication. If the hepatic vein occlusion is complete, death from hepatic failure may rapidly ensue.

In the more chronic form the patient presents with ascites, abdominal pain and fever. The liver is enlarged, hard and may be tender. If the inferior vena cava is affected, oedema of the legs occurs and distended superficial abdominal veins appear. There may be transient albuminuria. Pressure over the liver fails to fill the jugular veins. Splenomegaly and portosystemic collaterals develop as the increased pressure within the liver is transmitted to the portal system. Gradually a picture of chronic portal hypertension with hepatic damage may evolve, which may be compatible with survival for many years.

Laboratory findings

Standard biochemical tests for liver disease are often only slightly abnormal in chronic forms but reflect hepatic necrosis in acute cases. Prothrombin time is markedly prolonged in the acute forms (international normalized ratio >3), less in the chronic forms. Functional renal failure is present in acute cases and in many with severe chronic disease. Anaemia and thrombocytopenia are common. Ultrasonography provides useful diagnostic information. Absence of normal Doppler images of blood flow in the main hepatic veins is a helpful finding. Depending on the site of the lesion main hepatic veins may be obliterated or distended. The caudate lobe may be enlarged. The inferior vena cava may be partially or completely occluded. A technetium-99m colloid liver scan shows decreased isotope uptake, but if the venous drainage of the caudate lobe has been spared, uptake in this area is excellent. Computed tomography which with contrast injection shows mottled enhancement in the early phase and homogeneous opacification in the late phase, may be helpful if ultrasonographic findings are not classic. If a needle biopsy can be performed typical histological features will be seen, but confirmation of the diagnosis requires hepatic vein catheterization with pressure measurement and hepatic venography. A hepatic catheter cannot be passed even a short distance along the hepatic vein wedging within a few centimetres from the diaphragm. It is impossible to obtain a normal wedged hepatic venogram but abnormal lace-like venous collaterals may be demonstrated in chronic cases (Figure 22.2).

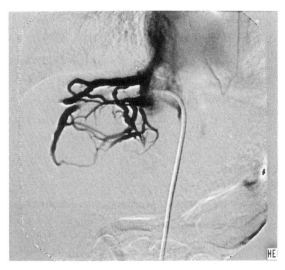

Figure 22.2 Hepatic venography demonstrating characteristic appearance of Budd-Chiari syndrome caused by hepatic vein thrombosis. There is no filling of normal hepatic veins but the typical appearance of hepatic vein collaterals is demonstrated

Inferior venacavography may be necessary to establish the patency of the inferior vena cava. The hepatic segment of the vein may be compressed from side to side due to the enlarged liver. The venacaval pressure may be greater than 15 mmHg. Portal pressure is usually considerably higher. The venacaval-atrial pressure gradient is high. Constrictive pericarditis is excluded by normal pressures in the right heart. Appropriate investigations are necessary to exclude underlying disease considered in aetiology.

Treatment

In the absence of a surgically treatable cause such as a web in the inferior vena cava or constrictive pericarditis, therapy is symptomatic. Treatment of thrombogenic conditions may prevent further thrombosis. In patients with intractable ascites, marked hepatomegaly or alimentary bleeding, palliative surgical treatment should be considered. The objective is to transform the portal vein into an outflow tract. A portocaval anastomosis, if there is a sufficient portocaval gradient, relieves liver congestion and some of the complications of portal hypertension. Liver function may improve. If there is occlusion or high pressure in the inferior vena cava a porto- or mesoatrial shunt via a prosthesis may be effective. There are considerable acute and chronic complications of these procedures. In a recent report of 22 children with Budd-Chiari syndrome, 18 of whom were treated surgically, only six of the 12 surviving, were symptom free. Liver transplantation is required for patients presenting with fulminant liver failure and for cirrhosis if a hypercoagulable state is excluded. Whatever form of surgery is used postoperative long-term anticoagulation should be considered. Symptomatic measures for fluid retention and alimentary bleeding are also necessary. There is no evidence that anticoagulants such as heparin, or agents to lyse clots, such as streptokinase, are helpful.

Veno-occlusive disease of the liver

This is a particular form of hepatic vein obstruction which occurs more commonly in children than in other age groups, and is the most frequent cause of hepatic vein obstruction in children. It is characterized by occlusion of the centrilobular venules or sublobular hepatic veins. The sinusoidal lining cells may also be damaged primarily. In cases reported from the Middle East there is frequently thrombosis of larger veins with stenosis. It was first recognized in Jamaica but subsequently has been shown to occur in other parts of the world such as South Africa, India, Dominica, Columbia, Venezuela and in Israel.

Pathology

The disorder starts in the endothelium of the small branches of the hepatic vein. The initial lesion is of endothelial oedema followed by marked fibroblastic proliferation, leading to phlebosclerosis with occlusion of the vessel lumen. There is secondary sinusoidal congestion and necrosis of hepatic cells leading to a progressive fibrosis and ultimately cirrhosis.

Aetiology

The condition is thought to be caused by ingestion of herbal infusions. The following plants have been implicated: *Senecio, Crotalaria, Borrago officinales, Cordia alba* and *Helitropicum indicum*. A herbal tea ingested throughout pregnancy as an expectorant was associated with this disorder in a neonate. Pyrrolizidine alkaloids and other toxins are also considered to be causes. Similar pathological changes have followed irradiation and/or cytotoxic drug-induced injury to the liver.

Clinical features

The clinical features are those of the Budd-Chiari syndrome. The maximum age incidence is between 1 and 6 years. The syndrome starts with the sudden onset of abdominal distension and pain due to hepatomegaly and ascites in up to 70% of cases. The reported outcome varies. In South America approximately 20% of patients die in the acute stage, while 30% develop chronic liver disease with cirrhosis and portal hypertension; 50% gradually recover over the course of 4 to 6 weeks. In Egypt the majority die within 1 year but a few survive and develop cirrhosis and portal hypertension after 2 or 3 years. There is no specific treatment.

Veno-occlusive disease after bone marrow transplantation

Veno-occlusive disease been reported in up to 28% of bone marrow transplantation patients, with a mortality of 47 to 52%. It is characterized clinically by jaundice, hepatomegaly, right upper quadrant pain and unexplained weight gain and/or ascites with 30 days of grafting. Shulman and Hinterberg (1992) showed that 13 of 32 patients with typical liver histology had no clinical features. Liver failure contributes to death in 50%. Diagnosis requires exclusion of other causes of liver disease. A rise in the serum concentration of the aminopropeptide of collagen type III (PIIINP) to a level more than eight times the normal standard deviation value for age is strongly suggestive of the diagnosis. Liver biopsy is frequently not possible because of the deranged clotting. Early treatment with plasminogen activator or prostaglandin E2 has been advocated. Prophylactic low dose heparin may prevent the condition (Attal *et al.*, 1992).

Chronic constrictive pericarditis

Hepatic effects

Chronic constrictive pericarditis causes an increase in pressure within the hepatic vein and liver damage similar to that of chronic Budd-Chiari syndrome.

Clinical features

Symptoms start insidiously. Fatigue, dyspnoea on effort but classically without orthopnoea, and massive abdominal swelling due to hepatomegaly, splenomegaly and ascites develop often over the course of 6 to 12 months. There may be noticeable facial oedema. Weight loss, failure to grow, and symptoms attributable to steatorrhoea and protein-losing enteropathy may also occur.

Diagnosis

The following cardiovascular abnormalities should suggest the diagnosis: persistently raised jugular venous pressure with absent hepatojugular reflux; poor pulse pressure with low blood pressure; and a quiet, inactive heart. On chest radiography pericardial calcification may be seen and on screening of the pericardium there is limited pulsation. The ECG classically shows flat or inverted 'T' waves and a QRS complex of reduced amplitude.

It must be noted, however, that many of the cardiac abnormalities may be minimal as indicated in the case history given in Figure 22.3.

The diagnosis may be suggested on the basis of ultrasonic examination of the liver showing distended hepatic veins. Liver biopsy will show loss of hepatocytes and collapse of the reticulin framework around the hepatic vein tributaries. This area will show dilated sinusoids with many red cells present. Ultrasonic echography may show a thickened, rigid pericardium. Confirmation of the diagnosis is by cardiac catheterization which confirms a high pressure in the right side of the heart with a characteristic appearance of the right atrial pulse wave, a steep Y descent being diagnostic. On angiography the right atrial wall is rigid and the tricuspid valve hypermobile.

Differential diagnosis

Difficulty may arise in distinguishing pericarditis from patients with chronic liver disease and much fluid retention.

Treatment

If the disorder is due to active tuberculosis it should be treated with antituberculous drugs and corticosteroids. If the disease is inactive, or the disorder is idiopathic, pericardectomy should be undertaken. Provided the underlying myocardial damage is not severe, there will be a gradual return of cardiac efficiency during the subsequent 24 months. The hepatic lesion regresses similarly.

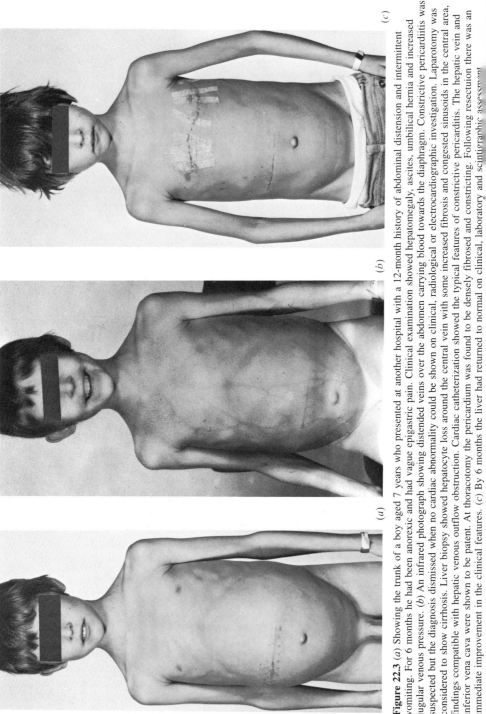

Figure 22.3 (*a*) Showing the trunk of a boy aged 7 years who presented at another hospital with a 12-month history of abdominal distension and intermittent vomiting. For 6 months he had been anorexic and had vague epigastric pain. Clinical examination showed hepatomegaly, ascites, umbilical hernia and increased jugular venous pressure. (*b*) An infrared photograph showing distended veins over the abdomen carrying blood towards the diaphragm. Constrictive pericarditis was suspected but the diagnosis dismissed when no cardiac abnormality could be shown on clinical, radiological or electrocardiographic investigation. Laparotomy was considered to show cirrhosis. Liver biopsy showed hepatocyte loss around the central vein with some increased fibrosis and congested sinusoids in the central area, findings compatible with hepatic venous outflow obstruction. Cardiac catheterization showed the typical features of constrictive pericarditis. The hepatic vein and inferior vena cava were shown to be patent. At thoracotomy the pericardium was found to be densely fibrosed and constricting. Following resection there was an immediate improvement in the clinical features. (*c*) By 6 months the liver had returned to normal on clinical, laboratory and scintigraphic assessment.

Investigation of a patient with suspected portal hypertension

In the patient presenting with alimentary bleeding the first priority is to assess and control it (see p. 387). In such patients and in patients presenting with splenomegaly, ascites or malabsorption a systematic approach is then required to confirm the presence of portal hypertension and to determine its cause (Table 22.5).

Table 22.5 Investigations in suspected portal hypertension

Liver function tests
Prothrombin time
Complete blood count
Reticuloycte count
Paul Bunnell test
Ultrasonic echography of the liver, biliary system,
    portal venous system and kidneys
Radioisotope imaging of liver and spleen
Endoscopy
Barium swallow
Investigation for causes of chronic liver disease
Liver biopsy

Investigations before surgery:
Demonstration of portal vein and its branches by
    splanchnic angiography, splenic venography or
    umbilical portography
In some instances cardiac catheterization, hepatic
    vein pressure measurements
Retrograde hepatic venogram
Inferior venacavogram
Percutaneous transhepatic portal venography

Initial investigations

A full blood count with red cell indices, morphology and reticulocyte count, a total and differential white blood count and platelet count should exclude primary haematological disorders. Abnormal white blood cell inclusions may be found in some storage diseases, e.g. mannosidosis. Abnormal biochemical tests of liver function are usually present in intrahepatic disorders, but in congenital hepatic fibrosis the only abnormality may be a raised alkaline phosphatase and even in cirrhosis the liver function tests may be normal. A prolongation of the prothrombin time by 3–5 seconds occurs in portal vein obstruction as well as in intrahepatic disease.

Ultrasonography performed by an experienced, careful observer is an extremely helpful investigation. The size of the portal vein may be determined and the velocity and direction of its blood flow determined by a Doppler probe. Retrograde flow is seen in severe intrahepatic fibrosis.

In portal vein thrombosis the portal vein is replaced with an echogenic mass through which channels can be visualized. A widening of the free border of the lesser omentum (which carries the left gastric vein) to a diameter more than 1.7 times that of the aorta at that level is a useful indicator of portal hypertension. Collaterals may also be demonstrated below the liver around the area of the portahepatis. Ultrasonography may also contribute to the assessment of the causes of the portal hypertension by demonstrating abnormalities in the biliary system or abnormal echo patterns within the liver. A plain film of the abdomen may occasionally contribute by confirming the size of the liver and spleen and by showing the presence of calcification in the splenic or portal veins. A barium study of the upper gastrointestinal tract may demonstrate subepithelial veins elevating the mucosa (Figure 22.4). These are characteristically serpiginous channels which change with respiration. They are usually best seen with a barium sulphate suspension which adheres to the mucosa in the distal oesophagus. Varices may also be seen in the stomach or duodenum. Peptic ulceration may be excluded. Retroperitoneal oedema, a feature complicating extrahepatic portal hypertension, but occasionally intrahepatic disease, may cause distortion of the duodenum.

Endoscopy is the most reliable method for detecting submucosal varices. Large varices, particularly if the overlying mucosa has red spots (varices on varices) or is darkened, are thought to carry particular risk of early bleeding. In children over the age of 9 years it may be possible to perform this investigation with the help of diazepam, but a general anaesthetic is required in younger children.

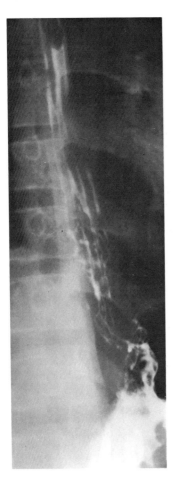

Figure 22.4 Barium swallow demonstrating oesophageal varices. These occupy the lower third of the oesophagus. The linear mucosal folds seen in the upper two-thirds are replaced by tortuous lines where the mucosa has been elevated by serpiginous subepithelial veins

If liver function tests are abnormal acute and chronic liver disease must be systematically investigated, including liver biopsy, in most cases.

Anatomical diagnosis

If surgical correction of the portal hypertension or liver transplantation are to be considered, further investigations are necessary to define the portal venous anatomy. The patency and calibre of the portal vein, splenic vein and superior mesenteric vein must be documented and directions of venous blood flow assessed. Ultrasonically directed Doppler investigations are very helpful in this regard.

Splanchnic angiography and/or splenic venography

The most useful investigation is a splanchnic angiogram performed by catheterizing the coeliac and superior mesenteric arteries, using catheters inserted percutaneously via the femoral arteries. Space-occupying lesions within the liver and abnormalities of the hepatic artery including arteriovenous fistulae can be demonstrated. Films taken during the venous phase outline the anatomy of portal venous system including the superior mesenteric and splenic veins (Figure 22.5).

The alternative is to perform a splenic venogram, which allows visualization of the splenic vein, portal vein and its intrahepatic branches if these are patent. If these are obstructed collateral vessels are shown as dilated, tortuous channels. There is poor hepatic sinusoidal filling. If cirrhosis is present, little contrast may enter the portal vein due to stagnant or reversed (hepatofugal) blood flow. The technique has the advantage over selective splanchnic angiograms in that it may more clearly show the splenic vein (Figure 22.6) and allow direct measurement of the intrasplenic pulp pressure, a measure of portal hypertension. Since intrasplenic pressure does not necessarily produce a reliable measure of portal hypertension and is unnecessary for clinical management, this investigation is rarely necessary. Further, its complications include subcapsular and intraperitoneal haemorrhage, sometimes leading to emergency splenectomy. While it provides a very clear picture of the collateral vessels running to the oesophagus, it may not demonstrate vessels such as the superior mesenteric vein which may be utilized for surgery. Splenic venography should not be performed unless splenectomy can be undertaken without jeopardy. Splanchnic angiography does carry the risks of arterial puncture, occasionally including thrombosis of the femoral artery, particularly if done in young infants. It gives less satisfactory radiological contrast in the splenic vein than splenic portography. It does demonstrate much more of the portal venous system. Occasionally, both investigations are necessary to give the surgeon optimum information on the venous system.

Computed tomography

This will allow visualization of the portal vein and of collaterals but is no better than ultrasonography with Doppler. It does require a general anaesthetic.

Digital subtraction angiography

This technique allows visualization of the hepatic artery, portal venous system and intrahepatic vessels with intravenous rather than intra-arterial or intersplanchnic injection of contrast. Complications are thus much less. Spatial resolution and details of anatomy may be less satisfactory than with conventional angiography.

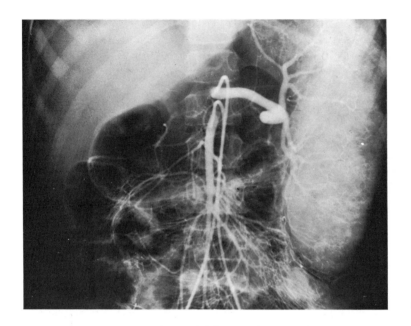

(a)

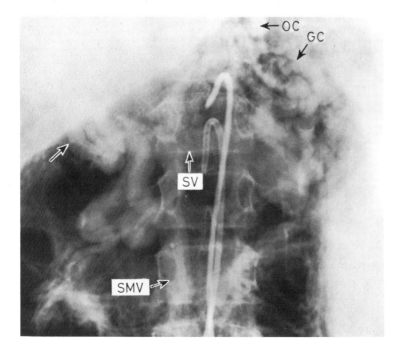

(b)

Umbilical portography

Umbilical portography, in which contrast is injected into the portal vein or its tributaries following catheterization of the umbilical vein, demonstrates the portal vein, its intrahepatic branches and the hepatic sinusoids. The umbilical vein is catheterized surgically in the mid-line 2–3 cm above the umbilicus. It may be used to evaluate portal hypertension in the rare instances when the above studies are inconclusive or contraindicated. In extrahepatic portal hypertension, in which the portal vein is usually involved, this technique rarely demonstrates the splenic vein. It will fail also if the umbilical vein has previously been transected at laparotomy or invaded by neoplasms. It does allow reliable measurement of portal venous pressure.

Percutaneous transhepatic portography

This technique in which a catheter is placed in an intrahepatic branch of the portal vein (see Chapter 23) and advanced along the portal vein or splenic vein, provides excellent visualization of the portal venous system. It is used mainly as a preliminary to transhepatic obliteration of varices but it may also be used where it is essential to confirm that the portal vein is not patent, e.g. in the child being considered for liver transplantation in whom the portal vein has not been demonstrated by other means. Its complication rate is greater than other procedures.

Hepatic vein pressure measurement

The free hepatic vein pressure is recorded with a catheter which lies in an unobstructed major hepatic vein branch. The pressures obtained must be considered in relation to the pressures recorded in the inferior vena cava and in the right atrium. The hepatic vein pressure is directly related to the measured portal vein pressure. A normal hepatic wedged pressure is about 5–6 mmHg. The values of approximately 20 mm Hg are found in patients with sinusoidal or postsinusoidal hypertension. In congenital hepatic fibrosis, schistosomiasis and hepatoportal sclerosis the gradient is between 1 and 10 mmHg. In extrahepatic portal vein block, both the wedged pressure and the free hepatic vein pressure are normal. Ascites can produce falsely high values. The main value of this investigation is in indicating the presence of significant intrahepatic disease when other more definitive tests are contraindicated. In most instances a percutaneous liver biopsy will give much more information at little extra risk.

Figure 22.5 Arterial portogram of a patient with extrahepatic portal hypertension. This child developed umbilical sepsis in the neonatal period, followed by osteomyelitis and a parotid abscess. He was treated with vigorous antibiotic therapy. At the age of 7 years he had a haematemesis which had recurred on three occasions. On each occasion these had been preceded by viral infections which were treated with aspirin. Severe anaemia resulted. Physical examination showed a healthy looking child with a markedly enlarged spleen but no features of chronic liver disease. Laboratory investigations were unremarkable, except that the total white count was 3.8 × 10⁹/l with a platelet count of 80 × 10⁹/l. Liver function tests were normal and specific causes of liver disease in this age group were negative. (*a*) Shows an arterio-portogram carried out by simultaneous selective catheterization of the coeliac and superior mesenteric arteries, 30 ml of 45% Hypaque were injected into each catheter at a rate of 7.5 ml/second. (*b*) The portal vein is thrombosed and replaced by numerous large collaterals (→) running alongside it taking the venous flow from the patent superior mesenteric (SMV) and splenic (SV) veins. the diameter of the superior mesenteric vein was estimated at 1.0 cm, that of the splenic vein 0.8 cm. Gastric (GC) and lower oesophageal collaterals (OC) are visible. The patient was advised to avoid aspirin, and in the 20 years since investigation has not yet had further alimentary bleeding

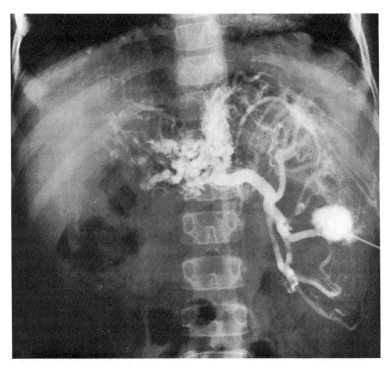

Figure 22.6 Splenic portogram in a girl aged 10 years with idiopathic extrahepatic portal hypertension. Contrast medium flows through a dilated splenic vein but at the mid-line is replaced by numerous collateral vessels which drain towards the portahepatis and to the gastric veins. These collaterals completely replace the portal vein

Intravenous pyelogram

This is an essential investigation to confirm the presence of functioning kidneys in patients who may require a shunt to a renal vein. It is also of value in assessing renal involvement in congenital hepatic fibrosis.

Further investigations in selected patients

Investigations occasionally required include inferior venacavography to detect partial or complete obstruction to the inferior vena cava or its compression by tumour or enlarged cardiac lobe; retrograde hepatic venography to demonstrate the Budd–Chiari syndrome; cardiac catheterization to identify constrictive pericarditis or cardiomyopathy; percutaneous transhepatic venography using a contrast medium injected directly into the portal or hepatic vein through the hepatic substance. This technique has been used largely in adults as an aid to a therapeutic measure in which a fine catheter is passed in a retrograde fashion along the portal vein into its coronary tributaries which are then occluded by fibrin plugs.

Liver biopsy

In intrahepatic disease the diagnosis and prognosis is largely dependent on the liver biopsy findings. These may be entirely morphological but on occasions biochemical studies will also be necessary.

Treatment of portal hypertension

Alimentary bleeding

Alimentary bleeding requires emergency treatment. As soon as the patient is haemodynamically stable an experienced endoscopist should confirm the source of bleeding and commence sclerotherapy, currently the best measure to prevent further bleeding. Preferably this should be done in a unit with full facilities and staff who are familiar with the whole range of measures required to manage the causes of portal hypertension in children. In patients with cirrhosis who continue to bleed following two or more attempts at endoscopic therapy, surgery should be considered at the earliest opportunity to prevent the inevitable rapid deterioration in the clinical condition that occurs with ongoing haemorrhage. Judicious use of balloon tamponade and drugs with a vasoconstrictive effect on the splanchnic circulation as adjuvants to sclerotherapy may be life-saving.

Initial management

However small the bleed, the child should be admitted immediately to the nearest hospital with blood transfusion facilities. Slow ooze with melaena or anaemia may become a brisk bleed with sudden haematemesis and shock requiring rapid blood transfusion to prevent death. Bleeding by causing anaemia and hypotension impairs hepatic perfusion, causes deterioration of liver function precipitating jaundice, ascites and encephalopathy. Blood in the gut contributes to the latter.

On admission the priorities are to make a baseline assessment of the clinical, haematological and biochemical state, cross-match whole blood, establish a secure intravenous infusion line in a peripheral vein and to ascertain that intravenous pitressin or somatostatin and a Sengstaken-Blakemore tube of suitable size are available if needed. Depending on the condition of the child, intensive care may be required. In the clinical assessment the cardiovascular and neurological status are important as are features of causes and complications of alimentary bleeding.

Haemoglobin, red blood cell indices, reticulocyte count, total and differential white blood count, platelet count, prothrombin time and standard biochemical tests of liver function should be determined. Close observation is essential to detect the presence and severity of continuing bleeding. This requires regular monitoring of the pulse, blood pressure, urinary output, stool appearance and haemoglobin concentration. Gastric aspiration with a fine nasogastric tube can be useful in detecting continual oozing.

If the blood volume is depleted, transfusion of fresh whole blood or packed cells to which fresh frozen plasma has been added must be given at a rate which will maintain a normal blood pressure and adequate tissue perfusion. Overtransfusion should be avoided since it may precipitate further bleeding by distending the varices. If cirrhosis is suspected hepatic encephalopathy must be anticipated. Sedatives should take the form of small doses of diazepam. Neomycin or lactulose should be given by nasogastric tube. If portal hypertension is known to be due to extrahepatic causes, sedation may be more generous since encephalopathy is not a high risk. Ranitidine should be given intravenously to reduce the risk of bleeding from the gastric erosions. If the prothrombin time is prolonged, intravenous vitamin K should be given.

As soon as the initial assessment is complete and these emergency measures instituted, it is essential to contact a unit with full facilities and skills to manage the causes and complications of portal hypertension in children. The transfer to such a unit should be arranged as soon as the child's condition is stable enough to travel and there is an adequate supply of cross-matched blood available.

Endoscopy   Endoscopy is essential to confirm the presence of varices and to ascertain the cause of bleeding. This latter is important since patients with portal hypertension may bleed from gastric erosions or peptic ulceration. Ideally, diagnostic endoscopy should be combined with injection sclerotherapy. The timing of endoscopy may thus be dictated by the experience of the operator available as well as by the continuation of bleeding after admission. The varices may not be seen on endoscopy if the blood volume is very depleted.

Vasopressin (pitressin)   If bleeding continues, the portal venous pressure may be lowered by this drug which causes constriction of the splanchnic arterial bed. A dose of 0.33 units/kg intravenously over a period of 20 minutes, followed by the same amount per hour by continuous infusion, frequently arrests bleeding. An effective dose usually causes skin pallor, abdominal colic and evacuation of the bowels. If bleeding continues the dose may be increased up to threefold. In adults it has been found that using it concomitantly with nitroglycerine (0.4 mg subcutaneously or 40–400 µg/minute intravenously) minimizes the rise in blood pressure and coronary artery constriction with a subsequent reduction in side-effects and increased efficacy. Glypressin (triglycyl lysine vasopressin) is an expensive inactive precursor of pitressin; 30 µg/kg repeated every 4 to 6 hours in combination with a vasodilator such as nitroglycerine in the form of a 10 mg patch which reduces the haemodynamic complications has proved useful in adults.

Somatostatin or its longer acting analogue octreotide have a major splanchnic vasoconstrictor effect with few adverse consequences on systemic or pulmonary circulations would appear to be the drugs of choice for pharmacological therapy. Somatostatin in a dose of 250 µg as a bolus followed by the same dose hourly, by continuous infusion, appears to be effective in adults. Octreotide 25 µg/hour IV or 50–150 µg subcutaneously 8 hourly is also effective. Neither have been systematically evaluated in children.

Sengstaken–Blakemore tube   If the above measures fail to control bleeding, consideration must be given to the use of balloon tamponade with a paediatric Sengstaken–Blakemore tube. This is a complex three or four-lumen tube, one lumen of which communicates with the stomach. A second lumen connects with the stomach balloon, which when well within the stomach is filled with weak radio-opaque solution and with gentle traction is retracted well into the fundus of the stomach (Figure 22.7). This will frequently control bleeding. If it does not the third lumen is used to inflated the oesophageal balloon with air to a pressure of between 20 and 30 mmHg. This should compress oesophageal varices. A fourth tube is essential to allow continuous aspiration of the pharynx (Figure 22.8).

These tubes are very successful in controlling bleeding from varices but they do have many complications and should only be used for those patients who are at immediate risk of exsanguination while preparing for sclerotherapy or more definitive surgical management. An anaesthetist with full resuscitation equipment must be present when the tube is inserted. Full anaesthesia is necessary and kinder for many children. The

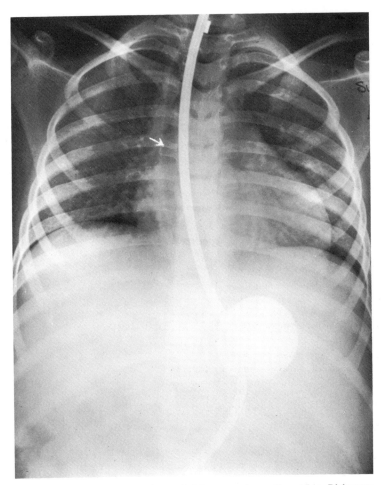

Figure 22.7 Radiograph of the chest and abdomen to show a Sengstaken–Blakemore tube *in situ* in a patient bleeding form oesophageal varices. The gastric balloon is well placed in the fundus of the stomach. The arrow indicates the air-filled oesophageal balloon

complications of the tube include malpositioning of the various balloons leading to asphyxia and aspiration of secretions into the lungs and oesophageal perforation. Erosions at pressure points also occur. Considerable nursing skill is required to manage such complicated situations.

Direct obliteration of varices

Endoscopic sclerotherapy

Of the techniques now available to prevent recurrence of bleeding this is the most efficacious for both intrahepatic disease and portal vein obstruction. There are many

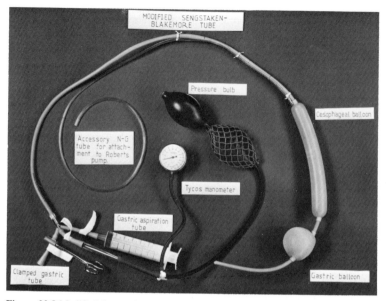

Figure 22.8 Modified Sengstaken–Blakemore tube and accessories. Note the nasogastric (N–G) tube which as been added to allow continuous aspiration of the pharynx

variations in the details of the procedure. The varix is identified endoscopically and obliterated or the overlying mucosa thickened. Usually this is achieved by injecting 1–5 ml of sclerosant in and around the varices just above the cardia. Three or four varices will be injected. Alternatively, up to 40 injections of small volumes (0.5 ml) of sclerosant are made along either side of the major varices starting at the oesophageal-gastric junction and continuing up the lower half of the oesophagus. This produces a fibrous layer of mucosa which covers but does not occlude the underlying varix. Such injections are best done when bleeding has stopped. In the presence of active bleeding accurate placement of the sclerosant is difficult. Endoscopy is repeated and further injections made at 1–4-week intervals until the varices are hidden by the thickened mucosa or are obliterated, being replaced by white fibrous cords.

Injections are usually performed with the assistance of a flexible endoscope. Old fashioned rigid endoscopes are now rarely used except in the face of active bleeding in which they have the advantage of compressing many of the varices and providing a wider channel for suction. The most favoured sclerosants with perhaps fewer side-effects than others are 5% ethanolamine and polidocanol.

The most frequent complication is mild chest discomfort and fever lasting for 24–48 hours after injection. There may be bacteraemia or septicaemia. Other complications fall into three main categories. Most common are oesophageal ulcers (14%) and strictures which can be easily dilated by bougies (9%).

Sucralfate minimizes the risk of such ulceration and deals with coincidental duodenal ulceration, without the risk of gastric colonization by *Pseudomonas aeruginosa* as may occur with H_2 antagonists. Other complications are rare. Among oesophageal ones are decreased motility, rupture with mediastinitis, increased gastro-oesophageal reflux and dysplastic or even carcinomatous change (Kukodo *et al.*, 1990). Among a range of pulmonary/pericardial problems is adult respiratory distress syndrome. Thromboembolic/ anaphylactic problems include permanent spinal cord damage. Newer endoscopic techniques such as the injection of tissue adhesives, thrombin and/or banding ligation of varices may replace the injection of sclerosing agents.

Results   Randomized control trials in adults with intrahepatic disease have shown both a reduction in the frequency of the bleeding and a prolongation of survival (Westaby, 1992). No such trials have been reported in children. The results in 82 children with portal vein thrombosis followed-up for periods ranging from 6 months to 11 years are encouraging. There were no deaths and only three re-bled, one having bled from oesophageal varices. In 30 children with intrahepatic disease 9% had late bleeds and a further 10% recurrence of varices which were easily obliterated by further injections. Eight of the children died because of progression of the intrahepatic disease (Howard *et al.*, 1988).

Endoscopic sclerotherapy thus seems to be a useful palliative measure in controlling bleeding oesophageal varices in children. It does have the advantage that it does not in itself cause diminution of liver blood flow. In patients in whom liver transplantation may be required later, it does not make this more difficult as would occur if intra-abdominal shunt surgery had been performed. It does have the consequence of repeated anaesthesia. Further follow-up will be required to demonstrate its long-term effectiveness. More studies are required to determine the best technique.

Surgical procedures in portal hypertension

The place of surgical procedures in management remains controversial. At present four measures, currently advocated largely on the basis of observations in adult patients with cirrhosis, require consideration. For the patient with severe intrahepatic disease liver transplantation must be considered but it is preferable to delay transplantation until bleeding has stopped.

Surgical portosystemic shunts

Portosystemic shunts decompress the portal venous system and greatly reduce the risk of alimentary bleeding. All shunting procedures (Figures 22.9a and b) sooner or later cause a decrease in portal vein blood flow, decrease hepatic perfusion and carry the risk of accelerating hepatic deterioration and the onset of portosystemic encephalopathy. This is so irrespective of the aetiology of the chronic liver disease. The distal splenorenal shunt (Figure 22.9c) does maintain hepatic inflow from the superior mesenteric vein initially but new transgastric, pancreatic and colonic collaterals develop and within 1 year the hepatic blood flow is decreased to the same degree as occurs following total portal diversion. Rapid deterioration may occur even when the hepatic state before surgery is satisfactory as assessed by Child's criteria (Child, 1964). The more severe the liver disease before surgery the greater is the risk of this occurring. It is however impossible to predict which child will tolerate shunting without deterioration of the liver function.

Randomized controlled trials in adult patients have not shown any significant prolongation of survival with conventional portosystemic anastomosis or with distal splenorenal shunts. No randomized controlled trials have been reported in children. Shunting procedures with dissection in or near the portahepatis may make subsequent

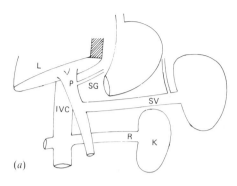

(a)

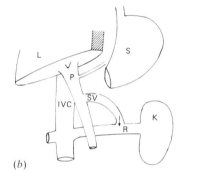

(b)

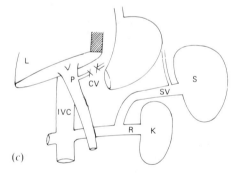

(c)

Figure 22.9 Diagrammatic representation of: (*a*) normal anatomy in portal hypertension; (*b*) lieno-renal shunt and (*c*) distal selective lieno-renal shunt showing liver (L), spleen (S), kidneys (K), portal vein (P), splenic vein (SV), renal vein (R), and inferior vena cava (IVC). In the selective lieno-renal shunt vessels draining into varices such as the coronary vein (CV) and the right gastric right gastroepiploic are ligated. The short gastric veins are preserved in the hope that retrograde flow from the varices will occur

liver transplant more difficult. This is particularly so if the shunt or the portal venous system thromboses. This is an increased risk following splenectomy. Splenectomy also predisposes to fulminant septicaemia. Shunt procedures may be required for patients with extrahepatic disease who develop persistent alimentary bleeding from gastric or intestinal varices.

Shunting procedures may have to be considered in children living in an area with limited facilities for blood transfusion or expert medical care during acute bleeding episodes and where there is limited access to an endoscopist experienced in performing endoscopic sclerotherapy. The shunt chosen will depend on what vessels are available and the preference of the operator. Other surgical measures should be considered.

Sugiura procedure

This is a major two-step procedure which combines splenectomy and devascularization of the upper part of the stomach with transection of the oesophagus and devascularization of its lower third. Through a left thoracotomy the oesophagus is devascularized from the left lower pulmonary vein to the diaphragm ligating some 30–40 collaterals joining the perioesophageal and intraoesophageal varices. The oesophagus is divided at the gastro-oesophageal junction and reanastomosed with multiple fine sutures. In the second stage the spleen is removed and the upper third of the stomach devascularized. A pyloroplasty is performed. Over 700 such procedures have been reported mainly in Japanese adults with cirrhosis, with an operative mortality of only 5%, a re-bleeding rate of 4% and no encephalopathy. Further evaluation of this operation in children would seem desirable.

Transgastric oesophageal transection with gastro-oesophageal devascularization

Transthoracic oesophageal transection to control variceal bleeding has a high mortality and at best a very transient effect in preventing re-bleeding. Its use has been largely abandoned. The development of a mechanical apparatus which allows rapid transection and resection of a ring of oesophagus at the same time performing a safe anastomosis has renewed interest in this procedure. The apparatus is placed inside the oesophagus through a transgastric incision. A ligature is tied around the lower oesophagus to invaginate a ring of oesophagus into the apparatus before it is activated. If this is accompanied by oesophago-gastric devascularization and a splenectomy, a prolonged bleeding-free period is achieved.

Transjugular intrahepatic portocaval stent shunting (TIPSS)

In this procedure a needle passed via the jugular vein is used to develop a tract between a major hepatic vein branch and a related portal vein branch. The tract is further dilated by a balloon and kept patent by a stent. It has been used effectively in critically ill adults to decrease portal pressure, but over 60% occlude within 1 year. This technically difficult procedure has not so far been reported in children.

Circumstances requiring special consideration

Schistosomiasis

Portosystemic surgical shunts in this condition are frequently complicated by hepatic encephalopathy. Both selective splenorenal shunts and Sugiura procedures have been advocated but neither have been assessed by randomized controlled trials.

Congenital hepatic fibrosis

Effective portal decompression in this condition controls further alimentary bleeding; in follow-up for up to 9 years it is unassociated with hepatic encephalopathy. Early death may occur.

Portal vein obstruction

In children with obstruction of the portal vein alone, a peripheral shunt may be fashioned using the splenic or superior mesenteric veins. A mesocaval shunt with jugular vein interposition, avoiding the risks of splenectomy, is preferable.

If splenectomy is performed it should be preceded by pneumococcal vaccination and requires prophylactic penicillin long-term postoperatively. Bernard and co-workers (1985) have emphasized that the risks of encephalopathy are negligible, finding no evidence of encephalopathy in 41 patients followed for a mean of 6 years, three being followed beyond 15 years after shunting. On the other hand, will such surgery accelerate the onset of portosystemic encephalopathy which occurs in up to one-third of adults with this disorder (Webb and Sherlock, 1979)? Although it must be admitted that many of these patients had unsuccessful attempts at shunting.

With diffuse thrombosis of the portal system shunt procedures are impossible. Endoscopic sclerotherapy or the Suguira procedure are the only options. The latter may be technically very difficult because of the large number of collaterals present, described as cavernous transformation of the peritoneum (Franco and Smadja, 1985).

Splenic vein obstruction

Isolated splenic vein obstruction which may be caused by most of the factors resulting in portal vein obstruction, frequently causes large varices in the fundus of the stomach and lower oesophagus. If bleeding occurs splenectomy is usually curative.

Hepatic arterial-portal venous fistulae

Portal hypertension is caused by the increased portal venous inflow but frequently the portal zones show increased fibrosis. The fistulae should be obliterated by selective non-invasive embolization or removed surgically. If portal hypertension persists the measures considered above may be required.

Medical management to prevent bleeding and re-bleeding

Beta-adrenergic blockers, both non-selective, such as propranolol and selective β_1 antagonists such as atenolol, reduce hepatic arterial and/or portal vein blood flow. Propranolol has been intensively studied in adults with portal hypertension. In patients in whom the hepatic vein pressure gradient is reduced to less than 12 mmHg bleeding does not occur. For reason that are unknown between 30 and 50% of patients do not have such a fall in pressure. Its efficacy in preventing recurrence of alimentary bleeding in adults is at least as good as sclerotherapy. Although advocated by some workers for the prevention of recurrence of bleeding in portal hypertension in children, a variable effect on splenic pressure was noticed in the single short-term study in children with portal hypertension. What effect these drugs have on the long-term prognosis of the underlying liver disease is unknown. At present it would seem wise to limit their use to well organized controlled studies in carefully documented patients. An even newer approach has been the use of pharmacological agents which increase the lower oesophageal sphincter pressure thereby reducing the inflow of blood into the submucous venous plexus of the oesophagus and hence into the varices. With both metoclopramide and domperidone moderate reductions of azygous blood flow has been noted. Therapeutic benefit will have to be demonstrated in appropriate controlled clinical trials.

Bibliography and references

Alagille, D., Carlier, J. C., Chiva, M., Ziade, R., Ziade, M. and Moy, F. (1986) Long term neuropsychological outcome in children undergoing portal systemic shunts for portal vein obstruction without liver disease. *J. Pediatr. Gastroenterol. Nutr.*, **5**, 861–866

Alvarez, F., Bernard, O., Brunnelle, F. *et al.* (1983a) Portal obstruction in children. 1. Clinical investigation and haemorrhage risk. *J. Pediatr.*, **103**, 696

Alvarez, F., Bernard, Brunnelle, F. *et al.* (1983b) Portal obstruction in children. 2. Results of surgical portosystemic shunt. *J. Pediatr.*, **103**, 703

Atkinson, J. B. and Woolley, M. M. (1983) Treatment of oesophageal varices by sclerotherapy in childhood. *Am. J. Surg.*, **146**, 103

Bernard, O., Alvarez, F., Brunnelle, F., Hadchouel, P. and Alagille, D. (1985) Portal hypertension in children. *Clin. Gastroenterol.*, **14**, 33

Bilodeau, M., Rioux, L., Willems, B. and Pomier-Layrargues, G. (1992) Transjugular intrahepatic portacaval stent shunt as a rescue treatment for life threatening variceal bleeding in a cirrhotic patient with severe liver failure. *Am. J. Gastroenterol.*, **87**, 369–371

Bismuth, H. and Franco, D. (1976) Portal diversion for portal hypertension in early childhood. *Ann. Surg.*, **83**, 439

Bordas, J. M., Feu, F., Vilella, A. and Rodes, J. (1989) Anaphylactic reaction to ethanolamine oleate injection in sclerotherapy of esophageal varices. *Endoscopy*, **21**, 50

Burroughs, A. K. and Bosch, J. (1991) Clinical manifestations and management of bleeding episodes in cirrhotics. In: *Textbook of Clinical Hepatology* (eds McIntyre, N., Benhamou, J.-P., Bricher, J., Rizzetto and Rodes, J.). Oxford Medical, Oxford, pp. 408–425

Caletti, G. C., Brocchi, E., Labriola, E., Gasbarrini, G. and Barbara, L. (1990) Pericarditis: a probably overlooked complication of endoscopic variceal sclerotherapy. *Endoscopy*, **22**, 144–145

Carson, J. A., Tunell, W. P., Barnes, P. and Altshuler, B. (1981) Hepato-portal sclerosis in childhood: A mimic of extrahepatic portal hypertension. *J. Pediatr. Surg.*, **16**, 291

Chaudhary, A., Tatke, M. and Aranya, R. C. (1990) Endoscopic sclerotherapy: the far and near effects. *Br. J. Surg.*, **77**, 963

Child, C. G. (1964) *The Liver and Portal Hypertension*, Philadelphia, Saunders, p. 50

Coran, A. G., Wesley, J. R. and Weintrub, W. H. (1980) A central spleno-renal shunt for portal hypertension in children. Experience with 8 consecutive patient anastomoses. *J. Pediatr. Surg.*, **15**, 827

Franco, D. and Smadja, C. (1985) Prevention of variceal bleeding: surgical procedures. *Clin. Gastroenterol.*, **14**, 233

Gauthier, F., De Dreuzy, O., Valayer, J. and Montupet, P. (1989) H-type shunt with an autologous venous graft for treatment of portal hypertension in children. *J. Pediatr. Surg.*, **24**, 1041–1043

Grauer, S. E. and Swartz, S. R. (1979) Extrahepatic portal hypertension: a retrospective analysis. *Ann. Surg.*, **189**, 566

Hassall, E., Berquist, W. E., Ament, M. E., Vargas, J. and Dorney, S. (1989) Sclerotherapy for extrahepatic portal hypertension in childhood. *J. Pediatr.*, **115**, 69–74

Howard, E. R., Stamatakis, J. D. and Mowat, A. P. (1984) Management of oesophageal varices in children by injection sclerotherapy. *J. Pediatr. Surg.*, **19**, 2

Howard, E. R., Stringer, M. D. and Mowat, A. P. (1988) Assessment of injection sclerotherapy in the management of 152 children with oesophageal varices. *Br. J. Surg.*, **75**, 404–408

Kavetz, D., Bosch, J., Teres, J. *et al.* (1984) Comparison of intravenous somatostatin and vasopressin infusions in treatment of acute variceal haemorrhage. *Hepatology*, **4**, 442

Kokudo, N., Sanjo, K. and Umekita, N. (1990) Squamous cell carcinoma after endoscopic injection sclerotherapy for esophageal varices. *Am. J. Gastroenterol.*, **85**, 861–865

Maksoud, J. G., Goncalves, M. E. P., Porta, G., Miura, I. and Velhote, M. C. P. (1991) The endoscopic and surgical management of portal hypertension in children: analysis of 123 cases. *J. Pediatr. Surg.*, **26**, 178–181

Maksoud, J.-G. and Mies, S. (1982) Distal splenorenal shunts in children. *Ann. Surg.*, **195**, 401

Mentha, G., Huber, O., Meyer, P., Le Coultre, C. and Rohner, A. (1989) L'hypertension portale hemorragique: une place pour la transplantation hepatique? *Gastroenterol. Clin. Biol.*, **13**, 318–319

Morikawa, S., Kumada, K., Fukui, K., Moriyasu, F., Kawasaki, T. and Ozawa, K. (1989) Closure of interposition mesocaval shunt reversed encephalopathy in a case of idiopathic portal hypertension. *Am. J. Gastroenterol.*, **84**, 548–551

Mowat, A. P. (1986) Prevention of variceal bleeding. *J. Pediatr. Gastroenterol. Nutr.*, **5**, 679

Odievre, M., Pige, G. and Alagille, D. (1977a) Congenital abnormalities associated with extrahepatic portal hypertension. *Arch. Dis. Childh.*, **52**, 383

Odievre, M., Chaumont, P., Montagne, J.-P. and Alagille, D. (1977b) Anomalies of intrahepatic portal venous system in congenital hepatic fibrosis. *Radiology*, **122**, 427

Ohnishi, K. *et al.* (1987) Portal haemodynamics in idiopathic portal hypertension (Banti's syndrome). Comparison with chronic persistent hepatitis and normal subjects. *Gastroentrology*, **92**, 751–758

Paquet, K.-J. (1985) Ten years experience with paravariceal injection sclerotherapyh of oesophageal varices in children. *J. Pediatr. Surg.*, **20**, 109

Premkumar, A., Berdon, W. E., Levy, J., Amodio, S. J. and Newhouse, J. H. (1988) The emergence of hepatic fibrosis and portal hypertension in infants and children with autosomal recessive polycystic disease. *Pediatr. Radiol.*, **18**, 123–129

Psacharopoulos, H. T., Howard, E. R., Portmann, B. *et al.* (1981) Hepatic complications of cystic fibrosis. *Lancet*, **ii**, 78

Reiley, J. J., Schade, R. and Van Thiel, D. H. (1984) Oesophageal function after injection sclerotherapy: pathogenesis of oesophageal stricture. *Ann. J. Surg.*, **147**, 85

Roy, C. C., Weber, A. M., Morgan, C. L. *et al.* (1982) Hepatobiliary disease in cystic fibrosis: A survey of current issues and concepts. *J. Pediatr. Gastroenterol. Nutr.*, **1**, 469

Sarin, S. K., Sasan, S. and Nigam (1992) Portal vein obstruction in children leads to growth retardation. *Hepatology*, **15**, 229–233

Sarin, S. K., Sreenivas, D. V., Lahoti, D. and Saraya, A. (1992) Factors influencing development of portal hypertensive gastropathy in patients with portal hypertension. *Gastroenterology*, **102**, 994–999

Seidman, E., Weber, A. M., Morgan, C. L. *et al.* (1984) Spinal cord paralysis following sclerotherapy for oesophageal varices. *Hepatology*, **4**, 970

Sorensen, T., Burcharth, E., Pederson, M. L. *et al.* (1984) Oesophageal stricture and dysphagia after endoscopic sclerotherapy for bleeding varices. *Gut*, **25**, 437

Stringer, M. D., Howard, E. R. and Mowat, A. P. (1989) Endoscopic sclerotherapy in the management of esophageal varices in 61 children with biliary atresia. *J. Pediatr. Surg.*, **24**, 438–442

Stringer, M. D. and Howard, E. R. (1991) The role of endoscopic injection sclerotherapy in the management of portal hypertension in children. In: *Surgery of Liver Disease in Children* (ed. Howard, E. R.). Bujtterworth-Heinemann, Oxford, pp. 157–170

Valayer, J. (1991) Portosystemic shunt surgery. In: *Surgery of Liver Disease in Children* (ed. Howard, E. R.). Butterworth-Heinemann, Oxford, pp. 171–180

Webb, L. J. and Sherlock, S. (1979) The aetiology, presentation and natural history of extrahepatic portal venous obstruction. *Q. Jl. Med.*, **48**, 627

Westaby, D. (1992) *Management of Variceal Bleeding*. W. B. Saunders, Philadelphia

Budd-Chiari syndrome

Attal, M., Huguet, F., Rubie, H. *et al.* (1992) Prevention of hepatic veno-occlusive disease after bone marrow transplantation by continuous infusion of low-dose heparin: a prospective randomized trial. *Blood*, **79**, 2834–2840

Baglin, T. P., Harper, P. and Marcus, R. E. (1990) Veno-occlusive disease of the liver complicating allogeneic bone marrow transplantation successfully treated with recombinant tissue plasminogen activator. *Bone Marrow Transplant*, **5**, 439–441

Gentil-Kocher, S., Bernard, O., Brunelle, F. *et al.* (1988) Budd-Chiari syndrome in chkldren: report of 22 cases. *J. Pediatr.*, **113**, 30–38

Gluckman, E., Jolivet, I., Scrobohaci, M. L. *et al.* (1990) Use of prostaglandin E1 for prevention of liver veno-occlusive disease in leukaemic patients treated by allogeneic bone marrow transplantation. *Br. J. Haematol.*, **74**, 277–281

Jones, R. J., Lee, K. S. K., Beschorner, W. E. *et al.* (1987) Veno-occlusive disease of the liver following bone marrow transplantation. *Transplantation*, **44**, 778–783

Kage, M., Arakawa, M., Kojiro, M. and Okuda, K. (1992) Histopathology of membranous obstruction of the inferior vena cava in the Budd-Chiari syndrome. *Gastroenterology*, **102**, 2081–2090

Petersen, C., Zimmermann, H. and Mildenberger, H. (1991) Occlusion of liver veins (Budd-Chiari syndrome) in childhood: a case report. *Eur. J. Pediatr. Surg.*, **1**, 369–371

Roulet, M., Laurini, R., Rivier, L. and Calame, A. (1988) Hepatic veno-occlusive disease in newborn infant of a woman drinking herbal tea. *Clin. Lab. Observ.*, **112**, 433–436

Shulman, H. M. and Hinterberg, W. (1992) Hepatic veno-occlusive disease – liver toxicity syndrome after bone marrow transplantation. *Bone Marrow Transplant.*, **10**, 197–214

Vella, D., Dhumeaux, D., Babany, G. *et al.* (1987) Hepatic Vein Thrombosis in paroxysmal nocturnal haemoglobinuria. *Gastroenterology*, **3**, 87–93

Unusual causes

Barsky, M. F., Rankin, R. N., Wall, W. J., Ghent, C. N. and Garcia, B. (1989) Patent ductus venosus: problems in assessment and management. *Can. J. Surg.*, **32**, 271–275

Keller, E. S., Rosch, J. and Dotter, C. T. (1980) Bleeding from oesophageal varices exacerbated by splenic AV fistula. *Cardiovasc. Intervent. Radiol.*, **3**, 97

Madsen, M. S., Peterson, T. H. and Sommer, H. (1986) Segmental portal hypertension. *Ann. Surg.* **204**, 72–77

Roulet, M., Laurini, R., Rivier, L. and Calame, A. (1988) Hepatic veno-occlusive disease in newborn infant of a woman drinking herbal tea. *Clin. Lab. Observ.*, **112**, 433–436

Sutton, J. P., Yarborough, D. Y. and Richards, J. T. (1970) Isolated splenic vein occlusion,. *Arch. Surg.*, **100**, 623

Vanway, C., Crane, J. M., Riddle, D. H. and Foster, J. H. (1971) Arterio-venous fistulae in the portal circulation. *Surgery,* **78**, 876

Medical management to prevent re-bleeding

Mastai, R., Grande, L., Bosch, J. *et al.* (1986) Effects of Metoclopramide and Domperidone on azygous venous blood flow in patients with cirrhosis and portal hypertension. *Hepatology,* **6**, 1244

Navasa, M., Bosch, J. and Rodes, J. (1991) Pharmacological agents and portal hypertension. In: *Portal Hypertension – Clinical and Physiological Aspects* (eds Okuda, K. and Benhamou, J. P.). Springer, Berlin, pp. 35–50

Qzsoylu, S., Kocak, N. and Yuce, A. (1985) Propranolol therapy for portal hypertension in children. *J. Pediatr.*, **106**, 312

Villeneuve, J.-P., Pomier-Layrargues, G., Infante-Rivard, C. *et al.* (1986) Propranolol for the prevention of recurrent variceal haemorrhage: a controlled trial. *Hepatology,* **6**, 1239

Chapter 23

Liver tumours

Introduction

Primary liver tumours are rare, accounting for between 0.5 and 2% of paediatric malignancies, including leukaemia and lymphomas. They occur with approximately one-tenth of the frequency of nephroblastoma and neuroblastoma. Of the malignant tumours (Table 23.1), hepatoblastoma is the most frequent. Rhabdomyosarcoma, sarcoma, mesenchymal and yolk sac tumours are very rare, as is hepatocellular carcinoma except in areas where many children are infected by hepatitis B virus. Exact diagnosis is essential since combined treatment with new chemotherapeutic regimens which are specific for particular types of tumour and radical surgery have produced a considerable improvement in prognosis. Approximately one-third of primary hepatic tumours are benign. Tumours usually present with abdominal distension. Pain, fever, pallor, anaemia or jaundice occasionally occur. Rare complications found with liver tumours are listed in Table 23.2.

Malignant hepatic tumours (see Table 23.1)

Hepatoblastoma

Hepatoblastomas are single large tumours that arise in and distort an otherwise normal liver. The majority occur in the right lobe. Characteristically they are supplied by large

Table 23.1 Malignant liver tumours

Hepatoblastoma
Hepatocellular carcinoma
 Fibrolamellar variant
Mesenchymal tumours
 Embryonal rhabdomyosarcoma
 Angiosarcoma
 Undifferentiated or embryonal sarcoma
 Occult hepatic sinusoidal tumour
Yolk sac tumours
Teratocarcinoma
Cholangiocarcinoma
Malignant histiocytoma
Non-Hodgkin's lymphoma
Histiocytosis X (Langerhaus cell histiocytosis)

Table 23.2 Complications associated with liver tumours

Angiomata	Hypofibrinogenaemia
	Angiopathic haemolytic anaemia
	Thrombocytopenia
	Congestive cardiac failure
Solid tumours	Osteomalacia
	Polycythaemia
	Sexual precocity
	Cystathionuria
	Hypercalcaemia
	Hyperglycaemia
	Hyperlipidaemia

vessels and have many dilated sinusoidal channels. The cut surface is green, yellow or white. The tumour spreads within the liver and to adjacent tissues and metastasizes to lymph nodes, lungs, central nervous system and rarely, to bone and other tissues.

Microscopically the tumour is often heterogeneous with epithelial cells resembling liver cells in some area, while other areas appear fetal, embryonal or anaplastic. In 50% of cases there is mesenchymal tissue with ductular elements and up to 40% have osteoid cartilage and bone.

Clinical features

Over 75% of cases occur before the age of 3 years, the majority by 1 year. Tumours have been detected antenatally by ultrasound. The male to female ratio is 2:1. The commonest presentation is abdominal distension, with or without malaise, weight loss and pallor. Rarely, there may be vomiting and abdominal pain. On clinical examination the liver is found to be enlarged and there may be a palpable mass. Splenomegaly is frequently found. As soon as malignancy is suspected examination of the abdomen should be restricted because of the risk of causing dissemination of malignant cells. A striking complication is marked osteoporosis leading to pathological fracture occurring in up to 35%. Precocious puberty is another distinctive complication. Hepatoblastoma may complicate the disorders listed in Table 23.3. By far the strongest association is with familial adenomatous

Table 23.3 Hepatoblastoma

Familial adenomatous polyposis
Gardner's syndrome
Beckwith's syndrome
Fetal alcohol syndrome
Wilm's tumour
Renal dysplasia or absence
Adrenal absence
Hemi-hypertrophy

polyposis (FAP) on its own or with extra-intestinal lesions (Gardner syndrome). FAP, an autosomal dominant disorder, is caused by at least six mutations of a gene on chromosome 5q21. It causes thousands of colorectal adenomata in adolescence and early adult life. If prophylactic colectomy is not performed colorectal carcinoma will develop by the fifth decade. Based on a study of 167 FAP families and seven cases of hepatoblastoma the relative risk of hepatoblastoma increased 847-fold with an incidence rate of hepatoblastoma by the fifth birthday of 1 in 305 person-years (Giardiello *et al.*, 1991). Survivors of hepatoblastoma and parents of patients with hepatoblastoma should be examined for FAP.

Diagnosis (Figure 23.1)

The diagnosis is based on the radiographic appearances, high serum alpha-fetoprotein and ultimately the histological appearances. The main disorders to be considered in differential diagnosis are neuroblastoma, nephroblastoma, gastrointestinal malignancy or other forms of benign or malignant liver tumour. Ultrasonography of the liver, spleen,

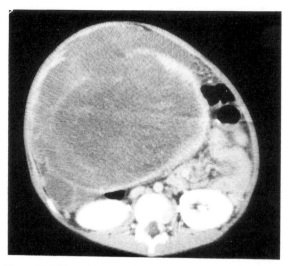

Figure 23.1 Hepatoblastoma. Computed tomography of the liver with intravenous contrast demonstrating a large low density tumour (hepatoblastoma) within the right lobe of the liver, with peripheral enhancement. There is displacement of normal viscera laterally

intra-abdominal blood vessels, kidneys and adrenal glands should be the initial investigation. Further investigations to be considered are given in Table 23.4.

An intravenous pyelogram, to exclude a right-sided Wilms' tumour or neuroblastoma pushing the liver forward, is essential in nearly all cases. Liver function tests are usually normal unless jaundice is present. Anaemia is present in the majority and over 35% have thrombocytosis. The serum alpha-fetoprotein which is often >10 000 ng/dl is elevated in up to 95% cases. A high serum cholesterol is associated with a poor prognosis (Muraji *et al.*, 1985). Hepatic arteriography is essential to determine whether resection is possible. It will show displacement and dilatation of the supplying vessels and an abnormally increased sinusoidal circulation appearing as an amorphous blush on the radiograph. The radiological appearance may be mimicked by focal nodular hypoplasia. Computed tomography with contrast injection gives a cleared indication of tumour size than ultrasonography (see Figure 23.1). Magnetic resonance imaging can provide valuable information on segmental and vascular involvement. It also provides clear caval imaging without the risks of tumour dislodgement as can occur with venacavography.

Liver biopsy should not be performed until there has been very careful consideration of all other data and only when its results could assist in planning management. Its only value if the alpha-fetoprotein is positive is in excluding yolk sac tumours. Percutaneous liver biopsy directed at the major ultrasonographic or arteriographic lesion may occasionally be indicated where more than one lesion appears to be present but is probably best postponed until laparotomy, It may also have a place in young infants with diffuse hepatic enlargement in which neuroblastoma stage IVa may be the diagnosis. It must be remembered, however, that biopsy may cause dissemination of the tumour both along the needle track and more distally. It may also produce marked haemorrhage. These risks must be weighed very carefully against the advantages of establishing the correct histological diagnosis before operative treatment.

Table 23.4 Investigation of liver tumour

Standard liver function tests
Full blood count
Prothrombin time
Blood group
Ultrasonic scan of liver, kidneys and adrenal glands
Intravenous pyelogram
Serum alpha-fetoprotein
Urinary vanillylmandelic acid excretion
X-ray of abdomen, chest and long bones
Computed tomography of liver, abdomen, chest and skull
Hepatic arteriography
Radionucleotide bone scan

Selected cases
Serum transcobalamin
Neurotensin
Testosterone
Human chorionic gonadotrophin
C-reactive protein
Intravenous pyelogram,
Inferior venacavogram,
Magnetic resonance imaging
Laparotomy
Bone marrow examination

Treatment

Patients with suspected hepatic tumours should be referred to centres with experience in the diagnosis and management of such lesions. The only effective treatment is total resection usually combined with chemotherapy. *Resection* can involve removing up to 85% of the liver. With infusions of 5 to 10% dextrose and albumin with fresh frozen plasma given every 12 hours for 48 hours hypoglycaemia and coagulopathy can usually be avoided. Selective angiography, computed tomography and nuclear magnetic resonance imaging are invaluable in delineating the location and extent of the tumour and in determining its blood supply prior to laparotomy. In some instances resectability can only be assessed at laparotomy. Intraoperative ultrasonography which defines the relationship of the tumour to segmental vessels and ducts, allows maximum preservation of unaffected tissue. The use of an ultrasonic surgical dissector and fibrin sealant minimizes bleeding and bile leaks from the cut surface of the liver. In the majority it should be performed during a course of chemotherapy which reduces tumour mass, making resection less hazardous. Primary surgery is possible in less than 50% and curative at best in only 60% of those. Resection is possible if there is no extrahepatic direct spread or distant metastasis, no invasion of the main portal and hepatic veins and viable hepatic segments can be preserved. Rarely liver transplantation is required.

Chemotherapy   Cisplatin and doxorubicin are the most effective agents, often producing a dramatic decrease in size of both primary and secondary tumours with a progressive fall in serum alpha-fetoprotein concentration. Cisplatin in a dose of $50–100 \, mg/m^2$ and doxorubicin $50–60 \, mg/m^2$ are given by continuous infusion over a 72-hour period at 3-weekly intervals, for a total of six courses. Hydration at a rate of 125 ml/h commences 12 hours before cisplatin and continues for 24 hours after completion. This minimizes the risks of cardiomyopathy, renal failure and high tone hearing loss. Some investigators add ifosphamide as an additional agent. With such therapies a 35–95% reduction in tumour mass was achieved in a recent series of 15 children (Filler *at al.*, 1991). Up to 85% of tumours become resectable after, usually, four courses of the therapy. Some children require surgical removal of pulmonary secondaries. Disease-free survival for more than 2 years has been reported in over 70% of patients, including those whose lesions were initially unresectable. There is yet no consensus as to what chemotherapy should be given to patients whose tumour is well localized and resectable at presentation. Since the 2-year survival rate for such patients is only 70%, some chemotherapy would appear to be advisable.

If there is no regression carboplatin, $550\,mg/m^2$/day at 3-weekly intervals may be tried and if regression is apparent after two courses continued for five courses. If carboplatin is ineffective etoposide $200mg/m^2$/day for 5 days may be tried.

If the tumour cannot be resected orthotopic liver transplantation is the only option. Six of 12 children were reported to be alive with no evidence of recurrence 24 to 70 months after transplantation (Koneru *et al.*, 1991). Six died, three of tumour recurrence. Unifocal tumours with no extrahepatic spread had a better prognosis than multifocal or metastatic lesions. Serial serum alpha-fetoprotein determination is helpful in assessing the response to chemotherapy, falling to normal with complete resection but rising if metastases develop.

Hepatocellular carcinoma

Hepatocellular carcinoma is less common than hepatoblastoma except in areas in which there is a high prevalence of hepatitis B virus infection in childhood (Chen *et al.*, 1988). The two ages of peak incidence are early infancy and between the ages of 10 and 15 years.

Hepatocellular carcinoma frequently starts in a liver with underlying cirrhosis (Table 23.5). The tumour is often multicentric. The tumour cells are polygonal, of varying size, with a hyperchromatic nucleus, and show frequent mitosis. Some secrete bile. They invade both hepatic and portal vein branches. It is important to distinguish the *fibrolamellar* variant which has cells with voluminous, deeply acidophilic cytoplasm and prominent nucleoli compartmentalized by bands of lamellar collagen.

Table 23.5 Disorders predisposing to hepatocellular carcinoma

Tyrosinaemia
Galactosaemia
Wilms' tumour
Glycogen storage diseases I, III, VI, IX
Alpha-1 antitrypsin deficiency
Wilson's disease
Thalassaemia
Ataxia telangiectasia
Hepatitis B virus infection
? Hepatitis C virus infection
Primary sclerosing cholangitis
Extrahepatic biliary atresia
Familial cholestatic jaundice
Cholangiodysplastic pseudocirrhosis
Di-Soto's cerebral giantism
Fanconi's anaemia

The clinical and biochemical features are similar to those of hepatoblastoma, except that they may reflect the underlying primary disease process. Fever, weight loss and jaundice are more common. Serum alpha-fetoprotein is positive in 60–80%. Osteoporosis is rarely seen. Serum transcobalamin II and neurotensin may be elevated but alpha-fetoprotein is negative in fibrolamellar tumours.

The investigation and management of hepatocellular carcinoma in childhood is as outlined for hepatoblastoma. Treatment is less satisfactory. In a review of 71 cases of whom 12 had chemotherapy there were only two long-term survivors (Ni *et al.*, 1991). Chemotherapeutic regimens used for hepatoblastoma should be tried since they can be dramatically effective. Resection is rarely possible but long-term survival (>5 years) has been reported following both resection and transplantation in approximately 10% in a recent large, largely adult series (Iwatsuki *et al.*, 1991). Early stages of hepatocellular carcinoma arising in a cirrhotic liver and fibrolamellar lesions are highly represented in the survivors. With the fibrolamellar variant the course is often slower and disease-free survival to 20 years has been reported.

Malignant mesenchymal tumours

Rhabdomyosarcoma

This rare tumour usually arises from the common bile duct but can occur in the common hepatic duct or even within the liver. The bile duct wall becomes thickened by a polypoid tumour which grows along it and encroaches on the lumen with grape-like extensions. The tumours commonly undergo necrosis and are the sites of bleeding. Bile duct rupture may occur. It may extend up into the liver or down to the pancreas and adjacent tissues. Histologically, the features are those of a sarcoma with, in some cells, cross-striations appearing.

The clinical features are jaundice with pruritus, fever, malaise, abdominal pain, often leading to a clinical diagnosis of infective hepatitis until negative serological tests or a relatively high serum alkaline phosphatase concentration prompts ultrasonography. An apparent choledochal cyst but containing intraluminal matter is demonstrated.

The age at onset ranges from 1–9 years, but usually is between 4 and 5 years. The diagnosis may be suspected on the basis of the ultrasonic and computed tomography findings. Cholangiography should be delayed until laparotomy, when it is useful in defining the extent of the tumour. Treatment is by resection followed by multiple drug chemotherapy but the optimum regimen is as yet uncertain and few have been reported to survive more than 2 years.

Mesenchymal sarcoma (mesenchymoma)

These rare tumours consisting of sarcomatous cells with frequent mitosis and areas of necrosis produce space-occupying hypovascular lesions usually in the right lobe of the liver. The tumour may contain malignant endothelial elements. The median age of presentation is 9 years. Treatment by resection and chemotherapy usually in the form of vincristine and actinomycin D gives a survival rate of almost 40% (Leuschner *et al.*, 1990).

Primary malignant germ cell (yolk sac) tumours

Primary malignant germ cell tumours can very rarely arise in the liver (Mann *et al.*, 1990). They produce alpha-fetoprotein with a different glycosylation pattern from that of liver-

Table 23.6 Benign hepatic tumours in childhood

Infantile haemangioendothelioma	Lymphangioma
Cavernous haemangioma	Teratoma
Mesenchymal hamartoma	Cysts: parasitic and non-parasitic
Focal nodular hypoplasia	Abscess
Adenoma	

derived alpha-fetoprotein. Human chorionic gonadotrophin is made by 20% of tumours. Carboplatin, etoposide and bleomycin combined are often effective chemotherapeutic measures if followed by surgical resection of residual tumour (Pinkerton *et al.*, 1990).

Benign hepatic tumours (Table 23.6)

Benign tumours usually present with hepatomegaly, abdominal distension or abdominal discomfort. Rarely they may be the sites of infection or bleeding into the peritoneum. Very infrequently they cause jaundice due to bile duct obstruction. Features of infantile haemangioendotheliomata, mesenchymal hamartomata, and focal nodular hypoplasia are considered in detail below.

Diagnosis of benign tumours is based on ultrasound, computed tomography, angiography and histological assessment. Often a frozen section biopsy obtained at laparotomy will be required. Treatment is by resection.

Mesenchymal hamartoma

These are usually multi-loculated cystic tumours containing a variable amount of connective tissue and dysplastic bile ducts, with liver cells in the surrounding solid structure. The cysts usually contain clear serous material. Rarely the lesion may be solid. In most instances these present as a mass in the upper abdomen often without symptoms other than epigastric fullness. Large lesions cause respiratory and nutritional difficulties. CT scanning may give a typical picture (Figure 23.2). Selective hepatic arteriography is

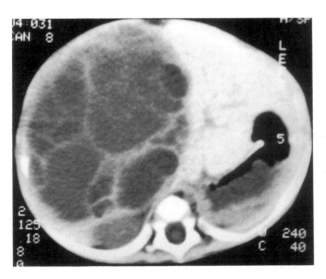

Figure 23.2 Mesenchymal hamartoma. Axial CT scan of the liver demonstrating multicystic tumour within the right lobe of the liver, with normal liver architecture demonstrated in the lateral segment of the left lobe. The multicystic nature of the tumour is characteristic of a mesenchymal hamartoma

a most informative investigation showing an abnormal blood supply to the tumour but without the characteristic blush of a malignancy. Diagnosis requires biopsy. When the tumour is large resection is necessary.

Angiomatous malformation of the liver

Two forms of these vascular tumours may be distinguished histologically. The capillary haemangioma-endothelioma has small interconnecting vascular channels lined by epithelial cells several layers thick at the periphery of the lesion, but in the centre the separation of vessels is less clear-cut. Cavernous haemangiomata have larger blood-filled spaces lined by plump endothelial cells with a stroma of single plates of hepatocytes with or without varying amounts of fibrous tissue. Both forms may be present in one tumour. In over 30% of patients more than one tumour is identified. Tumours may undergo

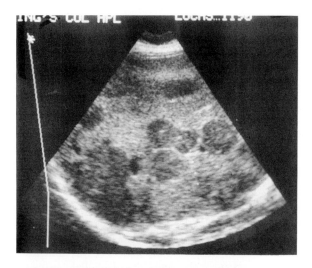

Figure 23.3 Ultrasound of liver showing multiple haemangiomata. The lesions appear as clearly defined poorly reflective lesions within an otherwise normal liver

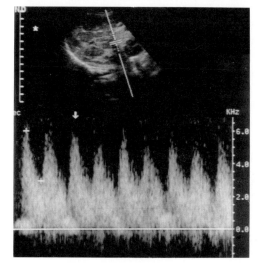

Figure 23.4 Doppler ultrasound of the hepatic artery in a patient with multiple hepatic haemangio-endotheliomata. The lesions have large shunts. There is therefore very fast blood flow in the hepatic artery throughout the cardiac cycle

spontaneous regression by thrombosis and scarring, but in later infancy the cavernous form, particularly, may grow rapidly. Both tumours, if large, are supplied by wide blood vessels taking a large proportion of the cardiac output (Figures 23.3 and 23.4).

Clinical features

These tumours most commonly present in the first 3 months of life and rarely after the age of 2 years. Characteristically there is hepatic enlargement which may be focal and associated with a systolic bruit. Over 60% have cutaneous haemangiomata.

The most common complication is high output congestive cardiac failure and failure to thrive. Intraperitoneal haemorrhage and a haemorrhagic diathesis with hypofibrinogenaemia or platelet sequestration in the tumour, may also be life-threatening. Obstructive jaundice, portal hypertension and alimentary bleeding and intestinal obstruction are occasional associated features. *Angiosarcoma* developing at the age of 4 years has also been reported as a complication (Kirchner *et al.*, 1981).

Investigation

Ultrasonography shows clearly defined cystic spaces surrounded by echogenic tissue with posterior enhancement, a pulsatile hepatic artery with increased blood flow and usually dilated hepatic veins. These findings are confirmed by angiography which shows widely dilated supplying blood vessels leading to a very vascular tumour through which the radio-opaque material passes very quickly and a narrow distal aorta because of tumour 'steal' of blood flow (Figure 23.5) or enhanced CT scan (Figure 23.6).

Management

Since even large tumours may resolve spontaneously, if no complications are present a period of observation is advocated. If cardiac failure develops in an infant of less than 6 weeks, the mortality is more than 50% unless treated by hepatic artery ligation. Diuretics and digoxin should be given prior to surgery. In patients of more than 5 weeks, a 2-week course of prednisolone in a dose of 2.5 mg/kg/day may accelerate spontaneous resolution of the lesion. If there is no response, hepatic artery ligation should be performed. In experienced hands, hepatic artery ligation is a safer procedure than embolization which may be complicated by liver necrosis in 20–50% of cases (Weber *et al.*, 1990), renal failure, sepsis and pulmonary embolism. Localized lesions may be treated by hepatic resection or by ligating the branch of the hepatic artery supplying the tumour.

Focal nodular hyperplasia

This is a rare, slow growing, benign tumour of hepatic parenchyma, characterized pathologically by a central dense fibrous scar from which radiate septa containing proliferating bile ducts and blood vessels, often with medial and intimal hypertrophy.

Figure 23.5 Aortic angiogram study in an infant aged 3 months who had presented with congestive cardiac failure. Two superficial haemangiomata were present on the trunk. A haemic murmur was heard over the liver. The angiogram (*a*) shows that much of the contrast in the upper abdominal aorta passes into large blood vessels supplying the liver. (*b*) the capillary phase of the angiograms shows marked opacification of the hepatic parenchyma due to stasis of contrast material in angiomatous transformation within the liver. Following hepatic artery ligation the congestive cardiac failure was easily controlled with digoxin. This was withdrawn 5 months after surgery. The patient is now aged 12 years and has no clinical or laboratory features of cardiovascular or hepatic disease. The haemangiomata on the skin regressed completely by the age of 4 years

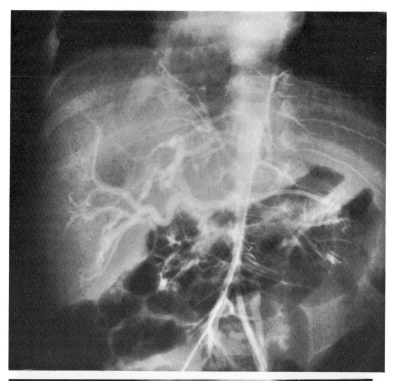

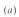

(a)

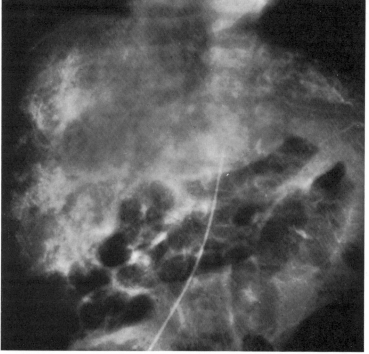

(b)

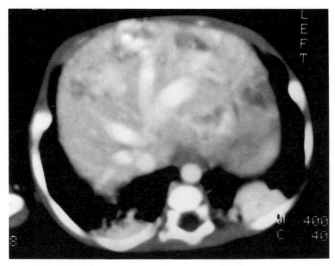

Figure 23.6 Haemangio-endiothelioma of the liver. Enhanced CT scan of the liver demonstrating contrast filling vascular spaces within a large liver. There is gross dilatation of the hepatic veins indicative of a large hepatic artery to hepatic vein shunt, characteristic of this benign tumour

Between the septa there are normal hepatocytes. The exact nature of this well demarcated tumour is still debated. It may be a precursor of fibrolamellar hepatoma (Shortell and Schwarz, 1991).

Clinical features and treatment

It presents as a hard hepatic mass which, in childhood, may be very large. There may be some abdominal discomfort but rarely other symptoms. Ultrasonic and angiographic features are those of hepatocellular carcinoma or hepatoblastoma but no filling defect may be seen on technetium-99m colloid scintigraphy. Small lesions require no treatment; in larger lesions resection has usually been advocated, but ligation of the supplying blood vessels should be considered if lobectomy is thought to carry a risk of mortality.

Rare tumours

Hepatocellular adenoma, adenoma of the bile ducts, true teratoma, peliosis hepatis and solitary non-parasitic cysts are all rare benign tumours. They present as a hepatic mass with or without abdominal pain or bile duct obstruction. Treatment is by resection. Rare malignant tumours are listed in Table 23.1.

Bibliography and references

General

Brock, P., Casteel, M., Desmet, V. *et al.* (1991) Primary malignant liver tumors. In: *Hepatobiliary Surgery in Childhood* (eds Schweizer P. and Schier, F.). Schattauer, Stuttgart, pp. 75–141

Chen, W. J., Lee, J. C. and Hung, W. T. (1988) Primary malignant tumour of liver in infants and children in Taiwan. *J. Pediatr. Surg.*, **23**, 457–461

Dehner, L. P. (1978) Hepatic tumours in the paediatric age-group: a distinctive clinico-pathological spectrum. *Perspect. Pediatr. Pathol.*, **14**, 217

Edoute, Y., Ben-Haim, S. A., Brenner, B. and Malberger, E. (1992) Fatal hemoperitoneum after fine-needle aspiration of a liver metastasis. *Am. Gastroenterol.*, **87**, 358–360

Gauthier, F., Valayer, I., Le Thai, B. *et al.* (1986) Hepatoblastoma and hepatocarcinoma in children. *J. Pediatr. Surg.*, **21**, 424

Giacomantonio, M., Ein, S. H., Mancer, K. and Stevens, C. A. (1984). Thirty years of experience in paediatric primary malignant liver tumours. *J. Pediatr. Surg.*, **19**, 523

Gururangan, S., O'Meara, A., MacMohan, C. *et al.* (1992) Primary hepatic tumours in children: a 26-year review. *J. Surg. Oncol.*, **50**, 30–36

Haas, J. E., Muczynski, K. A., Krailo, M. *et al.* (1989) Histopathology and prognosis in childhood hepatoblastoma and hepatocarcinoma. *Cancer*, **64**, 1082–1095

Howard, E. R. and Heaton, N. D. Benign and malignant tumours. In: *Surgery of Liver Disease in Children* (ed. Howard, E. R.). Butterworth-Heinemann, Oxford, pp. 126–142

Mann, J. R., Kasthuri, N., Raafat, F. *et al.* (1990) Malignant hepatic tumours in children: incidence, clinical features and aetiology. *Paediatr. Perinat. Epidemiol.*, **4**, 276–289

Pritchard, J. (1991) Chemotherapy of malignant liver tumours. In: *Surgery of Liver Disease in Children* (ed. Howard, E. R.). Butterworth-Heinemann, Oxford, pp. 143–148

Schmidt, D., Harmns, D. and Lang, W. (1985) Primary malignant hepatic tumours in childhood. *Virchows. Arch.*, **47**, 387

Tagge, E. P., Tagge, D. U., Reyes, J. *et al.* (1992) Resection, including transplantation, for hepatoblastoma and hepatocellular carcinoma: impact on survival. *J. Pediatr. Surg.*, **27**, 292–297

Weinberg, A. G. and Finegold, M. J. (1983) Primary hepatic tumours of childhood. *Hum. Pathol.*, **14**, 512

Hepatoblastoma

Amendola, M. A., Blane, C. E., Amendola, A. E. *et al.* (1984) CT findings in hepatoblastoma. *J. Comput. Assist. Tomogr.*, **8**, 1105

Bernstein, I. T., Bulow, S. and Mauritzen, K. (1992) Hepatoblastoma in two cousins in a family with adenomatous polyposis. *Dis. Colon Rectum*, April, 373–374

Conran, R. M., Hitchcock, C. L., Maclawiw, M. A., Stocker, J. M. and Ishak, K. G. (1992) Hepatoblastoma: the prognostic significance of histologic type. *Pediatr. Pathol.*, **12**, 167–183

Cross, S. S. and Variend, S. (1992) Combined hepatoblastoma and yolk sac tumor of the liver. *Cancer*, **69**, 1323–1326

Dehner, L. P. and Manivel, J. C. (1988) Hepatoblastoma: an analysis of the relationship between morphologic subtypes and prognosis. *Am. J. Pediatr. Hematol. Oncol.*, **10**, 301–307

Filler, R. M., Ehrlich, P. F., Greenburg, M. L. and Babyn, P. S. (1991) Preoperative chemotherapy in hepatoblastoma. *Surgery*, **110**, 591–597

Giardiello, F. M., Offerhaus, J. A., Krush, A. J. *et al.* (1991) Risk of hepatoblastoma in familial adenomatous polyposis. *J. Pediatr.*, **119**, 766–768

Hata, Y. (1990) The clinical features and prognosis of hepatoblastoma: follow-up studies done on pediatric tumours enrolled in the Japanese Pediatric Tumor Registry between 1971-1980, part 1. *Jap. J. Surg.*, **20**, 498–502

Honzumi, M., Miura, T., Fujino, I. and Suzuki, H. (1990) Hepatoblastoma in neonates: a report of a case and review of the Japanese literature. *Jap. J. Surg.*, **20**, 331–334

Kingston, J. E., Herbert, A., Draper, G. J. and Mann, J. R. (1984) Association between hepatoblastoma and polyposis coli. *Arch. Dis. Childh.*, **53**, 959

Koneru, B., Flye, M. W., Busuttil, R. *et al.* (1991) Liver transplantation in Hepatoblastoma. *Ann. Surg.*, **213**, 118–121

Krush, A. J., Traboulsi, E. I., Offerhaus, J. A., Maumenee, I. H., Yardley, J. H. and Levin. L. S. (1988) Hepatoblastoma, pigmented ocular fundus lesions and jaw lesions in gardner syndrome. *Am. J. Med. Genet.*, **29**, 323–332

Lack, E. E., Neave, C. and Vawter, O. F. (1982) Hepatoblastoma: A clinical and pathological study of 54 cases. *Am. J. Surg. Pathol.*, **6**, 693

MacPherson, A. J. S., Bjarnason, I. and Forgacs, I. (1992) Discovery of the gene for familial adnomatous polyposis. *Br. Med. J.*, **304**, 858–859

Muraji, T., Woolley, M. M., Sinatra, F. *et al.* (1985) The prognostic implications of hypercholesterolaemia in infants and children with hepatoblastoma. *J. Pediatr. Surg.*, **20**, 228

Nakagawara, A., Ikeda, T., Tsuneyoshi, M. *et al.* (1985) Hepatoblastoma producing both alphafetoprotein and human chorionic gonadotrophin. Clinico-pathological analysis of 4 cases and review of the literature. *Cancer*, **56**, 1636

Pierro, A., Langevin, A. M., Filler, R. M., Liu, P., Phillips, M. J. and Greenberg, M. L. (1989) Preoperative chemotherapy in "unresectable" hepatoblastoma. *J. Pediatr. Surg.*, **24**, 24–29

Reynolds, M., Douglass, E. C., Finegold, M., Cantor, A. and Glicksman, A. (1992) Chemotherapy can convert unresectable hepatoblastoma. *J. Pediatr. Surg.*, **27**, 1080–1084

Shneider, B. L., Haque, S., van Hoff, J., Touloukian, R. J. and West, A. B. (1992) Familial adenomatous polyposis following liver transplantation for a virilizing hepatoblastoma. *J. Pediatr. Gastroenterol.*, **15**, 198–201

Takayama, T., Makuuchi, M., Takayasu, K. *et al.* (1990) Resection after intraarterial chemotherapy of a hepatoblastoma originating in the caudate lobe. *Surgery*, **107**, 231–235

Hepatocellular carcinoma

Behrens, R., Wagner-Thiessen, E. and Stehr, K. (1984) Cholangiodysplastic pseudocirrhosis. *Clin. Klin. Pädiat.*, **196**, 398

Conti, J. A. and Kemeny, N. (1992) Type Ia glycogenosis associated with hepatocellular carcinoma. *Cancer*, **69**, 1320–1322

Fletman, D., Rosenberg, H. K. and Evans, A. E. (1984) Hepatocellular carcinoma in an infant presenting with a calcified soft tissue mass. Case report on 25 year experience. *Clin. Pediatr.*, **23**, 643

Hsu, H. C., Wu, M. Z., Chang, M. H., Su, I. J. and Chen, D. S. (1987) Childhood hepatocellular carcinoma develops exclusively in hepatitis B surface antigen carriers in three decades in Taiwan: a report of 51 cases strongly associated with rapid development of liver cirrhosis. *J. Hepatol.*, **5**, 260–267

Iwatsuki, S., Starzl, T., Sheahan, D. G. *et al.* (1991) Hepatic resection versus transplantation for hepatocellular carcinoma. *Ann. Surg.*, **214**, 221–229

Kovalic, J. J., Thomas, P. R. M., Beckwith, J. B., Feusner, J. H. and Norkool, P. A. (1991) Hepatocellular carcinoma as second malignant neoplasms in successfully treated Wilms' tumor patients. *A National Wilms' Tumor Study Report*, **67**, 342–344

Lack, E. E., Neave, C. and Vawter, G. F. (1983) Hepatocellular carcinoma. A review of 32 cases in childhood and adolescence. *Cancer*, **52**, 1510

Lee, F. Y., Lee, S. D., Tsai, Y. T., Wu, J. C., Lai, K. H. and Lo, K. J. (1989) Serum C-reactive protein as a serum marker for the diagnosis of hepatocellular carcinoma. *Cancer*, **63**, 1567–1571

Ni, Y.-H., Chang, M.-H., Hsu, H.-Y. *et al.* (1991) Hepatocellular carcinoma in childhood: clinical manifestations and prognosis. *Cancer*, **68**, 1737–1741

Trounce, J. Q., Flower, A. J. E., Shannon, R. F. and Tanner, M. (1985) A case of hepatocellular carcinoma complicating hepatitis B infection in a 9-year-old boy. *Q. Jl. Med.*, **57**, 791

Wee, A., Ludwig, J., Coffey, R. J. *et al.* (1985) Hepatobiliary carcinoma associated with primary sclerosing cholangitis and chronic ulcerative colitis. *Hum. Pathol.*, **16**, 719

Weinstein, S., Scottolini, A. G., Loo, S. Y. T. *et al.* (1985) Ataxia telangiectasia with hepatocellular carcinoma in a 15-year old girl and studies of kindred. *Arch. Pathol. Lab. Med.*, **109**, 1000

Yen-Hsuan, N., Mei-Hwei, C., Hong-Yuan, H. *et al.* (1991) Hepatocellular carcinoma in childhood: clinical manifestations and prognosis. *Cancer*, **68**, 1737–1741

Rhabdomyosarcoma

Anon. (1989) Prognostic factors in childhood rhabdomyosarcoma. *Lancet*, **ii**, 959–960

Arnaud, O., Bosq, M., Asquier, E. and Michel, J. (1987) Embryonal rhabdomyosarcoma of the biliary tree in children: a case report. *Pediatr. Radiol.*, **17**, 250–251

Dodd, S., Malone, M. and McCullough, W. (1989) Rhabdomyosarcoma in children: a histological and immunohistochemical study of 59 cases. *J. Pathol.*, **158**, 13–18

Geoffrey, A., Couanet, D., Montagne, J. P., Lectere, J. and Flamant, F. (1987) Ultra-sonography and computer tomography for diagnosis and follow-up of biliary duct rhabdomyosarcoma. *Pediatr. Radiol.*, **17**, 127–131

Maurer, H. M., Beltangady, M., Gehan, E. A. *et al.* (1988) The intergroup rhabdomyosarcoma study-1: a final report. *Cancer*, **61**, 209–220

Ruymann, M. B., Raney, R. B., Cristie, W. M. *et al.* (1985) Rhabdomyosarcoma of the biliary tree in childhood. A Report from the Inter-Group Rhabdomyosarcoma Study. *Cancer*, **56**, 575

Rare malignant tumours

Chou, P., Mangkornkanok, M. and Gonzales-Crussi, F. (1990) Undifferentiated (embryonal) sarcoma of the liver: ultrastructure, immunohisto-chemistry and DNA ploidy analysis of two cases. *Pediatr. Pathol.*, **10**, 549–562

Czaga, M. J., Goldfarb, G. P., Cho, K. C. *et al.* (1985) Bile duct carcinoma in an adolescent. *Am. Gastroenterol.*, **80**, 486

Danhaive, O., Ninane, J., Sokal, E. *et al.* (1992) Hepatic localization of a fibrosarcoma in a child with a liver transplant. *J. Pediatr.*, **120**, 434–437

Horowitz, M. E., Etcubanas, E., Webber, B. L. *et al.* (1987) Hepatic undifferentiated (embryonal) sarcoma and rhabdomyosarcoma in children and adults. *Cancer*, **59**, 396–402

Hsu, W., Deziel, D. J., Gould, V. E., Warren, W. H., Gooch, G. T. and Staren, E. D. (1991) Neuroendocrine differentiation and prognosis of extrahepatic biliary tract carcinomas. *Surgery*, **110**, 604–611

Hsu, W., Deziel, D. J., Gould, V. E., Warren, W. H., Gooch, G. T. and Staren, E. D. (1991) Neuroendocrine differentiation and prognosis of extrahepatic biliary tract carcinomas. *Surgery*, **110**, 726–735

Leuschner, I., Schmidt, D. and Harms, D. (1990) Undifferentiated sarcoma of the liver in childhood: morphology, flow cytometry and literature review. *Human Pathol.*, **21**, 68–76

Miller, S. T., Wollner, N., Meyers, P. A. *et al.* (1983) Primary hepatic or hepatosplenic non-Hodgkin's lymphoma in children. *Cancer*, **52**, 2285

Noronha, R. and Gonzalez-Crussi, F. (1984) Hepatic angiosarcoma in childhood. *Am. Surg. Pathol.*, **8**, 863

Pinkerton, C. R., Broadbent V., Horwich, A., Levitt, G., McElwain, T. J., Melloer, S. T. *et al.* (1990) A carboplatin based regimen for malignant germ cell tumours in children. *Brit. J. Cancer.*, **62**, 257–262

Platt, M. S., Agamanolis, D. P., Trill, C. E. *et al.* (1983) Occult hepatic sinusoid tumour of infancy simulating neuroblastoma. *Cancer*, **52**, 1183

Soares, F. A., Landell, G. A., Peres, L. C., Oliveira, M. A., Vicente, Y. A., Tone, L. G. (1989) Liposarcoma of hepatic hilum in childhood: report of a case and review of the literature. *Med. Pediatr. Oncol.*, **17**, 239–243

Benign liver tumours

Chandra, R. S., Kapur, S. P., Kelleher, J. *et al.* (1984) Benign hepatocellular tumours in the young. *Arch. Pathol. Lab. Med.*, **108**, 168

Ehren, H., Hossein-Mahour, G. and Isaacs, H. (1983) Benign liver tumours in infancy and childhood. Report of 48 cases. *Am. J. Surg.*, **145**, 325

Heller, K., Markus, B. H. and Waag, K.-L. (1992) Central hamartoma of the liver in a child. *Eur. J. Pediatr. Surg.*, **2**, 108–109

Schweizer, P. (1991) Benign liver tumors. In: *Hepatobiliary Surgery in Childhood* (eds Schweizer, P. and Schier, F.). Schattauer, Stuttgart, pp. 145–151

Wheeler, D. A., Edmondson, H. A. and Reynolds, T. B. (1985) Spontaneous liver cell adenoma in children. *Am. J. Clin. Pathol.*, **85**, 6

Williams, J. G., Newman, B. M., Sutphen, J. L., Madison, J., Frierson, H. and McIlhenny, J. (1990) Hepatobiliary cystadenoma: a rare hepatic tumor in a child. *J. Pediatr. Surg.*, **25**, 1250–1252

Yandza, T. and Valayer, J. (1986) Benign tumours of the liver in children: an analysis of 20 cases. *J. Pediatr. Surg.*, **21**, 419

Haemangiomas

Burrows, P. E., Rosenberg, N. C. and Chuang, H. S. (1985) Acute hepatic haemangiomas: percutaneous transcatheter embolization with detachable silicone balloons. *Radiology*, **156**, 85

Fellows, K. E., Hoffer, F. A., Markowitz, T\R. I. and O'Neill, J. A. (1991) Multiple arteriovenous malformations: effect of embolization. *Radiology*, **181**, 813–818

Howard, E. R. and Heaton, N. D. Haemangiomas. In: *Surgery of Liver Disease in Children* (ed. Howard, E. R.). Butterworth-Heinemann, Oxford, pp. 115–125

Kirchner, S. G., Heller, R. M., Kasselberg, A. P. and Green, H. L. (1981) Infantile hepatic haemangio-endothelioma with subsequent malignant degeneration. *Pediatr. Radiol.*, **11**, 42

Larcher, V. F., Howard, E. R. and Mowat, A. P. (1981) Hepatic haemangiomata: diagnosis and management. *Arch. Dis. Childh.*, **56**, 7

Stanley, P., Geer, G. D., Miller, J. H., Gilsanz, V., Landing, B. H. and Boechat, I, M. (1989) Infantile hepatic haemangiomas: clinical features, radiologic investigations and treatment of 20 patients. *Cancer*, 936–949

Weber, T. R., Connors, R. H., Tracy, T. F. and Bailey, P. V. (1990) Complex hemangiomas of infants and children: individualized management in 22 cases. *Arch. Surg.*, **125**, 1017–1021

Mesenchymal hamartomata

Ankalay, A. L., Puri, A. R., Pomerance, J. J. *et al.* (1985) Mesenchymal hamartomata of the liver responsive to cyclophosphamide therapy: therapeutic approach. *J. Pediatr.*, **20**, 125

Smithson, W. A., Telander, R. L. and Carney, J. A. (1982) Mesenchymoma of the liver in childhood: five-year survival after modality treatment. *J. Pediatr. Surg.*, **17**, 70

Stanley, R. J., Hall, T. R., Woolley, M. M., Diament, M. J., Gilsanz, V. and Miller, J. H. (1986) Mesenchymal hamartomas of the liver in childhood sonographic and CT findings. *Am. J. Roentgenol.*, **147**, 1035–1039

Focal nodular hyperplasia

Atkinson, G. O., Kodroff, M., Sones, P. I. and Gay, B. B. (1980) Focal nodular hypoplasia of the liver in children. A report of 3 new cases. *Radiology*, **137**, 171

Lee, M. J., Saini, S., Hamm, B. *et al.* (1991) Focal nodular hyperplasia of the liver: MR findings in 35 proved cases. *Am. J. Roentgenol.*, **156**, 317–320

Mowat, A. P., Jutjhar, P., Portmann, B., Dawson, J. L. and Williams, R. (1976) Focal nodular hypoplasia of the liver: a rational approach to treatment. *Gut*, **17**, 492

Shortell, C. K. and Schwartz, S. I. (1991) Hepatic adenoma and focal nodular hyperplasia. *Surg. Gynecol. Obstetr.*, **173**, 426–431

Infantile peliosis hepatis

Cragg, A., Casteneda-Zuniga, W., Lund, G. *et al.* (1984) Infantile peliosis hepatis. *Pediatr. Radiol.*, **14**,

Solitary liver cysts

Byrne, W. I. and Fonkelsrud, E. W. (1982) Congenital solitary non-parasitic cysts of the liver: a rare cause of a rapid enlargement of abdominal mass in infancy. *J. Pediatr. Surg.*, **17**, 316

Chapter 24

Disorders of the gall bladder and biliary tract

Congenital abnormalities of the biliary tree

Abnormalities may predispose to stasis, inflammation and cholelithiasis, but often are asymptomatic and of no clinical importance. A knowledge of their occurrence is, however, important to radiologists, ultrasonographers and to surgeons operating on the biliary system. The hepatic artery is particularly variable calling for careful surgical dissection in this area. When abnormalities occur they may do so in isolation, but they are often associated with other congenital lesions such as polycystic disease and cardiac defects. All the abnormalities are rare. Only the least rare will be mentioned.

Absence of the gall bladder

This may occur as an isolated asymptomatic abnormality. It is often associated with other anomalies such as direct entry of the hepatic ducts into the duodenum with absence of the common bile duct. Failure of vacuolization of the gall bladder, which persists in its solid state, has been reported. This is usually associated with atresia of the extrahepatic bile ducts. Whether this really does occur as a congenital abnormality or is an acquired condition. is considered elsewhere (see p. 80). It should be noted that the gall bladder may not be immediately obvious at operation if it is intrahepatic, buried in extensive fibrous tissue or atrophied because of previous cholecystitis. Such abnormalities are most commonly seen in childhood in association with cystic fibrosis.

Double gall bladder and anomalies of the cystic duct

Double gall bladders are usually recognized at cholecystography. The second gall bladder varies considerably in size and has an anomalous association with the biliary system; joining it within the hepatic substance, at the common bile duct via its own cystic duct, or emptying directly into the duodenum. A double gall bladder may be confused with a bilobe gall bladder in which the gall bladder appears to form two distinct and separate fundi, having a common cystic duct. In up to 20% of subjects the cystic duct lies parallel to the common hepatic duct for a few centimetres, encased in a common sheath.

Accessory bile ducts

An additional bile duct may leave the right lobe of the liver, draining directly to the common hepatic duct, to the cystic duct, the gall bladder or even the duodenum. In addition, accessory ducts may join the liver directly to the gall bladder or stomach. Bronchobiliary fistulae may cause respiratory problems.

Choledochal cyst

Choledochal cysts are dilatations of all or part of the extrahepatic biliary system. The dilatation may be fusiform (the ratio of the width to the length being less than one-third) or cystic. If unrecognized these cysts may be complicated by progressive biliary obstruction leading to biliary cirrhosis, cholangitis and carcinoma.

Three distinct varieties with differing clinicopathological consequences are recognized (Figure 24.1):

(1) Cystic or fusiform dilatations of the bile duct, commonly extending from just below the bifurcation to a narrow or obliterated distal common bile duct 1–3 cm from the duodenum. Rarely there may be dilatation of the common hepatic duct. There may be cystic or fusiform dilatation of intrahepatic bile ducts, affecting both lobes or limited to the left lobe, in up to 70% of patients.
(2) A pedunculated diverticulum from the lateral wall of the common bile duct.
(3) Herniation of the terminal end of the common duct into the duodenum associated with the formation of a small cyst, usually termed a 'cholecystocele' or 'choledochocele' (analogous to a ureterocele). There is little proximal bile duct dilatation. The cyst may obstruct the pancreatic duct causing pancreatitis.
(4) A fourth composite variety takes the form of multiple communicating cystic or fusiform dilatations of both the intrahepatic and the extrahepatic ducts. Rarely, single intrahepatic cysts coexist with single cysts of the common bile duct.

Pathology

The cyst wall which varies from 0.2 to 10 mm in thickness is composed of dense fibrous tissue with little elastic or muscle tissue and often no epithelial lining. The distal common bile duct may be narrowed or obliterated. The cyst volume ranges from 5 ml to more than 3 litres. Carcinoma develops in the cyst wall with a frequency which has ranged from 17% (Todani et al., 1987) to 28% (Nagorney et al., 1984). This can happen as early as 12 years of age with two-thirds occurring by 40 years.

Secondary changes occur within the liver. The hepatic architecture is maintained but portal tracts enlarge showing bile duct reduplication with inflammatory cell infiltrate and ever-increasing fibrosis. The picture in young infants may be similar to that seen in biliary atresia. If obstruction persists biliary cirrhosis and its complications will develop. Following surgical correction such abnormalities regress. Interestingly, some patients with dilated intrahepatic bile ducts show minimal changes in the hepatic parenchyma.

Aetiology

The aetiology is unknown. The estimated incidence ranges from 1 in 13 000 live births in Japan to 1 in 200 000 in Europe. Approximately 80% of cases occur in females. There is no increased familial incidence. The disorder may be diagnosed ultrasonically as early as 17 weeks' gestation. It has been suggested that bile duct damage may be initiated by pancreatic enzymes gaining access to the biliary system.

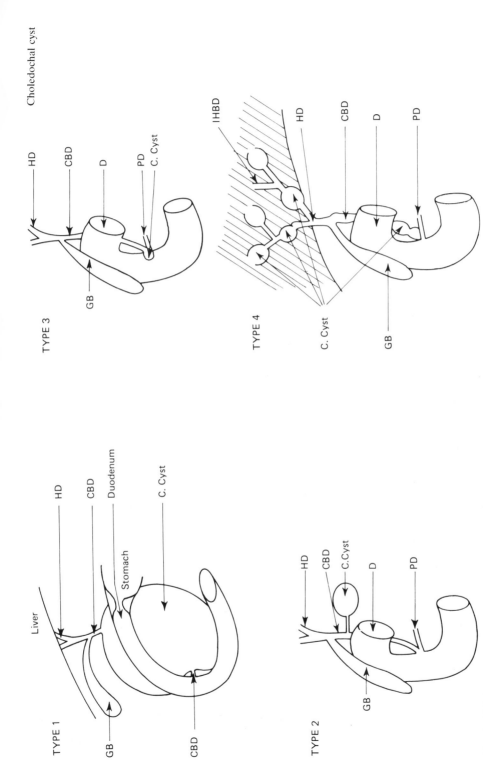

Figure 24.1 Choledochal cyst types 1, 2, 3 and 4. Abbreviations: HD = hepatic duct; CBD = common bile duct; GB = gall bladder: D = duodenum; PD = pancreatic duct; IHBD = intrahepatic bile duct

Pancreatic enzymes are sometimes detected in choledochal cysts. In up to 70% of cases the common bile duct and the pancreatic duct share a long common pathway, with the ducts joining at a less acute angle than normal in up to one-third of cases. It is suggested that such abnormalities may facilitate a mixture of bile and pancreatic enzymes with activation of proteolytic enzymes, lipases and phospholipases with the production of tissue damaging substances such as lysolecithin. In a review of almost 1600 endoscopic cholangiograms 18 of 24 with a long common pathway had a choledochal cyst (Yamauchi *et al.*, 1987). Other postulated aetiological mechanisms include a congenital weakness of the muscle wall, congenital inflammation or valvular obstruction occurring in the ampulla of Vater or excessive proliferation of the epithelial cells of the primitive choledochus which leads to biliary dilatation when canalization occurs. Since choledochal cysts may occur in association with congenital hepatic fibrosis it is sometimes classified with the fibropolycystic disorders considered in Chapter 16.

Clinical features

Twenty five percent present in the first year of life with 40–90% in varying series presenting by 10 years of age. The disorder may be recognized ultrasonically in utero or may not be recognized until the eighth decade.

The classic triad of features suggesting the diagnosis of choledochal cyst is intermittent obstructive jaundice, abdominal pain and a cystic abdominal mass. Unfortunately these are rarely present early in the course and are found in less than 10% of cases in recently reported series. In most series, jaundice occurred in 60–90% of cases. It may be intermittent initially but with progressive liver damage may become persistent. Pruritus may develop. The abdominal pain is often poorly localized but it may be felt principally in the right upper quadrant or referred to the back. If the diagnosis is considered it is prudent not to try to detect the cyst clinically and await ultrasonography rather than cause its rupture. In infants the features are frequently those of biliary atresia although abdominal distension, fever, vomiting and failure to thrive may be more common. The infant may be irritable. The cyst is rarely palpable.

In most cases, symptoms will have occurred for the first time between the ages of 1 and 3 years but, unfortunately, 75% of the cases are unlikely to be diagnosed before the age of 10 years, during which time progressive hepatocellular change leading to cirrhosis may have occurred. Complications are listed in Table 24.1.

Diagnosis

Careful ultrasonic examination of the biliary tree is the most helpful investigation demonstrating a cystic dilatation of the common bile duct without gall bladder dilatation although the intrahepatic bile ducts may be widened (Figure 24.2). Ultrasonography also

Table 24.1 Complications of choledochal cyst

Recurrent ascending cholangitis
Biliary cirrhosis
Rupture with bile peritonitis
Pancreatitis
Portal vein thrombosis
Hepatic abscess
Carcinoma of cyst wall
Gall-stones

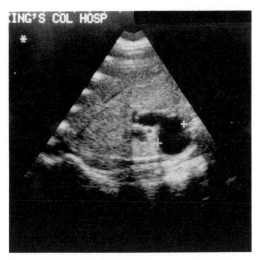

Figure 24.2 Ultrasound appearance of a choledochal cyst. There is a circular dilatation of the extrahepatic bile duct (+ to +) and moderate fusiform dilatation of the intrahepatic duct. The hepatic artery and portal vein are seen posterior to the dilated duct

shows the degree of displacement of adjacent structures such as the duodenum or portal vein. In patients with pancreatitis computed tomography scanning is helpful. CT scanning also clarifies the relationship of the cyst to other structures (Figure 24.3) and can detect carcinomatous change. If there is any doubt that the cyst is in the biliary system this can be confirmed by scintiscanning following intravenous injection of technetium-99m tagged iminodiacetic acid derivatives such as methylbromo-iminodiacetic acid (MBrIDA). The isotope is seen to be concentrated in the dilated biliary system. Percutaneous liver biopsy, percutaneous transhepatic or endoscopic cholangiography should not be attempted because of the risks of causing a bile leak or pancreatitis. The diagnosis is confirmed at laparotomy. An operative cholangiogram through the gall bladder is necessary to define the severity of other abnormalities in the biliary system. Endoscopy with inspection of the ampulla of Vater is helpful if a type 3 lesion is present.

Differential diagnosis

In infancy the main differential diagnosis is biliary atresia or hepatitis syndrome (Chapters 4 and 5). Ultrasonography cannot distinguish between a choledochal cyst and a cyst in the extrahepatic biliary duct associated with biliary atresia. Since both require skilled surgical management this is only important in prelaparotomy counselling of parents. In the older child the differential diagnosis will include chronic hepatitis and, if abdominal pain is marked, pancreatitis. Serum amylase may be elevated. Intra-abdominal neoplasms must also be considered.

Treatment

The best results are obtained if there is accurate preoperative diagnosis. The treatment of choice is radical excision of the cyst with hepatico-jejunostomy or porto-jejunostomy to

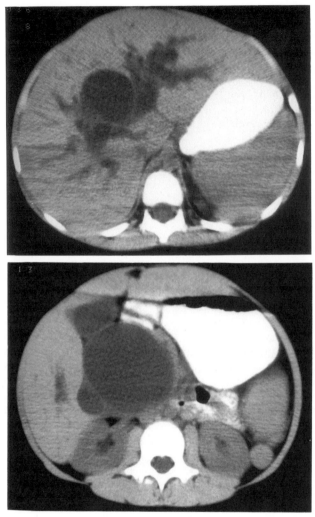

Figure 24.3 Unenhanced computed tomography, with oral contrast, demonstrating dilatation of the intrahepatic bile ducts with a large cystic lesion arising at the level of the hilum (*a*). Lower cuts demonstrate close apposition of the choledochal cyst to a normal gall bladder (*b*)

a Roux-en-Y loop. Excision eliminates the reservoir of bile stasis with the attendant risks of ascending cholangitis and biliary cirrhosis. It also removes the dangers associated with malignant change in the cyst wall and spontaneous rupture with biliary peritonitis. If excision is not feasible because the cyst is adherent to vital structures such as the portal vein, or because of the large number of portosystemic collaterals developing because of portal hypertension, choledochocyst-jejunostomy to a Roux-en-Y loop should be performed and later excision planned. With retropancreatic or infraduodenal cysts, endocystic removal of the internal wall of the cyst obliterating the cyst lumen but leaving its external walls *in situ*, may avoid damage to adjacent vital structures. A hepatico-jejunostomy is performed above the cyst remnant (Saing *et al.*, 1985). With effective bile drainage and the avoidance of cholangitis intrahepatic damage is arrested and there may be complete reversal of established biliary cirrhosis (Yeong *et al.*, 1982). Dilatation of the intrahepatic bile ducts decreases in the vast majority of cases (Ohi *et al.*, 1985).

Because of the risks of ascending cholangitis, strictures developing at the bile duct–bowel anastomosis, cholelithiasis and possible malignant change in the intrahepatic ducts (Iwai *et al.*, 1992) it is essential that patients be reviewed regularly throughout childhood and adult life.

Spontaneous perforation of the bile duct in infancy

In the first 3 years of life spontaneous biliary peritonitis may develop due to a leakage of bile from the junction of the cystic duct and the common hepatic duct. It is commonest between the ages of 1 week and 2 months. More than 80 cases have been reported.

Pathology

Although the site of perforation is constant, its cause is unknown. Operative cholangiography frequently shows an obstruction to bile flow at the lower end of the common bile duct, but the nature of the obstruction is difficult to determine. This is an area which is not explored at surgery. Mucus plugs and gall-stones have been responsible in individual cases. In other infants there is permanent obstruction with apparent fibrosis. In some the distal bile duct appears to be normal.

The intrahepatic changes are minimal unless there is secondary ascending cholangitis. The bile initially causes little peritoneal reaction but later bacterial peritonitis may develop.

Clinical features

Birth and the immediate neonatal period are usually unremarkable. Signs usually appear by 8 weeks of age but may occur as late as 30 months. The initial features are of mild jaundice, failure to gain weight and, sometimes, vomiting. The stools are pale or acholic and the urine is persistently yellow. Ascites causes abdominal distension, hydroceles and inguinal or umbilical hernia which typically are bile stained (Figure 24.4). Death occurs from malnutrition or sepsis.

Laboratory investigations

The total serum bilirubin is usually less than 8 mg/100 ml (135 μmol/litre) with between 40 and 90% conjugated. The gamma-glutamyl transpeptidase and serum alkaline phosphatase levels are raised but transaminase levels may be normal. The prothrombin time may be prolonged but corrects immediately with parenteral vitamin K. Ultra-sonography may show an echogenic mass around the common bile duct. Early MBrIDA scans may show isotope accumulating in this area before spreading in the ascitic fluid. Abdominal paracentesis confirms the presence of bile-stained ascites.

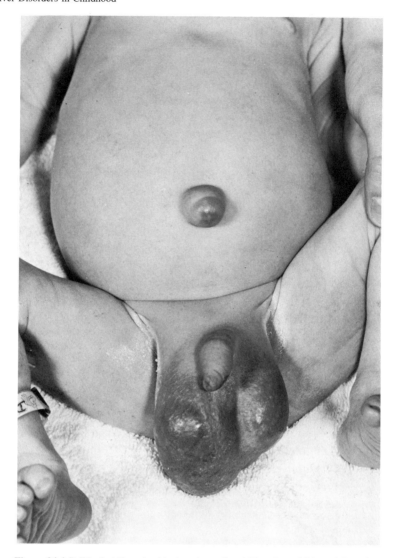

Figure 24.4 Strikingly bile-stained hydroceles and umbilicus in a child aged 7 weeks who had been juandiced since the age of 14 days. The stools were acholic, weight gain had been poor. At laparotomy there was clear bile-stained ascites and a large bile-containing cyst of the lower sac; the gall bladder was distended with bile. The liver was normal macroscopically, and subsequent histological examination showed no abnormality

Treatment

Surgical treatment is essential. Laparotomy and operative cholangiography through the gall bladder shows leakage of contrast from the junction of the cystic duct and the common hepatic duct (Figure 24.5). If there is free drainage of contrast into the duodenum, the perforation should be sutured and the area of leakage drained. If there is

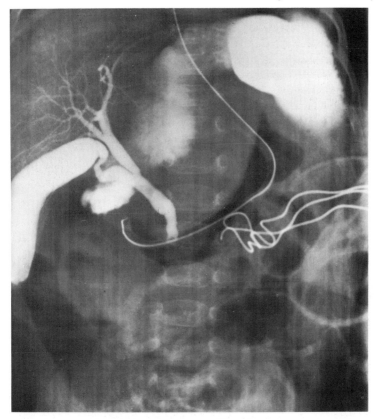

Figure 24.5 Operative cholangiogram (in the case shown in Figure 24.4) performed
through the gall bladder showed normal intrahepatic biliary tree but with no flow
from the distal common bile duct. The gall bladder was anastomosed to a Roux-en-Y
loop of jejunum into the duodenum. Contrast medium leaked from the perforation at
the junction of the cystic duct and common bile duct. Postoperative progress has
been uneventful and at the age of 2 years the child is clinically well and liver
function tests are normal

obstruction to the common bile duct a T tube may be placed in the perforation. This
decompresses the biliary system and allows the perforation to heal if there is no permanent
distal obstruction. If there is a permanent obstruction a cholecyst-jejunostomy to a Roux-
en-Y loop of jejunum should be constructed. With such management the prognosis is
excellent although ascending cholangitis may occur.

Gall-stones

Definition

Gall-stones are amorphous or crystalline material which has precipitated in bile. Their
pathological effects include obstruction to bile flow, cholecystitis, cholangitis and, rarely,
rupture of the biliary tree.

Types of gall-stones

The most common type is a so-called mixed gall-stone. It contains cholesterol, bile pigment, calcium and an organic or protein matrix. Such gall-stones are usually multiple with faceted surfaces and contain enough calcium to be radio-opaque.

Pure cholesterol stones are usually rounded single stones which are not radio-opaque. However, when secondary infection occurs in the gall bladder a layer of radio-opaque calcium is deposited, giving a radio-opaque ring appearance on the radiograph.

Black bile pigment stones are usually small, hard and amorphous. In addition to bile pigment they contain a variable amount of calcium and organic matter. They are usually associated with chronic haemolysis and are radio-opaque. Brown pigment stones are associated with recurrent infection in the biliary system.

Aetiology

Gall-stones occur more commonly in adult life than in childhood. The pathogenesis of their formation has been the subject of extensive studies in the last decade. Many aspects of their aetiology remain unknown. The unusual physicochemical properties of bile, and the nature of the lipids in bile, are now recognized as being very important contributory factors. Approximately 8% of the lipid in bile is in the form of cholesterol and between 15 and 20% in the form of phospholipid. Both are virtually insoluble in water but are held in solution in bile by virtue of the detergent action of bile salts. Events which influence the relative concentrations of these substances may be of crucial importance in their solubility. Cholesterol and phospholipid are kept in solution in the biliary system in two physicochemical forms. The bile salt micelle which makes extremely efficient use of the detergent properties of bile salts to keep phospholipid and cholesterol in solution is the predominant form in the gall bladder. In hepatic bile cholesterol and phospholipid is held mainly in uni- or multilamellar vesicles. When bile salts are present in high concentrations cholesterol moves from vesicles to micelles. When the molar ratio of cholesterol to phospholipid approaches 1, microcrystals of cholesterol form. Biliary apolipoproteins, mucus, glycoproteins and mucosal prostaglandins may have a role in promoting and inhibiting crystallization.

Table 24.2 Pathological mechanisms in cholelithiasis

Formation of abnormal bile due to primary liver disease
Decreased biliary bile salt concentration
Increased biliary cholesterol concentration
Ileal pathology causing reduced enterohepatic circulation of bile salts
Abnormality of gall bladder function:
    Impaired emptying causing reduction in bile salt recycling
    Excessive concentration of bile
    Hyperconcentration of bile at mucosal level
Abnormal bile constituents:
    Excess bilirubin in haemolytic disease
    Abnormal mucoprotein in cystic fibrosis
    Bacteria
    Parasites, e.g. *Ascaris, Clonorchis sinensis*
    Cell debris
Stasis due to obstruction of bile duct
Statis due to abnormality of bile duct
Drugs or toxins causing cholestasis, increased biliary cholesterol or bile salt depletion

Table 24.3 Contributory factors in cholelithiasis

Cholecystitis
Liver disease
Ileal disease or resection
Haemolytic disorders
Cystic fibrosis
Obesity
Intra-abdominal infection
Intra-abdominal surgery
Family history of liver or gall bladder disease
Parenteral nutrition ± frusemide
Cholestyramine therapy
Selective IgA deficiency

Micelles are thought to be formed in the bile canaliculi as bile is produced. In the gall bladder much liquid is absorbed from the bile causing an increase in micelle size. In patients without disorders predisposing to gall-stone formation it is unclear whether the primary abnormality causing gall-stone formation lies in the gall bladder or in bile formation.

Pathological mechanisms predisposing to gallstone formation in children are shown in Table 24.2, while specific causes are listed in Table 24.3.

Thus, any condition *causing reduced bile acid excretion*, whether due to primary liver disease or from a reduced enterohepatic circulation of bile salts, may predispose to gall-stone formation. Further evidence for the key role of bile acid metabolism in gall-stone formation is the observation that in humans oral administration of the bile salt chenodeoxycholic acid causes gradual dissolution of small gall-stones.

Bacterial infection may also play a part in gallstone formation, by bacterial action on the components of micelles. Deconjugation of bile acids and diffusion of the free bile acids through the gall bladder wall may shift the concentration from the critical micellar phase. Similarly, the conversion of lecithin to lysolecithin and fatty acids may cause a precipitation of cholesterol.

Bacterial beta-glucuronidase may have a role in the production of bile pigment stones, causing the deconjugation of bilirubin glucuronide to insoluble bilirubin which may provide a pigment nucleus for gall-stone formation. This mechanism may operate also in *haemolytic disorders* such as sickle cell anaemia, or acholuric jaundice, in which bilirubin excretion is excessive. It should be remembered, however, that such excretion is in a soluble form and therefore some additional factor is necessary to promote gall-stone formation. It should also be noted that pigment gallstones occur in patients with idiopathic cirrhosis.

In *cystic fibrosis* the factors leading to gall-stone formation are complex. It seems likely that in many instances bile salt excretion in duodenal juice and in the stools may be reduced. The bile may contain abnormal mucin which provides a nucleus for gall-stone formation. The gall bladder is frequently small and the extrahepatic circulation of bile salts may be deranged. Finally, cirrhosis complicating the cystic fibrosis may produce secondary changes in bile salt secretion.

Total parenteral nutrition, vagotomy, spinal injury and octreotide may contribute to gall-stone formation by causing bile stasis. In infants receiving total parenteral nutrition infections and dietary factors may also contribute.

Clinical features

The vast majority of stones are found in the gall bladder, less than 6% occluding the cystic duct or common bile duct. In many instances gall-stones are asymptomatic, being discovered unexpectedly during investigation for problems seemingly unrelated to biliary tract disease. They may occur at any age, even in fetal life, but the majority in children are found at about the time of puberty. In early childhood the sex incidence is equal, but towards adolescence females predominate.

Where symptoms occur they take the form of intermittent abdominal pain of mild or marked severity usually peri-umbilical in site, but occasionally localized to the right upper quadrant. In infants, the pain cannot be localized and irritability may be the most marked feature. Vomiting is a frequently reported complaint in all age groups. On examination tenderness localized to the right upper quadrant may be observed.

Laboratory investigations

Laboratory investigations are not particularly helpful, but an elevation of alkaline phosphatase or gamma-glutamyl transpeptidase, without similar elevation in bilirubin or aspartate aminotransferase, should suggest biliary tract disease. Plain radiographs of the gall bladder region may show calculi. Ultrasonography is up to 95% sensitive in detecting stones in the gall bladder or cystic duct. Oral cholecystography may be necessary in rare instances.

Complications

Gall-stones predispose to cholecystitis and biliary obstruction which can even lead to biliary cirrhosis. Perforation of the gall bladder has been reported. They may also predispose to carcinoma of the gall bladder in adult life.

Treatment

Careful investigation to exclude persisting treatable contributory factors such as liver disease or bile duct abnormality is essential. For the patient with symptoms or those with a non-functioning gall bladder treatment is surgical with operative or laparoscopic cholecystectomy. If there is suspicion of common bile duct stones, operative chole-cystectomy and cholangiography are probably advisable but in some instances saline irrigation performed during percutaneous cholangiography may be effective (Pariente *et al.*, 1989). In uncomplicated cases the prognosis seems excellent, with common bile duct stenosis a very infrequent problem. In adults percutaneous cholecystolithotomy and laser contact lithotripsy have been used but since both leave a diseased gall bladder their role in paediatrics must be limited.

For the asymptomatic patient with normal liver function tests, the case for surgery is less clear-cut. Spontaneous resolution may occur in infants. In adults ursodeoxycholic acid 10 mg/kg/day produces gradual dissolution of cholesterol stones of less than 3 mm extending up to 20 mm if combined with extracorporeal shock-wave lithotripsy. Cholecystectomy may reasonably be carried out at the same time as splenectomy in a patient with microspherocytosis. For the patient with cystic fibrosis the hazards of general anaesthesia and the risks of exacerbation of respiratory infection in the postoperative period are such that cholecystectomy would be ill-advised. In yet less clear-cut circumstances, clinical judgement must be made assessing the risks of the procedure against the risks of the complications which may arise and the overall prognosis related to the underlying disease.

If surgery is not undertaken, the patient should be told to report to the physician as soon as symptoms start so that cholecystectomy may be performed as early as possible to minimize the morbidity and mortality from acute cholecystitis.

Stones in the common bile duct

Stones in the common bile duct cause bile duct obstruction, cholangitis, intrahepatic abscesses and pancreatitis. Stones may develop primarily in the common bile duct when it is dilated but frequently they represent stones which have migrated from the gall bladder or dilated intrahepatic ducts. These ducts may be dilated due to congenital anomalies or sclerosing cholangitis or from previous trauma including surgery.

Clinical features and investigation findings

The classic clinical features are the acute onset of jaundice with dark urine, pale stools, pruritus, abdominal pain and fever which may be accompanied by rigors. Rarely painless jaundice without fever may be due to common bile duct stones. Standard biochemical tests of liver function are abnormal. There may be leucocytosis. Blood cultures frequently reveal bacteraemia caused by intestinal organisms or anaerobes. The diagnosis may be suspected when an X-ray shows calculi in the gall bladder or medially and posteriorly in the common bile duct. Computed tomography may also reveal the stones in the bile duct. Ultrasound is notoriously ineffective in identifying stones at or near the ampulla of Vater. Endoscopic retrograde cholangiography or percutaneous cholangiography are frequently required to identify the cause of the obstruction and related abnormalities in the biliary tree.

Treatment

Acutely ill patients require broad spectrum antibiotic cover pending the results of bacterial investigation. Percutaneous decompression of dilated ducts should be considered if the patient is hypotensive, acidotic or thrombocytopenic. When the patient's general condition is satisfactory the stone must be removed surgically or endoscopically, and any underlying disorder managed appropriately. This should include cholecystectomy if the source of the stones is the gall bladder. Endoscopic removal following sphincterotomy of the ampulla of Vater is being increasingly used in adults. The stone may be passed spontaneously or be pulled out using specially designed baskets. YAG lasers have also been used to fragment stones too large to pass spontaneously. The long-term effects of sphincterotomy are unknown.

Calculous cholecystitis

Definition

Calculous cholecystitis is an acute or chronic inflammation of the gall bladder associated with the presence of gall-stones in the gall bladder. In the acute form the cystic duct is commonly obstructed by the stone.

Pathogenesis

A combination of increased pressure in the gall bladder and bacterial action is required to cause cholecystitis. Vascular compression and ischaemia follow and may lead to infarction and gangrene. Except in rare instances bacteria appear to play no part in the initiation of the cholecystitis although within 24 hours of the onset of an attack, intestinal organisms such as *E. coli*, anaerobic streptococci, and lactobacilli are frequently recoverable from the gall bladder wall, gall bladder bile and liver substance. An important initiating factor is impaction of a stone in the cystic duct. Bacterial infection certainly contributes to the condition both by release of bacterial endotoxins and from the action of bacteria on bile salts which become deconjugated into more toxic forms.

In many instances chronic cholecystitis follows one or more attacks of acute cholecystitis, but it may also occur insidiously, presumably due to recurrent damage to the gall bladder mucosa produced by the gall-stones. In addition, bile may have a direct toxic effect on areas of the gall bladder mucosa, such as the Rolitansky-Aschoff sinuses in which inspissated bile accumulates. However, these are rarely found in children.

Pathology

The pathological changes in acute cholecystitis range from small focal lesions that heal with little scarring, to widespread haemorrhagic necrosis with perforation and peritonitis.

The wall may be thin, but more commonly it is somewhat thickened and often has a reddish-brown colour. The mucosa will show small areas of necrosis, and occasionally intramural abscesses are to be seen. Thrombi will be seen occluding some of the arterioles, leading in severe cases to a gangrenous cholecystitis. The gall bladder content may appear frankly purulent; in most cases the content is not true pus but bile thickened by a mixture of inflammatory exudate and precipitated cholesterol and calcium carbonate. Regional lymph glands are enlarged.

In the second week of the illness the neutrophil infiltrate in the gall bladder wall increases, to be replaced in the third week by lymphocytes, plasma cells and macrophages, eventually leading to more or less extensive fibrosis of the wall of the gall bladder with destruction of its muscle coat. In chronic cholecystitis the mucosa is thin and flat and the wall contracted. There are commonly adhesions to adjacent structures.

Clinical features

The majority of childhood cases are in females, with a mean age of 12 years. An almost constant feature is the acute onset of a constant colicky pain in the right upper quadrant. In the young child it may be difficult to localize. Occasionally, the pain may be felt in the epigastrium or peri-umbilical region. Rarely, it may be referred to the right scapula or shoulder. Vomiting occurs in about 75% of cases. An equal percentage have nausea. Chills and rigors are not infrequent but fat intolerance is rarely reported.

Fever is usual. Half are jaundiced. The abdomen moves poorly with respiration. Palpation elicits tenderness and guarding in the right upper quadrant but a mass is rarely felt.

Appendicitis, acute pancreatitis, intussusception, and bowel perforation are the conditions which may be confused with acute cholecystitis. Rarely, right basal pneumonia with diaphragmatic involvement may cause diagnostic difficulties.

Laboratory investigations

The total white blood count may be normal initially but usually rises in the second or third day with a predominance of polymorphonuclear neutrophil leucocytes. Serum bilirubin may be elevated, together with the alkaline phosphatase. The serum amylase may also be elevated. The finding of a calcified area in the gall bladder region on anteroposterior or lateral radiographs of the abdomen should suggest the diagnosis. Oral cholecystograms are rarely helpful. Biliary isotope scans may show a malfunctioning gall bladder.

Treatment

Because of the rarity of the disorder and the difficulty in differential diagnosis, early laparotomy is usually undertaken at a time when cholecystectomy is a relatively simple procedure. If the child has fever, tachycardia, poor peripheral circulation, hypotension or peritonitis a cholecystotomy should be performed and the patient treated vigorously with intravenous fluids, analgesics, and broad spectrum antibiotics. Cefoxitin and gentamicin should be used until bacterial culture results are available. Insertion of a drainage tube through which cholangiography can be performed to exclude stones in the common bile duct is a necessary part of the procedure. Cholecystectomy should be performed 4–6 weeks later, provided signs of acute inflammation have settled and the liver function tests have returned to normal. The prognosis following surgery is excellent except where there is significant underlying disease such as cirrhosis. (Cystic fibrosis, see p. 357; sickle cell disease, see p. 363.)

Non-calculous cholecystitis

Definition

Non-calculous cholecystitis is an acute inflammatory disease of the gall bladder in the absence of cholelithiasis.

Aetiology

Acute cholecystitis may occur as part of a systemic infection. It is increasingly recognized in intensive care units following multiple injuries, burns and severe sepsis. It can occur with enteric infections caused by *Salmonella typhi*, or *Shigella* and in viral gastroenteritis. Other specific disorders which have been associated are scarlet fever and leptospirosis.

Parasitic infections with *Giardia*, *Ascaris* and, in the Orient, *Clonorchis* are rare causes.

Salmonella typhi and *Clonorchis* can both cause chronic cholecystitis. The other aetiological factors in non-calculous cholecystitis are congenital abnormalities of the gall bladder which result in bile stasis. This presumably causes the formation of inspissated bile with chemical injury to the gall bladder mucosa and subsequent cholecystitis.

Pathology

The pathological changes depend on the underlying cause. Many of the infections are self-limiting. The chronic ones have been referred to above. There is no acute distension of the gall bladder, so that the risks of perforation are less than in the calculous cholecystitis.

Clinical aspects

The clinical features, diagnosis and management are similar to that of calculous cholecystitis.

Non-calculous distension of the gall bladder (acute hydrops)

Definition

This is a rare, self-limiting disorder in which there is acute distension of the gall bladder in the absence of any mechanical obstruction to the cystic duct. It may complicate Kawasaki disease (see below).

Aetiology and pathogenesis

The aetiology is unknown. In 13 of 25 cases (Chamberlain and Hung, 1970) there was a generalized mesenteric adenitis involving glands near the cystic duct. Although these lymph glands may be large there is no mechanical compression, although associated hyperaemia may cause mucosal oedema and thus obstruct the cystic duct lumen. No specific infectious agent has been incriminated as causing the adenitis, although a history of upper respiratory tract infection is frequently obtained. Some reports suggest that the hepatitis A virus may be implicated in that previous infectious hepatitis occurred in one patient, two were in contact with acute hepatitis and three were jaundiced, and a further three had abnormal liver function tests at the time of presentation.

Pathology

There are few reports on excised gall bladders. These show either normal or oedematous mucosa with fibrous thickening of the gall bladder wall and cellular infiltration. One patient with cystic fibrosis had areas of infarction and fibrinoid necrosis in the arterioles. There are no reports of histological changes in the cystic duct.

The bile is reported to be green or yellow in the majority of cases. In a minority it is white, while small numbers have had turbid or brown bile. Where the bile has been examined it is often reported to be sterile, alkaline, with no protein and scant leucocytes, but in 15 of 31 patients in which the bile was cultured a variety of pathogens were isolated.

Clinical features

A period of preceding illness is present in up to 60% of cases. Age distribution ranges from 1 month to 15 years, the male-to-female ratio is 5:2. The principal feature is abdominal pain, most commonly severe and of sudden onset. Occasionally it is intermittent, suggesting an intussusception. Fever is rare but anorexia, nausea and vomiting are prominent.

There is a marked tenderness on palpation of the right upper quadrant but a mass is rarely palpable except under general anaesthesia. Jaundice is unusual but has been reported.

Diagnosis

Liver function tests are rarely recorded in case reports of this condition and laboratory investigations do not appear to have contributed to the diagnosis, which is most frequently made at laparotomy carried out to exclude intussusception or appendix abscess, although occasionally cholecystitis will be the pre-laparotomy diagnosis.

Treatment

Cholecystostomy is the treatment of choice. It is important to perform a postoperative cholangiogram to exclude an obstructive lesion in the biliary tree. Since the majority of patients can be expected to make a complete recovery with normal biliary tract function, cholecystectomy, which was often used as the initial therapy in earlier reported cases, should be reserved as a secondary procedure to be used only when indicated as a result of cholangiography.

Kawasaki disease (mucocutaneous lymph node syndrome)

This is an acute self-limiting diffuse vasculitis of medium and small blood vessels of unknown cause. It affects most frequently children under the age of 5 years. The cardinal features are fever lasting 5 days or more, reddening and oedema followed by desquamation of the extremities, a polymorphous exanthema, bilateral conjunctival congestion and oral reddening seen in 90% of patients with 50–70% having cervical lymphadenopathy. The major complications are cardiac with up to 20% of untreated cases having coronary artery aneurisms. The mortality is 2%. There are no specific investigative findings. A platelet count of >400 $\times$ 10^9/l and an erythrocyte sedimentation rate of >50 mm are typically found in the second week of the illness. Immune complexes in serum and a decreased T8$^+$ and increased T4$^+$ helper lymphocyte count provide support for the diagnosis.

Hepatobiliary features

Kawasaki disease is often complicated by hepatobiliary abnormalities. Biochemical tests for liver were abnormal in 31% with 15% having hepatomegaly (Burns et al., 1991) and 13.7% of 117 had hydrops of the gall bladder on ultrasonography (Suddelston et al., 1987). Acute hydrops of the gall bladder, with thickening of the gall bladder wall, may be the presenting feature. Liver biopsies in five cases have shown a polymorphonuclear and eosinophilic infiltrate around and involving bile ducts in widen portal tracts, with conspicuous bile duct injury or necrosis. At autopsy additional features include vasculitis, inflammatory cell infiltrate in the sinusoids and Kupffer cell proliferation. Hepatic involvement is self limiting. Hydrops may require drainage as detailed above. Aspirin (100 mg/kg/day for 14 days) and (immunoglobulin 400 mg/Kg/day for 4 days) may prevent coronary aneurysm but its effect on the liver involvement is unknown.

Bibliography and references

Suddleson, E. A., Reid, B., Woolley, M. M. and Takahashi, M. (1987) Hydrops of the gall bladder associated with Kawasaki syndrome. J. Ped. Surg. 22, 956–959

Congenital abnormalities of the biliary tree

Chang, C. C. N. and Giullian, B. B. (1985) Congenital broncho-biliary fistula. *Radiology*, **156**, 52

Flannery, M. G. and Caster, M. P. (1956) Congenital abnormalities of the gallbladder; review of 101 cases. *Surg. Gynec. Obstet.*, **103**, 439

Kanematsu, M., Imaeda, T., Seki, M., Goto, H., Doi, H. and Shimokawa, K. (1992) Accessory bile duct draining into the stomach: case report and review. *Gastrointest. Radiol.*, **17**, 27–30

Kassner, E. G. and Klotz, D. H. (1975) Cholecystitis and calculi in a diverticulum of the gallbladder. *J. Pediatr. Surg.*, **10**, 967

Maingot, R. (1964) Anomalies of the gallbladder, bile ducts, and arteries. In: *Surgery of the Gallbladder and Bile Ducts* (eds Smith, R. and Sherlock, S.). Butterworths, London, p. 12

Muller, H., Greiner, P., Salm, R., Wenz, W. and Fielder, L. (1988) Post hepatitic cholestasis due to anomalies of the pancreatico-biliary tract in the young child. *Monatsschr. Kinderheilkd.*, **136**, 640–643

Pinter, A., Pilaszanowich, I., Schaffer, J. and Weisenbach, J. (1975) Membranous obstruction of the common bile duct. *J. Pediatr. Surg.*, **10**, 839

Udelsman, R. and Sugarbaker, P. H. (1985) Congenital duplication of the gallbladder associated with an anomalous right hepatic artery. *Am. J. Surg.*, **149**, 812

Yasbeck, S., Grignon, A. and Boisvert, J. (1985) A pseudo-choledochal cyst. *J. Can. Assoc. Radiol.*, **36**, 74

Choledochal cyst

Bova, J. G., Dempsher, C. J. and Sepulveda, G. (1983) Cholangiocarcinoma associated with Type 2 choledochal cyst. *Gastrointest. Radiol.*, **8**, 41

Eliscu, E. H. and Weiss, G. M. (1988) Hemobilia due to a pseudoaneurysm complicating a choledochal cyst. *Am. J. Radiol.*, **151**, 783–784

Howard, E. R. (1989b) Choledochal cysts. In: *Maingot's Abdominal Operations*, 9th edition (eds Schwartz, C. and Ellis, H.). Appleton-Lange, East Norwalk, Connecticut, pp. 1365–1379

Howard, E. R. (1991) Choledochal cysts. In: *Surgery of Liver Disease in Children* (eds. Howard, E. R.). Butterworth-Heinemann, Oxford, pp. 78–90

Iwai, N., Yanagihara, J., Tokiwa, K., Shimotake, T. and Nakamura, K. (1992) Congenital choledochal dilatation with emphasis on pathophysiology of the biliary tract. *Ann. Surg.*, **215**, 27–30

Komi, N., Tamara, T., Tsuge, S., Miyoshi, Y., Udaka, H. and Takehara, H. (1986) Relation of patients age to premalignant alterations in choledochal duct epithelium: histochemical and immunohistochemical studies. *J. Pediatr. Surg.*, **21**, 430–433

Komi, N., Takehara, H. and Kunitomo, K. (1989) Choledochal cyst: Anomalous arrangement of the pancreatico-biliary ductal system and biliary malignancy. *J. Gastroenterol. Hepatol.*, **4**, 63–74

Manning, P. B., Pooley, T. Z. and Oldham, K. T. (1990) Choledochocoele: An unusual form of choledochal cyst. *Pediatr. Surg. Int.*, **5**, 22–26

Nagorney, D. M., McIlbraith, D. C. and Adson, M. A. (1984) Choledochal cysts in adults: clinical management. *Surgery*, **96**, 656–663

Ng, W. D., Liu, K., Wong, M. K. *et al.* (1992) Endoscopic sphincterotomy in young patients with choledochal dilatation and a long common channel: a preliminary report. *Br. J. Surg.*, **79**, 550–552

Ohi, R., Taoita, S., Kamiyama, T., Ibrahim, H., Hayashi, Y. and Chiba, T. (1990) Surgical treatment of congenital dilatation of the bile duct with special reference to late complications after total excision. *J. Pediatr. Surg.*, **25**, 613–617

Ohi, R., Koike, N., Matsumoto, Y. *et al.* (1985) Changes of intrahepatic bile duct dilatation after surgery for congenital dilatation of the bile ducts. *J. Pediatr. Surg.*, **20**, 138

Saing, H., Tam, P. K. H., Lea, J. M. H. and Nyun, P. (1985) Surgical management of choledochal cysts: a review of 60 cases. *J. Pediatr. Surg.*, **20**, 443

Serradel, A. F., Linares, E. S. and Goepfert, R. H. (1991) Cystic dilatation of the cystic duct: a new type of biliary cyst. *Surgery*, **109**, 320–332

Tan, K. C. and Howard, E. R. (1988) Choledochal cyst: a fourteen year surgical experience with 36 patients. *Br. J. Surg.*, **75**, 892–895

Todani, T., Watanabe, Y., Toki, A. and Urushihara, N. (1987) Carcinoma related to choledochal cysts with internal drainage operations. *Surg. Gynaecol. Obst.*, **164**, 61–64

Todani, T., Watanabe, Y. and Toki, A. (1988) Reoperation for congenital choledochal cyst. *Ann. Surg.*, **207**, 142–147

Todani, K., Yatanabe, Y., Fuji, T. and Uemura, S. (1984) Anomalous arrangement of the pancreatobiliary duct system in patients with a choledochal cyst. *Am. J. Surg.*, **147**, 672

Venu, R. P., Geenen, J. E., Hogan, W. J. *et al.* (1984) The role of endoscopic retrograde pancreaticography in the diagnosis and treatment of choledochocele. *Gastroenterology*, **87**, 1144

Yamaguchi, M. (1980) Congenital choledochal cyst. Analysis of 1433 patients in the Japanese literature. *Am. J. Surg.*, **140**, 653

Yamashiro, Y., Miyano, T., Siruga, K. *et al.* (1984) Experimental study of the pathogenesis of choledochal cyst and pancreatitis, with special reference to the role of bile acids and pancreatic enzymes in the anomalous choledocho-pancreatico junction. *J. Pediatr. Gastroenterol. Nutr.*, **3**, 721

Yamauchi, S., Koga, A., Matsumoto, S., Tanaka, M. and Nakayama, F. (1987) Anomalous junction of pancreatico-biliary duct without choleductal cyst: possible risk factor for gallbladder cancer. *Am. J. Gastroenter.*, **82**, 20–24

Yeong, M. L., Nicholson, G. I. and Lee, S. P. (1982) Regression of biliary cirrhosis following choledochal cyst drainage. *Gastroenterology*, **82**, 332

Spontaneous perforation of the bile duct

Bahia, J. O., Boal, D. K. B., Karl, S. R. and Gross, G. W. (1986) Ultrasonic detection of spontaneous perforation of the extrahepatic bile ducts in infancy. *Pediatr. Radiol.*, **16**, 157

Davenport, M., Heaton, N. D. and Howard, E. R. (1991) Spontaneous perforation of the bile ducts in infants. *Br. J. Surg.*, **78**, 1068–1070

Fitzgerald, R., Parbhoo, K. and Guiney, E. (1978) Spontaneous perforation of the bile ducts in neonates. *Surgery*, **83**, 303

Haller, J. O., Condon, V. R., Berdon, W. E. *et al.* (1989) Spontaneous perforation of the common bile duct in children. *Radiology*, **172**, 621–624

Howard, E. R., Johnston, D. I. and Mowat, A. P. (1976) Spontaneous perforation of the common bile duct in infants. *Arch. Dis. Childh.*, **59**, 883

Gall-stones

Akierman, A., Elliott, P. D. and Gall, D. G. (1984) Association of cholelithiasis with total parenteral nutrition and fasting in the preterm infant. *Can. Med. Soc. J.*, **131**, 272

Boyle, R. J., Sumner, T. E. and Volberg, F. M. (1983) Cholelithiasis in a 3-week-old small premature infant. *Pediatrics*, **71**, 967

Danon, Y. L., Dinari, G., Garty, B.-Z. *et al.* (1983) Cholelithiasis in children with immunoglobulin A deficiency: a new gastroenterological syndrome. *J. Pediatr. Gastroenterol. Nutr.*, **2**, 663

Davidoff, A., Branum, G. D., Murray, E. A. *et al.* (1992) The technique of laparoscopic cholecystectomy in children. *Ann. Surg.*, **215**, 186–191

Descos, B., Bernard, O., Brunelle, F. *et al.* (1984) Pigment stones of the common bile duct in infancy. *Hepatology*, **4**, 687

Hofmann, A. F. (ed.) (1984) Physical chemistry of bile in health and disease. *Hepatology*, **4**, No. 5 (Supplement)

Howard, E. R. (1991) Gallbladder disease and cholelithiasis. In: *Surgery of Liver Disease in Children* (ed. Howard, E. R.). Butterworth-Heinemann, Oxford, pp. 102–106

Jacir, N. N., Anderson, K. D., Eicherberger, M. and Guzzetta, P. C. (1986) Cholelithiasis in infancy: resolution of gallstones in 3 of 4 infants. *J. Pediatr. Surg.*, **20**, 567–569

Klingensmith, W. C. and Cioffi-Ragan, D. T. (1988) Fetal gallstones. *Radiology*, **167**, 143–144

Lilly, J. (1980) Common bile duct calculi in infants and children. *J. Pediatr. Surg.*, **15**, 577

Ljung, R., Ivarsson, S., Nilsson, P. *et al.* (1992) Cholelithiasis during the first year of life: case reports and literature review. *Acta Paediatr.*, **81**, 69–72

Mahmoud, H., Schell, M. and Pui, C. H. (1991) Cholelithiasis after treatment for childhood cancer. *Cancer*, **67**, 1439–1442

Megison, S. M. and Votteler, T. P. (1992) Management of common bile duct obstruction associated with spontaneous perforation of the biliary tree. *Surgery*, **111**, 237–239

Pariente, D., Bernard, O., Gautier, F., Brundelle, F. and Chaumont, P. (1989) Radiological treatment of common duct lithiasis in infancy. *Pediatr. Radiol.*, **19**, 104–107

Robertson, J. F. R., Carachi, R., Sweet, E. M. and Raine, P. A. M. (1988) Cholelithiasis in childhood: a follow-up study. *J. Pediatr. Surgery*, **23**, 246–249

Saing, H., Tam, P. K. H., Choi, T. K. and Wong, J. (1988) Childhood recurrent pyogenic cholangitis. *J. Pediatr. Surg.*, **23**, 424–429

Strasberg, S. M. and Clavien, P. A. (1992) Cholecystolithiasis: lithotherapy for the 1990s. *Hepatology*, **16**, 820–839
Takiff, H. and Fonkelsrud, F. W. (1984) Gallbladder disease in childhood. *Am. J. Dis. Child.*, **138**, 565
Teele, R. L., Nussbaum, A. R., Wyly, J. B., Allred, E. N. and Emans, J. (1987) Cholelithiasis after spinal fusion for scoliosis in children. *J. Pediatr.*, **111**, 857–860
Treem, W. R., Malet, P. F., Gourley, G. R. and Hyams, J. S. (1989) Bile and stone analysis in two infants with brown pigment stones and infected bile. *Gastroenterology*, **96**, 519–523
Whittington, P. F. and Black, D. D. (1980) Cholelithiasis in premature infants treated with parenteral nutrition and frusemide. *J. Pediatr.*, **97**, 647

Cholecystitis

D'Alonzo, W. A. and Hayman, S. (1985) Biliary scintigraphy in children with sickle cell anaemia and acute abdominal pain. *Pediatr. Radiol.*, **15**, 395
Piereti, R., Aldisu, A. W. and Stevens, C. A. (1975) Acute cholecystitis in children. *Surg. Gynecol. Obstetr.*, **440**, 16
Pokorny, W. J., Saleem, M., O'Gorman, R. B., McGill, C. W. and Harberg, F. J. (1984) Cholelithiasis and cholecystitis in childhood. *Am. J. Surg.*, **148**, 472
Traynelis, V. C. and Harabovsky, E. E. (1985) Acalculous cholecystitis in a neonate. *Am. J. Dis. Child.*, **139**, 893

Non-calculous distension of the gall bladder

Benichou, J. J. and Labrune, B. (1985) Hydrops of the gallbladder in children. *Arch. Fr. Pediatr.*, **42**, 125
Chamberlain, J. W. and Hung, D. W. (1970) Acute hydrops of the gallbladder in children. *Surgery*, **68**, 899
Peevy, K. J. and Loisman, H. J. (1982) Gallbladder distension in septic neonates. *Arch. Dis. Childh.*, **57**, 75

Kawasaki disease

Bader-Meunier, B., Hadchouel, M., Fabre, M., Arnoud, M. D. and Dommergues, J. P. (1992) Intrahepatic bile duct damage in children with Kawasaki disease. *J. Pediatr.*, **120**, 750–752
Bissenden, J. G. and Hall, S. (1990) Kawasaki Syndrome: lesson for Britain. *Br. Med. J.*, **300**, 1025–1026
Burns, J. C., Mason, W. H., Glode, M. P. *et al.* (1991) Clinical and epidemiological characteristics of patients referred for evaluation of possible Kawasaki disease. *J. Pediatrics*, **118**, 680–686
Gear, J. H. S., Meyers, K. E. C. and Steele, M. (1992) Kawasaki disease manifesting with acute cholecystitis. *South Afr. Med. J.*, **81**, 31–33
Suddleson, E. A., Reid, B., Woolley, M. M. and Takahashi, M. (1987) Hydrops of the gall bladder associated with Kawasaki syndrome. *J. Ped. Surg.*, **22**, 956–959
Wirth, S., Baumann, W., Keller, K. M., Dittrich, M. and Montfering, M. (1985) Kawasaki's disease with acute hydrops of the gallbladder. Report of a case and review of the literature. *Klin. Pädiat.*, **197**, 68

Chapter 25

Liver transplantation

Introduction

Orthotopic liver transplantation (OLT) is a therapeutic option which should be considered at an early stage in any child with a life-threatening liver disease. The majority of recipients can now expect to enjoy a good quality of life with normal growth and development. The role of OLT has expanded from the treatment of chronic liver disorders to include an increasing range of liver-based metabolic disorders and selected cases of acute liver failure and, rarely, liver tumours. It has sometimes been used for children with chronic cholestatic disorders in whom the quality of life is severely impaired by pruritus or osteopenia although the severity of liver damage is not considered to be life threatening (Table 25.1). Results have improved to such an extent that careful consideration is required if children with liver disease are to be subjected to surgical procedures in the upper abdomen which might prejudice the outcome of OLT.

Liver transplantation remains a formidable surgical procedure. The recipient is likely to have one or more life-threatening complications in the perioperative or early postoperative period. Carefully supervised life-long immunosuppressive therapy is required. Close medical and surgical supervision is necessary to minimize complications. Between 10 and 20% die in the first year. The later annual death rate is estimated to be 1–2%. The longest survivor to date remains well 22 years after transplant but the longer-term prognosis is unknown. Lack of donor livers matched for size, blood group and cytomegalovirus (CMV) status remains a major difficulty with the increasing requirment for liver transplantation. The majority of paediatric recipients are less than 2 years of age. Another important limiting factor is scarcity of intensive care facilities and trained nursing staff. The precise indications, timing, optimum management of some of the intraoperative and postoperative problems, including the control of rejection remain subjects of ongoing research and assessment.

Table 25.1 Circumstances in which orthotopic liver transplantation should be considered

Chronic end-stage liver disease
Acute liver failure
Handicapping liver-based metabolic disorders
Liver tumours not treatable by hepatectomy
Poor quality of life due to chronic liver disorders

Results

Orthotopic liver transplantation was first performed in humans in 1963 but the first successful OLT was in a child of 18 months with hepatocellular carcinoma who survived for 12 months before dying of disseminated malignancy (Starzl et al., 1968). Through the 1970s major technical difficulties and problems with infection and rejection resulted in much morbidity and a high early mortality with the 1-year survival rate rarely exceeding 30%. In the 1980s, the reported 1-year survival usually exceeded 60%. In the early 1990s up to 80% of recipients with chronic liver disorders or metabolic disorders can expect to enjoy a good quality of life with normal growth and development. The steadily improving survival rate following OLT stems from technical advances, improvements in immuno-suppression, intensive care and in the management of complications and also from the increased availability of donor organs as a result of reduction hepatectomy (see below). In the Cambridge/King's College Hospital liver transplantation programme, for example, analysis of the first 100 children transplanted between December 1983 and March 1990 (Salt et al., 1992) gave an overall survival rate of 65% but in the last 2 years the 1-year survival rate was 86%. Five-year survival rates ranging from 64–78% have been reported. Even in infants under 12 months of age 1-year survival figures of 65% have been achieved although with considerable morbidity. The use of reduction hepatectomy in which a part of the right or left lobe from an older child or even an adult is used to replace the diseased liver has decreased the chances of death while waiting for a donor of similar size and blood group. In the UK in 1991 over 25% of children listed for transplantation waited more than 3 months. In North America, Australia and Japan *segmental grafts from living relatives* have been used to decrease the waiting time and allow OLT before the child's condition deteriorates substantially. Survival rates of 90% have been reported in infants in whom portoenterostomy for biliary atresia had been unsuccessful (Broelsch et al., 1991). The outcome of grafting in acute liver failure is less satisfactory with survival rates in the region of 70%. Mortality is higher because of deaths from acute cerebral oedema, infection, from multi-organ failure and, rarely, from recurrence of the primary disease.

The majority of recipients can expect to enjoy a good quality of life with normal growth and development (Stewart et al., 1991). For children who avoid complications, liver function tests return to normal and serious long-term effects of liver disease gradually regress. They show a marked increase in energy and activity and frequently good catch-up growth. Educational difficulties requiring skilled assessment and teaching are particularly frequent in those recipients with a history of cholestatic liver disease starting in infancy.

The recipient operation

The operating theatre team comprises surgeons, anaesthetists, nurses and specialized technicians with much complex monitoring and resuscitative equipment. The abdomen is opened through a bilateral subcostal incision with a vertical extension in the mid-line up to the xiphisternum. With meticulous haemostasis the hepatic artery, portal vein, bile duct and inferior vena cava below the liver are identified and separated from surrounding structures. The right lobe of the liver is turned forward and the vena cava above the liver identified. Hepatic arteries and the portal vein are ligated and divided as close to the liver as possible, leaving as much of the vessel as feasible for anastomosis. The common hepatic duct is divided near the liver. The inferior vena cava is clamped first below then above the liver and the liver removed.

During this anhepatic phase blood from the portal vein and the femoral veins are delivered to the left axillary vein using a partial cardiopulmonary bypass technique in older children, but this is not required in infants or young children.

After securing complete haemostasis the new liver is inserted with the anastomoses being completed and clamps removed in the following order: suprahepatic vena cava, portal vein, vena cava below the liver and finally the hepatic artery. Following the first two the liver is flushed to allow free egress of air, retained potassium and hydrogen ions through the other open vessels. The biliary anastomosis is then completed over a T tube or stent by direct duct to duct anastomosis if possible. If there is marked discrepancy in the size of the ducts, if they are small or if the recipient's distal duct is destroyed as in biliary atresia, a choledocho-jejunostomy in a Roux-en-Y fashion is constructed over a stent.

Lack of size-matched donor livers for children has led to the use of parts of liver from larger, older donors. Three types of reduced grafts are possible: right lobe (segments V-VIII), left lobe (segments II-IV) and left lateral (segments II-III). For the latter two the recipient's inferior vena cava is left *in situ* to provide a venous outflow. Additional vascular grafts may be required. The survival rate with such reduction hepatectomies is similar to that with full-sized grafts. Bleeding from the cut surface is a frequent problem. On the other hand hepatic artery thrombosis is be rarer. The left lateral lobe is transplanted from living donors. Complications are less frequent in recipients of such grafts perhaps because the donor liver is in better condition, there is less rejection and the procedure is performed electively. Split-liver transplantation in which the right lobe is used for one recipient and left lateral segments for another is likely to have an increasing role.

Auxiliary liver transplantation

Auxiliary transplantation, both heterotopic and orthotopic, in which the left lobe is replaced, has the advantage that the residual liver may have sufficient function to maintain life if the graft fails. A major problem is that the graft atrophies unless it receives sufficient portal blood flow and trophic factors. There are many technical difficulties. Full immunosuppression is required. In acute liver failure the technique has allowed the native liver to recover. In cirrhosis heterotopic grafting can be successful but leaves the patient at risk of malignancy. In a 13-year-old with Crigler-Najjar syndrome auxiliary orthotopic auxiliary grafting, initially from a living donor and subsequently from a cadaver, combined with portal vein banding reduced the bilirubin from over 700 μmol/litre to 70 μmol/litre despite chronic rejection of the left lobe (Whittington *et al.*, 1993).

Donor operation

The donor must be of similar size and ABO blood group. Brain death should have occurred without major hypoxia or hypotension, usually being caused by trauma, major intracranial haemorrhage or tumour. Ventilation is sustained mechanically. Biochemical tests of liver function should be normal. Ventilation and circulation (at or near normal blood pressure) must be maintained with infusions of blood and plasma as required throughout the removal. The liver is isolated and perfused *in situ* with Hartmann's solution at 4°C, then flushed with plasma-protein fraction. It is then removed with its complete arterial supply including, in children, part of the aorta, and as much of the portal vein and infrahepatic vena cava as possible. The suprahepatic vena cava is removed at its insertion into the right atrium taking with it a cuff of diaphragm. After further flushing with plasma-protein fraction the liver is placed in a bag of ice-cold saline and transported on ice to the recipient. For optimum functioning the graft should be revascularized within 6 hours but liver function may be maintained for up to 24 hours if University of Wisconsin preservation solution is used. If the liver is being reduced in size ultrasonic dissection minimizes bleeding from the cut surface.

Postoperative management

Intensive postoperative care with respiratory support to maintain good tissue oxygenation is required in all cases. The duration depends on the preoperative state and the nature and severity of the postoperative complications. The median stay in intensive care was 7 (range one to 80) days with ventilation being required for more than 1 day in over 80% of recipients in a recent series (Salt *et al.*, 1992). If the graft is successful liver function is rapidly restored as evidenced by bile production, a normal serum bicarbonate concentration with a fall in serum potassium with the international normalized ratio (INR) falling progressively from 12 hours post-transplantation to normal in 2–3 days. The aspartate transaminase falls from levels of 1000 IU/litre in whole grafts and up to 3000 IU/litre in reduced grafts on the second day to normal levels within 1 week. As soon as the ileus clears oral feeding can begin. Broad spectrum antibiotics are given for 48 hours. In the immediate postoperative period inevitable areas of concern as well as graft function are sepsis, fluid balance, blood loss, coagulation, blood glucose, pulmonary, renal and gastrointestinal dysfunction, haematological and electrolyte abnormalities and hypertension. Alimentary bleeding and cardiac arrhythmias are also common. Central nervous system status is of particular concern in patients transplanted for acute liver failure or if there is severe graft dysfunction, caused, for example, by hepatic artery and portal vein block, after transplantation. Intravenous feeding is commenced on the second postoperative day and continued until oral feeding is possible. The haematocrit is maintained at around 30% since higher values may be associated with hepatic artery thrombosis. Physiological monitoring is continuous with laboratory investigations at 1, 4 or 24 hourly intervals. Drains, catheters and venous lines are removed as early as possible, the tips being sent for bacterial cultures together with secretions, discharges and urine. Adequate sedation and analgesia is essential at all times.

On returning to the wards monitoring is less intense. Liver function tests, clotting screens, electrolyte determination and drug concentrations are checked less frequently. The interval can usually be extended to weekly by 2 months if there have been no major problems.

Immunosuppression

A combination of three or four immunosuppressants are used to achieve optimum immunosuppression with minimal side-effects. Cyclosporin A and corticosteroids with or without azathioprine, antilymphocytic globulins, including monoclonal anti-T cell antibodies (OKT3), are used to prevent or control rejection. The exact details of anti-rejection regimens vary from centre to centre. *Cyclosporin* is the mainstay of maintenance immunosuppression. It causes a reversible inhibition of T lymphocyte-mediated immune responses by suppression of interleukin-2 production. It has no effect on phagocytes or on haemopoiesis. Dose or tissue concentration-related side-effects of cyclosporin include acute and chronic renal failure, hepatic dysfunction, hypertension, fluid retention, convulsions, tremor, gastrointestinal disturbance, paraesthesia in the hands and feet, hirsutism, haemolysis and thrombocytopenia. The propensity to hepatic or kidney damage is potentiated by other noxious factors such as ischaemia or nephrotoxic antibiotics. In

North America and much of Europe cyclosporin is administered 12 hours before grafting and continued thereafter. In the UK cyclosporin is usually first used on the second post-transplant day because of the high incidence of acute renal failure when used earlier. Cyclosporin A is given intravenously until intestinal absorption is established. The aim is to maintain the concentration within a 'therapeutic' range which depends on the method of measurement used. The optimum blood level of cyclosporin to give maximum immunosuppression with the least risk of long-term side-effects has still to be established. Normal liver and renal function with no side-effects are the immediate clinical objectives.

High doses of prednisolone are given intraoperatively and continued in the immediate postoperative period. Long-term azathioprine is started immediately postoperatively. Antilymphocytic globulin, if used, is given from day 2 to 12. In the early weeks there is a very slender margin of safety between giving too much immunosuppressive therapy with an enhanced risk of infection and other toxic effects and giving too little and incurring rejection. Gradually over a period of weeks the dose of prednisolone is reduced while liver function tests remain normal.

Complications

Complications are those of major surgery with multiple vascular and biliary anastomosis, of rejection and side-effects of long-term anti-rejection drugs (see above). In the *immediate postoperative period* problems include bleeding from the liver bed, respiratory difficulties associated with massive infusions during the operative period, particularly if there is a degree of renal failure.

There may be primary graft failure. Technical imperfections may lead to leaks from vascular or biliary anastomoses. Hepatic artery and/or portal vein thrombosis and bile duct obstruction may occur. There may be massive losses of ascitic fluid. *Graft failure* with deteriorating liver function may be due to rejection, infection of the liver including hepatitis B, C and non-A,B,C hepatitis, sepsis, bile duct obstruction, hepatic artery and portal vein thrombosis or hepatic ischaemia. Up to 40% of recipients require regrafting for primary non-function, vascular thrombosis or chronic rejection.

The patient is at risk from longer-term surgical complications affecting the anastomosed channels (stenosis and leaks) and medical complications, particularly related to the life-long requirement for immunosuppression. The emotional strain on the family is immense. The child is likely to experience a number of life-threatening complications, particularly in the immediate postoperative weeks. Periods of elation and exhilaration may be followed by periods of despair and sadness as new complications develop. In older children anxiety and depression can be major problems. In many countries the family will face hugh costs for the procedure, for long-term supervision and for drugs.

Specific complications

Infection

Viral, bacterial, fungal or protozoal infections cause significant morbidity and mortality. Although cytomegalovirus, Enterobacteriaceae, *Candida* or *Aspergillus* species and *Pneumocystis carinii* are the organisms within these classes of pathogens most frequently causing problems virtually any organism may be pathogenic. The frequency and severity of infection is increased by poor pre-transplantation nutritional status, high doses of corticosteroids, the use of antilymphocyte antibodies, intra-abdominal bleeding, poor graft perfusion and bile stasis. Infections develop as a result of invasion by endogenous organisms, activation of latent infections, particularly viral, or are introduced with the allograft, blood products or through intravenous lines, catheters or drains. The incidence is very high early in the course when immunosuppressive therapy is most intense and technical complications are most common and also in the patient with chronic rejection. Opportunistic infections and community-acquired infections are always a danger. Septicaemia, pneumonia, abscess formation, cholangitis, disseminated viral infection and opportunistic bacterial and fungal infections may occur at any time in the course. Specific antimicrobial treatment is determined by isolating the pathogen, often difficult with invasive fungi. In life-threatening visceral or cerebral viral infections, e.g. adenovirus type 5, immunosuppression must be stopped.

To minimize infection full immunization, including *S. pneumoniae, H. influenzae varicella*, prior to grafting is desirable. In CMV negative recipients the donor organ and blood products should be CMV negative. If not ganciclovir (5 mg/kg twice daily) from 7 to 28 days after transplantation appears to minimize serious infection. The place of prophylactic hyperimmune globulin is more contentious. Selective bowel decontamination for 3 weeks following grafting, with tobramycin and amphotericin, appears to reduce endogenously derived infections. Acyclovir decreases herpetic infections and controls herpes zoster infections. Prolonged co-trimoxazole prevents *Pneumocystis carinii* infections. Over 80% of patients grafted for chronic HBV infection become chronic carriers, with up to 40% losing the graft from a rapidly progressive fibrosing cholestatic hepatitis, acute hepatitis or chronic hepatitis. Curiously coexistent HDV infection appears to be relatively protective. Hyperimmune globulin in the anhepatic phase and continued for up to 12 months appears to delay the appearance of HBV infection and reduce its impact on the graft but its role is still being evaluated.

A worrying complication is Epstein-Barr virus-related lymphoproliferative disease which is frequently fatal unless immunosuppressive drugs are stopped. In one paediatric series an incidence of over 2.8% per year was reported (Malatak *et al.*, 1991). This has been reported as a complication with the most recently introduced immunosuppressive agent FK 506. Lymphoma and other malignant disease may be more common in recipients of anti-rejection drugs than in the normal population.

Rejection

Rejection takes three forms: hyperacute or fulminant rejection, acute cellular rejection and chronic rejection (also called ductopaenic or irreversible). *Hyperacute* or *fulminant* rejection is very rare, is thought to be antibody mediated, occurs within 1–3 days or transplantation and can only be treated by regrafting. *Acute cellular rejection* episodes are particularly frequent early in the course after liver transplantation before host macrophages and dendritic cells replace those of the donor in the hepatic sinusoids. Clinically significant episodes, characterized by fever, malaise or asymptomatic rise in aspartate transaminase or gamma-glutamyl transpeptidase levels, occur between 4 and 14 days after grafting in up to 70% of recipients. Rejection must be suspected in any patient with deteriorating liver function.

Distinguishing acute rejection, which is treated with increased doses of corticosteroids and/or antilymphocytic antibodies, from systemic or hepatic infection (viral, bacterial, fungal and/or protozoal) is a major challenge. The differential diagnosis includes major complications requiring surgical management such as bile duct obstruction, hepatic artery thrombosis and/or portal vein thrombosis. Ultrasonographic and invasive imaging techniques may be required to demonstrate patency of these vessels. Drug toxicity or graft-versus-host disease must also be considered.

Liver biopsy is necessary for diagnosis and to exclude other causes of acute graft dysfunction. The immunological reaction in rejection appears to be directed against bile duct epithelial cells and vascular endothelium rather than towards the hepatocytes. In acute rejection the liver biopsy shows a mixed portal tract infiltrate with bile duct damage and an endothelitis of hepatic and/or portal vein branches.

Treatment   Episodes of rejection are treated with methyl prednisolone (500 mg/m^2/day or 125 mg/10 kg) for 3 days followed by prednisolone 2 mg/kg/day reducing by 0.25 mg/kg every 3 days. Steroid resistant episodes are treated with antilymphocytic immunoglobulin (OKT3). Intensified immunosuppression reverses rejection in up to 80% of cases but the remainder will go on to chronic rejection unless there is further intensification of immunosuppression which currently entails the replacement of cyclosporin by the newer agent FK 506, an antifungal antibiotic with impressive immunosuppressive properties. Its clinical efficacy and toxicity are currently being assessed in prospective studies largely in adults. It is available for children in Europe on a named patient basis only. Other immunosuppressive agents currently being assessed include rapamycin, RS-61443, deoxyspergualin, thalidomide, and prostaglandin analogues, all of which affect a number of aspects of lymphocyte function, and monoclonal antibodies against proinflammatory cytokines or intercellular adhesion molecules.

Chronic rejection (also called ductopaenic or irreversible rejection) is characterized by progressive loss of interlobular bile ducts and arteriopathy with occlusion of arteries by foamy cell infiltrate of the intima. It may follow episodes of acute rejection or occur indolently with progressive deterioration in liver function tests. There is destruction of liver tissue for which regrafting is usually required although in a few patients the process can be arrested with FK 506.

Factors affecting the outcome of transplantation

Contraindications

Contraindications for transplantation are in a state of constant flux as medical and surgical advances overcome particular problems. At present metastatic malignancy, intractable extrahepatic sepsis, particularly fungal and permanent neurological damage, are considered absolute contra-indications. Relative contraindications include complex congenital heart disease, major intra-abdominal vascular anomalies, advanced renal or lung disease and severe short bowel syndrome. The place of transplantation in patients with cirrhosis due to hepatitis B is controversial since the recurrence of viral infection, with a high incidence of liver damage, cannot be reliably prevented. Its onset can be delayed by hyperimmune gamma-globulin. Preliminary studies suggest that hepatitis C will behave similarly. The position of liver transplantation in the patient who is positive for HIV is even more contentious.

Age

Successful liver transplant has been reported in the first month of life but results in infancy are less satisfactory (1-year survival rates of 60–70%) than in older children in whom results are better than in adults.

Portal vein obstruction

If the portal vein or its main branches are occluded liver transplantation is impossible unless the obstruction can be overcome by disobliteration or by grafting. This has been done but is associated with an increased incidence of postoperative complications.

Prior intra-abdominal surgery

Intra-abdominal surgery in patients with cirrhosis is usually associated with the development of fragile, ectopic portosystemic shunts around adhesions. These add to the difficulties of surgery particularly if they are in the area of the portahepatis. Such surgery has proved a major problem in adults and older children but its deleterious effect is less clear in the young child.

Bleeding oesophageal varices

Variceal bleeding should if possible be controlled by injection sclerotherapy prior to transplantation to prevent bleeding in the immediate post-transplant period.

Evaluation of candidates for liver transplantation

As soon as an infant or child is recognized to have a life-threatening acute and chronic liver disorder referral to a paediatric hepatologist working with a children's liver transplantation service is advisable. With early referral less hazardous treatment may be possible, potential complications may be minimized and more time is available to find a suitable donor and to help the family to prepare for the procedure. The paediatric hepatologist's responsibility is to confirm the primary diagnosis and to estimate its severity and likely evolution with other forms of therapy. For many liver disorders there is a relatively small data base on which to base an estimate of the relative risk of OLT versus non-transplant management. Developing such criteria is a major challenge. Hepatology units should be seen as serving an academic function which will include the development of the data base which allows more precise determination of the exact indications for transplantation. Nevertheless at present a rational plan can be developed for most patients on the basis of current knowledge, the anticipated availability of donors and transplant facilities.

If transplantation requires serious consideration full assessment is essential (Table 25.2). The surgical, anaesthetic and intensive care team will assess the particular operative risks for the patient. Evaluation by the nutritionist, psychologist, nurse specialist, social worker and transplantation coordinator is also essential. The whole procedure and its known complications will be repeatedly discussed with the parents (Table 25.3). Before reaching a decision the parents must be fully advised of known short-term risks of this procedure, the necessity for time-consuming, invasive and frequently painful investigations, both before and after transplant, the necessity for life-long medical and surgical supervision because of possible problems with anastomoses and to supervise life-long immunosuppressive therapy. They must know that the long-term prognosis is uncertain. Particular social difficulties likely to be encountered by the family are identified and minimized by social work. These may include problems with finance, employment, accommodation, travel and care for other family members. Anxieties are identified and discussed. In this way the family and the support team become better equipped to cope

Table 25.2 Assessment of potential liver transplant recipients

Review of medical/surgical record, histology and radiology
Complete history and physical examination
Height/weight/skinfold thickness, mid-upper arm circumference, head, chest, abdominal circumference
Clinical photograph
Laboratory data:
   Biochemical tests of liver function, bilirubin, total and direct, cholesterol, ammonia, creatinine, urea,
      sodium, potassium, calcium, phosphate, magnesium, zinc, uric acid
   Prothrombin time, full blood count, blood group
   HLA status
   Urinalysis
   Bacterial cultures: skin, nose, throat, urine and blood
   Viral serology and culture (if relevant) for CMV, EBV, HIV, hepatitis B and C, herpes simplex, chicken
      pox, measles
   Toxoplasma, aspergillosis antibody
   Specific diagnostic tests for causes of liver disorder
   Vitamin E concentration
   Blood gas
   Lung function studies if relevant
Scanning and radiological investigations:
   Chest, wrist and abdominal X-ray
   Ultrasonography of the portal vein and biliary system
   Coeliac and superior mesenteric angiography in suspected portal vein obstruction and combined with
      venacavography in biliary atresia with sub-diaphragmatic anomalies, particularly polysplenia
   Abdominal and chest CT scan (not all cases)
ECG
Endoscopy for oesophageal varices
Lung function studies
Social and psychiatric assessment

Table 25.3 Factors to be considered by parents contemplating liver transplantation

(1) Known short-term risks
(2) Repeated time-consuming, frequently painful investigations
    which are sometimes potentially dangerous, both before and
    after transplant
(3) Life-long medical and surgical supervision for:
      control of immunosuppressive therapy and its side-effects
      complications of vascular and biliary anastomosis
      recurrence of primary diseases
(4) Unknown long-term prognosis

with the stresses associated with liver transplantation and its acute short-term complications.

Timing of transplantation

The timing of liver transplantation is determined by consideration of the child's prospects with other forms of treatment, the anticipated availability of a donor and of transplant facilities and the likely outcome of OLT. The results are better in children transplanted after 1 year of age (or >10 kg) and if the procedure is done electively rather than as an emergency. Recipients who are less growth-retarded have fewer serious infections, surgical complications and require fewer re-transplantations and have a lower mortality than children with severe growth retardation. To operate on a patient with chronic liver disease near death and requiring intensive care increases the already high operative risks. On the other hand, unsuccessful transplantation at the onset of hepatic decompensation may deprive the child of many years of normal activity. The course of many liver disorders may be unpredictably punctuated by life-threatening complications which require very expert management if full recovery is to occur. Selecting the appropriate time for surgery is difficult in any of the four categories of liver disease in which liver grafting is now an option. Some guides to prognosis in particular liver disorders are given below.

Timing of transplantation in particular disorders

Liver transplantation in cirrhosis

Liver transplantation should be considered at the first appearance of complications or the abnormalities in liver function tests listed in Table 25.4 in any child with cirrhosis, irrespective of the cause.

Table 25.4 Indications for liver transplantation in chronic liver disease

Ascites refractory to fluid restriction and diuretics
Alimentary bleeding not controlled by sclerotherapy or propranalol
Spontaneous bacterial peritonitis
Growth retardation
Loss of muscle bulk
Hepatic encephalopathy
Hypoxia due to pulmonary shunt
Prothrombin ratio (international normalized ratio [INR]) >1.4
Cholesterol <2.6 mmol/l (100 mg/dl)
Indirect bilirubin >102 μmol/l (6 mg/dl)
Impaired lidocaine metabolism to MEGX (monoethylglycinexylidide) [<10 μg/L 30 mins. after IV 1 mg/kg]

In the following disorders additional factors require consideration.

Extrahepatic biliary atresia

Biliary atresia accounts for 50–70% of children transplanted in most centres. If, following portoenterostomy, infants remain icteric the rate at which cirrhosis and its complications develop varies from case to case with a mean age at death of 14 months. Transplantation should be undertaken as soon as growth arrest resistant to comprehensive dietary support occurs or at the earliest signs of complications of cirrhosis. Transplantation may be required for refractory cholangitis. Transplantation may be impossible if the inferior vena cava is absent or if there are major vascular anomalies affecting the portal vein. Prior surgery at the portahepatis does make transplantation more difficult but the results of liver grafting in biliary atresia are probably no different from those in children transplanted for other reasons. This in part may be because after unsuccessful portoenterostomy these children face certain death from liver disease and are transplanted before decompensation of cirrhosis is as severe as in other conditions in which the prognosis is less clear or in which spontaneous arrest of cirrhosis may occur. Nevertheless, complicated modification of portoenterostomy and repeated surgery at the portahepatis should be avoided.

Biliary hypoplasia

Cirrhosis is a rare complication particularly in the syndromic form. The majority of those transplanted have had inappropriate portoenterostomy performed in the mistaken belief that the patient had biliary atresia. There is no good evidence of increase growth rate following OLT in this condition.

Acute liver failure

The management of fulminant hepatic failure or late onset hepatic encephalopathy or severe acute liver failure with no encephalopathy but severe coagulopathy (prothrombin ratio >4) should include consideration of liver transplantation since the mortality without transplantation is over 70% (except when due to galactosaemia or fructosaemia). Referral as soon as it is confirmed that the prothrombin is prolonged by more than 6 seconds is essential even if the severity of encephalopathy seems mild. Other elements in management include an accurate diagnosis of the liver disorder and the encephalopathy with skilled intensive care to minimize the aggravating factors and control complications, particularly cerebral oedema, circulatory and renal failure and infections.

Who will benefit from OLT for fulminant hepatic failure and when to transplant

Liver transplantation must take place against a background of full intensive care including measurement of systemic and pulmonary blood pressure and intracranial pressure and maintenance of a normal cerebral perfusion. In analysis of children treated at King's College Hospital in the last decade those aged less than 2 years or with an INR ratio of >4 had a 90% mortality without transplantation. Such children should be listed for grafting irrespective of the degree of encephalopathy or apparent cause of liver disease. In studies of patients of all ages at King's College Hospital those with grade 3 or 4 encephalopathy due to drugs or non-A, non-B hepatitis and those with subacute hepatic failure have survival rates without transplantation ranging from 10–20% (O'Grady et al., 1989). Patients with type A hepatitis had a 66% recovery rate and those with hepatitis B a 40% recovery rate. With cerebral oedema, cerebral oedema associated with renal failure or metabolic acidosis the survival rates were lower. Patients with a INR ratio of 4 or more should be transplanted if any of three of the following are present transplantation is indicated:

(1) age 2 to 10 years,
(2) non-A, non-B or drug hepatitis,
(3) jaundiced encephalopathy interval >7 days,
(4) serum bilirubin of >300 μmol/litre.

Liver-based metabolic disorders

In those disorders causing liver damage (Table 25.5a) the indications for transplantation are similar to those in any other form of cirrhosis or fulminant liver failure, with the exceptions referred to below. Note that disorders which are lysosomal or haemopoietic, such as erythropoietic porphyria, are not arrested by OLT.

Table 25.5 Liver transplantation for metabolic disorders

(a) *End stage liver disease or premalignant changes*
Alpha-1 antitrypsin deficiency
Wilson's disease
Tyrosinaemia
Galactosaemia
Haemochromatosis
Glycogen storage disease, IV
Cystic fibrosis
Defects of fatty acid oxidation
Glycogen storage disease types 1 and 3

(b) *for major extrahepatic features*
Familial hypercholesterolaemia
Primary hyperoxaluria
Crigler-Najjar syndrome
Factor VIII deficiency
Protein C deficiency
Tyrosinaemia
Urea cycle defects
Glycogen storage disease type 1

Wilson's Disease

Patients with fulminant liver failure or with decompensated cirrhosis and a hepatic prognostic index of >8 (see Chapter 17) do not survive with penicillamine therapy alone and should be transplanted as soon as a donor becomes available. Those with an index of 5 to 8 should be treated with penicillamine and zinc sulphate, 6 hours apart, at 12-hourly interval and transplanted unless the index, checked at weekly intervals, has fallen to 5 before a donor becomes available. Those with an index of 5 survive with medical management but may require skilled care of cirrhosis for up to 6 months. Liver function tests may take 4 to 5 years to return to normal. Transplantation is necessary in adolescents who relapse because chelation therapy has been stopped.

Tyrosinaemia

Hereditary tyrosinaemia is considered in detail in Chapter 15. Unless the disease is controlled by diet and nitro-trifluoromethylbenzoyl-cyclohexanedione (Lindstedt *et al.*, 1992) progressive hepatocellular damage is associated with a high propensity to hepatoma formation by 5 years of age. Approximately 60% of those presenting by 2 months of age are dead by 12 months. In these OLT should be performed as soon as possible if liver failure is severe or when growth arrest occurs, usually between 3 and 8 months of age. For those with onset between 2 and 6 months similar considerations are pertinent since 25% are dead by 1 year. In the more chronic forms liver transplantation should be considered by the second birthday because of the high risk of hepatic malignancy spreading to tissues outside the liver. If the ultrasound and CT scan are normal transplantation can be delayed. It is frequently impossible to differentiate between malignant transformation as opposed to regeneration nodules in the liver of a child with tyrosinaemia by ultrasound, CT scanning or angiography.

Hepatocellular carcinoma may be present with the alpha-fetoprotein concentration normal; conversely high serum concentrations are present with no malignancy in the resected liver. A sharp rise in concentration has been considered an indicator of malignancy but this is not invariably true. OLT may be necessary also in patients with recurrent episodes of acute liver insufficiency or for repeated neurological crises. Combined liver and renal transplantation is advised if there is severe glomerular failure with a glomerular filtration rate $<40 \, ml/min/1.73 \, m^2$. Liver transplantation allows the patient to take a normal diet, prevents further neurological crises but does not correct the excessive urinary excretion of succinylacetone which is presumed to be renal in origin. It is not clear whether such patients are more prone to progressive renal failure than other OLT recipients receiving cyclosporin A.

Alpha-1 antitrypsin deficiency, PIZZ

Rarely transplantation is required for progressive cholestasis in infancy. In the majority of infants jaundice clears. Half of those with cirrhosis die in the first decade. OLT must be considered when jaundice recurs or there is a fall in albumin although the interval to death may be as long as four years (Psacharopoulos et al., 1983). Whether OLT will prevent emphysema is unknown but in one patient followed for 15 years it had not appeared.

Cystic fibrosis

The results of liver transplantation in over 30 patients with *predominantly liver involvement* appear to be as good as in other liver disorders with as yet no evidence that infective complications other than *Pseudomonas* and aspergillosis are particular problems. Some recipients experience a significant improvement in pulmonary function. Since there is some epidemiological evidence suggesting that cirrhosis may cause early death from lung failure OLT should be considered at the onset of complications of cirrhosis.

Cholesteryl ester storage disease

Liver transplantation undertaken for uncontrollable bleeding from oesophageal varices in a 14-year-old with cholesteryl ester storage disease failed to prevent elevation of serum triglycerides. Prolonged follow-up will be required to assess its effect on pulmonary, vascular or renal complications of this condition.

Progressive familial intrahepatic cholestasis

These presumed genetic disorders of unknown pathogenesis cause death from cirrhosis or from heart failure. In one subset the low serum apolipoprotein A-1 concentration is corrected by OLT.

Haemochromatosis

Haemochromatosis of the idiopathic adult HLA-related form is controlled by venesection but this may not decrease the risk of hepatocellular carcinoma for which OLT may be indicated. It is rarely required for end-stage liver disease. In neonatal haemochromatosis excess iron is deposited in the same tissues as in the adult form. It is often rapidly fatal. It may represent a number of disorders with different pathogenesis with possibly differing response to OLT.

Glycogen storage diseases

Liver transplantation corrects the metabolic and growth effect of these disorders. It should be considered in infants with very severe GSD type I disease which cannot be controlled by diet and in adults with malignant disease confined to the liver. Its role in those with adenomata, which may be stable for up to 5 years, has not been defined. In type IV disease which is characterized by cirrhosis with or without evidence of cardiac or brain involvement, transplantation at 20–46 months of age appeared to prevent accumulation of amylopectin-like polysaccharide in the transplanted livers, decreased amylopectin in myocardial biopsies and no progression of cardiac disease up to 6 years later. In contrast death from heart failure developing at 15 months of age occurred in an infant grafted at 9 months.

Survival to the age of 13 years with a good quality of life and no complications of cirrhosis provides further evidence of the heterogeneity of this condition.

Transferase deficiency galactosaemia galactose-1-phosphate uridyl transferase deficiency

A few patients with very advanced cirrhosis because of late diagnosis become candidates for liver transplantation in childhood or early adult life.

Transplantation in disorders causing no liver damage but irreversible injury to other vital organs.

Where the liver is structurally normal but the patient with a liver-based metabolic disorder is at risk from irreparable damage to vital tissue, i.e. the brain, heart or kidneys, transplantation should be undertaken when it is clear that less hazardous therapy will fail (Table 25.5b). Here the hepatologist will need guidance from colleagues specializing in metabolic disorders.

Primary hyperoxaluria type I

Primary hyperoxaluria type I is an autosomal recessive disorder with deficient peroxisomal alanine:glyoxylate aminotransferase (EC 2.1.44) activity leading to renal and cardiovascular damage. There is both genetic and phenotypic heterogeneity. Initially renal transplantation was attempted for this disorder but calcium oxalate caused early graft failure. This led to the introduction of liver and kidney grafting which has proved successful. Another approach is to perform a liver transplantation then to proceed to renal transplantation when the oxalate pool is diminished so as to avoid renal allograft failure.

Unfortunately severe bone disease may develop in the interval. It is important that transplantation be performed before severe cardiovascular disease arises due to systemic oxalosis. It essential to maintain a very high urinary output for the first few days post-transplant when the renal oxalate load is still very high.

Crigler-Najjar type I

Crigler-Najjar Type I is a heterogeneous disorder characterized by a complete failure of bilirubin glucuronide formation in the liver. Severely affected patients develop kernicterus unless this is prevented by exchange transfusion in the neonatal period and by phototherapy given for up to 12 hours each night. As the child gets older phototherapy becomes less effective and OLT becomes necessary to prevent brain damage which can occur at any age during exacerbations of hyperbilirubinaemia associated with intercurrent infections. OLT should be considered before phototherapy ceases to be practical, effective or the jaundice socially unacceptable, possibly about 4 years of age.

Primary hypercholesterolaemia

Primary hypercholesterolaemia caused by homozygous deficiency of low-density lipoprotein (LDL) receptors treated by diet, drugs, LDL plasmapheresis or ileal bypass may still progress to intractable myocardial ischaemia. In such patients liver transplantation produces an 80% decrease in lipids but usually the patient also requires cardiac transplantation or coronary artery bypass.

Coagulopathies

Haemophilia A, haemophilia B and protein C deficiency have all been treated successfully by liver transplantation. In haemophilia OLT has been undertaken for end-stage liver disease induced by viral contaminated blood products.

Urea cycle disorders

Urea cycle disorders show considerable genetic and phenotypic variability with a continuous spectrum of clinical expression. Those with neonatal onset frequently die or develop mental retardation before liver transplantation is considered or becomes a reasonable prospect with current techniques. Cases of later onset have a better prognosis with strict dietary and drug control. OLT has been performed in such cases when it is clear that dietary management is ineffective but there is no significant brain damage. OLT prevents hyperammonaemic crises but arginine and citrulline supplements may be required.

Malignant liver tumours

Patients with suspected hepatic tumours should be referred to centres with experience in the diagnosis, chemotherapeutic and surgical management of such lesions. Total resection, usually in conjunction with a course of chemotherapy is the only effective treatment for malignant lesions (Chapter 23). If hepatic lobectomy is not possible even after cytotoxic administration, liver transplantation should be considered provided metastases cannot be demonstrated outside the liver using scintigraphy, CT scanning, arteriography and laparotomy. Even if these investigations are negative metastases may appear. Six of 12 children with hepatoblastoma were reported to be alive with no evidence of recurrence 24 to 70 months after transplantation. Six died, three of tumour recurrence. A 50% 5-year survival was noted in another study. Unifocal tumours with no extrahepatic spread had a better prognosis than multifocal or metastatic lesions. Serial serum alpha-fetoprotein determination is helpful in assessing the response to chemotherapy, falling to normal with complete resection but rising if metastases develop.

With hepatocellular carcinoma treatment is even less satisfactory. The average duration of disease from diagnosis to death was 4.2 months in a recent series. Resection is rarely possible but long-term survival (>5 years) has been reported following both resection and transplantation in 10–18% in two recent large series, predominantly in adults. Early stages of hepatocellular carcinoma arising in a cirrhotic liver and fibrolamellar lesions are highly represented in the survivors.

Transplantation because of poor quality of life but with no life-threatening complications

In some infants and children with chronic cholestatic disorders constant pruritus interfering with play, study and sleep makes life miserable for the child and his family. If the pruritus cannot be relieved by cholestyramine, ursodeoxycholic acid, rifampicin and other enzyme inducers or by light therapy consideration should be given to partial bile drainage as an alternative to transplantation. Symptoms may be so severe that parents opt for liver transplantation even with a full knowledge of its current risks. Osteopenia with frequent painful fractures despite of meticulous dietary supplements and control of calcium and phosphate metabolism may provoke the same response.

In patients with good synthetic function and no problems from portal hypertension it is easier to advocate OLT if the disorder is considered likely to progress to decompensated cirrhosis at a later date. In the more common disorder syndromic paucity of the interlobular bile ducts in which death from liver disease occurs in less than 20% the decision is more contentious, particularly since transplantation is unlikely to increase growth rate, another major parental concern in this condition.

Improving the outcome of liver transplantation

Paediatricians have a key role in the early recognition and referral of infants and children with life-threatening acute and chronic liver disorders. With early referral less hazardous treatment may be possible, potential complications may be minimized and more time is available to find a suitable donor. Prior to transplantation a full programme of immunization against viruses, *Strep. pneumoniae* and *Haemophilus influenza* should be instituted. Avoiding unnecessary hospitalization and/or antimicrobials before transplantation will reduce the risk of being colonized by resistant organisms. Expert care of complications of cirrhosis such as bleeding varices and ascites will help to bring the patient to transplantation in better shape and minimize postoperative problems. Nutritional support in the form of calories, proteins, vitamin supplements if necessary given by nasogastric feeding and rarely intravenously may allow the patient to tolerate transplantation more satisfactorily. Every effort should be made to avoid intra-abdominal surgery in patients who are potential candidates. Surgery in the area of the porta hepatis causes particular difficulties. The parents and, as far as possible, the child should be fully informed of the likely course and possible problems so that they and the family can make the appropriate plans. Post-transplantation early treatment of bacterial, fungal and viral infections such as herpes, chicken pox and cytomegalovirus is essential, however small the dose of immunosuppressives. Scarcity of donors is still a major obstacle to optimizing this therapy in infants and young children. Paediatricians and workers in the intensive care facilities must recognize that organ donation is a potentially positive step for some donors' families as well as being life saving for the recipient. Advances in surgical techniques, donor organ preservation, immunosuppressive regimens and antimicrobial measures are subjects of ongoing research which will continue to improve outcome.

Bibliography and references

General

Burdelski, M., Oellerich, M., Lamesch, P. *et al.* (1987) Evaluation of quantitative liver function tests in liver donors. *Transplant. Proc.*, **19**, 3838–3839

Calne, R. Y. (ed.) (1987) *Liver Transplantation – The Cambridge/Kings Experience*, 2nd edn. Grune and Stratton, New York

Iwatsuki, S., Starzl, T. E., Todo, S. *et al.* (1988) Experience in 1,000 liver transplants under Cyclosporin-steroid therapy: A survival report. *Transplant. Proc.*, **20S**, 498–504

Kalayoglu, M., Sollinger, H. W., Stratta, R. J. *et al.* (1988) Extended preservation of the liver for clinical transplantation. *Lancet*, **ii**, 617–619

Kawasaki, S., Makuuchi, M., Ishizone, S., Matsunami, H., Terada, M., Kawarazaki, H. (1992) Liver regeneration in recipients and donors after transplantation. *Lancet*, **339**, 580–581

Lindstedt, S., Holme, E., Lock, E. A., Hjalmarson, O. and Strandvik, B. (1992) Treatment of hereditary tyrosinaemia by inhibition of 4-hydroxyphenylpyruvate dioxygenase. *Lancet*, **340**, 813–817

National Institute of Health Consensus Development Conference statement (1984) Liver transplantation – 20–23 June, 1983. *Hepatology*, **4**(suppl.), 107–110

Potter, D., Peachey, T., Eason, J., Ginsburg, R. and O'Grady, J. (1989) Intracranial pressure monitoring during orthotopic liver transplantation for acute liver failure. *Transplant Proc.*, **21**, 3528

Psacharopoulos, H. T., Mowat, A. P., Cooke, P. J. L., Carlile, P. A., Portmann, B. and Rodeck, C. H. (1983) Outcome of liver disease associated with alpha-1 antitrypsin deficiency. Implications for genetic counselling and antenatal diagnosis. *Arch. Dis. Childh.*, **58**, 882–887

Shaw, B. W., Wood, R. P., Stratts, R. J., Pillen, T. J. and Langnas, A. N. (1989) Stratifying the causes of death in liver transplant recipients. An approach to improving survival. *Arch. Surg.*, **124**, 895–900

Starzl, T. E., Groth, C. T., Brettschneider, L. *et al.* (1968) Orthotopic homotransplantation of the human liver. *Ann. Surg.*, **168**, 392

Starzl, T. E., Demetris, A. J. and Van Thiel, D. (1989) Liver Transplantation. *N. Engl. J. Med.*, **321**, 1014–1021, 1092–1099

Todo, S., Fung, J. J., Starzl, T. E. *et al.* (1990) Liver, kidney and thoracic organ transplantation under FK 506. *Ann. Surg.*, **212**, 295–307

Ventataramanan, R., Jain, A., Warty, V. S. *et al.* (1991) Pharmacokinetics of FK 506 in transplantation patients. *Transplant Proc.*, **23**, 2736–2740

Paediatric

Baker, A., Ross-Russell, R. and Mowat, A. P. (1992) Intensive care management of children following orthotopic liver transplantation. *Br. J. Intens. Care*, **2**, 229–240

Bhaduri, B. R., Tan, K. C., Humphreys, S. *et al.* (1990) Graft-versus-host disease after orthotopic liver transplantation in a child. *Transplant. Proc.*, **22**, 2378–2380

Busuttil, R. W., Seu, P., Millis, J. M. *et al.* (1991) Liver transplantation in children. *Ann. Surg.*, **213**, 48–57

Chiyende, J. and Mowat, A. P. (1992) Liver Transplantation in children. *Arch. Dis. Child.*, **67**, 1124–1127

Lloyd-Still, J. D. (1991) Impact of orthotopic liver transplantation on mortality from pediatric liver disease. *J. Pediatr. Gastroenterol. Nutr.*, **12**, 305–309

Moukarzel, A. A., Najm, I., Vargas, J., McDairmid, J., Busuttil, R. W. and Ament, M. E. (1990) Effect of nutritional status on outcome of orthotopic liver transplantation in pediatric patients. *Transplant. Proc.*, **22**, 1560–1563

Mowat, A. P. (1993) Indications for liver transplantation in childhood. *J. Transplant.* (in press)

Otte, J. B., Yandza, T., De Ville de Goyet, J., Tan, K. C., Salizzoni and De Hemptinne, B. (1988) Pediatric liver transplantation: report on 52 patients with a 2-year survival of 86%. *J. Pediatr. Surg.*, **23**, 250–253

Paradis, K. J. G., Freese, D. K. and Sharp, H. L. (1988) A pediatric perspective on liver transplantation. *Ped. Clin. N. Am.*, **35**, 409–433

Salt, A., Noble-Jamieson, G., Barnes, N. D. *et al.* (1992) Liver transplantation in 100 children: The Cambridge and King's College Hospital Series. *Br. Med. J.*, **304**, 416–421

Sokal, E. M., Veyckemans, F., De Ville de Goyet, J. *et al.* (1990) Liver transplantation in children less than 1 year of age. *J. Pediatr.*, **17**, 205–210

Sommerauer, J., Gayle, M., Frewen, T. *et al.* (1988) Intensive care course following liver transplantation in children. *J. Pediatr. Surg.*, **23**, 705–708

Spolidoro, J. V. N., Berquist, W. E., Pehlivanoglu, E. *et al.* (1988) Growth acceleration in children after orthotopic liver transplantation. *J. Pediatr.*, **112**, 41–44

Stewart, S. M., Hiltebeitel, C., Nici, J., Waller, D. A., Uauy, R. and Andrews, W. S. (1991) Neuropsychological outcome of Pediatric liver Transplantation. *pediatrics*, **87**, 367–376

Stewart, S. M., Uauy, R., Waller, D. A., Kennard, B. D., Benser, M. and Andrews, W. S. (1989) Mental and motor development, social competence and growth one year after successful pediatric liver transplantation. *J. Pediatr.*, **114**, 574–581

Whitington, P. F. and Balistreri, F. (1991) Liver transplantation in pediatrics: Indications, contraindications, and pretransplant management. *J. Pediatr.*, **118**, 169–177

Woodle, E. S., Thistlethwaite, J. R., Emond, J. C. *et al.* (1990) Successful hepatic transplantation in congenital absence of recipient portal vein. *Surgery*, **107**, 475–479

Zitelli, B. J., Miller, J. W., Gartner, J. C. *et al.* (1988) Changes in life-style after liver transplantation. *Pediatrics*, **82**, 173–180

Infections

Cames, B., Rahier, J., Burtomboy, G. *et al.* (1992) Acute adenovirus hepatitis in liver transplant recipients. *J. Pediatr.*, **120**, 33–37

Castaldo, P., Stratta, R. J., Wood, R. P. *et al.* (1991) Clinical spectrum of fungal infections after orthotopic liver transplantation. *Arch. Surg.*, **126**, 149–156

Fagan, E., Yousef, G., Brahm, J. *et al.* (1990) Persistence of Hepatitis A Virus in Fulminant Hepatitis and after Liver Transplantation. *J. Med. Virol.*, **30**, 131–136

Feray, C., Samuel, D., Thiers, V. *et al.* (1992) Reinfection of liver graft by hepatitis C virus after liver transplantation. *J. Clin. Invest.*, **89**, 1361–1365

McGregor, R. S., Zitelli, B. J., Urbach, A. H., Malatack, J. J. and Cartner, J. C. (1989) Varicella in paediatric orthotopic liver transplant recipients. *Pediatrics*, **83**, 256–261

Malatack, J. J., Gartner, J. C., Urbach, A. H. and Zitelli, B. J. (1991) Orthotopic liver transplantation, Epstein-Barr virus, cyclosporin, and lymphoproliferative disease: a growing concern. *J. Pediatr.*, **118**, 667–675

Markin, R. S., Stratta, R. J. and Woods, G. L. (1990) Infection after liver transplantation. *Am. J. Surg. Pathol.*, **14**, 64–78

Martin, M., Kusne, S., Alessiani, M., Simmons, R. and Starzl, T. E. (1991) Infections after liver transplantation: risk factors and prevention. *Transplant. Proc.*, **23**, 1929–1930

Michaels, M. G., Green, M., Wald, E. R. and Starzl, T. E. (1992) Adenovirus infection in pediatric liver transplant recipients. *J. Infect. Dis.*, **165**, 170–174

O'Grady, J. G., Smith, H. M., Davies, S. E. *et al.* (1992) Hepatitis B virus reinfection after orthotopic liver transplantation. Serological and clinical implications. *J. Hepatol.*, **14**, 104–111

Pereira, B. J. G., Milford, E. L., Kirkman, R. L. and Levey, A. S. (1991) Transmission of hepatitis C virus by organ transplantation. *New Engl. J. Med.*, **325**, 454–460

Pohl, C., Green, M., Wald, E. R. and Ledesma-Medina, J. (1992) Respiratory synctial virus infections in pediatric liver transplant recipients. *J. Infect. Dis.*, **165**, 127–133

Rubin, R. H. (1988) Infectious disease problems. In: *Transplantation of the Liver* (ed. Maddrey, W. C.) *Current Topics in Gastroenterology Series.* Elsevier Press, New York, pp. 279–308

Shaefer, M. S., Stratta, R. J., Markin, R. S. *et al.* (1991) Ganciclovir therapy for cytomegalovirus disease in liver transplant recipients. *Transplant. Proc.*, **23**, 1515–1516

Wajszczuk, C. P., Dummers, S., Ho, M. *et al.* (1985) Fungal infections in liver transplant recipients. *Transplantation*, **40**, 347–353

Wiesner, R. H. (1991) Selective bowel decontamination for infection prophylaxis in liver transplantation patients. *Transplant. Proc.*, **23**, 1927–1928

Rejection

Adams, D. H. and Neuberger, J. M. (1992) Treatment of acute rejection. *Sem. Liver Dis.*, **12**, 80–88

Britton, P. D., Lomas, D. J., Coulden, R. A., Farman, P. and Revell, S. (1992) The role of hepatic vein doppler in diagnosing acute rejection following paediatric liver transplantation. *Clin. Radiol.*, **46**, 38–42

Gubernatis, G., Kemnitz, J., Bornscheuer, A., Kuse, E. R. and Pichlmayr, R. (1989) Potential various appearances of hyperacute rejection in human liver transplantation. *Langenbecks Arch. Chir.*, **374**, 240–244

Vierling, J. M. (1992) Immunological mechanisms of hepatic allograft rejection. *Sem. Liver Dis.*, **12**, 16–27

Metabolic disorders

Brudelski, M., Rodeck, B., Latta, A. *et al.* (1991) Treatment of inherited metabolic disorders by liver transplantation. *J. Inher. Met. Dis.*, **14**, 604–618

Casella, J. F., Lewis, J. H., Bontempo, F. A., Zitelli, B. J., Markel, H. and Starzl, T. (1988) Successful treatment of Homozygous Protein C deficiency by hepatic transplantation. *Lancet*, **i**, 435–437

Cohen, A., O'Grady, J., Mowat, A. P. and Williams, R. (1989) Liver transplantation for metabolic disorders. In: *Bailliere's Clinical Gastroenterology*, (eds Creutzfeldt, W. and Pichlmayr, R.), **3**, 767–786

Cohen, A. T., Mowat, A. P., Bhaduri, B. H. *et al.* (1991) Liver transplantation for inborn errors of metabolism and genetic disorders; Experience in the King's Cambridge Liver transplantation program. In: *Inborn Errors of Metabolism* (eds Schaub, J., Van Hoof, F. and Vis, H. L.). Nestle Nutrition Workshop Series Vol. 24, Raven Press, New York, pp. 213–222

Hardy, L., Hansen, J. L., Kushner, J. P. and Knisely, A. S. (1990) Neonatal Haemochromatosis. Genetic analysis of Transferrin-receptor, H-apoferritin, and L-apoferritin Loci and of the human leucocyte antigen Class 1 region. *Am. J. Path.*, **137**, 149–153

Herbert, A., Corbin, D., Williams, A., Thompson, D., Buckels, J. and Elias, E. (1991) Erythropoietic protoporphyria: Unusual skin and neurological problems after liver transplantation. *Gastroenterology*, **100**, 1753–1757

Kirschner, B. S., Baker, A. L. and Thorp, F. K. (1991) Growth in Adulthood after liver transplantation for GSD Type 1. *Gastroenterology*, **1**, 238–241

Largilliere, C., Houssin, D., Gottrand, F. *et al.* (1989) Liver transplantation for ornithine transcarbamylase deficiency in a girl. *J. Pediatr.*, **115**, 415–417

Latta, K. and Brodehl, J. (1990) Primary hyperoxaluria type 1. *Eur. J. Pediatr.*, **149**, 518–522

Mowat, A. P. (1992) Liver transplantation in the management of metabolic disorders. *Eur. J. Paediatr.*, **151**, S32–S38

Mowat, A. P. (1991) Prospects for the management of inborn errors of Metabolism. In *Inborn Errors of Metabolism* (eds Schaub, J., Van Hoof, F. and Vis, H. L.). Nestle Nutrition Workshop Series, Vol. 24, Raven Press, New York, pp. 207–211

Noble-Jamieson, G., Barnes, N., Thiru, S. and Mowat, A. P. (1990) Severe hypertension after liver transplantation in children with alpha-1-antitrypsin deficiency. *Arch. Dis. Childh.*, **65**, 1217–1221

Otto, G., Herfarth, C., Senninger, N., Feist, G. and Post Gmelin, K. (1989) Hepatic transplantation in Galactosaemia. *Transplantation*, **47**, 902–903

Paradis, K., Weber, A., Seidman, E. G. *et al.* (1990) Liver transplantation for hereditary tyrosinaemia: the Quebec experience. *Am. J. Hum. Gen.*, **47**, 338–342

Pett, S. and Mowat, A. P. (1987) Crigler-Najjar Syndrome Types I and II. Clinical experience – King's College Hospital 1972–1987. Phenobarbitone, Phototherapy and liver Transplantation. *Molecular Aspects of Medicine*, **9**, 473–482

Selby, R., Starzl, T. E., Yunis, E. *et al.* (1991) Liver transplantation for Type IV glycogen storage disease. *New Engl. J. Med.*, **324**, 39–42

Sokal, E. M., Hoof, F. V., Alberti, D., de Ville de Goyet, J., de Barsy, T. and Otte, J. B. (1992) Progressive cardiac failure following orthotopic liver transplantation for type IV glycogenosis. *Eur. J. Pediatr.*, **151**, 200–203

Todo, S., Starzl, T. E., Tzakis, A. *et al.* (1992) Orthotopic liver transplantation for urea cycle enzyme deficiency. *Hepatology*, **15**, 419–422

Van der Zee, D. C., Van Melkebeke, E., de Goyet, J., de Ville *et al.* (1991) Indications and timing of liver transplantation in metabolic disorders. In: *Inborn Errors of Metabolism*, Vol. 24 (eds Schaub, J., Van Hoof, F. and Vis, H. L.). Vevey/Raven Press Ltd, New York, pp. 263–274

Witzleben, C. L. and Uri, A. (1989) Perinatal hemochromatosis: entity or end result? *Human Pathol.*, **20**, 335–340

Williams, S. G. J., Westaby, D., Tanner, M. S. and Mowat, A. P. (1992) Liver and biliary problems in cystic fibrosis. *Br. Med. Bull.*, **48**, 877–892

Acute liver failure

Bismuth, H., Samuel, D., Gugenheim, J. *et al.* (1987) Emergency liver transplantation for fulminant hepatitis. *Ann. Intern. Med.*, **107**, 337–341

DeVictor, D., Desplanques, L., Debray *et al.* (1992) Emergency liver transplantation for fulminant liver failure in infants and children. *Hepatology*, **16**, 1156–1162

Emond, J. C., Aran, P. P., Whitington, P. F., Broelsch, C. E. and Baker, A. L. (1989) Liver transplantation in the management of fulminant hepatic failure. *Gastroneterology*, **96**, 1583–1588

Mondragon, R., Mieli-Vergani, G., Heaton, N. D. *et al.* (1992) Results of liver transplantation for fulminant hepatic failure in children. *Transplant. Int.*, **5**, S206–S208

O'Grady, J. G., Alexander, G. J. M., Hayllar, K. and Williams, R. (1989) Early indicators of prognosis in fulminant hepatic failure. *Gastroenterology*, **97**, 439–445

Pinson, C. W., Daya, M. R., Benner, K. G. *et al.* (1990) Liver transplantation for severe Amanita phalloides mushroom poisoning. *Am. J. Surg.*, **159**, 493–499

Shaefer, M. S., Edmunds, A. L., Markin, R. S., Wood, R. P., Pillen, T. J. and Shaw, B. W. Jr (1990) Hepatic failure associated with imipramine therapy. *Pharmacotherapy*, **10**, 66–69

Stampfl, D. A., Munoz, S. J., Moritz, M. J. *et al.* (1990) Heterotopic liver transplantation for fulminant Wilson's disease. *Gastroenterology*, **99**, 1834–1836

Reduced liver graft

Badger, I. L., Czerniak, A., Beath, S. *et al.* (1992) Hepatic transplantation in children using reduced size allografts. *Br. J. Surg.*, **79**, 47–49

Broelsch, C. E., Emond, J. C., Thistlethwaite, J. R. *et al.* (1988) Liver transplantation, including the concept of reduced-size liver transplants in children. *Ann. Surg.*, **208**, 410–420

Otte, J. B., de Ville de Goyet, J., Sokal, E. *et al.* (1990) Size reduction of the donor liver is a safe way to alleviate the shortage of size-matched organs in pediatric liver transplantation. *Ann. Surg.*, **211**, 146–157

Living related donors

Broelsch, C. E., Whitington, P. F., Edmond, J. C. *et al.* (1991) Liver transplantations in children from living related donors. Surgical techniques and results. *Ann. Surg.*, **214**, 428–439

Whitington, P. F., Emond, J. C. and Broelsch, C. E. (1991) Rediced-size liver transplantation in infants using living related donors. *Hepatology*, **12**, 870

Malignant disease

Iwatsuki, S., Starzl, T., Sheahan, D. G. *et al.* (1991) Hepatic resection versus transplantation for hepatocellular carcinoma. *Ann. Surg.*, **214**, 221–229

Koneru, B., Flye, M. W., Busuttil, R. *et al.* (1991) Liver transplantation in Hepatoblastoma. *Ann. Surg.*, **213**, 118–121

Penn. I. (1991) Hepatic Transplantation for primary and metastatic cancers of the liver. *Surgery*, 110, 726–735

Auxiliary liver transplantation

Metselaar, H. J., Hesselink, E. J., DeRave, S. *et al.* (1990) Recovery of failing liver after auxiliary heterotopic liver transplantation. *Lancet*, **335**, 1156–1157

Terpstra, O. T., Schalm, S. W., Weimar, W. *et al.* (1988) Auxiliary partial liver transplantation for end-stage chronic liver disease. *N. Engl. J. Med.*, **319**, 1507–1511

Whitington, P. F., Emond, J. C., Heffron, T. and Thistlewaite, J. R. (1993) Severe familial nonhemolytic jaundice (Crigler-Najjar syndrome type 1) treated with orthotopic auxiliary liver transplantation. (Submitted for publication)

Chapter 26

Laboratory assessment of hepatobiliary disease

Laboratory investigations are usually essential to establish or confirm a clinical diagnosis. They are of value in monitoring the progress of disease. They are also important in excluding hepatic disease, for example, in acute unexplained coma in childhood which might suggest a diagnosis of Reye's syndrome, or in the assessment of possible hepatotoxic effects of new drugs.

The relative importance of specific investigations in the diagnosis of particular disorders is considered throughout the text. The most useful are those which identify specific aetiological factors, for example, alpha-1 antitrypsin deficiency, type PIZ; or hepatitis B surface antigen and e antigen. Tests which give anatomical or histological information, for example, splenic angiography or liver biopsy, are often invaluable in diagnosis and in assessing severity of liver damage.

Laboratory tests for liver disease

Standard, routinely available, automated laboratory investigations for liver disease will usually verify or exclude the presence of significant hepatobiliary disease. These investigations should include at least serum (or plasma) total bilirubin, an aminotransferase, gamma-glutamyl transpeptidase, alkaline phosphatase, total protein and albumin. The results are of value in monitoring the progress of disease and in the assessment of possible hepatotoxic effects of new drugs. They are particularly important in identifying hepatic disease in the patient with no jaundice or other clinical features of liver disease. Abnormal results might lead to consideration of Reye's syndrome in acute unexplained coma. In such circumstances a blood ammonia, which is rarely routinely available and must be measured promptly, can be invaluable in directing attention to disorders such as urea cycle defects. The results of these investigations are frequently influenced by many non-hepatic factors. Note that elevated serum activities of single enzymes may occur in children with no disease (Schoenau et al., 1986; Perrault et al., 1990). It is unfortunate that none of the automated investigations are specific for liver disease. The direct bilirubin test is specific but is less rigorously standardized than the above tests. It is no more specific, and much more expensive, than the underused urine test strips, impregnated with diazo reagent, which detect as little as 1 μmol of bilirubin per litre. Serum bile salt concentrations are also relatively specific but are no more sensitive than the batch of routinely available investigations prompted by the clinician's request for 'liver function tests'. None test liver function! Only a prolonged prothrombin time (international normalized ratio, INR) or reduced factor V concentration indicate the severity of acute hepatic damage. Too often these tests are forgotten. Their concentrations can be decreased by intravascular coagulation.

Aminotransferases

Aminotransferases (transaminases) are intracellular enzymes found in nearly all tissues with the greatest activity in liver, heart, skeletal muscle, adipose tissue, brain and kidney. Increases in serum activities of *aspartate aminotransferase* or transaminase (AsAT or AST, L-aspartate-2-oxaloglutarate aminotransferase (EC 2.6.1.1), formerly serum glutamic-oxalo-acetic transaminase, SGOT) and *alanine aminotransferase* or transaminase (AsAt or ALT). L-Alanine-2-oxaloglutarate aminotransferase (EC 2.6.1.2), formerly serum glutamic-pyruvic transaminase, SGPT) are sensitive indicators of hepatocellular necrosis. Leakage from damaged tissues is thought to be the main reason for the rise rather than impaired clearance by hepatic endothelial cells. ALT is more sensitive and liver specific than AST which has advantages in epidemiological studies but in paediatric clinical practice AST is as useful. Increases in serum values occur in all types of liver disease. The activity is a poor guide to possible pathology. Levels may be normal in cirrhosis. Elevations may also occur in severe cardiac or skeletal muscle damage, pancreatitis, infarction of the kidney, brain or lung and in haemolytic anaemia. There are a number of different techniques for measuring transferases. These can be influenced by the conditions under which the assay is performed. The clinician, therefore, must always be aware of the normal range of values relevant to the method used in the laboratory in which the test was done.

Other enzyme activities which can be determined in serum and have been correlated with hepatocellular necrosis include sorbitol dehydrogenase, isocitrate dehydrogenase, lactic acid dehydrogenase and leucine aminopeptidase. There seems little evidence that these add significantly to the information obtained from the more commonly measured transaminases.

Serum alkaline phosphatase

Isoenzymes of alkaline phosphatase (EC 3.13.1, orthophosphoric monoester phosphohydrolase, ALP) are found in the liver, bone, kidney, intestines and placenta. In the liver they are located mainly on canalicular microvilli but are also present on the sinusoidal border of the hepatocytes where they increase in experimental bile duct ligation. Serum concentrations are increased in many types of liver disease particularly if there is impaired bile production. The degree of elevation is of no value in distinguishing between intrahepatic or extrahepatic disease. An increased ALP, with other tests normal, may occur in malignant and benign infiltrations of the liver, including liver abscess and in congenital hepatic fibrosis. Elevations occur in disorders with no liver involvement and as a familial trait.

In the first month of life, the alkaline phosphatase is usually raised to between 70 and 210 IU/litre, but by the age of 1 month the range is usually between 30 and 200 IU/litre. During puberty, levels of up to 290 IU/litre occur without disease being detected.

Gamma-glutamyl transpeptidase

Gamma-glutamyl transpeptidase (γ-GT) is present throughout the hepatobiliary tree and in other organs such as the heart, kidney, lungs, pancreas and seminal vesicles. Enzymatic activity is increased by enzyme-inducing drugs in the absence of other evidence of liver disorder. The finding of elevated serum γ-GT activity is thus of limited use. In patients with known hepatobiliary disorders it may serve to follow the course of these disorders or indicate recrudescence of disease in the anicteric patient when the AST/ALT are still normal. Conversely values may become more abnormal for some months when all other features of liver disease are improving. In the individual patient the activity frequently correlates with that of alkaline phosphatase. The activity levels do not help in identifying the nature of the hepatobiliary pathology in hepatitis syndrome in infants (Manolaki *et al.*, 1983). A persistently normal value in the presence of other clinical and laboratory evidence of chronic liver disease is found in a proportion of infants with progressive intrahepatic cholestasis. Normal levels can occur in benign recurrent cholestasis however (Maggiore *et al.*, 1991).

Enzymatic activity is less than 40 IU/litre from the age of 1 year, but in the newborn period the upper limit of normal may be three times this value, the activity falling gradually during infancy.

5'-Nucleotidase

5'-Nucleotidase (5'-ribonucleotide phosphohydrolase, EC 3.1.3.5) is an enzyme which has a similar distribution within the hepatocytes as alkaline phosphatase, and may play a role in membrane-mediated transport. Although present in bone, its concentration does not change with growth. Its main role may be in distinguishing between hepatic and non-hepatic causes of the raised serum alkaline phosphatase. Normal values at all ages are less than 15 IU/litre. There are technical difficulties in analysis.

Serum protein determination

Serum albumin is formed by the liver. Hypoalbuminaemia is found in advanced chronic liver diseases. This may be due to decreased synthesis or increased degradation but may also be due to an increased plasma volume. It is a useful but imprecise index of severity of liver damage. It is of little value in predicting the patient's prognosis or response to surgery such as portosystemic shunting. Temporary low levels are found in extrahepatic portal hypertension following alimentary bleeding. In acute disease hypoalbuminaemia is less striking, perhaps because of the long half-life of albumin (about 20 days).

Serum gammaglobulins are composed of immunoglobulins produced in the reticulo-endothelial system. Elevations of serum immunoglobulins IgG, IgA and IgM may be found in chronic liver disease. IgM is raised in viral hepatitis. Very high levels of IgG are commonly found in autoimmune chronic hepatitis and in primary sclerosing cholangitis in children. Abnormally low levels of IgA and complement component C4 are found in some patients with autoimmune chronic active hepatitis. In Wilson's disease all serum immunoglobulins may be elevated. The caeruloplasmin is low in 70–95% of cases.

Non-organ-specific autoantibodies

The presence in serum of non-organ-specific autoantibodies directed against elements in the subcellular organelles indicates an underlying genetic predisposition to autoimmune disorders. High levels of antinuclear factor and/or smooth muscle antibodies are found in children with primary sclerosing cholangitis, autoimmune chronic active hepatitis and less commonly in Wilson's disease. Liver-kidney microsomal or cytosolic antibodies are found in categories of autoimmune chronic active hepatitis.

Prothrombin time: international normalized ratio (INR)

The liver is the site of synthesis of many coagulation factors. The half-life of these varies from a few hours to 4 days. Thus a decrease in hepatic synthesis due to acute liver dysfunction is rapidly reflected in a decrease in the plasma levels of these factors (I, II, V, VII, IX and X). All except factor I require vitamin K for synthesis and activation. The one-stage prothrombin time with standardized substrate and expressed as INR (international normalized ratio) is a widely available test of these factors and fibrinogen.

An increased INR which is rapidly corrected to normal following intramuscular injection of vitamin K, indicates vitamin K malabsorption due to reduced bile secretion without marked synthetic impairment. Vitamin K-resistant increased INR indicates severe hepatic disease or disseminated intravascular coagulation. Such increases are commonly found in fulminant hepatic failure, metabolic disorders, severe chronic active hepatitis and in decompensated cirrhosis. An INR of 1.3–1.5 is present in the majority of patients with portal vein obstruction.

Urinary bilirubin

Bilirubin in the urine may be the first indication of hepatobiliary disease in patients who are not overtly jaundiced. In jaundiced patients it indicates the presence of conjugated bilirubin in the serum, a sign of hepatocellular parenchymal damage or bile duct obstruction (Mowat, 1990). Commercially prepared bilirubin testing strips, detect as little as 1 μmol/litre. Urine that has been standing at room temperature for several hours may give a false-negative test. Beeturia and chlorpromazine metabolites in the urine may interfere with the test.

Serum cholesterol

Cholesterol is synthesized in the liver and intestinal wall. Esterification occurs in the liver. Low serum values of cholesterol and its esters are found in acute and chronic liver diseases. Very low values (< 2 μmol/litre) in chronic disease indicate a poor prognosis (Ballin, 1986). Very high serum cholesterol values (six times normal) are found in patients with chronic biliary problems, particularly paucity of intrahepatic bile ducts.

Normal cord serum cholesterol is between 50 and 150 mg/100 ml (1.29–3.8 mmol/litre). This increases to from 90 to 200 mg/100 ml (3.0–5.16 mmol/litre) by the age of 6 weeks, and in children over the age of 1 year it is between 120 and 160 mg/100 ml (3.1–4.13 mmol/litre). Adult values range from 120 to 250 mg/100 ml (3.1–6.4 mmol/litre). Such normal values, however, may vary from community to community, depending on dietary habits.

Ammonia

The concentration of blood ammonia is primarily regulated by the liver. Endogenous ammonia is produced in the colon by the action of bacterial urease or is synthesized in the liver, kidney or small intestine. Exogenous sources include dietary protein and amino acids.

Ammonia may be raised in acute and chronic hepatic encephalopathy. In these circumstances diagnosis and monitoring of the patient's progress can usually be determined in other ways (Mowat, 1991 and 1993). The main role of blood ammonia determination is in the investigation of unexplained neurological dysfunction. A value above 130 μmol/litre should prompt full investigation to exclude inherited errors of metabolism but values up to 300 μmol/litre may occur in any severe illness (Clayton, 1991).

Serum bile salts

Primary bile salts are synthesized and conjugated in the liver and secreted in the bile. Over 95% are reabsorbed from the intestine and are efficiently extracted from the portal blood into the hepatocytes to be recirculated. As hepatic extraction becomes less efficient the plasma concentration of bile salts rises. Thus a raised serum bile salt concentration is specific for hepatobiliary disease. The maximum values are found 2 hours after a meal. The test is no more sensitive than a combination of the standard laboratory tests for liver damage. The lack of a reliable automated method of analysis has prevented the widespread introduction of this test. A further problem is that serum values rise in healthy children in the first week of life and remain above normal adult values until 4 to 8 years of age. The normal bile salt levels found in genetic disorders of bilirubin metabolism, as opposed to raised values found with hyperbilirubinaemia caused by hepatobiliary disease, are the best example of the value of bile acids in specific diagnosis.

Urinary bile salts

Bile salts in urine reflect those in serum. The absence of primary salts and the presence of abnormal C24 bile salt derivatives, detected by gas chromatography-mass spectrometry, is diagnostic of inherited abnormalities of bile salt metabolism (Clayton, 1991).

Quantification of liver function

As mentioned above albumin and the INR are the only commonly available tests of liver synthetic function. Test of hepatic clearance of substances from the circulation (a measure of perfusion, uptake and/or metabolism) using dyes such as indocyanine green or sulphobromophthalein have been largely replaced in clinical practice by radionucleotides.

Sulphobromophthalein sodium may cause systemic allergic or anaphylactic reactions which may be fatal (Bar-Meir et al., 1986). Caffeine clearance from serum or saliva (Lewis and Rector, 1992) and lidocaine metabolite formation (Oellerich et al., 1990) provide a practical means of estimating microsomal function. Both are being evaluated for their prognostic significance but have not yet been introduced as routine clinical tests.

Specific investigations

Caeruloplasmin and copper studies

Caeruloplasmin is a copper-binding protein which possesses copper oxidase enzymatic activity. In Wilson's disease caeruloplasmin may be absent or present in very low concentrations in 70–95% of cases. In fulminant hepatic failure or subacute hepatic necrosis low levels may be found, returning to normal if the liver recovers. In most other forms of liver disease the caeruloplasmin concentration is high. Low values are found in the nephrotic syndrome and protein-losing enteropathy. The normal range is from 20 to 40 mg/100 ml (1.25–2.5 μmol/litre), much lower values are found in cord blood and in the first 2 months of life. An increased 24 hour urinary copper excretion particularly with a penicillamine challenge (0.5 g at 0 and 12 hours) is more specific for the diagnosis of Wilson's disease (Da Costa *et al.*, 1992). Values above 25 μmol/24 hours are highly specific except in acute liver disease.

Alpha-1 antitrypsin deficiency, PIZ

The genetic variant of alpha-1 antitrypsin associated with liver disease, protease inhibitor genotype ZZ (PIZZ), is most easily identified by isoelectric focusing complemented by immunofixation procedures. Serum levels do not identify all PIZ individuals. In advanced liver disease some PIZZ sera may be identified as SZ. Parental PI studies or DNA techniques using genotype-specific oligonucleotide probes clarify the phenotype in these circumstances.

Alpha-fetoprotein

Alpha-fetoprotein is synthesized by embryonic or poorly differentiated liver cells. In intrauterine life it is the major serum protein. It reaches its highest levels in serum between 13 and 20 weeks' gestation after which it declines gradually. In the newborn the mean value is approximately 50 000 ng/ml falling to 2500, 325, 90 and 12.5 ng/ml at 1, 2, 3 and 6 months respectively. High levels of alpha-fetoprotein concentrations are found in infants with intrahepatic cholestatic syndromes in the first 10–20 weeks of life (Johnston *et al.*, 1976). Patients with extrahepatic biliary atresia have levels which tend to be slightly lower but there is a large overlap between the values found in these two conditions, and alpha-fetoprotein determination cannot be recommended as a method for distinguishing the two conditions. In this age group elevated levels of up to 150 times normal may be found in the presence of benign liver tumours.

Very high levels of alpha-fetoprotein are very useful markers of hepatoblastoma or hepatocellular carcinoma, being found in the serum of up to 90% of cases. If positive, it is also a useful test for assessing whether surgical removal has been complete and in monitoring the effects of chemotherapy. Approximately one-third of children with embryonal teratoblastoma have elevated alpha-fetoprotein in the blood. Yolk sac tumours also produce elevated levels. Levels of greater than 100 ng/ml may occur in patients recovering from fulminant hepatic failure.

Diagnostic imaging of the liver, biliary tree and portal venous system

Grey scale ultrasonography, radionuclide and radiological imaging, with or without computed tomography, are complementary techniques which provide information on hepatobiliary structure, function and blood flow. Since ultrasonography is painless, involves no irradiation, utilizes equipment which is portable and requires no anaesthesia, it should be the first mode of imaging in infants and children. Optimum visualization of pathology in the hepatobiliary system requires an appreciation of the type of information available from different imaging modalities. Interpretation of the information requires an understanding of the pathological processes involved. Close liaison between the clinician, pathologist and the imaging specialist is essential if these aids to diagnosis and management are to be exploited correctly.

Plain abdominal X-ray

This is of little diagnostic value other than demonstrating calcification in the liver, spleen, gall bladder or biliary system, pancreas or adrenals. Calcification in the liver may be due to primary or secondary tumour, chronic infections or granulomata. It has been reported in patients on dialysis. It may be found in apparently normal neonates. Between 10 and 60% of gall-stones calcify. Adrenal calcification is a feature of Wolman's disease, pancreatic of chronic pancreatitis. Gas in branches of the portal vein is a feature of intra-abdominal sepsis particularly necrotizing enterocolitis. Biliary gas is seen when there is an abnormal connection between the biliary system and the gut, usually following biliary surgery.

Ultrasonography

Grey scale ultrasonography is an extremely efficient anatomical imaging technique allowing resolution of structures as small as 1–2 mm. It can provide essential information in all forms of chronic or complicated acute liver disease. Although easy to use, interpretation is extremely dependent on the operator's skill and knowledge.

Ultrasound may be used to determine accurately the size of the spleen, portal vein and gall bladder. It is particularly useful in demonstrating dilated ducts associated with choledochal cysts, distal strictures, inspissated bile, or tumours in the biliary tree. Gall bladder calculi, sludge and polyps in the gall bladder are easily visualized. In cholecystitis the gall bladder wall may be seen to be thickened. It is also effective in demonstrating focal liver lesions including hypertrophy and/or atrophy of lobes. Cysts appear as echo-free structures with posterior enhancement. Abscesses and necrotic primary or secondary tumours typically appear as irregular cavitating lesions. Solid tumours appear as focal areas of low reflectivity with posterior acoustic shadowing. Cavernous haemangiomata are echogenic with posterior acoustic enhancement and have irregular echo-free cavities.

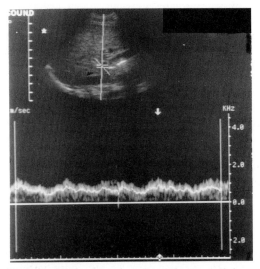

Figure 26.1 Normal hepatic vein and Doppler tracing. There is flow away from the transducer with marked decelerations during the cardiac A and V waves

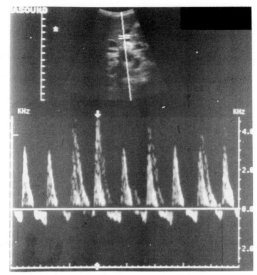

Figure 26.2 Doppler ultrasound showing abnormal hepatic vein tracing. The A and V wave pulsations have been obliterated by a stiff liver

Blood vessels supplying and draining tumours may be seen to be enlarged and blood flow is increased.

Demonstrating the portal vein, hepatic veins, hepatic artery, their tributaries and branches or the inferior vena cava requires more skill. Cavernous transformation of the portal vein, periportal, subhepatic and umbilical collaterals and the main portal vein and its branches can be identified. With an ultrasonically localized Doppler probe and computer analysis, blood flow velocity in the portal vein, hepatic artery and hepatic veins can be assessed. In advanced cirrhosis reversed flow in the portal vein, an increased pulsatility in the hepatic artery with, in extreme cases, reversed flow in diastole may be observed. With less severe pathological change liver 'stiffness' causes decreased pulsatility of the hepatic vein. The prognostic significance of this change is not yet known (Figures 26.1 and 26.2).

Intravascular tumour may be identified in hepatic and portal veins.

Ultrasound is imprecise in estimating liver size. The findings in diffuse liver disease are non-specific. Increased reflectivity may be due to fat or fibrosis. High reflectivity suggests a storage disease. A nodular surface and/or parenchyma implies cirrhosis. It does not distinguish regeneration nodules from malignant ones. Apart from detecting choledochal and other cysts it is of very limited value in assessing the biliary system in hepatitis syndrome of infancy. It is very difficult to visualize the lower bile duct because of overlying gas.

Computed tomography

Computed tomography, like ultrasound, demonstrates anatomical features. Interpretation is more straightforward. The patient must be still during the procedure, so general anaesthesia is usually required in infants and young children. The liver is represented as a series of transverse slices approximately 1 cm thick.

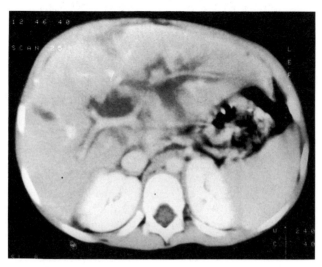

Figure 26.3 Computed tomography scan after intravenous contrast injection showing massive areas of hypoperfusion of the liver in acute hepatic necrosis 8 days following liver transplantation

A detailed three-dimensional picture of hepatic anatomy or of focal lesions can be built up particularly with the use of radio-opaque material to define the gastrointestinal tract, blood vessels, bile ducts or kidneys. This is particularly useful when planning possible surgical resection, in tumour staging and in assessing the response to chemotherapy. It has the advantage over ultrasound in that it is not affected by gas and can show other intra-abdominal pathology (Figure 26.3). Cysts are clearly defined. Abscesses appear as low density areas which may be confused with haematomas or cystic degeneration of tumours. Tumours appear as areas of low attenuation particularly after contrast injection. Haemangiomata may have increased attenuation. Adenomata and focal nodular hyperplasia may be undetected. A diffuse increase in attenuation is seen in haemochromatosis and has been reported in some patients with glycogen storage disease and following intravenous feeding. Decreased attenuation occurs with fatty infiltration. In biliary disease CT scanning is better than ultrasound scanning demonstrating lesions at the level of the ampulla of Vater.

The place in clinical assessment of magnetic resonance imaging (MRI) and the newer techniques of nuclear magnetic resonance spectroscopy and single photo-emission computed tomography remains to be defined. MRI based on imaging of protons allows much clearer imaging in the coronal and sagittal plains and provides excellent images of blood vessels without contrast injection. It may be of value in discriminating between malignant and non-malignant nodules in tyrosinaemia. Cavernous haemangiomata have very long T2 relaxation times compared with other masses.

Radioisotope imaging

Radioisotopes are useful in demonstrating morphological and functional changes in the liver and biliary system. Two types of radiopharmaceuticals are used: chemicals actively transported by the hepatocytes into bile and colloid preparations taken up by Kupffer cells.

They are given intravenously tagged to a gamma-emitting isotope usually technetium-99m and the tissue distribution monitored by a gamma camera.

Technetium-99 labelled iminodiacetic acid (IDA) derivatives have replaced ^{131}I-labelled Rose Bengal in demonstrating hepatic uptake and biliary excretion. Following intravenous injection, these agents rapidly enter the hepatocytes and are secreted into and concentrated in the biliary system and gall bladder before appearing in the bowel. The technique thus reflects hepatic function as well as biliary pathology. Computers linked to gamma cameras allow more precise analysis of the rate of uptake and secretion and may thus be used as a measure of hepatic function. It is essential to use IDA derivatives such as methylbromoIDA (MBrIDA) or diisopropylIDA (DISIDA) which have a relatively poor renal uptake and good hepatic uptake.

These images are particularly valuable in demonstrating bile duct patency in infants with suspected extrahepatic biliary atresia. Discrimination from intrahepatic cholestasis is enhanced if the infants are pretreated with phenobarbitone (5 mg/kg for at least 3 days). Repeated imaging up to 24 hours after injection may be required to demonstrate isotope in the biliary system or gut. Equally effective discrimination may be achieved by computer analysis of distribution within 10 minutes of intravenous injections (El Tumi *et al.*, 1987). In acute cholecystitis there is no uptake in the gall bladder but the rest of the biliary system is normal. Dilated ducts may be demonstrated with this technique but it is no better than ultrasonography (Figure 26.4).

Technetium-99 sulphur colloid imaging reflects reticulo-endothelial function and intrahepatic blood flow. Colloid imaging is less specific than ultrasound in the assessment of focal lesions and has a declining place in practice as the role of ultrasound becomes more clearly established. The scan visualizes organ size, shape, uniformity of isotope uptake and the relative uptake in the liver, spleen and bone marrow. The normal liver uptake is most dense over the right lobe, isotope uptake decreasing evenly towards the

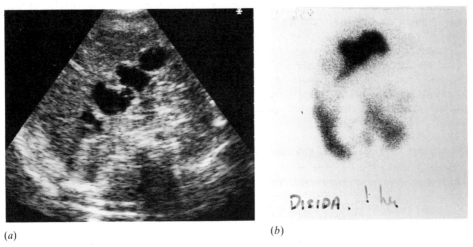

(*a*)   (*b*)

Figure 26.4 Complementary use of ultrasonic and radiopharmaceutical imaging in an infant of 11 months with intrahepatic bile duct dilatation in association with Jeune's syndrome (asphyxiating thoracic dystrophy). (*a*) Ultrasound scan showing four large intrahepatic cysts; (*b*) complementary intense concentration of isotope 1 hour after intravenous injection of ⁹⁹ᵐTc DISIDA confirms their connection with the biliary tree. The liver outline is faintly seen, the isotope having not yet been completely cleared from the hepatic parenchyma. Isotope is seen concentrated in the bowel

liver margin which may show an indentation at the site of the gall bladder. Splenic uptake is minimal. No bone marrow uptake is seen.

In diffuse liver disease there is decreased and often patchy uptake in the liver, increased uptake in the spleen and if liver function is severely impaired, uptake in the bone marrow. Liver uptake may be particularly poor in Wilson's disease. Good uptake in the caudate lobe with poor uptake elsewhere in the liver is seen in the Budd-Chiari syndrome. The relative uptake in the liver and spleen may be used to assess progression of disease and response to therapy.

Percutaneous liver biopsy

Microscopic examination of liver tissue often provides invaluable information for the management of the child with liver disease, providing evidence which is not available by other means (Table 26.1). It can also provide material for bacterial and viral culture, analysis of enzymatic activity, chemical content as well as histochemical, immuno-fluorescent and electron microscopy studies. Such special studies require planning with the staff who will perform the analysis. The technique does carry a slight but definite morbidity and even mortality. It can therefore only be justified when it is necessary to know the nature and severity of liver disease more precisely than can be assessed by less invasive techniques, and where the information sought may be crucial in modifying management. Certain contraindications should be observed and complications anticipated.

The procedure should be performed by physicians who have had adequate instruction and supervision by others who have frequently performed this procedure. Except in elucidating poorly characterized metabolic disorders and in identifying chronic intra-hepatic infection such as candidiasis in immunosuppressed patients, a percutaneous liver biopsy obtained with a sharp Menghini needle will provide sufficient material for full diagnosis. Interpretation is a task for the specialist. Misdiagnoses are particularly liable to occur with small biopsies particularly if there is failure to obtain sufficient portal tracts. Ultrasonography directed biopsies may increase the yield in focal lesions.

Percutaneous liver biopsy may be done under local anaesthesia in young infants and in cooperative children over the age of 6 years. In most children between the age of 6 months and 6 years, a brief general anaesthetic is preferable to the very deep sedation necessary to ensure the child's compliance during the procedure. Preoperative preparation should include haematocrit, blood count, platelet count, prothrombin time and blood group

Table 26.1 Indications for percutaneous liver biopsy

Differentiation of conjugated hyperbilirubinaemia in infancy
Investigation of obscure hepatomegaly
Chronic hepatitis
Chronic or recurrent conjugated hyperbilirubinaemia
Investigation of portal hypertension
Diagnosis of Wilson's disease
Diagnosis of metabolic or storage disorders
Reye's syndrome
Drug, toxic or irradiation hepatitis
Pyrexia of uncertain origin
Staging of lymphoma

Table 26.2 Contraindications to liver biopsy

Purpura or a prothrombin time prolonged by more than
   three seconds compared with the control, or a platelet
   count of less than $40 \times 10^9/l$
Extreme dyspnoea
Hydatid disease in the right lobe of the liver
A pyogenic abscess in the right lobe of the liver
Biliary tract infection
Infection of the peritoneum, right pleura or lung
Angiomatous malformation of the liver
Alpha-fetoprotein-positive suspected primary hepatic
   tumour
Suspected extrahepatic bile duct obstruction with possibly
   dilated biliary tree (ultrasonography or percutaneous
   cholangiography are better investigations)
Ascites

---

determination and an ultrasound scan to exclude filling defects within the right lobe of the liver. Contraindications are given in Table 26.2.

Menghini technique

An aspiration biopsy, using the Menghini needle, is safest since the needle is in the liver for only a very short time and is thus less likely to tear the liver capsule if the patient breathes. It often bypasses fibrous structures and thereby reduces the risk of damage to large intrahepatic blood vessels or bile ducts. It may underestimate the severity of hepatic fibrosis.

The Menghini needle is hollow – 40, 70, or 120 mm in length and 1.0, 1.2 and 1.4 mm in diameter. The tip is bevelled at 45 degrees and flat ground. A square 'nail' or obturator measuring 10 or 40 mm and having a flattened head is inserted into the proximal end of the needle before assembly with the syringe. The obturator prevents aspiration of the specimen into the syringe. Sharp disposable needles are now available. A 1.4 mm diameter needle is used in most instances.

The patient is placed in a supine position on a firm bed with the right flank exposed and the right arm drawn up beside the head. The point of entry of the needle into the liver is then selected. The upper limit of liver dullness is determined by percussion in the anterior axillary line. The biopsy is taken from one intercostal space below. It usually lies in the seventh and eighth intercostal space. The point of entry of the needle should be marked by applying tincture of iodine to the point or using an indelible marker.

The operator then prepares for the procedure by washing his hands and donning surgical gloves. The area of the biopsy is cleaned with chlorhexidine solution. The needle tract is anaesthetized down to the liver capsule with local anaesthetic. While this is taking effect, the Menghini needle, obturator and 10 ml syringe containing approximately 2 ml of sterile normal saline solution, is assembled. The system should be checked for leaks by occluding the biopsy needle opening with a gloved fingertip and retracting the plunger of the syringe The connection of the needle and syringe must be adjusted until a 'leak-proof' system is achieved. A small nick is then made in the skin with a small-bladed scalpel. A trocar is then passed through the intercostal muscles to form a track for the biopsy needle. This step is unnecessary when disposable needles are used. It should follow an imaginary line that will place the needle at right angles in the liver surface. The Menghini needle on its syringe is then introduced as far as the intercostal ligament which can often be felt to give way on penetration. A few drops of normal saline solution are then expressed through the needle to clear debris from the tip. With the patient's breath in expiration and the syringe barrel in full suction, the needle is rapidly advanced into the liver 2–5 cm and immediately withdrawn. At all times the needle is directed at right angles to the liver surface.

In young infants, the procedure should be done 4 hours after the last feed. The baby will normally be fractious during the preparation period, and can usually be soothed by means of a 'dummy' or comforter. This is withdrawn after the needle tip has been cleared of any debris. The infant will then usually cry vigorously and, during the expiratory cry, the biopsy can be performed safely.

Following the procedure, the patient should lie on the right side for 4 hours. The pulse and respiration should be monitored at 15 minute intervals for 2 hours, and thereafter at 30 minute intervals for a further 6 hours. The abdomen should be gently palpated 6 hours after the procedure for signs of peritoneal irritation.

Complications

Complications are likely to be minimal if careful consideration is given to the contraindications listed and if the procedural details for performing the biopsy are followed. They appear to occur in less than 1:1000 biopsies. The more common complications are local pain and infection, subcapsular and intrahepatic haematomata. Rarely there may be capsular, intrathoracic or intrapulmonary bleeding or haemobilia. Pleural pain, pneumothorax, intraperitoneal bile leaks and penetration of other abdominal organs may occur. Arteriovenous fistula can develop. Deaths have usually occurred because of delay in management of arterial bleeding, surgically or by embolization, or in repair of a punctured viscus. Problems are most likely to arise if the puncture is made low; the needle then transverses the thinnest part of the right lobe of the liver and may impinge on the gallbladder and structures in the portahepatis.

Tru-cut liver biopsy

With the availability of disposable sharp Menghini needles it is very rarely necessary to use this needle which causes complications much more frequently. The Tru-cut needle consists of a sharp, pointed needle with a 2 cm notch and cutting sleeve. The patient is prepared as for aspiration biopsy, including the injection of local anaesthetic down to the capsule of the liver. The skin is nicked.

Respiration is arrested in expiration. The needle with the sleeve advanced is introduced just within the liver capsule. The needle alone is then advanced into the liver, the sleeve advanced to close over the notch, to cut and trap a cylinder of liver within the lumen of the needle, and the needle and sleeve are withdrawn together immediately. This technique is thus much more complicated than for a Menghini needle biopsy. It involves three distinct manoeuvres while the needle is within the liver. Inexperienced operators frequently pull the needle back within the liver, rather than advancing the sleeve. The author's technique is to introduce the needle and sleeve with the right hand, to advance the needle with the left hand, placing the fifth finger of the left hand on the surgical drape, to ensure that the left hand does not move, and then to advance the sleeve with the right hand. It is clearly important that this technique be perfected in the autopsy room.

Transjugular liver biopsy

A transjugular biopsy technique may be used in patients with impaired coagulation, or with thrombocytopenia. The liver biopsy is taken through the hepatic vein via a catheter which is passed through the internal jugular vein into the right lobe of the liver. The size of the biopsy may be inadequate for diagnosis. Provided this technique is used by those experienced in cannulation of the hepatic veins it is relatively safe but traversing the liver surface is a hazard. It appears to have a limited role in paediatric practice.

Handling the tissue

The liver tissue is removed from the Menghini needle by expelling a little saline, or by dismantling the syringe and pushing the core of tissue out, using a fine trocar. The material should be transferred into the embedding or fixative material as quickly as possible. This is particularly important if histochemical studies or electron microscopy is to be performed. Embedding in slowly frozen OTC embedding solution maintains tissue integrity and enzymatic activity. It is important not to use forceps to manipulate the biopsy as these squeeze and distort the tissue. In general, it is best not to apply the tissue to filter paper or other mounting material provided one can guarantee to get the material to the laboratory without undue shaking and fragmentation of the tissue. Relatively normal liver appears as a homogeneous cord 1–4 cm in length and weighing 1–0 mg. Fatty liver is pale yellow or greasy and floats in formal-saline. Cholestatic livers are green. The core of a cirrhotic liver has an irregular outline and the intensity of colour is variable throughout its length. It frequently fragments. Malignant deposits are dull white.

Laparoscopy

Laparoscopy combined with biopsy may have a role in the investigation of focal lesions. It is so rarely required in paediatric practice that a mini-laparotomy may be preferable in the rare focal neoplastic or infective disorders causing diagnostic difficulty. Although it allows confirmation of macronodular cirrhosis in the rare instances that it cannot be inferred from clinical examination and be missed on liver biopsy, the prognostic value of this information may be outweighed by the risk of penetrating portosystemic collaterals in the abdominal wall.

Upper gastrointestinal endoscopy

Diagnostic endoscopy is invaluable in identifying bleeding points, confirming peptic ulceration and oesophageal varices. It may be combined with sclerotherapy if these have bled.

Cholangiography

Endoscopic retrograde cholangio-pancreatography (ERCP) provides good definition of the extrahepatic and intrahepatic bile ducts. The procedure is performed under general anaesthetic. Its most important role is in defining unusual extrahepatic biliary obstruction and in the diagnosis of sclerosing cholangitis. It also has a role in detecting stones in the common bile duct but small stones may be obscured by contrast. Using prototype instruments it is useful in demonstrating bile duct patency and thus excluding atresia in a small proportion of completely cholestatic infants with Alagille's syndrome in whom the liver biliary appearances are not diagnostic (Wilkinson *et al.*, 1991). Cannulation of the pancreatic duct but failure to opacify the biliary system implies biliary atresia. It may demonstrate a long common channel in patients with choledochal cysts and/or recurrent pancreatitis. Complications include cholangitis, bacteraemia, raised serum amylase concentration, pancreatitis, biliary leak, haemobilia, duodenal perforation and damage to the ampulla. ERCP may be combined with a variety of endoscopic therapeutic procedures such as sphincterotomy, extraction of stones from the biliary system, the insertion of transbiliary prostheses and balloon dilatation of strictures.

Percutaneous transhepatic cholangiography is undertaken to demonstrate the site of extrahepatic obstruction of the biliary tree or obstruction to the bile ducts within the liver. It is important to visualize both right and left hepatic ducts. General anaesthesia is required. It may have the therapeutic effect of clearing biliary sludge and relieving obstruction (Figure 26.5).

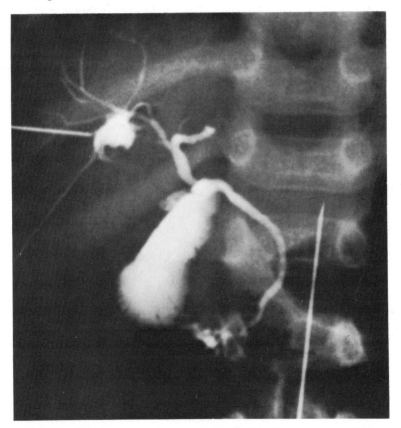

Figure 26.5 Percutaneous cholangiogram using the flexible Okuda needle in a child aged 21 months. The child had had three episodes of jaundice, had persistent pruritus and rickets. Liver biopsy findings did not exclude bile duct obstruction. The tip of the Okuda needle is obscured by a pool of contrast medium within the hepatic parenchyma. Contrast medium has entered fine normal distal bile ducts in the right lobe of the liver and opacified the main right and left hepatic ducts. The common hepatic duct, cystic duct, gall bladder and common hepatic bile duct are normal in calibre. Contrast is seen in the duodenum, excluding the obstruction

It may be combined with balloon dilatation of postsurgical strictures or insertion of a polyethylene endoprosthesis inserted over the guidewire and advanced through the obstruction. The procedure has three major complications: bacteraemia or septicaemia sometimes complicated by shock if the bile ducts are infected, bile leakage and haemorrhage from the liver substance. Prophylactic antibiotics, e.g. gentamicin and cefoxitin, must be given intravenously at the time of the procedure.

Operative cholangiography via the gallbladder or cystic duct at laparotomy may be helpful in unusual choledochal cysts or tumours of the bile duct. With the above techniques, modern ultrasound scanning, radioisotopic imaging and skilful interpretation of percutaneous liver biopsies it has a declining place in practice. Even experienced operators find that laparotomy and cholangiographic findings may give misleading results, leading to incorrect diagnosis of biliary atresia and inappropriate hepatic portoenter-ostomy (Markowitz *et al.*, 1983). In exceptional circumstances it may assist in the diagnosis of syndromic intrahepatic bile duct hypoplasia at the stage when the liver biopsy shows bile duct proliferation and radioisotope studies have shown complete cholestasis. In such infants it is frequently difficult to fill the proximal biliary tree and intrahepatic bile ducts, leading to the false diagnosis of biliary atresia. Methylene blue cholangiography (0.1%) in such infants provides a rapid means of visualizing the proximal extrahepatic bile ducts as bright blue structures when they cannot be identified by contrast cholangiography (Schwartz, 1985). Operative cholangiography does assist in identifying additional stones in patients with gall-stones. T tube cholangiography following biliary surgery or liver transplantation provides an excellent way of visualizing the biliary system. *Oral cholecystography* which detects gall bladder disease by assessing the ability of the gall bladder to concentrate the radio-opaque medium and to contract following a fatty meal has little place in paediatric practice. *Intravenous cholangiography* has been replaced by ultrasound scanning and isotope or CT imaging.

Angiography

Splanchnic angiography performed by catheterizing the coeliac and superior mesenteric arteries, via the femoral arteries, helps in the definition of space-occupying lesions within the liver and identifying anomalies of the hepatic artery. Films taken during the venous phase outline the anatomy of portal venous system including the superior mesenteric and splenic veins more completely than a splenic venogram. *Splenoportography (percuta-neous trans-splenic portal venography)* is of value when it demonstrates portal vein patency. It is of less value in attempting to define the site of obstruction to portal blood flow when planning surgery for portal hypertension since the portal vein may fail to opacify because of retrograde flow as well as occlusion. It may not visualize vessels such as the superior mesenteric vein which could be utilized for surgery. Contraindications are those of liver biopsy and allergy to contrast media. The procedure should not be done unless removal of the spleen can safely be performed if the procedure causes splenic rupture or persisting intraperitoneal haemorrhage. Occasionally, both investigations are necessary to give the surgeon optimum information on the venous system. Both require skilled personnel and appropriate radiological equipment.

Digital subtraction angiography allows visualization of the hepatic artery, portal venous system and intrahepatic vessels with intravenous rather than intra-arterial or intersplanchnic injection of contrast. Complications are thus much less. Spatial resolution and details of anatomy may be less satisfactory than with conventional angiography.

Transhepatic portography in which the portal and splenic veins are visualized via a catheter, passed through a needle placed in an intrahepatic division of the portal vein, and advanced along the main portal vein into the splenic or superior mesenteric vein. Its main use in paediatrics is in confirming that the portal vein is truly occluded in candidates for liver grafting in whom other techniques have failed to demonstrate patency. It may be combined with balloon dilatation of stenotic segments of portal vein.

Hepatic vein catheterization, pressure measurement and venography   Hepatic vein pressure measurement, recorded with a catheter which lies in an unobstructed major hepatic vein branch, is directly related to the measured portal vein pressure. A normal hepatic wedged pressure is about 5–6 mmHg. The values of approximately 20 mmHg are found in patients with sinusoidal or postsinusoidal hypertension. In congenital hepatic fibrosis, schistosomiasis and hepatoportal sclerosis the gradient is between 1 and 10 mmHg. In extrahepatic portal vein block, both the wedged pressure and the free hepatic vein pressure are normal.

The main value of this investigation is in indicating the presence of significant intrahepatic disease when other more definitive tests are contraindicated. In most instances a percutaneous liver biopsy will give much more information at little extra risk. It is most useful when the biopsy has features of hepatic vein outflow block. Then it must be combined with retrograde hepatic venography to exclude hepatic vein obstruction and with intracardiac pressure measurement to exclude constrictive pericarditis or cardio-myopathy. Intrasplenic pressure measured at the time of splenic venography does not necessarily produce a reliable measure of portal hypertension and is rarely necessary. Inferior venacavography is occasionally required to detect partial or complete obstruction to the inferior vena cava or its compression by tumour or enlarged caudate lobe.

Bibliography and references

General

Gilmore, I. T. (1986) Modern methods of diagnosis in liver disease. *J. R. Coll. Physicians, London*, **22**, 201
McIntyre, N., Benhamou, J.-P., Bircher, J., Rizzetto, M. and Rodes, J. (eds) (1991) *Oxford Textbook of Clinical Hepatology*, Oxford University Press, Oxford
Millward-Sadler, G. H., Wright, R. and Arthur, M. J. P. (1992) *Wright's Liver and Biliary disease*, 3rd Edn, Saunders, London
Pain, J. and Karani, J. (1991) Investigation of the hepatobiliary tract. In: *Surgery of Liver Disease in Children* (ed. Howard, E. R.). Butterworth-Heinemann, Oxford, pp. 27–35

Serum enzymes

Deritis, F. and Cacciatore, L. (1983) Differential diagnosis of liver diseases by the enzyme pattern. In *Clinical Hepatology* (eds Csomos, G. and Thaler, H.). Berlin, Springer Verlag, p. 16
Knight, J. A. and Hammond, R. E. (1981) Gammaglutamyl transphorase and alkaline phosphatase activities compared in serum of normal children and children with liver disease. *Clin. Chem.*, **27**, 48
Kruse, K. (1983) Inherited isolated hyperphosphatasaemia. *Acta Paediatr. Scand.*, **72**, 833–835
Lackmann, G. M. and Tollner, U. (1992) Enzymaktivitaten im serum gesunder neugeborener. *Monatssch. Kinderheilk.*, **140**, 171–176
Maggiore, G., Bernard, O., Hadchouel, M., Lemonnier, A. and Alagille, D. (1991) Diagnostic value of serum gamma-glutamyl transpeptidase activity in liver disease in children. *J. Pediatr. Gastroenterol. Nutr.*, **12**, 21–26
Manolaki, N., Larcher, V. F., Mowat, A. P. *et al.* (1983) Pre-laparotomy diagnosis of extrahepatic biliary atresia. *Arch. Dis. Childh.*, **58**, 591
Perrault, J., O'Brien, J. F. and Tremaine, W. J. (1990) Macrotransaminase of aspartate aminotransferase (AST): a benign cause of elevated AST activity. *J. Pediatr.*, **117**, 444–445

Reichling, J. J. and Marshall, M. K. (1988) Clinical use of serum enzymes in liver disease. *Dig. Dis. Sci.*, **33**, 1601–1614

Schoenau, S., Herzog, K. H. and Boehles, H. J. (1986) Fragmented isoenzymes of alkaline phosphatase in the diagnosis of transient hyperphosphatasemia. *Clin. Chem.*, **32**, 2211–2213

Wiedemann, G., Armann, O., Reinhardt, M. and Biesenbach, R. (1989) Untersuchungen zur ermittlung von referenzbereichen der serumenzyme alaninamino-transferase (ALAT), aspartatamino-transferase (ASAT), gamma-glutamyltransferase (CGT), lactatdehydrogenase (LDH) and creatinkinase (CK) fur kinder vom 2 bis 7 lebensjahr. *Z. Klin. Med.*, **44**, 1059–1065

Proteins, immunoglobulins and tissue autoantibodies

Aksu, F. and Mietens, S. T. (1984) Serum immunoglobulin levels in acute viral hepatitis in childhood. *Klin. Padiatr.*, **196**, 83

Aledort, L. M. (1976) Blood clotting abnormalities in liver disease. In: *Progress in Liver Disease*, Volume 5 (eds Popper, H. and Schaffner, F.). Grune and Stratton, New York, p. 350

Alpert, C. A. (1974) Plasma protein measurement as a diagnostic aid. *New Engl. J. Med.*, **291**, 287

Bernuau, J., Rueff, B. and Benhamou, J. P. (1986) Fulminant and subfulminant liver failure: definition and causes. *Sem. Liver Dis.*, **6**, 97–106

Calcado, A., Trivedi, P., Portmann, B. and Mowat, A. P. (1991) Serum concentrations of extracellular matrix components: novel markers of metabolic control and hepatic pathology in glycogen storage disease. *J. Pediatr. Gastroenterol. Nutr.*, **13**, 1–9

Liedman, H. A., Fure, B. C. and Fure, B. (1982) Hepatic vitamin K-dependent carboxylation of blood-clotting proteins. *Hepatology*, **2**, 488

Mieli-Vergani, G., Lobo-Yeo, A., McFarlane, B. M., McFarlane, I. G., Mowat, A. P. and Vergani, D. (1989) Different immune mechanisms leading to autoimmunity in primary sclerosing cholangitis and autoimmune chronic active hepatitis of childhood. *Hepatology*, **9**, 198–203

Alpha-fetoprotein and other tumour markers

Johnson, P. J. and Williams, R. (1980) Serum alphaferoprotein estimations in doubling time in hepatocellular carcinoma: influence of therapy and possible value in early detection. *J. Natl. Cancer Inst.*, **64**, 1329

Johnston, D. I., Mowat, A. P., Orr, H. and Kohn, J. (1976) Serum alphafetoprotein levels in extrahepatic biliary atresia, idiopathic neonatal hepatitis and alpha-1 antitrypsin deficiency (PiZ). *Acta Paediat. Scand.*, **65**, 623

Maeda, M., Tozuka, S., Kanayama, M. and Uchida, T. (1988) Hepatocellular carcinoma producing carcinoembryonic antigen. *Dig. Dis. Sci.*, **33**, 1629–1631

Motohara, K., Endo, F., Matsuda, I. and Iwasama, T. (1987) Acarboxy prothrombin: a marker for hepatoblastoma in infants. *J. Pediatr. Gastroenterol. Nutr.*, **6**, 42–45

Vajro, P., Fontanella, A., de Vincenzo, A. *et al.* (1991) Monitor of serum alpha-fetoprotein levels in children with chronic hepatitis B virus infection. *J. Pediatr. Gastroenterol. Nutr.*, **12**, 27–32

Caeruloplasmin and copper studies

da Costa, C. M., Baldwin, D., Portmann, B., Lolin, Y., Mowat, A. P. and Mieli-Vergani, G. (1992) The value of urinary copper excretion after penicillamine challenge in the diagnosis of Wilson's disease. *Hepatology*, **15**, 609–615

Gibbs, K. and Walshe, J. M. (1979) A study of the caeruloplasmin concentrations found in 75 patients with Wilson's disease, their kinships and various control groups. *Q. Jl. Med.*, **48**, 447

Ritland, S., Steinnes, E. and Skrede, S. (1977) Hepatic copper content. Urinary copper excretion and serum caeruloplasmin in liver disease. *Scand. J. Gastroenterol.*, **12**, 81

Spechler, S. J. and Koff, R. S. (1980) Wilson's disease: diagnostic difficulties in the patient with chronic hepatitis and hypocaeruloplasminemia. *Gastroenterology*, **78**, 103

Alpha-1 antitrypsin deficiency

Cox, D. W. (1989) Alpha1-antitrypsin deficiency. In: *The Metabolic Basis of Inherited Disease*, 6th Edn (eds Scriver, C. R., Beautt, A. L., Sly, W. S., Valle, D.), McGraw-Hill, New York. pp. 2409–2437

Frants, R. R. and Eriksson, A. W. (1978) Reliable classification of 6 PiM sub-types by separator isoelectric focusing. *Hum. Hered.*, **28**, 212

Hussain, M., Mieli-Vergani, G. and Mowat, A. P. (1991) Alpha-1-antitrypsin Deficiency and Liver Disease: Clinical presentation, diagnosis and treatment. *J. Inher. Metabol. Dis.*, **14**, 497–511

Povey, S. (1990) The genetics of alpha-1-antitrypsin deficiency in relation to neonatal liver disease. *Mol. Biol. Med.*, **7**, 161–172

Cholesterol

Ballin, J. A. (1986) Lipid metabolism in relation to liver physiology and disease. In: *Liver Annual*, Volume 5 (eds Arias, I. M., Frenkel, M. and Wilson, J. H. P.). Amsterdam, Elsevier, p. 22

Tsang, R. C., Fallat, R. W. and Grueck, C. J. (1974) Cholesterol at birth. Comparison of normal and hypercholesterolaemic neonates. *J. Pediatr.*, **58**, 458

Ammonia

Green, A. (1988) When and how should we measure plasma ammonia? *Ann. Clin. Biochem.*, **25**, 199–209

Kvamme, E. (1983) Ammonia metabolism in the central nervous system. *Prog. Neurobiol.*, **20**, 109

Mowat, A. P. (1991) Acute liver failure. *Current Paediatrics*, **1**, 218–223

Mowat, A. P. (1993) Hepatic encephalopathy: Acute and Chronic. In: *Coma* (ed. J. A. Eyre) Bailliere's Clinical Paediatrics. Bailliere Tindall, London

Ratnaike, R. N., Battray, C. E., Malden, L. T. *et al.* (1983) Erythrocyte ammonia in live disease. *Scand. J. Gasroenterol.*, **18**, 103

Vilstrup, H., Gluud, C., Hardt, F. *et al.* (1990) Branched chain enriched amino acid versus glucose treatment of hepatic encephalopathy. A double-blind study of 65 patients with cirrhosis. *J. Hepatol.*, **10**, 291–296

Bile salts

Clayton, P. T. (1991) Inborn Errors of bile acid metabolism. *J. Inher. Met. Dis.*, **14**, 478–496

Matsui, A., Psacharopoulos, H. T., Mowat, A. P. *et al.* (1982) Radioimmunoassay of serum glycocholic acid. Standard laboratory tests of liver function and liver biopsy findings: comparative study of children with liver disease. *J. Clin. Pathol.*, **35**, 1011

Setchell, K. D. R., Piccoli, D., Heubi, J. and Balistreri, W. F. (1992) Inborn errors of bile acid metabolism. In: *Paediatric Cholestasis. Novel approaches to treatment* (eds Lentze, M. J. and Reichen, J.). Kluwer, London, p. 153

Vierling, J. M., Berk, P. D., Hofmann, A. F. *et al.* (1982) Normal fasting-state levels of serum cholyl-conjugated bile acids in Gilbert's syndrome: an aid to diagnosis. *Hepatology*, **2**, 340

Bilirubin

Blankaert, N. and Heirwegh, K. P. M. (1986) Analysis and preparation of bilirubins and Biliverdins. In: *Bile Pigments nad Jaundice Molecular, Metabolic and Medical Aspects* (ed. Ostrow, J. D.). Marcel Dekker, New York, Ch. 3, pp. 31–80

Mair, B. and Klempner, L. B. (1987) Abnormally high values in Direct Bilirubin in the Serum of Newborns as measured with the DuPont aca Analyser. *Am. J. Clin. Path.*, **87**, 642–644

Mowat, A. P. (1990) Urine Analysis in the assessment of Jaundiced Infants. In: *Clinical Urinalysis* (eds Newall, R. G. and Howell, R.). Ames Division, Miles Ltd, Stoke Poges. pp. 74–82

Rosenthal, P., Blanckaert, N., Kabra, P. M. and Thaler, M. M. (1986) Formation of Bilirubin Conjugates in Human Newborns. *Paediatr. Res.*, **20**, 947–950

Ultrasonography

Dicks-Mireaux, C. (1993) The paediatric liver. In: *Abdominal and General Ultrasound*, Vol. 1 (eds Cosgrove, D., Meire, H., Dewbury, K. and Farrant, P.). Churchill Livingstone, Edinburgh, pp. 439–451

Meire, H. B. and Farrant, P. (1993) The paediatric biliary system. In: *Abdominal and General Ultrasound*, Vol. 1 (eds Cosgrove, D., Meire, H., Dewbury, K. and Farrant, P.). Churchill Livingstone, Edinburgh, pp. 419–438

Traynor, O., Castaing, D. and Bismuth, H. (1988) Peroperative ultrasonography in the surgery of hepatic tumours. *Br. J. Surg.*, **75**, 197–202

Liver biopsy

Cohen, M. B., A-Kader, H. H., Lambers, D. and Heubi, J. E. (1992) Complications of percutaneous liver biopsy in children. *Gastroenterology*, **102**, 629–632

Desmet, V. J. (1992) Pathology of paediatric cholestasis. In: *Paediatric Cholestasis* (eds Lentze, M. J. and Reichen, J.). Kluwer, Lancaster, pp. 55–74

Edoute, Y., Ben-Haim, S. A., Brenner, B. and Malberger, E. (1992) Fatal hemoperitoneum after fine-needle aspiration of a liver metastasis. *Am. J. Gastroenterol.*, **87**, 358–360

Furuya, K. N., Burrows, P. E., Phillips, M. J. and Roberts, E. A. (1992) Transjugular liver biopsy in children. *Hepatology*, **15**, 1036–1042

Gilmore, I. T., Bradley, R. D. and Thompson, R. T. H. (1977) Transjugular liver biopsy. *Br. Med. J.*, **2**, 100

Hegarty, J. E. and Williams, R. (1984) Liver biopsy: techniques. Clinical applications and complications. *Br. Med. J.*, **288**, 1254

Ishak, K. G. (1990) Pathology of inherited metabolic disoreders. In: *Pediatric Hepatology* (eds Balistreri, W. F. and Stocker, J. T.). Hemisphere Publishing Company, New York, pp. 77–158

Portmann, B., Mowat, A. P. and Williams, R. (1976) Liver histology in neonates with conjugated hyperbilirubinaemia. *Acta Paediatr. Belg.*, **29**, 139

Roschlau, G. (1978) *Leberbiopsie in Kindersalter*, 2nd Edn. UEB Gustav Fischer Verlag Jena,

Sherlock, S., Dick, R. and Van Leeuwen, D. J. V. (1985) Liver biopsy today – the Royal Free Hospital experience. *J. Hepatol.*, **1**, 75

Tobin, M. V. and Gilmore, I. T. (1989) Plugged liver biopsy in patients with impaired coagulation. *Dig. Dis. Sci.*, **34**, 13–15

Cholangiography

Chaumont, P., Martin, N., Riou, J. Y. and Brunelle, F. (1982) Percutaneous transhepatic cholangiography in extrahepatic biliary atresia in children. *Ann. Radiol. (Paris)*, **25**, 94

Howard, E. R. and Nunnerley, H. B. (1979) Percutaneous cholangiography in prolonged jaundice of childhood. *J. R. Soc. Med.*, **72**, 495

Markowitz, J., Daum, F., Kahn, E. I. *et al.* (1983) Arterio-hepatic dysplasia 1. Pitfalls in diagnosis and management. *Hepatology*, **3**, 74

Schwartz, M. Z. (1985) An alternative method for intraoperative cholangiography in infants with severe obstructive jaundice. *J. Pediatr. Surg.*, **20**, 440

Wilkinson, M. L., Mieli-Vergani, G., Ball, C., Portmann, B. and Mowat, A. P. (1991) Endoscopic retrograde cholangiopancreatography (ERCP) in infantile cholestasis. *Arch. Dis. Child.*, **66**, 121–123

Angiography

Brunelle, F., Garel, L., Harry, G. and Chaumont, P. L. (1979) Angiographie portale des tumeures de l'enfant. *Ann. Radiol.*, **22**, 142–149

Melham, R. E. and Rizk, G. K. (1970) Splenoportographic evaluation of portal hypertension in children. *J. Pediatr. Surg.*, **5**, 522

Reynolds, T. B., Ito, S. and Iwaksuki, S. (1970) Measurement of portal pressure and its clinical applications. *Am. J. Med.*, **49**, 649

Smith-Lane, G., Camilo, N., Dick, R. *et al.* (1980) Percutaneous transhepatic portography in the assessment of portal hypertension. *Gastroenterology*, **78**, 197

Radionucleotides

El Tumi, M. A., Clarke, M. B., Barrett, J. J. and Mowat, A. P. (1987) A ten-minute radiopharmaceutical test in suspected biliary atresia. *Arch. Dis. Childh.*, **62**, 180

Tests of liver function

Bar-Meir, S., Bar-Tal, L., Papa, M. Z. and Peled, Y. (1986) Bromsulfophathalein clearance and minopyrine test in patients with Gilbert's syndrome. *Israel J. Med. Sci.*, **22**, 376–379

Lewis, F. W. and Rector, W. G. (1992) Caffeine clearance in cirrhosis: the value of simplified determinations of liver metabolic capacity. *J. Hepatol.*, **14**, 157–162

Oellerich, M., Burdelski, M., Lautz, H. U., Schulz, M., Schmidt, F. W. and Herrmann, H. (1990) Lidocaine metabolite formation as a measure of liver function in patients with cirrhosis. *Ther. Drug Monitor.*, **12**, 219–226

Index